Brain Edema

Proceedings of the Sixth International Symposium
November 7–10, 1984 in Tokyo

Edited by
Y. Inaba, I. Klatzo, and M. Spatz

With 427 Figures

Springer-Verlag
Berlin Heidelberg New York Tokyo

Prof. Dr. YUTAKA INABA
Department of Neurosurgery, Tokyo Medical and Dental University, Tokyo, Japan

Dr. IGOR KLATZO
Laboratory of Neuropathology and Neuroanatomical Sciences, National Institute of Neurological and Communicative Disorders and Stroke, National Institutes of Health, Bethesda, Maryland, USA

Dr. MARIA SPATZ
Laboratory of Neuropathology and Neuroanatomical Sciences, National Institute of Neurological and Communicative Disorders and Stroke, National Institutes of Health, Bethesda, Maryland, USA

ISBN-13: 978-3-642-70698-1 e-ISBN-13: 978-3-642-70696-7
DOI: 10.1007/978-3-642-70696-7

Softcover reprint of the hardcover 1st edition 1985

2121/3130-543210

Proceedings of the Sixth International Symposium on Brain Edema

Preface

The first International Symposium on Brain Edema was organized by Dr. Klatzo and Dr. Seitelberger and held in Vienna in 1965. The second Symposium was held in Mainz in 1972 and organized by Dr. H. J. Reulen and Dr. K. Schürmann, the third in Montreal in 1976 by Dr. H. M. Pappius, the fourth in Berlin in 1979 by Dr. J. Cervós-Navarro, and the fifth in Groningen in 1982 by Dr. K. G. Go.

This volume contains the papers presented at the 6th International Symposium on Brain Edema, held in Tokyo, Japan, November 7–10, 1984. The invited lectures by Dr. I. Klatzo, Dr. A. Hirano, Dr. S. I. Rapoport, Dr. B. K. Siesjö, Dr. H. M. Pappius, Dr. K. A. Hossmann, and Dr. D. M. Long are included as special chapters.

On behalf of the organizing committee, I wish to express my deep appreciation to all the participants for their contribution toward making this meeting so fruitful and significant. Moreover, the great success of this Symposium depended on the high quality of the invited lectures and presentations by experts in various fields, as well as on the free and enthusiastic discussion. I was deeply impressed with the papers presented by all the authors, who endeavored to elucidate their subjects. The editors have made only minor corrections and rearrangements, since prompt publication was considered to be important.

The most characteristic feature of this Symposium was the particular emphasis put on the poster session: the poster papers slide were shown by using a slide projector and discussed in the same hall where the oral presentations took place.

At the final advisory board meeting, all the members agreed that the 7th International Symposium on Brain Edema would be held in Baltimore in 1987, under the new chairman of the organizing committee, Dr. Donlin M. Long.

I would like to express my thanks to the authors, the editorial board, and all the coworkers for the realization of this publication. Particular gratitute must be expressed to Dr. Igor Klatzo and Dr. Maria Spatz for their precious and continuous support.

I am grateful to Springer-Verlag for technical aid in the preparation of this book and for its prompt publication.

Tokyo, September, 1985 YUTAKA INABA

Contents

Pathophysiology and BBB (I)

Morphology (II)

Pathophysiology and BBB (II)

Metabolism (II)

Invited Lecture (V)

Biochemistry

Invited Lecture (VI)

Ischemia

Diagnosis (I)

Therapy (I)

Invited Lecture (VII)

Diagnosis (II)

Therapy (II)

List of Abbreviations

AA	arachidonic acid
AIB	aminoisobutyric acid
ALB	albumin
AU	absorbance unit
BBB	blood-brain barrier
BLCL	bilateral carotid ligation
BP	blood pressure
CBF	cerebral blood flow
CBV	cerebral blood volume
CCA	common carotid artery
CCA	cardiocirculatory arrest
CEI	cerebral electrical impedance
CFY	nonspecific Sprague-Dawley strain
CT	computed tomography *or* X-ray computed tomography
DCR	direct cortical response
DM	dorsomedial nucleus of the hypothalamus
DSC	differential scanning calorimetry
EM	electron microscopy
FAG	fluorescein angiography
G	syringe needle gauge
GSH	reduced glutathione
GSSG	oxidized glutathione
HAM	human atheromatous material
HIH	hypertensive intracerebral hemorrhage
HPH	high-pressure hydrocephalus
HRP	horseradish peroxidase
5HT	5-hydroxytryptamine
IC	interendothelial cleft
ICP	intracranial pressure
KA	kainic acid
KK	kallikrein-kinin
λ	partition coefficient
lCBF	local cortical blood flow
lCGU	cortical local cerebral glucose utilization
$lCMRO_2$	local oxygen consumption
lOEF	local oxygen extraction fraction
MBRF	reticular formation of midbrain
MCA	middle cerebral artery
MDA	malonyldialdehyde
MORF	reticular formation of medulla oblongata
MP	methylprednisone
NE	norepinephrine
NMR	nuclear magnetic resonance
NPH	normal-pressure hydrocephalus
NTR	normotensive rat

OEF	oxygen extraction fraction
6-OHDA	6-hydroxydopamine
OβH	dopamine-β-hydroxylase
PFLD	perifocal low-density area
PG	prostaglandin
PTT	partial thromboplastin time
PVL	periventricular hypodensity
rCBF	regional cerebral blood flow
ROI	region of interest
SAP	systemic arterial pressure
SBTI	soybean-trypsin inhibitor
SG	specific gravity
SHR	spontaneously hypertensive rat/s
SHRSP	stroke-prone spontaneously hypertensive rat/s
SHRSR	stroke-resistant spontaneously hypertensive rat/s
SSS	superior sagittal sinus
SSSP	superior sagittal sinus pressure
T_1	longitudinal relaxation time
T_2	transverse relaxation time
$1/T_1$	longitudinal relaxation rate
$1/T_2$	transverse relaxation rate
TBA-RS	thiobarbituric acid response substances
TLC	temporal lobe contusion
TSI	thromboxane A_2 synthetase inhibitor
TXA_2	thromboxane A_2
VI	vasomotor index

Concepts of Ischemic Injury Associated with Brain Edema

I. KLATZO [1]

Key words: Cerebral ischemia, brain edema, selective vulnerability, cerebral blood flow, blood-brain barrier

During investigations of the complex pathophysiology of cerebral ischemia, several concepts determining some patterns of ischemic injury have been increasingly recognized. These are: (a) *selective vulnerability* with patterns of selective damage to various neuronal units following an ischemic insult; (b) *thresholds* with regard to various parameters of ischemic injury; (c) the *maturation phenomenon,* i.e., progressive development of the lesions following an ischemic insult, and related to it; and (d) *peripheral expansion* of the necrotic core of an infarction into the adjacent areas of penumbra. This last may lead to (e) a *vicious circle* – a synergistic, reciprocal relationship between regional increase in tissue pressure due to necrosis and edema and reduction of the regional cerebral blood flow (rCBF) to below critical levels for survival of the tissue in the adjacent areas.

Since edema constitutes an integral part of ischemic injury, its involvement and role in the patterns and concepts mentioned above deserve closer evaluation, which is attempted in this brief review.

Selective vulnerability of various neuronal units in the central nervous system has long been the subject of controversy between the proponents of two theories put forward in attempts to explain this phenomenon. One theory, proposed by Spielmeyer [17], ascribed the paramount role to a "vasal" factor and became known as the vascular theory of selective vulnerability. The other, promulgated by O. and C. Vogt [21], was based on the concept of pathoclisis and on the assumption of different intrinsic, physicochemical properties of various neuronal cell types, which would account for their different responses to various noxious factors.

The application of modern methods for regional mapping of the cerebral blood flow has provided considerable support for the basic tenet of Vogt and Vogt's theory of pathoclisis, which stated that sensitivity of neuronal units to injury must be related to intrinsic metabolic differences and not to rigid thresholds of blood perfusion levels. Thus, with the regional evaluations of blood flow in the studies of Suzuki et al. [18] no significant differences in the rCBF were observed among various sectors

---

[1] Laboratory of Neuropathology and Neuroanatomical Sciences, National Institute of Neurological and Communicative Disorders and Stroke, National Institutes of Health, Bethesda, Maryland 20205, USA

of hippocampus or other regions of the hemispheres affected by ischemia, and yet there was a striking selective vulnerability of the CA1 sector of the hippocampus with almost total destruction of neurons, occurring on the 3rd day after a 5-min ischemic insult. Otherwise, outside the hippocampus, the concept of pathoclisis appears to be applicable to observations on selective ischemic damage to small and medium-sized neurons of the striatum with preservation of large cells [14], which would be difficult to explain on the basis of differences in blood flow.

On the other hand, vascular factors could possibly play a role in the distribution and topography of ischemic lesions, such as intensely necrotic zones, observed in the locality of anatomic boundaries of blood supply by individual major arteries [6]. In these observations, relief of carotid occlusion was generally associated with a considerable drop in systemic blood pressure, and it can be speculated that in most peripheral zones of arterial blood supply the flow could be greatly reduced or completely cease (no reflux phenomenon). Also, in studies performed by Ito et al. [6] the laminar pattern of injury in the cerebral cortex could be related to compression of arterial branches penetrating from the surface to different cortical layers, which was due to edema associated with an increase in the intracranial pressure. Otherwise, it can be assumed that the distribution of individual foci of infarction which disregard borders of anatomic structures is determined by vascular factors related to the efficiency of collateral circulation.

The *concept of thresholds* for various parameters of ischemic injury, introduced in recent years by Symon and others [13, 19, 20], refers to the occurrence of various expressions of neuronal injury in relation to the degree of interference with blood perfusion. Thus, with a certain degree of rCBF reduction, the disturbances may be limited to failure of neuronal activity that is evident only in electrophysiological recordings; a more markedly compromised rCBF will induce interference with ionic pumps associated with cellular swelling, and finally, a severe CBF reduction (below 12 ml/100 g/min) will lead to irreversible neuronal death.

It is increasingly evident, however, that the concept of thresholds is closely related to selective vulnerability, since the thresholds for various expressions of ischemic damage are not based entirely on the levels of ischemic rCBF reduction but also on intrinsic properties of neuronal structures, as has been recently corroborated by comparative observations on the effects of ischemia in the adult (12- to 14-week-old) and young (3-week-old) gerbils. In these studies, bilateral occlusion of the common carotid arteries for 5 min resulted in selective destruction of the CA1 sector of the hippocampus in adult gerbils, whereas the young gerbils similarly treated showed no evidence of damage to the CA1 sector, although both groups of animals showed similar, very low, rCBF values during occlusion. Here again, the differences in neuronal damage could be best explained by differences in metabolic features between young and adult animals. Indeed, preliminary observations indicate that the high-energy metabolites are utilized at a significantly slower rate in young animals, and the young gerbils had considerably lower lactate levels at the end of the 5-min occlusion [12].

In recent years, it has been increasingly recognized that some mechanisms which decide neuronal survival or death become operative after an ischemic insult, and the effect of such postischemic pathophysiological events has been termed the *maturation phenomenon* [6, 8]. The main feature of this phenomenon appears to be the direct relationship between the intensity of an ischemic insult and the rate of maturation, a lesser intensity being associated with slower development of the lesions. The maturation of ischemic lesions can be recognized not only in morphological changes, but also in other parameters of ischemic injury, such as dysfunction of the BBB, biochemical changes, etc. [9]. It still remains a matter of conjecture which postischemic changes play an essential role in the development of ischemic lesions and which are merely coincidental. Postischemic pathomechanisms which have been implicated in development of the lesions are as follows: First, uncoupling between energy supply by blood flow and energy utilization can lead to the development of secondary postischemic hypoxia [5] and have a potentially damaging effect on brain tissue [11, 16]. Secondly, an abnormal entry of calcium into neurons has been suggested as the starting point of events leading to irreversible cell damage [3, 15]. Thirdly, a delayed entry of circulating biogenic amines [4] in cerebral ischemia may have a significant effect on CBF and metabolism. Otherwise, accumulation of free fatty acids, kinins, serotonin, and prostaglandins released from severely damaged tissue may contribute to the development of ischemic lesions [1].

All the postischemic changes mentioned have in common an association with *edema,* which first begins as an intracellular accumulation of water, promptly after an ischemic insult [2]. The main event in this water accumulation is a disturbance of cellular osmoregulation, which depends primarily on the Na^{+}-K^{+} exchange pump, with ATP as the energy source. Such cytotoxic edema is initially more pronounced in the gray matter than in the white matter, reflecting greater sensitivity of gray matter to ischemic injury. The initial cytotoxic edematous changes in transient and permanent cerebral ischemia take rather a dramatic turn with the opening of the BBB, which introduces the element of vasogenic edema.

A direct relationship between entry of serum proteins into extracellular spaces and an increase in the water content was recently demonstrated in the experimental model in which the opening of the BBB to proteins was not associated with any evidence of brain tissue injury [10]. In permanent arterial occlusion, the opening of the BBB to proteins is associated with severe ischemic tissue injury and it occurs after delay of hours or even days. In a temporary arterial occlusion, according to our recent studies [18, 22] there may be two independent BBB openings to proteins during postischemic periods. The first, occurring promptly after the relief of arterial occlusion, is associated with acute reactive hyperemia, which induces barrier opening by the hemodynamic effect of greatly increased intraluminal pressure in blood vessels that are maximally dilated owing to loss of autoregulation. The crucial factors in such hemodynamic barrier opening appear to be the amplitude and rapidity of reactive hyperemia and the density of the preceding ischemia. The second postischemic barrier opening occurs after some delay, which according to the principle of the maturation phenomenon is related to the intensity of ischemic insult [7], and it is likely to be associated with release of some substances that can affect the permeability of the BBB, such as the free fatty acids, kinins, serotonin, and prostaglandins already mentioned.

The necrotic changes in the severely injured tissue lead to infarction and provide such an area with a feature of self-propulsion and *peripheral expansion* into adjacent areas of penumbra. The extracellular compartment becomes rapidly enlarged in such irreversibly injured tissue, owing to rupture of the cellular membranes of dying cells. At the same time, the spillage of cellular contents into extracellular spaces and the catabolic products of cellular disintegration induce a pronounced increment in osmolality and a further significant increase in water content. The resulting marked regional increase in tissue pressure in such severely edematous foci significantly affects the microcirculation in the surrounding regions of penumbra. There, it may lead to depression of rCBF below the critical thresholds of viability, resulting in a further extension of territory with irreversible tissue damage – analogous to a forest fire engulfing the adjacent areas. Thus, the peripheral expansion of the ischemic lesions may develop into a *vicious circle* with a synergistic relationship between the regional increase in tissue pressure and the drop of circulatory blood supply below the critical levels for survival in the adjacent regions. In most cases, the progression of an ischemic lesion stops and it even recedes owing to factors engaged in the healing process. The regression is related to the most vigorous uptake of cellular debris and of extravasated proteins by cells of predominantly macrophagic origin, and to formation of a dense glial and mesodermal scar tissue. Unquestionably, when the pressure subsides the areas of penumbra affected by functional disturbances and swelling not amounting to irreversible neuronal damage promptly begin to recover, and this accounts for the remarkable clinical improvements observed in some stroke patients. The fact that the neurons in the areas of penumbra are capable of full restoration of function should stimulate further research directed at designing proper therapeutic measures facilitating and assuring such recovery.

Summary

In the pathophysiology of cerebral ischemia, several concepts and phenomena have been recognized, and this presentation represents an attempt to evaluate them, especially with regard to ischemic edema, which constitutes the integral and most important part of ischemic injury.

The phenomenon of selective vulnerability was first described long ago and it now appears to be firmly established that it is related to intrinsic, metabolic properties of individual neuronal units, confirming Vogt's theory of pathoclisis. Otherwise, selective vulnerability is closely connected with concept of thresholds for various forms of ischemic injury, since it is apparent that they are related not only to the levels of blood flow impairment but also to intrinsic metabolic properties of individual neuronal units.

The injury to the brain tissue does not stop with the cessation of an ischemic insult, and the postischemic development of ischemic lesions involving various pathomechanisms has been called the maturation phenomenon. Uncoupling of energy supply and utilization and abnormal entry and accumulation of noxious substances may play a significant role in such postischemic development of ischemic lesions.

Among the most important events in postischemic pathology is the onset of ischemic edema, which initially seems to be cytotoxic in type and after a certain duration and at a certain severity of ischemia is supplemented by vasogenic edema.

The peripheral extension of an ischemic lesion proceeds by interference with microcirculation in adjacent areas of the penumbra, leading occasionally to a vicious circle of self-propagation with grave clinical consequences.

References

1. Baethmann A (1978) Pathophysiological and pathochemical aspects of cerebral edema. Neurosurg Rev 1:85–96
2. Fujimoto T, Walker JT, Spatz M, Klatzo I (1976) Pathophysiologic aspects of ischemic edema. In: Pappius HM, Feindel W (eds) Dynamics of brain edema. Springer, Berlin Heidelberg New York, pp 171–180
3. Hass WK (1981) Beyond cerebral blood flow, metabolism and ischemic threshold: Examination of the role of calcium in the initiation of cerebral infarction. In: Meyer JS, Lechner H, Reivich M, Ott EO, Aranibar A (eds) Cerebral vascular disease, vol 3. Excerpta Medica, Amsterdam, pp 3–17
4. Hervonen H, Steinwall O, Spatz M, Klatzo I (1980) Behaviour of the blood-brain barrier toward biogenic amines in experimental cerebral ischemia. In: Eisenberg HM, Suddith RL (eds) The cerebral microvasculature. Plenum, New York, pp 295–305
5. Hossmann K-A, Lechtape-Gruther H, Hossmann V (1973) The role of cerebral blood flow for the recovery of brain after prolonged ischemia. Z Neurol 204:281–290
6. Ito U, Spatz M, Walker JT, Klatzo I (1975) Experimental cerebral ischemia in mongolian gerbils. I: Light microscopic observations. Acta Neuropathol (Berl) 32:209–223
7. Ito U, Go KG, Walker JT Jr, Spatz M, Klatzo I (1976) Experimental cerebral ischemia in mongolian gerbils. III: Behaviour of the blood-brain barrier. Acta Neuropathol (Berl) 34:1–6
8. Klatzo I (1975) Pathophysiologic aspects of cerebral ischemia. In: Tower DB (ed) The nervous system, vol 1. Raven, New York, pp 313–322
9. Klatzo I, Spatz M (1981) Cerebral ischaemia. In: Davison AN, Thompson RHS (eds) The molecular basis of neuropathology. Arnold, New York, pp 132–149
10. Kuroiwa T, Cahn R, Juhler M, Goping G, Campbell G, Klatzo I (1985) Role of extracellular proteins in the dynamics of vasogenic brain edema. Acta Neuropathol (Berl) (in press)
11. Levy D, Van Uitert R, Pike C (1979) Delayed post-ischemic hypoperfusion: a potentially damaging consequence of stroke. Neurology 29:1245–1252
12. Martinez H, Cahn R, Mrsulja BB, Klatzo I (1984) Reactivity of young gerbil brain to cerebral ischemia. J Neuropathol Exp Neurol (in press)
13. Moravetz RB, DeGirolami U, Ojeman RG, Marcoux FW, Crowell RM (1978) Cerebral blood flow determined by hydrogen clearance during middle cerebral artery occlusion in unanesthetized monkeys. Stroke 9:143–149
14. Pulsinelli WA, Brierley JB, Plum F (1982) Temporal profile of neuronal damage in a model of transient forebrain ischemia. Ann Neurol 11:491–498
15. Siesjo BK (1981) Cell damage in the brain: A speculative synthesis. J Cereb Blood Flow Metab 1:155–185
16. Snyder J, Nemoto E, Carroll R, Safar P (1975) Global ischemia in dogs: intracranial pressure, blood flow and metabolism. Stroke 6:21–27
17. Spielmeyer W (1925) Zur Pathogenese örtlich elektiver Gehirnveränderungen. Z Neurol Psychiatr 99:756–776
18. Suzuki R, Yamaguchi T, Kirino T, Orzi F, Klatzo I (1983) The effects of 5 minute ischemia in mongolian gerbils: I. Blood-brain barrier, cerebral blood flow and local cerebral glucose utilization changes. Acta Neuropathol (Berl) 60:207–216
19. Symon L, Brierley JB (1976) Morphological changes in cerebral blood vessels in chronic ischemic infarction: Flow correlation obtained by the hydrogen clearance method. In: Cervos-Navarro J (ed) The cerebral vessel wall. Raven, New York, pp 165–174
20. Symon L, Branston NM, Chikovani O (1979) Ischemic brain edema following middle cerebral artery occlusion in baboons: Relationship between regional cerebral water content and blood flow at 1 and 2 hours. Stroke 10:184–191
21. Vogt C, Vogt O (1922) Erkrankungen der Großhirnrinde im Lichte der Topistik, Pathoklise und Pathoarchitektonik. J Psychiatr Neurol 18:9–68
22. Wagner H, Cahn R, Kuroiwa T, Ting P, Yamaguchi T, Klatzo I (1983) Role of the blood-brain barrier opening to proteins in the pathophysiology of cerebral ischemia. J Cereb Blood Flow Metab [Suppl 1] 3:S417–S418

Edema and Myelin-Associated Extracellular Spaces

A. Hirano[1]

Key words: Extracellular space, myelinated axon, periaxonal space, Schmidt-Lanterman cleft, transverse bands

The white matter constitutes the major site of fluid accumulation in brain edema. The myelinated axon is one of the major elements in the white matter. It is associated with five extracellular compartments, which normally are not easily recognizable, but are clearly demonstrable in various edematous conditions.

The Extracellular Space Surrounding the Myelinated Axon

The most common type of brain edema is hematogenous or vasogenic brain edema. It is associated with injury, vascular lesion, brain tumor, inflammation, and other conditions in which the blood-brain barrier (BBB) is broken. The source of the edema fluid is blood plasma, which traverses the endothelial cells and spreads to the perivascular space. This hematogenous edema fluid infiltrates further into the brain parenchyma through the surrounding astrocytic perivascular foot processes. There are no tight junctions between the perivascular foot processes of the astrocytes, and they do not possess a barrier to certain protein molecules, such as horseradish peroxidase. The plasma protein is able to penetrate the astrocytic layer into the extracellular space.

The white matter contains large numbers of myelinated and unmyelinated axons. These fibers run in parallel fashion to form bundles as a tract. They do not have junctional apparatus between individual fibers. When the hematogenous edema fluid reaches the extracellular space in the white matter it spreads between the axons (Fig. 1).

In contrast, the gray matter has numerous synaptic connections between the neuronal processes and the soma. In addition, dendritic trees have their own individual spread and they usually do not run in parallel fashion. The astrocytes in the gray matter tend to form flattened and sheath-like expansions surrounding neuronal elements, and they have various junctional apparatus, such as punctate adhesions

[1] The Bluestone Laboratory of the Division of Neuropathology, Department of Pathology, Montefiore Medical Center, Albert Einstein College of Medicine, Bronx, New York 10467, USA

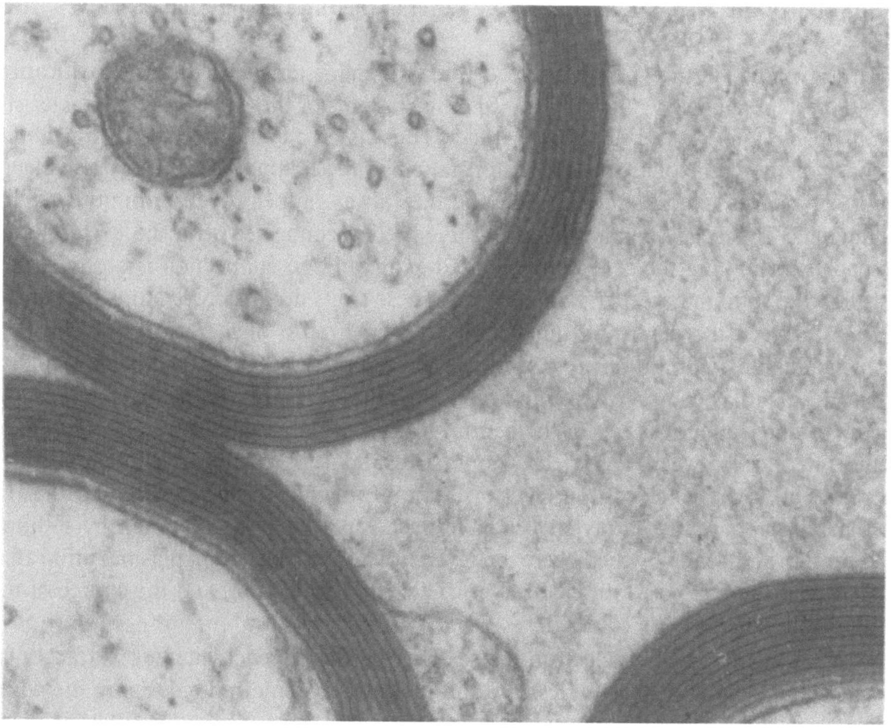

Fig. 1. Electron-dense edema fluid fills distended extracellular space among myelinated nerve fibers. ×94 000 [10]

and gap junctions. These adhesive devices maintain contact between adjacent cells and limit the expansion of the extracellular space.

The hematogenous edema fluid is similar in texture and density to blood plasma [10]. The fluid usually spreads around the fiber tracts and follows the anatomic arrangement of the axon. In this situation, the individual myelinated axons are widely separated from each other, and analysis of the individual nerve fibers is easier. The content of the extracellular fluid is also influenced by admixture with the fixative, which may dilute its appearance. It is important to note that in spite of various pathologic alterations associated with various causative factors, the individual myelinated axon retains its integrity remarkably well. The outer tongue is tightly adhered to the outermost myelin sheath, so that infiltration of the extracellular fluid into the myelin sheath does not usually occur. However, when disruption of the tight junction at the outer tongue and outermost myelin lamellae occurs or formation of this junction is immature, as it is in developing myelinated axons, regular separation of the myelin lamellae takes place, starting from the outer loop into the interior of the myelin sheath [2]. This type of regular separation of myelin is observed in experimental allergic encephalomyelitis and other pathologic conditions. The extracellular space in hematogenous edema is generally confined to the extracellular space between the myelinated axon and other cell processes [9].

Splitting of the Myelin Lamellae at the Level of the Intraperiod Line

Intramyelinic split at the intraperiod line is a characteristic feature of toxification with certain agents, e.g., triethyltin [3]. The contents of these splits are characteristically clear (Fig. 2), and the BBB is intact. There is no expansion of the extracellular space or the periaxonal space. The formation of these apparently empty and structureless spaces is focal and irregular, and they always appear deep within the myelin lamellae. This space has not been observed to be connected with the extracellular space surrounding the central myelinated axon, and no connection is observed between the split and the periaxonal space. These splits do not involve the area of the zone between the outer and inner loops, in which most of the central myelin falls into the same quadrant on cross section. Between these two loops there are regularly arranged radial components. These correspond to the orderly arrangement of the row of tight junctions [12]. In the central myelin, tight junctions are also present at the interface between the lateral loops. Thus, splitting of the myelin induced by triethyltin is prevented at the level of the tight junction of the myelin sheath. The clear and apparently empty spaces have been reported to be occupied by sodium, chloride, and water, which were believed to be derived from plasma infiltrates. However, there is no ruptured BBB in triethyltin toxification, and the source of the fluid still remains to be clarified.

When hematogenous electron-dense fluid in the parenchymatous extracellular space and clear and structureless fluid in the intramyelinic split coexist in the white matter, these two different edema fluids occupy two distinctly different compartments [11]. This situation can be created by IP injection of triethyltin acetate or sulfate and intracerebral implantation of the same substance in the experimental animal. The individual myelinated axon with intramyelinic split floats within the

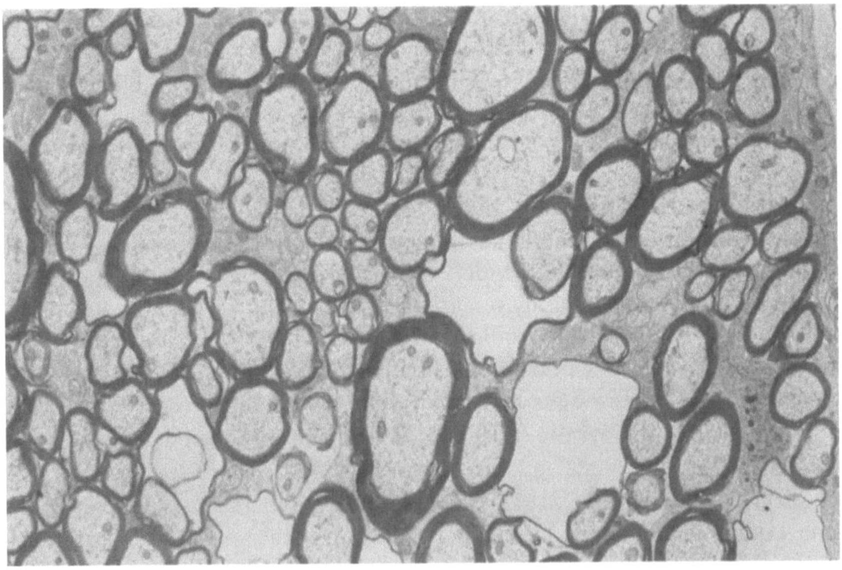

Fig. 2. Intramyelinic split in the optic nerve of a rat with triethyltin toxification. ×5000 [11]

electron-dense hematogenous edema fluid. The segregation of these two compartments is presumably due to the effective seal made by the tight junctions within the myelinated axon [6]. In contrast to the central nervous system, the peripheral nervous system remains intact without intramyelinic split in triethyltin toxification. A similar situation exists on a limited scale in other situations; but it is important to note that the intramyelinic split is one of the most common artifacts associated with various inadequate procedures for fixation. In the case of hexachlorophene intoxication, splitting of the myelin can be produced in both central and peripheral myelin in the developing animal.

The Periaxonal Space

The periaxonal space is a very narrow space less than 10 nm wide between the axon and the myelin-forming cell. This space is electron lucent, and there are no junctions between the axolemma and the plasma membrane of the myelin-forming cell.

The expansion of the axon or focal swelling of the myelin-forming cell should result in compression of the periaxonal space. However, the periaxonal space, surprisingly, maintains its usual width in such circumstances, suggesting that there is some material present between the two opposing membranes bordering the periaxonal space.

Sometimes shrinkage of the axon or distortion of the myelin results in substantial focal enlargement of the periaxonal space. The distended periaxonal space may or may not contain a dense material similar to the extracellular hematogenous edema fluid (Fig. 3). Even in these circumstances, when the axon and the inner cytoplasmic collar are preserved, the normal narrow distance between the axon and the myelin-forming cell is almost always retained in some areas, indicating remarkable maintenance of the intimate association between the axon and the myelin-forming cell. Focal distention of the periaxonal space occurs usually in the area close to the paranode, suggesting infiltration of the extracellular fluid at the interface between the lateral loop and axon. When the axon is completely surrounded by extracellular space, i.e., completely separated by the encircling myelin sheath, it implies severe destruction of the cytoplasmic area of the myelin-forming cell [5].

The Extracellular Spaces at the Schmidt-Lanterman Clefts and Paranodes

Electron-dense fluid has been observed in the extracellular spaces between adjacent cytoplasmic areas of the Schmidt-Lanterman clefts and between lateral loops at the paranodes (Fig. 4) [4]. They have been found in postmortem material of heavily myelinated fibers in the peripheral myelin sheaths. Similar dense fluid has also been observed in the extracellular spaces of the adjacent endoneurium and beneath the outer cytoplasmic collar of the Schwann cell. The dense fluid, however, did not infiltrate into the intraperiod line of the compact myelin. The fluid often reaches the periaxonal space, but wide separation of the periaxonal space usually does not occur. The lateral loops also usually remain in contact with the axon. Unmyelinated nerve fibers, thin myelinated fibers in the peripheral nervous system and central

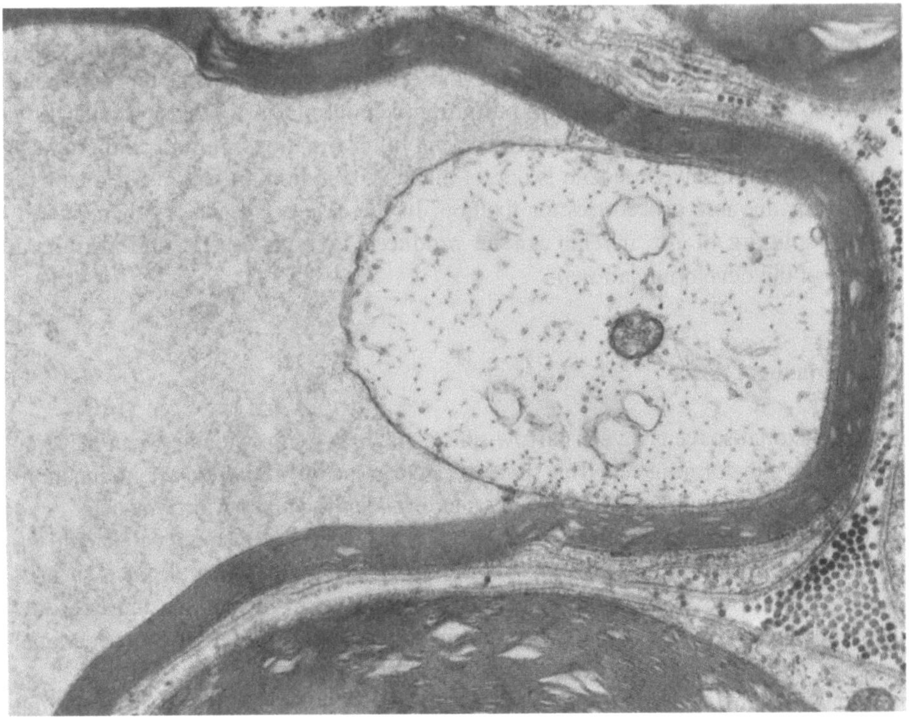

Fig. 3. Enlarged periaxonal space containing electron-dense fluid in an altered peripheral myelinated fiber in a mutant hamster. ×25 000 [5]

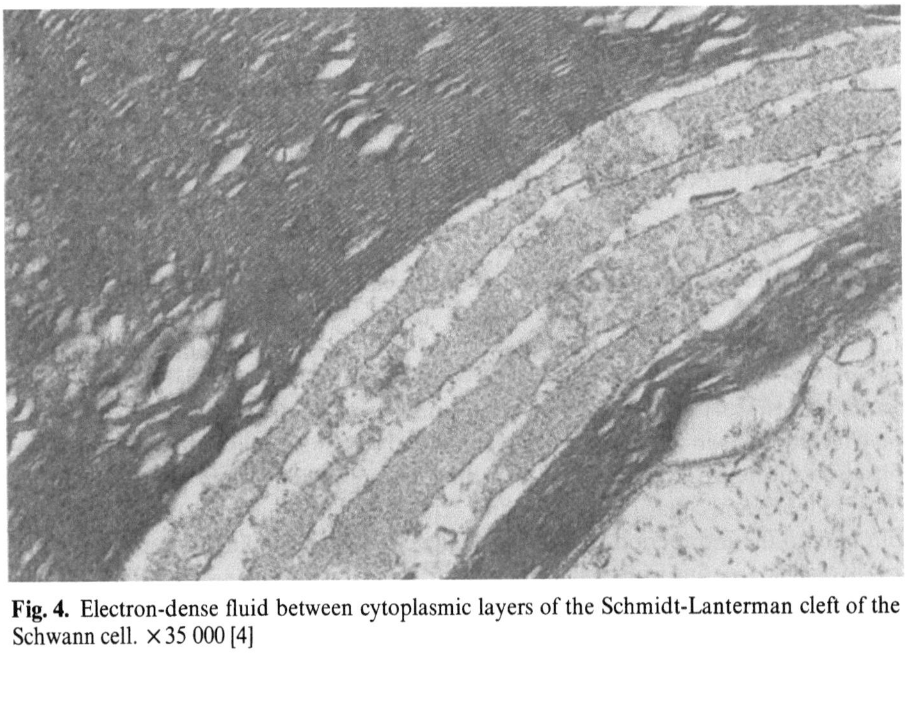

Fig. 4. Electron-dense fluid between cytoplasmic layers of the Schmidt-Lanterman cleft of the Schwann cell. ×35 000 [4]

myelin, are not associated with dense fluid, because these fibers do not usually contain Schmidt-Lanterman clefts. The origin and nature of the dense fluid is uncertain. Probably it originates in the extracellular space of the endoneurium and finds its way into the sheath after death. In the peripheral nervous system the tight junctions at the outer loops are occasionally absent, in contrast to their constant presence in the central nervous system. This may explain the infiltration of the fluid into the peripheral myelin seen in this situation.

The separation of the extracellular space between the Schmidt-Lanterman clefts has previously been reported in nonmanipulated peripheral nerves, and it has been shown to become especially wide in tissue exposed to hypotonic solutions [1, 14]. The electron-dense fluid described here is similar to the extracellular tracer lanthanum reported by Revel and Hamilton [13] and also by Hall and Williams [1]. This tracer material has been shown to infiltrate the extracellular spaces associated with the Schmidt-Lanterman clefts. Lanthanum, however, differs from the dense material reported here in that it also penetrates at least some of the intraperiod lines of the myelin sheath, particularly in the area near the periphery of the sheath [13]. The basis for the different capacities of lanthanum and the dense fluid described here for penetration are unclear. Perhaps electron-dense fluid is composed of higher molecular weight material than lanthanum, preventing it from penetrating to all the spaces accessible to lanthanum. Furthermore, lanthanum may be able to break junctions which are usually impermeable to most substances [7]. These observations suggest that a pathway exists between the extracellular spaces outside the heavily myelinated sheaths and the innermost portion of the sheath.

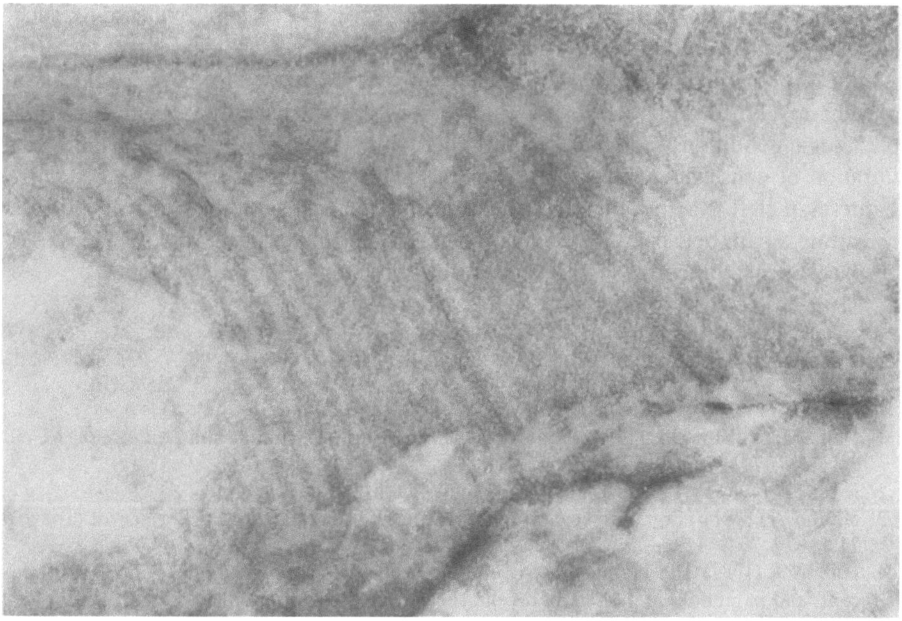

Fig. 5. Paranode of cerebral white matter of a lanthanum-treated rat. Spaces between transverse bands and lateral loops contain electron-dense deposits of lanthanum. ×112 400 [8]

The Extracellular Channels Between the Transverse Bands at the Paranode

The nodal regions of the myelinated fibers consist of a short length of axon exposed to the extracellular space, bounded on each side by the lateral loops of two neighboring myelin segments in the central nervous system. These loops are actually part of a continuous cytoplasmic rim, which traces a helical path around the axon. At the interface of the lateral loops and the axon, unique specializations of the external leaflet of the axonal membrane and the lateral loops of the oligodendroglial cell occur. These structures have been described as transverse bands. When lanthanum is injected into the extracellular spaces this tracer substance infiltrates the extracellular spaces [7]. It passes between the transverse bands at the paranode and appears within the periaxonal spaces (Fig. 5). The transverse bands have been found to be oriented both parallel to and at an angle to the spaces between the lateral loops [8].

The above-mentioned extracellular spaces surrounding myelinated axons are, for the most part, segregated by special junctional devices to give separate compartments.

Summary

The myelinated axon has five extracellular compartments, which normally are not easily recognizable but are clearly demonstrable in various edematous conditions. The extracellular space surrounding the myelinated axon is the major site of accumulation of hematogenous edema fluid. Accumulation of the edema fluid in this space is associated with breakdown of the BBB. The texture of edema fluid is electron-dense, similar to that of blood plasma. Splitting of the myelin lamellae at the level of the intraperiod line is the characteristic feature of certain toxifications, such as triethyltin. The interlamellar space content is characteristically clear and the BBB is intact. The periaxonal space is a very narrow extracellular space between the axon and the myelin-forming cell. Focal enlargement of this space may occur in certain pathologic conditions, and it is usually filled with hematogenous edema fluid. Infiltration of dense fluid may be observed selectively in the region of the Schmidt-Lanterman cleft. Narrow channels of extracellular spaces between transverse bands constitute a path between the parenchymatous extracellular space and the periaxonal space. Special junctional devices generally segregate these compartments.

References

1. Hall SM, Williams PL (1970) Studies on the 'incisures' of Schmidt and Lanterman. J Cell Sci 6:767–791
2. Hirano A (1981 a) A guide to neuropathology. Igaku-Shoin, Tokyo
3. Hirano A (1981 b) Some aspects of neuropathology of intoxications. Clin Neurol (Tokyo) 21:18–29
4. Hirano A (1982) The permeability of the extracellular spaces at the Schmidt-Lanterman clefts and paranodes in peripheral myelin sheaths. Acta Neuropathol (Berl) 58:34–38
5. Hirano A (1983) Reaction of the periaxonal space to some pathologic processes. In: Zimmerman HM (ed) Progress in neuropathology, vol 5. Raven, New York, p 99

6. Hirano A (1984) Nodes of Ranvier in pathological conditions. In: Zagoren JC, Fedoroff S (eds) Advances in cellular neurobiology, vol 6: The node of Ranvier. Academic, New York, p 213
7. Hirano A, Dembitzer HM (1969) The transverse bands as a means of access to the peri-axonal space of the central myelinated nerve fiber. J Ultrastruct Res 24:141–149
8. Hirano A, Dembitzer HM (1982) Further studies on the transverse bands. J Neurocytol 11:861–866
9. Hirano A, Llena JF (1983) Morphological aspects of brain edema. In: Federoff S, Hertz L (eds) Advances in cellular neurobiology, vol 4. Academic Press, New York, p 223
10. Hirano A, Zimmerman HM, Levine S (1965) The fine structure of cerebral fluid accumulation. IX. Edema following silver nitrate implantation. Am J Pathol 47:537–548
11. Hirano A, Zimmerman HM, Levine S (1968) Intramyelinic and extracellular spaces in triethyltin intoxication. J Neuropathol Exp Neurol 27:571–580
12. Nagara H, Suzuki K (1985) Radial component (interlamellar tight junctions) of central myelin in normal and mutant mice with myelin disorders. In: Adachi M, Hirano A, Aronson SM (eds) Pathology of the myelinated axon. Igaku-Shoin, New York, p 80
13. Revel JP, Hamilton DW (1969) The double nature of the intermediate dense line in peripheral nerve myelin. Anat Rec 163:7–16
14. Robertson JD (1958) The ultrastructure of Schmidt-Lanterman cleft and related shearing defects of the myelin sheath. J Biophys Biochem Cytol 4:39–46

Paracellular Pathway for the Resolution of Hydrocephalic Edema

Y. NAKAGAWA [1], J. CERVÓS-NAVARRO, and J. ARTIGAS

Key words: Hydrocephalus, blood-brain barrier, tight junction, paracellular pathway, ionic lanthanum

Materials and Methods

Wistar rats weighing 170–200 g were used in this study. To induce hydrocephalus, kaolin suspension was injected into the cisterna magna by the technique previously described [6]. At 1–4 weeks after kaolin injection thin needles were introduced into each lateral ventricle. Either HRP (Sigma type II, 0.5 mg/ml) or lanthanum chloride ($LaCl_3$; Sigma, 2–3 m*M*) dissolved in saline was perfused into the ventricle through one of the needles. The duration of lateral ventricle to lateral ventricle perfusion was 0.5–3 h at a pressure of 2–3 cmH_2O. Following the perfusion the brain was fixed by the transcardiac route, first with saline and then with mixture of 4% paraformaldehyde and 0.5% glutaraldehyde in 0.1 *M* phosphate buffer or sodium cacodylate buffer at pH 7.4 by means of an infusion at 120 cmH_2O. The brain was rapidly removed after transcardiac perfusion and sectioned with a Vibratome (Model 1000, Lancer USA) at a thickness of 50 μm. Some sections were then incubated for peroxidase activity by means of a two-step method [9]. Subsequently, portions of cerebral cortex containing subependymal and subcortical white matter were dissected out. The tissue blocks were rinsed and post-fixed in a buffered solution of 1% OsO_4 for 120 min, followed by dehydration in a graded series of acetone and embedding in Araldite (Merck). Ultrathin sections were examined in a Zeiss EM 10 electron microscope.

[1] Institute of Neuropathology, Free University Berlin, Hindenburgdamm 30, D-1000 Berlin 45
Present adress: Department of Neurological Surgery, School of Medicine, The University of Tokushima, Tokushima 770, Japan

Fig. 2. Hydrocephalic rat (2 weeks). Ependymal and subependymal areas of the lateral ventricle. HRP was demonstrated in the intercellular space between the ependymal cells, in the extracellular space around the neuropil, and in the basement membrane. Initial magnification ×8100

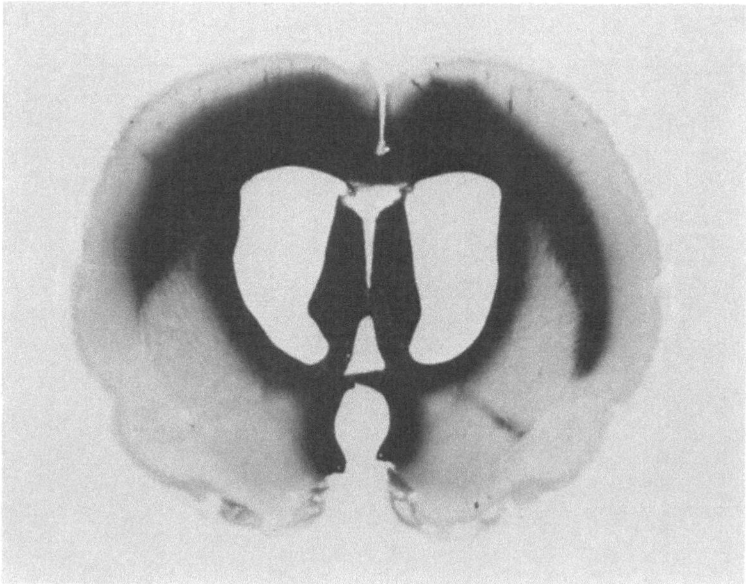

Fig. 1. Cerebral hemisphere in acute hydrocephalus (7 days after kaolin injection into cisterna magna). Dark reactive product of HRP was demonstrated only in the periventricular tissue and corpus callosum

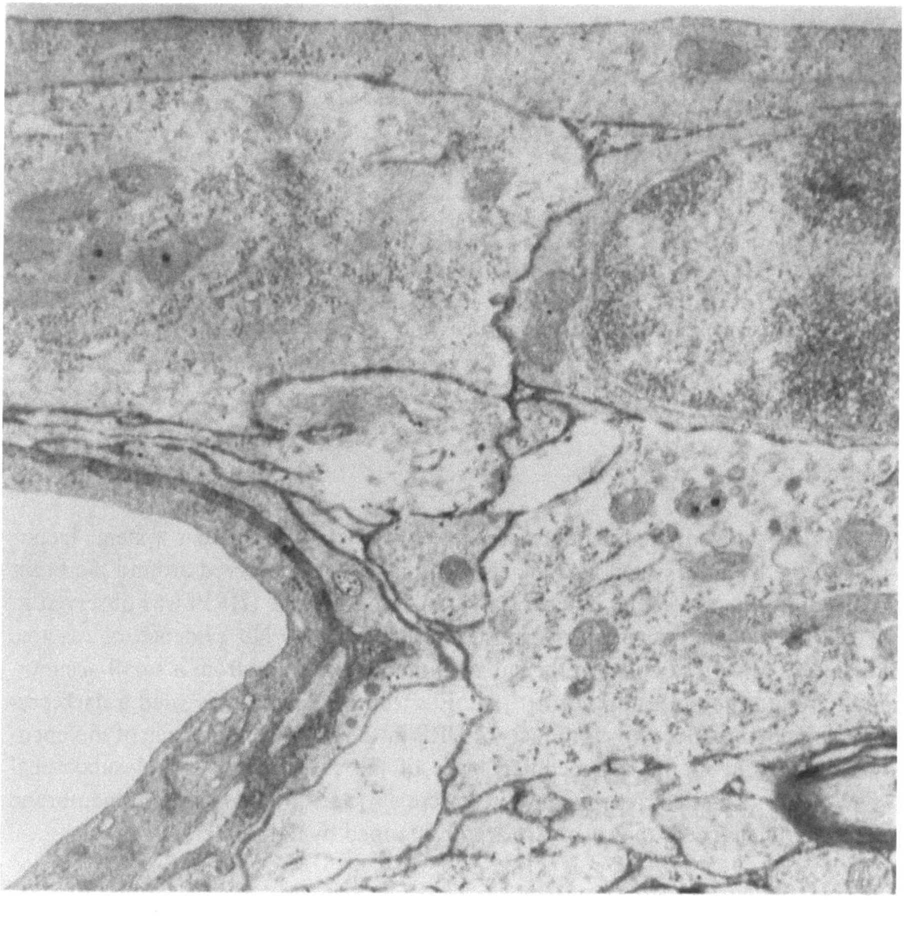

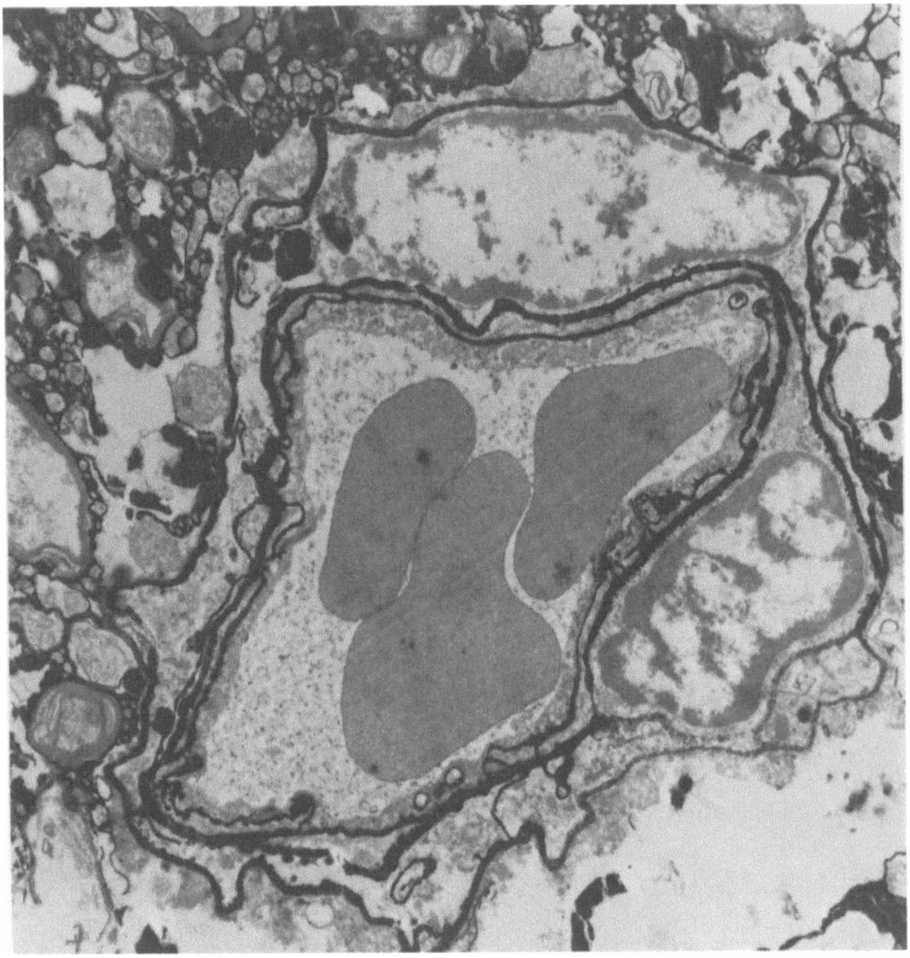

Fig. 3. Hydrocephalic rat (7 days). Electron-dense lanthanum was shown in the extracellular space in the basement membrane of the small arteriole. Lanthanum was also shown in the interendothelial cleft. Initial magnification ×3960

Results

All animals showed a moderately or markedly dilated ventricular system. Deposition of the kaolin injected into the cisterna magna was observed around the brain stem and in the chiasmatic cistern. Horseradish peroxidase (HRP) was observed in the periventricular tissues and corpus callosum (Fig. 1). No evidence of reactive products of HRP was noted in the subarachnoid space aside from a small accumulation around the perfusion needle tract. Electron microscopy revealed a dark precipitate made up of reactive products of HRP in the intercellular space of the ependymal cells and in the extracellular space of the subependymal and subcortical white matter. Although reactive products were also seen in the basement membrane of the endothelial cells they were apparently stopped by tight junctions.

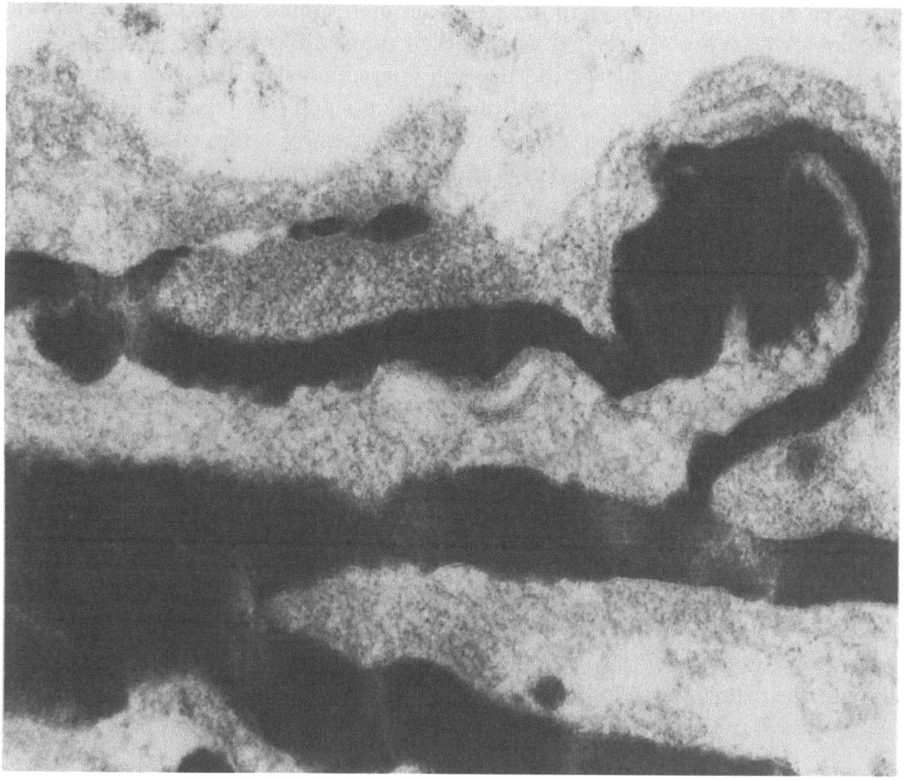

Fig. 4. Higher magnification of the interendothelial cleft. Lanthanum was demonstrated discontinuously in the individual components of intercellular space between the tight junctions. Initial magnification ×48 700

Lanthanum was also demonstrated in the subependymal and subcortical white matter, where it looked similar to HRP (Fig. 2). In addition, lanthanum was seen in the interendothelial cleft between the tight junctions (Fig. 3); it seemed to penetrate these and pass through the entire intercellular space to the lumen of the microvasculature (Fig. 4).

Discussion

Since the physiological study reported by Eisenberg et al. [3], it has been supposed that periventricular cerebrospinal fluid (CSF) or edema fluid in experimental hydrocephalus may not be absorbed into blood vessels in the periventricular white matter. In pathological studies the paracellular pathway for CSF was examined by means of various markers, such as HRP, microperoxidase, or ferritin, following intraventricular perfusion [1, 5, 7]. Although these substances penetrate the intercellular space between the ependymal cells and extend into the extracellular space up to the basement membrane, they are apparently restricted by the tight junction of the endothelium. Recently, however, the possibility of transventricular CSF absorption has been reported following studies based on metrizamide CT [4]. There are two principal mechanisms associated with tracer extravasation into the brain: passage through endothelial cytoplasm and through interendothelial spaces by penetration of tight junctions. It is supposed that this situation may be reversed in hydrocephalus. Those molecules perfused into the ventricle system pass through the intercellular space between the ependymal cells and move within the extracellular space up to the basement membrane. They diffuse through the endothelial cytoplasm, but most of them do not pass the tight junctions.

The permeability of the cell junctions was studied with fluorescent-labeled amino acids and synthetic or natural peptides by Simpson et al. [8]. They reported that molecules of up to 1200 daltons pass through the channels with velocities depending on molecular size, whereas molecules of 1900 daltons or greater do not pass through. Bundgaard and Cserr [2] used radiolabeled polyethylene glycols (900 and 4000 daltons) in the rat and the Atlantic hagfish in their studies. They suggested that there is a blood-brain barrier in both these vertebrates that is impermeable to hydrophilic molecules larger than 900 daltons.

According to the reports in the literature, the use of most substances that have molecules more than 1900 daltons in size may be limited to tracing the bulk flow of CSF or interstitial edema fluid. According to this and previous studies we postulate that in some of the conditions in which the BBB is open, such as hydrocephalus and water toxification, only small molecules penetrate the tight junctions and pass through the entire interendothelial space.

Summary

We studied the intracerebral movement of proteins and ionic lanthanum in experimental hydrocephalus. Hydrocephalus was induced by kaolin injection into the cisterna magna. After 1–4 weeks of hydrocephalus, horseradish peroxidase (HRP) or lanthanum chloride ($LaCl_3$) was perfused into the ventricular system. HRP was demonstrated mainly in the intercellular spaces between ependymal cells, in glial cells, and in perivascular spaces. Although the reactive products were also seen in the basement membrane of the endothelial cells they were apparently stopped by the tight junction. Ionic lanthanum (La^{3+}), however, was observed in the interendothelial cleft between the tight junctions. It seemed to penetrate the tight junctions and pass through the entire intercellular space to the lumen of the microvasculature.

References

1. Brightman MW (1965) The distribution within the brain of ferritin injected into cerebrospinal fluid compartments. J Cell Biol 26:99–122
2. Bundgaard M, Cserr HF (1981) Impermeability of hagfish cerebral capillaries to radiolabelled polyethylene glycols and to microperoxidase. Brain Res 206:71–81
3. Eisenberg HM, McLennan JE, Welch K (1974) Ventricular perfusion in cats with kaolin-induced hydrocephalus. J Neurosurg 41:20–28

4. Hiratsuka H, Tabata H, Tsuruoka S, Aoyagi M, Okada K, Inaba Y (1982) Evaluation of periventricular hypodensity in experimental hydrocephalus by metrizamide CT ventriculography. J Neurosurg 56:235–240
5. Milhorat TH, Davis DA, Hammock MK (1975) Experimental intracerebral movement of electron microscopic tracers of various molecular size. J Neurosurg 42:315–329
6. Nakagawa Y, Cervos-Navarro J, Artigas J (1984) A possible paracellular route for resolution of hydrocephalic edema. Acta Neuropathol (Berl) 64:122–128
7. Ogata J, Hochwald GM, Cravito H, Ransohoff J (1972) Distribution of intraventricular horseradish peroxidase in normal and hydrocephalic cats. J Neuropathol Exp Neurol 31:154–163
8. Simpson I, Rose B, Loewenstein WR (1977) Size limit of molecules permeating the junctional membrane channels. Science 195:294–296
9. Westergaard E, Deurs B, Bronsted HE (1977) Increased vesicular transfer of horseradish peroxidase across cerebral endothelium, evoked by acute hypertension. Acta Neuropathol (Berl) 37:141–152

Thermal Analysis of Edema Fluid and Electron Microscopic Studies in 6-ANA Brain Edema

H. Ishiguri[1], H. Kuchiwaki, N. Misu, S. Takada, S. Inao, J. Itoh, A. Ikeda, and N. Kageyama

Key words: Brain edema, electron microscopy, free and bound water, 6-aminonicotinamide (6-ANA), thermal analysis

Introduction

Some of the factors involved in the formation of brain edema are well known. Many previous papers in this field have suggested a mechanism for this formation of brain edema induced by cytotoxic, vasogenic, and other correlated factors [8, 12]. Although many important studies have been conducted using physiological, biochemical, and morphological methods, edema caused by cerebral ischemia has not yet been satisfactorily examined.

In a study of brain edema, Ambo [1] developed the idea of bound water and free water from an analysis of edema fluid. Furuse and the present authors [6, 13] stressed that the molecular aspects of edema fluid as estimated by the thermal method were an important factor in the causation of some kinds of brain edema.

In studies designed to increase their understanding of the pathogenesis of edema formation, the authors used a cytotoxic-type model of brain edema produced with 6-ANA (6-aminonicotinamide), which is a metabolic inhibitor [5]. In animals given 6-ANA edema formation is characteristically observed in the gray matter [3, 10, 11]. Using this model of brain edema we analyzed morphological changes by the thermal method and simultaneously by electron microscopy. We think that this use of two different techniques might be important for the understanding of brain edema at specific time points within this model.

Materials and Methods

Animal Preparation and Sampling

Wistar rats weighing 180–350 g and of both sexes were used in this experimental study. 6-Aminonicotinamide dissolved in distilled water was administered IP. The total dose was 120 mg/kg body weight for each animal. At 3, 6, 12, 24, 48, and 72 h after the administration of the drug the neurologic status of the animals was examined. Some were sacrificed for sampling at each experimental hour.

[1] Department of Neurosurgery, Nagoya University School of Medicine, Nagoya 466, Japan

Thermal Analysis with Differential Scanning Calorimetry

Approximately five experimental animals were anesthetized with ether and decapitated at each experimental hour. The brains were rapidly removed and sliced coronally with a sharp knife. Small pieces of these samples were taken from the cortex of the frontal region and from the basal ganglia, including the thalamus. The weight of the samples varied between 15 and 35 mg. They were rapidly enclosed in airtight and preweighed aluminium capsules (P/N 560-002: Daini Seikosha Co.). The capsules were reweighed and placed in the cell of a differential scanning calorimeter (DSC; SSC/560: Daini Seikosha Co.) for measurement of the free water content by freezing. In the present study, freezing was conducted at a constant rate of −10 °C/min from 20 °C to −50 °C. After freezing the capsules were reopened and replaced in the cell to be dried to a constant weight by heating to 150–200 °C at a rate of 50 °C/min followed by maintenance of this temperature for 6 min. After these measurements the relative amounts of free water (FW), total water (TW), and bound water (BW) were calculated. The equations for these calculations are given in Table 1.

Electron Microscopic Study

At each experimental hour, three or four of the rats were anesthetized by IP injection of pentobarbital sodium at a dose of 40 mg/kg body weight. As soon as the thoracic wall had been opened, the ascending aorta was cannulated via the left ventricle, and the right atrium was widely opened. Immediately after the blood had been completely washed out, 2.5% glutaraldehyde in 0.1 *M* phosphate buffer (pH 7.3) was infused for about 10–20 min at a pressure of about 150 cmH_2O.

The brains were removed after the perfusion, and small pieces of gray matter from the frontal region were sliced, fixed in the same solution for 2 h, and post-fixed in 2% osmium tetroxide for a further 2 h. The specimens were dehydrated in graded

Table 1. Calculation of water components

$$\text{Total water (mg)} = \text{Total weight (mg)} - \text{Dry weight (mg)}$$

$$\text{Water content (\%)} = \frac{\text{Total weight (mg)} - \text{Dry weight (mg)}}{\text{Total weight (mg)}} \times 100$$

$$\text{Free water (mg)} = \frac{\text{Calorific value (cal) (estimated in DSC freezing)}}{79.4\ \text{(cal/mg)}}$$

$$\text{Free water (\%)} = \frac{\text{Free water (mg)}}{\text{Total water (mg)}} \times 100$$

$$\text{Bound water (mg)} = \text{Total water (mg)} - \text{Free water (mg)}$$

$$\text{Bound water (\%)} = 100 - \text{Free water (\%)}$$

$$\text{Water binding to solid tissue component} = \frac{\text{Bound water (mg)}}{\text{Dry weight (mg)}}$$

Table 2. Neurological status after administration of 6-ANA (120 mg/kg)

Neurological status	Time course (h)						
	0	3	6	12	24	48	72
Normal	19						
Moderate paraparesis		4	6	4	1		
Severe paraparesis		1		1	2	2	
Tetraplegia					2	4	
Death							5
Total	19	5	6	5	5	6	5

ethanol and embedded in Epon 812. Sections were cut with glass knives on a Sorvall MT-1 ultramicrotome. Thin sections were placed on 200-mesh copper grids and photographed in an electron microscope (Hitachi H-500 and Nihondenshi JEM-100 CX).

Results

Neurologic Status

The neurological status of the animals (Table 2) was assessed in five categories: normal, moderate paraparesis, severe paraparesis, tetraplegia, and death. After the administration of 6-ANA the animals became hypoactive at 3 h and paraparetic at 6 h. Paraparesis gradually progressed with time. Of the five rats sacrificed at 24 h, one had moderate paraparesis, two severe paraparesis, and two tetraplegia. At 48 h four of the six rats were tetraplegic, lying on their sides and breathing irregularly. All five rats had died by 72 h. These results correlated well with the formation of brain edema detected by means of the other studies.

Thermoanalytic Studies

The mean TW content of the gray matter was 80.9% ± 0.1% (SE) in the control rats ($n = 79$), 92.6% ± 0.4% of this being FW. In the basal ganglia the mean TW content was 78.9% ± 0.2% and the FW accounted for 90.3% ± 0.7% of this. At no experimental hour was there any significant increase in TW compared with the control values, either in the gray matter or in the basal ganglia (Fig. 1).

In spite of the worsening of neurologic status, monitoring of TW content revealed no significant differences between the control stage and any other stage at any experimental hour.

In contrast, however, the FW content changed significantly over the course of the experiment. In the gray matter the percentage of FW increased gradually from the beginning of the 3rd hour and reached a peak value, 94.4% ± 0.7%, 12 h after toxifi-

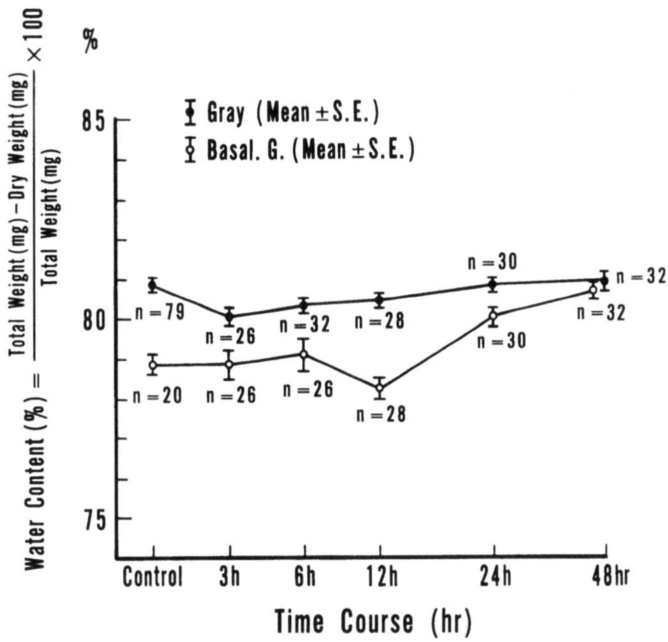

Fig. 1. Changes in TW content after the administration of 6-ANA. At no experimental hour was there any significant increase in TW compared with the control, either in the gray matter or in the basal ganglia

cation. Thereafter it decreased slightly, the decline being statistically nonsignificant. The FW fraction in the basal ganglia began to increase at 3 h, like that in the gray matter, and reached a maximum value, 92.9% ± 0.7%, at 12 h, which was also followed by a statistically nonsignificant decrease. The change in FW fraction followed a similar pattern in both regions (Fig. 2).

Morphological Studies

Minimal morphological changes were observed in the perivascular astrocytes, including neuropils (Fig. 3), even at 3 h. Swelling of the perivascular astrocytes had started to appear at 6 h and was manifestly clear by 12 h after the administration of 6-ANA (Fig. 3). From 12 h onward swollen oligodendrocytes with vacuolar degeneration were seen occasionally in the rough endoplasmic reticula. At 24 h after toxification the astrocytic processes became definitively swollen, in addition to the swelling of the perivascular astrocytes (Fig. 4a, b). At 48 h, the cytoplasm of the cell processes became more electron lucent and the intracellular structure became obscured by vacuolization (Fig. 4c, d).

Tissue degeneration in the gray matter progressed with time. This was mainly observed as swelling of the astrocytes.

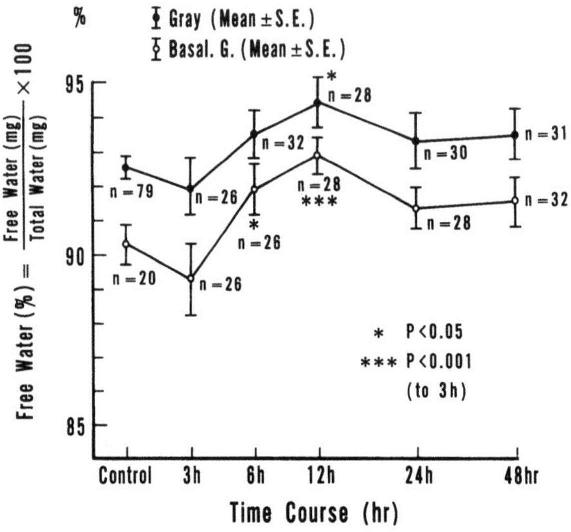

Fig. 2. Changes in FW fraction after the administration of 6-ANA. The FW fraction begins to increase at 3 h and reaches its peak at 12 h; there is a statistically significant difference both in the gray matter and in the basal ganglia between experimental and control values

Discussion

Since Klatzo's classification [12] of pathogenesis of brain edema, two types of categories, cytotoxic and vasogenic, have been thought to be important. This classification is based on the possibility of macromolecules permeating from the blood vessels. Edema formation of a cerebral infarction is studied by a similar pathogenesis. At one time such a classification seemed to be an aid to understanding of the pathogenesis of the brain edema. However, in the process of the formation of ischemic brain edema two different types appeared together in the case of brain swelling associated with a cerebral infarction. Schuier and Hossmann [19] reported that early ischemic brain edema following occlusion of the middle cerebral artery was of the cytotoxic type. However, other workers [8, 9] reported that the vasogenic factor was also related to the formation of ischemic brain edema.

We think that the process of ischemic edema formation is precipitated and maintained by a main cause and several other pathogenic factors. For the study of brain edema it is convenient to simplify the pathogenesis of edema formation.

The cytotoxic edema induced by the administration of 6-ANA has been evaluated previously [3, 10, 11, 17, 18]. Our experience demonstrates several particular features. 6-Aminonicotinamide, an antagonist of niacin [5], produces a typical edema in the gray matter of the brain [3, 10, 11]. Beathmann et al. [3] suggested that the mechanism of its action blocks the energy-producing mechanism and an inadequate supply of ATP to Na-K ATPase ultimately causes swelling of the glial cells owing to the influx of sodium and escape of potassium. In view of its mechanism of action [5] and the high activity of Na-K ATPase in gray matter [4], the cortex and the basal ganglia of rats were studied in these experiments. If triethyltin is used as

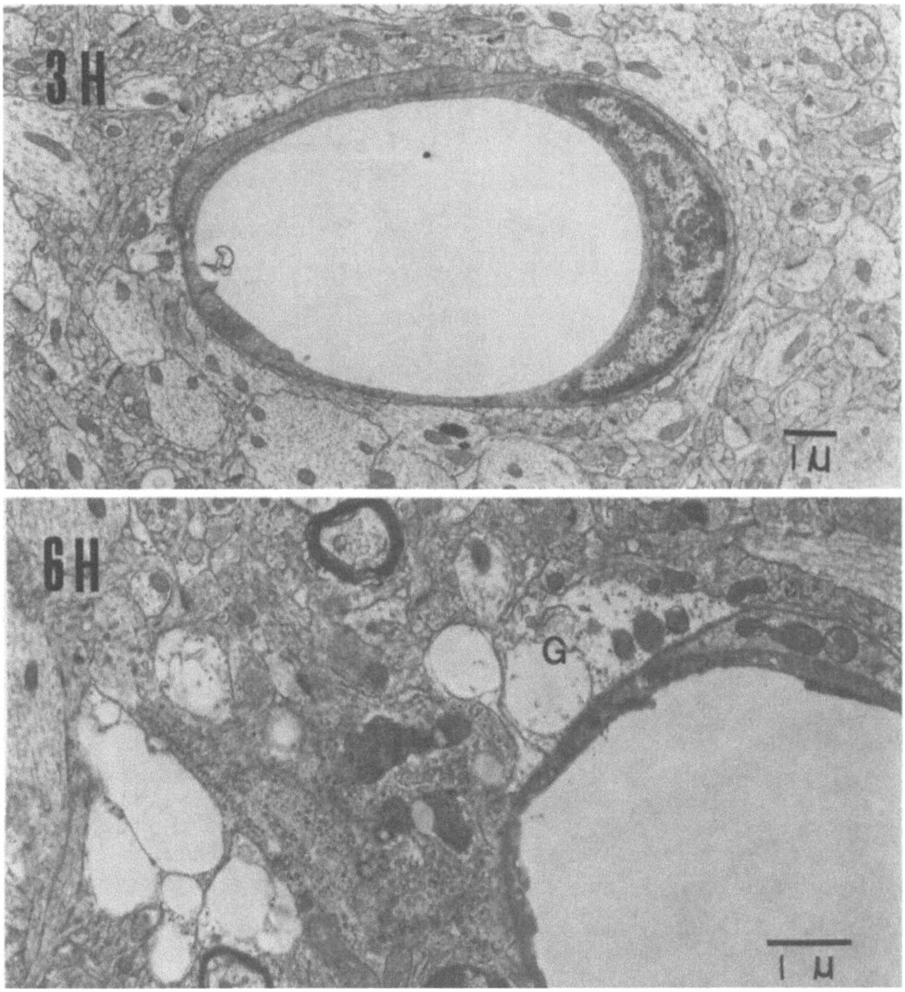

Fig. 3. Electron-microscopic findings at 3 h (*3H*), and at 6 h (*6H*). Morphologically minimal changes are observed at 3 h, but swelling of the perivascular astrocytes appears at 6 h. *G*, swollen perivascular astrocyte

the toxic agent rats are not suitable for these experiments, because it mainly affects the white matter [14], which is poorly developed in the rat.

The approach to edema analysis by a thermal method had been developed earlier in our laboratory. The changes in TW content determined by the method of dry-weight measurements provide little information. In recent years thermoanalysis and nuclear magnetic resonance (NMR) studies have provided information on the na-

Fig. 4a–d. Electron-microscopical findings at 24 h (*24H* **a, b**) and at 48 h (*48H* **c, d**). At 24 h, astrocytic processes become definitively swollen in the neuropil. At 48 h, the cytoplasm of the cell processes become more electron lucent and the intracellular structure becomes obscured by vacuolization

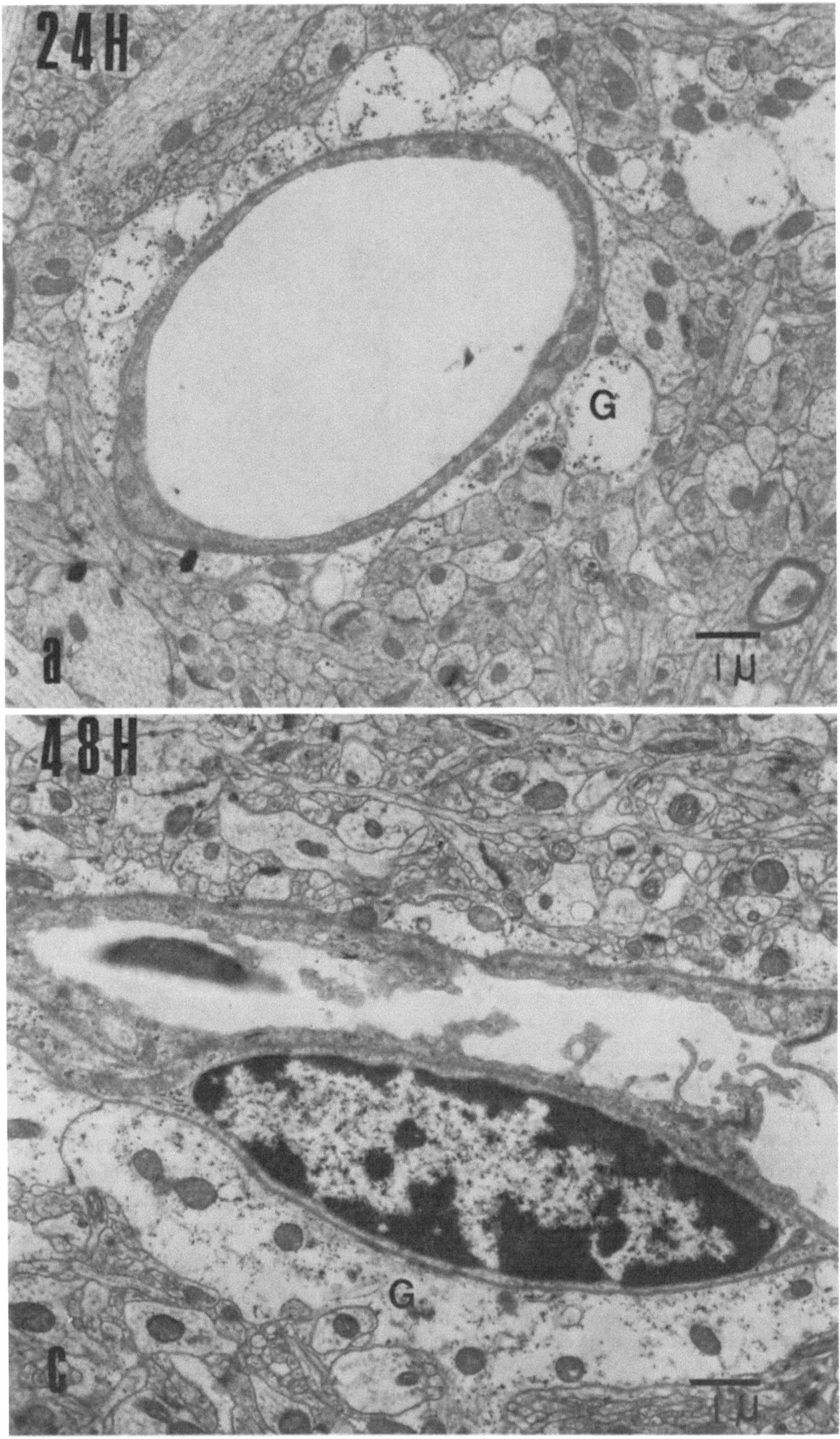
24 H
G
a
1 μ
48 H
G
c
1 μ

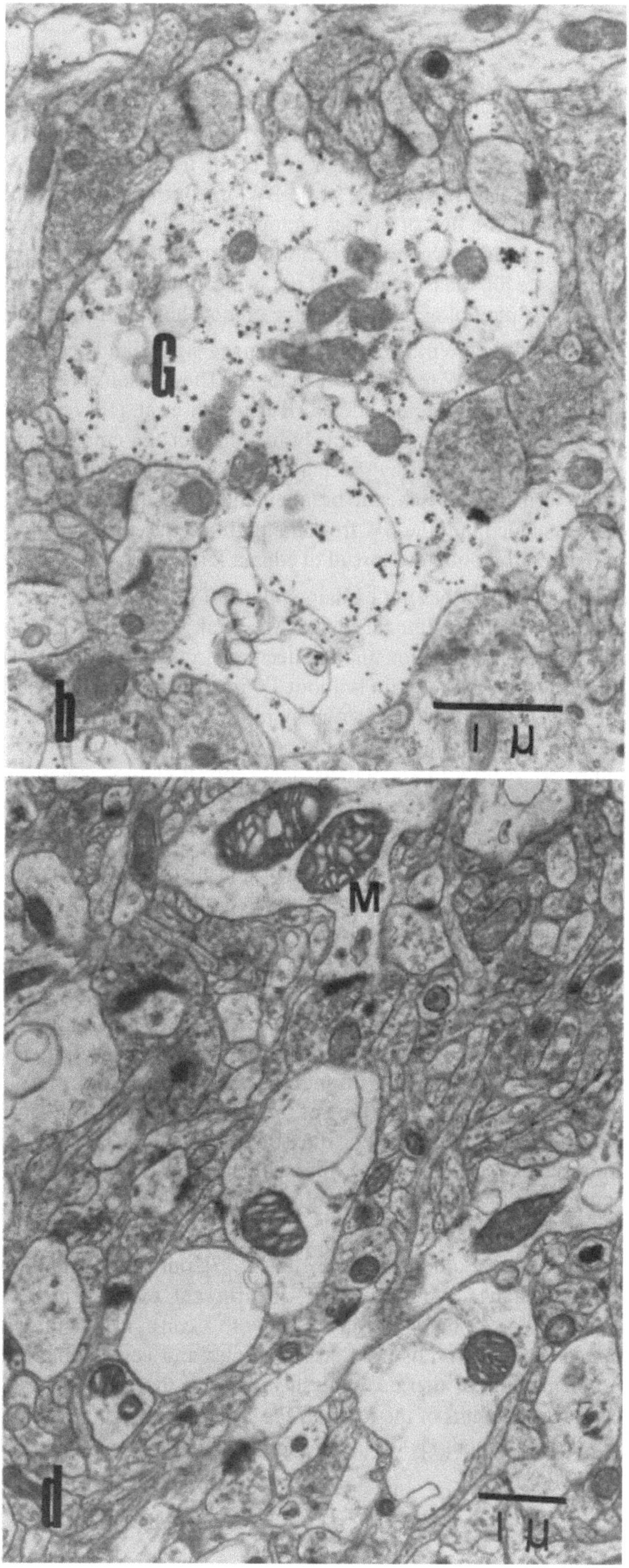
G
b
1 μ
M
d
1 μ

ture of the biomolecular activity of edema fluid [6, 13, 16]. The movements of edema water and its compositional changes have been more clearly demonstrated with these methods. The FW, a major part of the tissue water, can move freely across the various biological structures, while BW, in contrast, includes the structural water of the cell wall and that of various biological substances of high molecular weight, such as proteins and polypeptides. In addition, the BW fraction is larger in serum than in brain tissue [6]. Measurements of the two components can show the dynamics of water and the physiological significance of morphological changes.

In this study the fraction of FW changed significantly compared with that in controls, while the TW remained unchanged. These results are in contrast with those recorded in ischemic brain edema. Kuchiwaki et al. [13] reported that both FW and BW had increased simultaneously by 4 h after the embolization of the internal carotid artery in dogs. They speculated that an influx of BW played an important role in the formation of ischemic brain edema. They discussed the origin of edema fluid and concluded that the BW from the perifocal vascular bed induced high local tissue pressure, promoting the spread of edema formation.

However, this does not explain why the TW did not increase in the current experimental model of cytotoxic edema. We think the key to this question may be the increase in the FW fraction and the decrease in the BW fraction. The tissue–blood partition of water in the brain is about 1.0 in a normal physiological condition [20], and the movement of water is extremely rapid in biological tissue. The FW could be said to represent this rapidly movable portion of the TW in tissue. Thus, FW may be retained transiently in edematous tissue, but it cannot remain there for a long time and it might then be rapidly cleared from the edematous tissue through the surrounding vessels.

In the present study, the BW fraction decreased. This may mean a decrease in the amount of high-molecular substances bound and at the same time a decrease in the functional activity of tissue protein, e.g., such enzymes as polynucleosides.

6-Aminonicotinamide may interfere with cell metabolism and biosynthesis, resulting in the decrease of enzymatic activities and of synthetic products such as proteins, polypeptides, neurotransmitters, and other high-molecular substances. These chemical activities may be related to the morphological alteration in electrolucent cytoplasms, vacuolization of endoplasmic reticula, and morphological changes of the mitochondria. The swelling of the astrocytes was not equal to the increase in TW content. This swelling may be due solely to the movement of water, i.e., mainly FW, from the extracellular to the intracellular space. However, perfusion fixation might constitute a methodological problem by masking the extracellular space deformation in our study [3].

In contrast to other reports [3, 10, 11, 17], our results showed that the TW content did not change significantly. In the present experiment we used microsamples weighing 15–35 mg and heated rapidly to a constant weight. Other authors who obtained different results used large samples and conventional drying methods. One problem with our thermal analysis method is that such small samples demand precise measurements of the FW and the BW. To understand the discrepancies between the different methods the method of specific gravity should be used to reevaluate the results [8, 15].

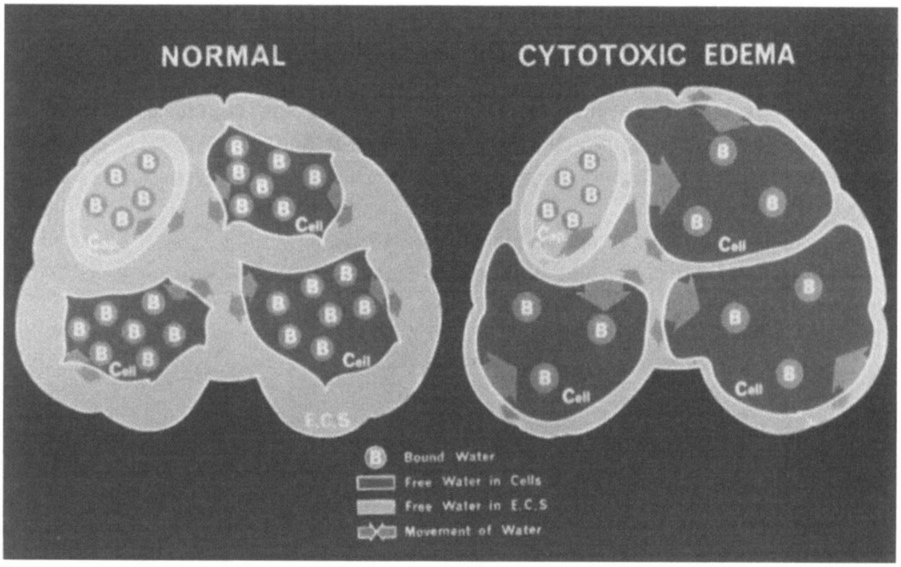

Fig. 5. Schematic illustrating the formation of cytotoxic edema

In this study morphological changes were not as severe as those in ischemic brain edema [2]. There was selective damage to neuroglial cells in the gray matter. However, neurons and endothelial cells were almost intact. In spite of the higher drug dose these findings are quite similar to morphological changes previously reported [3, 17, 18].

Figure 5 is a schematic illustrating the formation of cytotoxic edema which resulted from our model. The decrease in the extracellular space and swelling of the cells, especially astrocytes, is demonstrated. The rapid clearance of FW, which was expected to increase, in fact results in no water retention. An increase in pinocytotic vesicles was also found [17].

In conclusion, we believe that all these findings are characteristic of the cytotoxic edema produced by 6-ANA.

Summary

The increase of edema fluid and the progress of cytotoxic damage are important for understanding the pathogenesis of the formation of brain edema. The purpose of this study is to clarify the relationship of constitutional changes of edema fluid to the results of electron microscopic study of cellular damage.

Adult Wistar rats each received 120 mg/kg body weight 6-ANA (6-aminonicotinamide) by IP injection, and their neurologic status was examined after 3, 6, 12, 24, and 48 h. Constitutional changes in total water, free water, and bound water contents were analyzed at each experimental hour by a thermal method using differential scanning calorimetry (DSC). In the electron-microscopic studies cellular damage was also evaluated at various stages during the formation of the edema.

The neurologic status of the animals deteriorated after 3 h and became severely impaired by 48 h. The total water content did not increase, substantially, but the ratio of free water characteristically rose within 6 h, attaining a maximum value at 12 h. Bound water did not increase as much as in ischemic edema, as reported in our previous papers. Morphological studies have shown that perivascular astrocytes swell most remarkably at 48 h, which was somewhat later than the changes in the ratio of the water content. A rise in free water caused by cell damage in this model of cytotoxic brain edema increased the free water ratio.

However, total water content itself shows little change compared with ischemic brain edema.

References

1. Ambo H (1951) Experimental swelling of the brain and its bound water content. Acta Pathol Jpn 1:63–71
2. Arsenio-Nunes ML, Hossmann KA, Farkas-Bargeton E (1973) Ultrastructural and histochemical investigation of the cerebral cortex of cat during and after complete ischemia. Acta Neuropathol (Berl) 26:392–344
3. Beathmann A, Van Harreveld A (1973) Water and electrolyte distribution in gray matter rendered edematous with a metabolic inhibitor. J Neuropathol Exp Neurol 32:408–423
4. Bonting SL, Simon KA, Hawkins NM (1961) Studies on sodium-potassium activated adenosine triphosphatase: 1. Quantitative distribution in several tissues of the cat. Arch Biochem Biophys 95:416–423
5. Dietrich LS, Friedland IM, Kaplan LA (1958) Pyridine nucleotide metabolism: Mechanism of action the niacin antagonist, 6-aminonicotinamide. J Biol Chem 233:964–968
6. Furuse M, Gonda T, Kuchiwaki H, Hirai N, Inao S, Kageyama N (1984) Thermal analysis on the state of free and bound water in normal and edematous brain. In: Go G, Beathmann A (eds) Recent progress in the study and therapy of brain edema. Plenum, New York, p 293
7. Garcia JH, Kalimo H, Kamijyo Y, Trump BF (1977) Cellular events during partial cerebral ischemia. 1: Electron microscopy of feline cerebral cortex after middle-cerebral-artery occlusion. Virchows Arch [Cell Pathol] 25:191–206
8. Garcia HJ (1984) Experimental ischemic stroke: a review. Stroke 15:5–14
9. Hossmann K-A (1983) New trends for the evaluation of experimental brain edema. In: Ishii S, Nagai H, Brock M (eds) Intracranial pressure, vol V. Springer, Berlin Heidelberg New York, p 29
10. James HE, Laurin RA (1981) Intracranial hypertension and brain edema in albino rabbits: 1. Experimental models. Acta Neurochir 55:213–226
11. James HE, Bruce DA, Welsh F (1978) Cytotoxic edema produced by 6-aminonicotinamide and its response to therapy. Neurosurgery 3:196–200
12. Klazo I (1967) Neuropathological aspects of brain edema. J Neuropathol Exp Neurol 26:1–16
13. Kuchiwaki H, Furuse M, Gonda T, Hirai N, Inao S, Ikeyama A, Kageyama N (1984) Studies on changes in tissue water constitution and focal brain tissue pressure in experimental cerebral infarction. In: Go G, Beathmann A (eds) Recent progress in the study and therapy of brain edema. Plenum, New York, p 459
14. Lee JC, Bakay L (1965) Ultrastructural changes in edematous central nervous system: 1. Triethyltin edema. Arch Neurol 13:48–57
15. Marmarou A, Poll W, Shulman K, Bhagavan H (1978) A simple gravimetric technique for measurement of cerebral edema. J Neurosurg 49:530–537
16. Naruse S, Holicawa Y, Tanaka C, Hirakawa K, Nishikawa H, Yoshizaki K (1982) Proton nuclear magnetic resonance on brain edema. J Neurosurg 56:747–752

17. Sasaki S (1982) Brain edema and gliopathy induced by 6-aminonicotinamide intoxication in the central nervous system of rats. Am J Vet Res 43:1691–1695
18. Schneider H, Cervós-Navarro J (1974) Acute gliopathy in spinal cord and brain stem induced by 6-aminonicotinamide. Acta Neuropathol (Berl) 27:11–23
19. Schuier FJ, Hossmann K-A (1980) Experimental brain infarcts in cats, 2. Ischemic brain edema. Stroke 11:593–601
20. Ter-Pogossian MM, Eichling JO, Davis DO, Welch MJ, Metzger JM (1969) The determination of regional cerebral blood flow by means of water labeled with radioactive oxygen-15. Radiology 93:31–40

The Fine Structural Study of Brain Response to Intracerebral Infusion of Serum in the Cat

A. HIRANO [1], A. MARMAROU, T. NAKAMURA, and A. INOUE

Key words: Astrocytes, brain edema, extracellular space, phagocytosis, electron microscopy

Introduction

The mechanism of vasogenic edema resolution is unclear and is a subject of investigation at various laboratories, including our own. Our previous studies using the infusion model of brain edema indicated distinct differences between resolution after infusion of mock CSF and of serum, as evaluated by gravimetric assessment of the water content of the brain [6]. Rapid absorption of water to the normal level was achieved by 72 h in animals that received mock CSF, while those that received serum required 8 days for tissue water to return to normal levels. We now report on the morphological correlates to these studies.

Materials and Methods

A total of eight adult cats were studied: four were used as control; two were perfused immediately after serum infusion; one, 3 days after infusion; and one, 8 days after infusion. The method of infusion has been described in detail previously [6].

In this study, 0.5 mm^3 serum was infused into the left hemisphere. The animals were sacrificed by the perfusion technique [4]. They were anesthesized with an IP injection of Nembutal (35 mg/kg) and then given heparin (0.2 ml) IV. The animals were perfused with 4% paraformaldehyde in phosphate buffer, pH 7.4, for 5 min and switched to 5% glutaraldehyde in phosphate buffer, pH 7.4, for 10 min. After perfusion, the brain was removed and placed in 5% glutaraldehyde in phosphate buffer for 2–3 h, after which they were removed to buffer rinse with 70% sucrose overnight, 24–48 h. Blocks of tissue for electron microscopy sections were removed from the region in the left hemisphere with the aid of the dissecting microscope. The site of infusion, the white matter distal to the infusion, and the lateral corner of the frontal horn, including the ependymal lining, were sampled after slicing of each brain in the horizontal plane. The blocks of tissue were dehydrated after fixation in

---

[1] The Bluestone Laboratory of the Division of Neuropathology, Department of Pathology, Montefiore Medical Center, Albert Einstein College of Medicine, Bronx, New York 10467, USA

Dalton's osmium solution. The tissue was embedded in Epon. Thick sections from all the Epon-embedded material were stained with toluidine blue. After identification of the precise location thin sections were cut, stained with lead and uranyl salt, and examined with the electron microscope.

Results

The fine structure of normal gray and white matter in the untreated cat brain is essentially similar to that of other mammalian brains [2].

Changes Immediately After Infusion

The site of infusion and the adjacent white matter was characterized by markedly distended extracellular spaces in the white matter. These extracellular spaces were filled with electron-dense edema fluid (Fig. 1) essentially identical with those observed in the hematogenous edema fluid seen after silver nitrate implantation in the hemisphere. This electron-dense edema fluid separated individual myelinated and nonmyelinated axons, as well as glial cell processes. However, in the perivascular area, the vascular foot processes of astrocytes were continuous without separation. Junctional devices maintained contact between these cell processes. Astrocytic cytoplasm often showed various degrees of swelling. The ependymal layer was also saturated with edema fluid at the basal aspect. However, the junctional devices maintained connections between adjacent ependymal cells without separation in spite of large amounts of adjacent extracellular fluid.

In contrast to the white matter, the gray matter generally maintained relatively narrow and complicated extracellular spaces, even though similar electron-dense edema fluid infiltrated between the cells and cell processes. The presence of numerous synapses and other junctional apparatus and the complex arrangement of cell processes prevented the formation of ample extracellular spaces in the gray matter [1].

The astrocytes often contained membrane-bound vacuoles which were filled with granular substance of various densities, some of which were identical with the extracellular fluid (Fig. 2). In addition to the homogeneous electron-dense fluid there were markedly denser substances, often with globular configurations. Macrophages filled with many vacuoles containing various materials were often observed in the perivascular space. They were also occasionally present within the edematous extracellular space in the parenchyma. Oligodendroglial cells and axons were surrounded by the edema fluid. However, they were usually free of engulfed material. The neuronal soma in the adjacent gray matter was also devoid of membrane-bound edema fluid.

Changes 72 h After Infusion

Wide distention of the extracellular space persisted and morphological features were quite similar to those immediately after infusion. However, there were two dif-

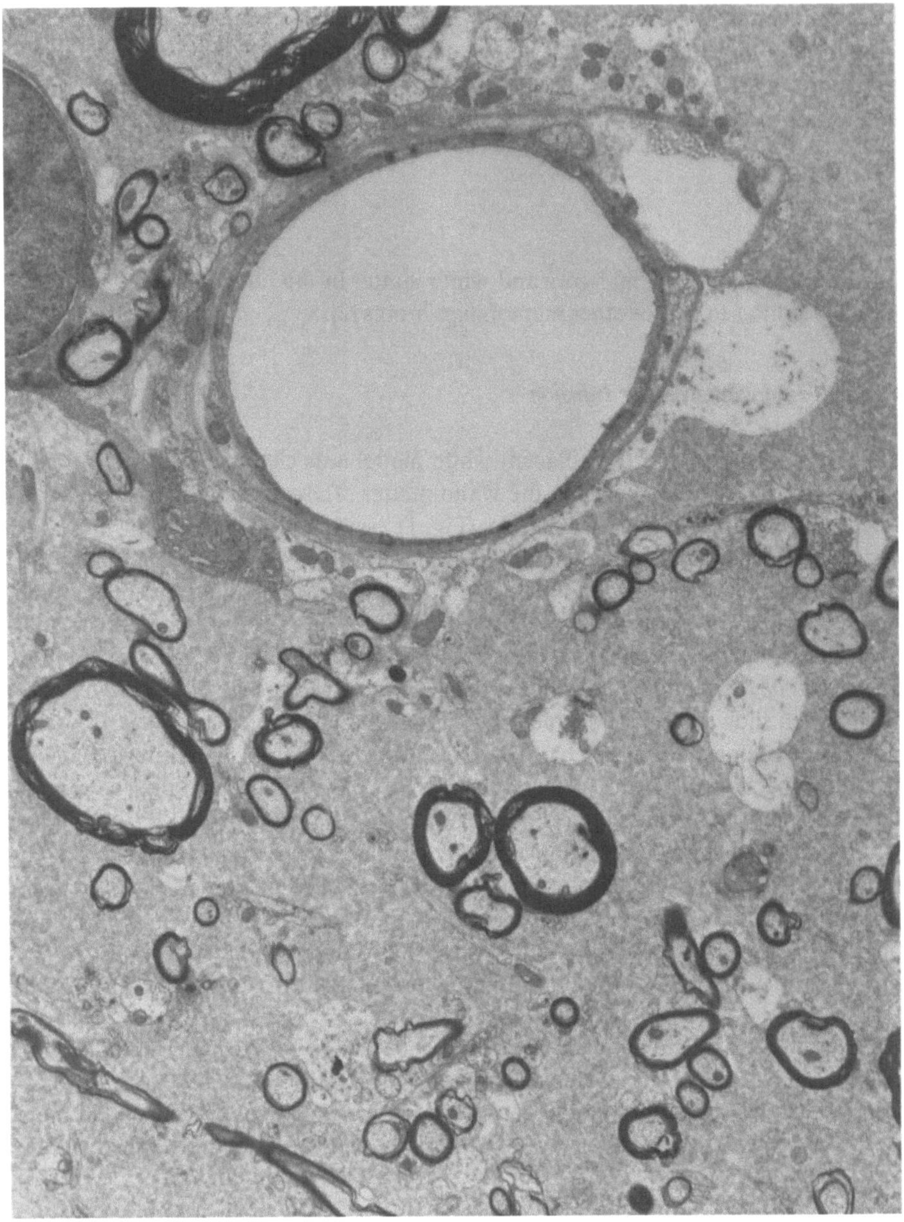

Fig. 1. Edematous white matter with markedly electron-dense material in the distended extracellular space immediately after infusion of serum. The blood vessel lumen is clear. ×5440

ferences. First, the density of the extracellular fluid was markedly reduced (Fig. 3). Even though the extracellular spaces contained an evenly distributed fine granular substance, their distribution was generally looser than that seen immediately after infusion. Another difference at this stage was the presence of swollen astrocytes and their cell processes, which contained numerous delicate glial fibrils (Fig. 4). The extracellular space was markedly reduced in some areas and hardly recognizable in

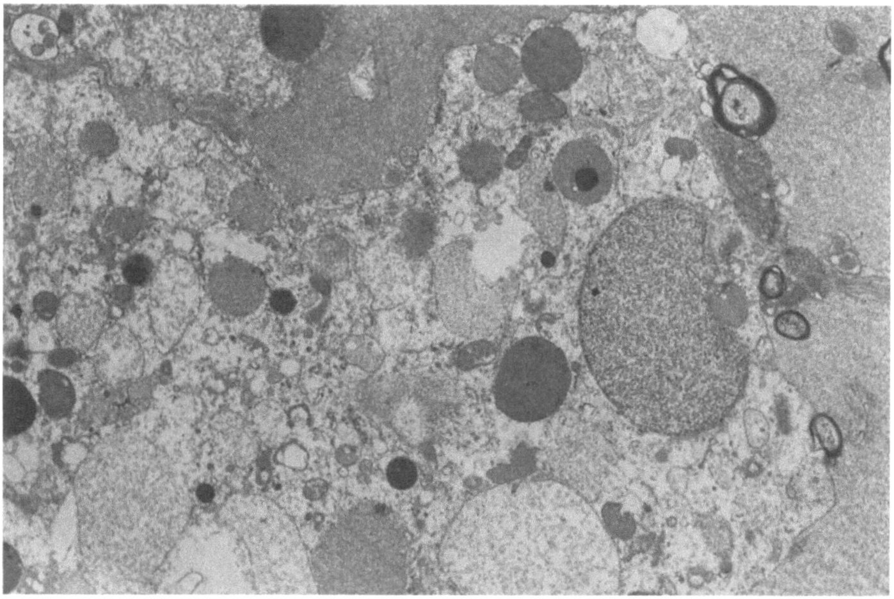

Fig. 2. Reactive astrocytes in the edematous white matter immediately after infusion of serum. There are many membrane-bound vacuoles containing material varying in electron density. ×5670

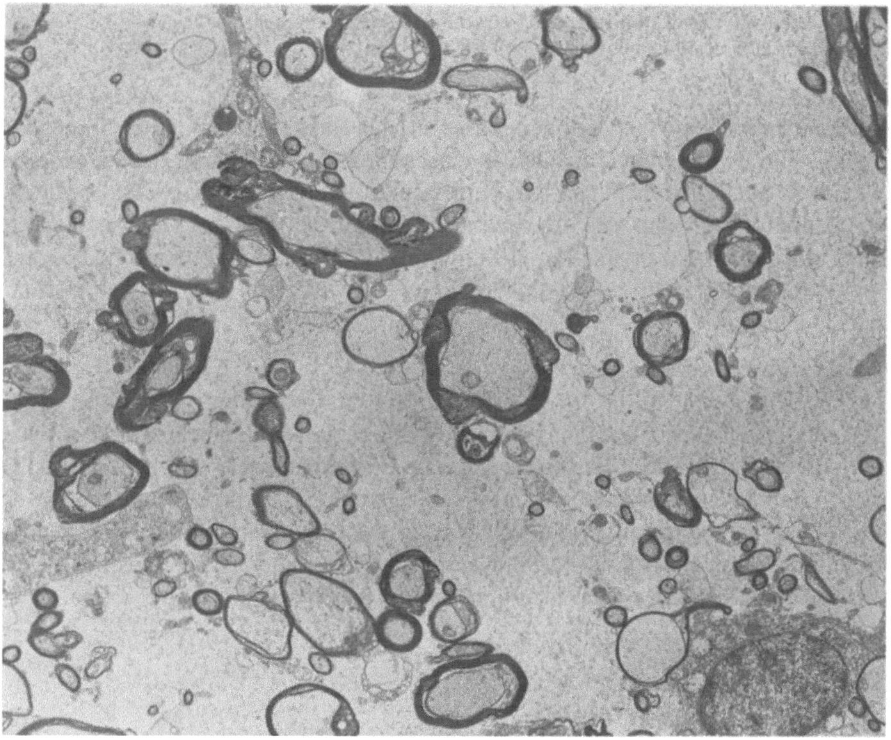

Fig. 3. Distended extracellular space in the edematous white matter 72 h after infusion of serum. Note less electron-dense edema fluid than in Fig. 1. ×3890

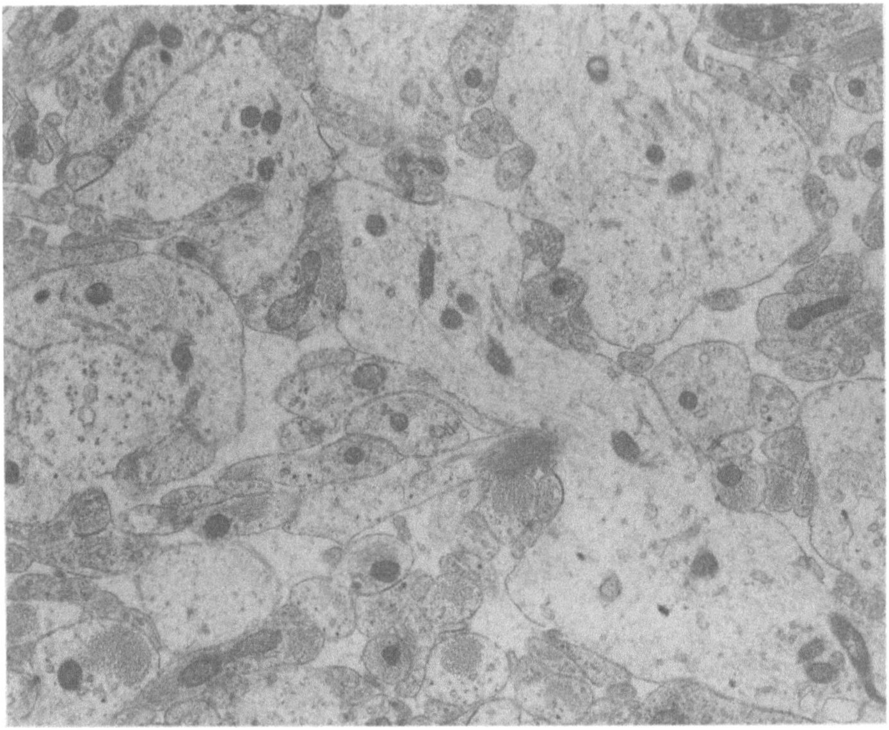

Fig. 4. Relatively small but distended extracellular space is evident between swollen glial cell processes 72 h after infusion of serum. ×9700

others, especially in the peripheral zone of the edematous area (Fig. 5). Macrophages filled with many vacuoles and occasional polymorphonuclear leukocytes were seen in the parenchymal and perivascular extracellular space. Wallerian degeneration of the axons was observed at the site of the infusion. These axons were filled with abnormal organelles, including many mitochondria, dense bodies, and vacuoles.

Changes 8 Days After Infusion

The extracellular space became very narrow at this state and appeared similar to the normal condition. The areas corresponding to the edema were replaced by reactive astrocytes filled with numerous glial fibrils. These areas included white matter, especially in the subependymal region (Fig. 6). Various membrane-bound vacuoles containing both electron-lucent and electron-dense material were frequently observed within the perivascular macrophages and astrocytes in the parenchyma.

Discussion

The extracellular space was markedly distended and filled with electron-dense fluid immediately after intracerebral infusion of serum. Accumulation of the fluid was

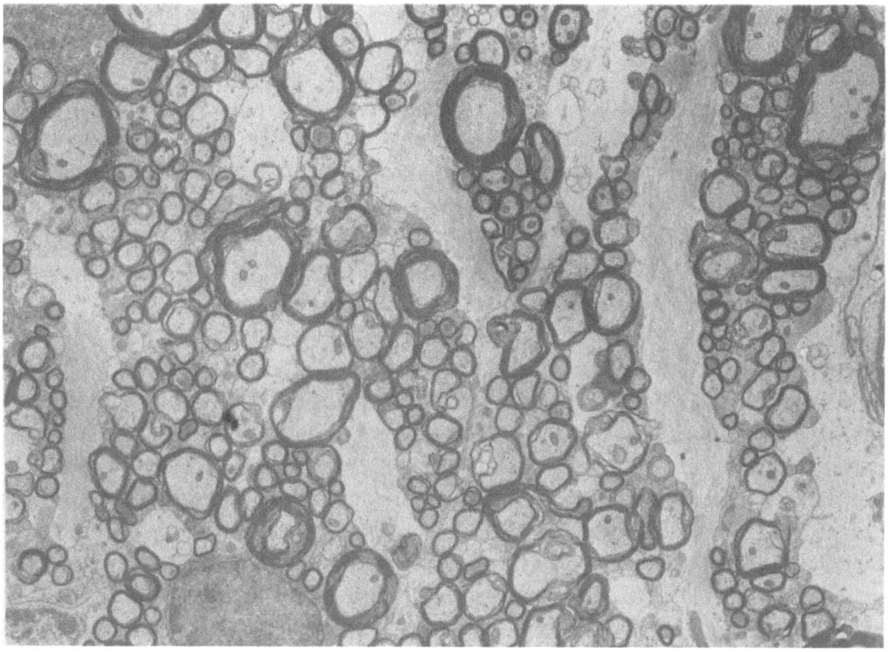

Fig. 5. White matter with swollen astrocytic processes 72 h after infusion of serum. The extracellular space is not distended. ×4050

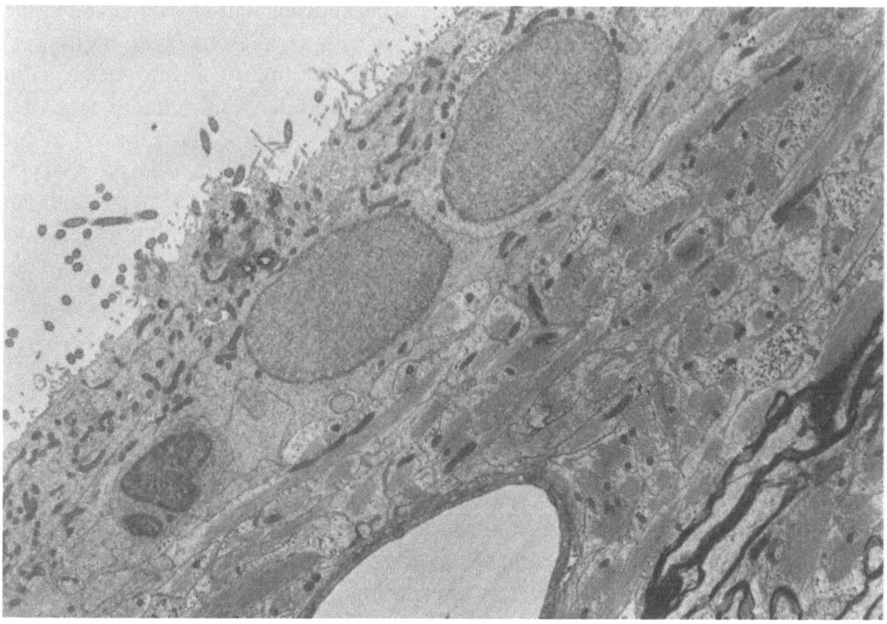

Fig. 6. Gliotic subependymal area 8 days after serum infusion. The extracellular space is not distended. Gliotic astrocytic processes are present. ×4050

generally confined to the white matter, and spread into distant areas including the subependymal region. The pool of edema fluid was bounded by astrocytic foot processes in the perivascular region and subpial region, by ependymal lining at the ventricle and by cortical gray matter. The effect of the parallel arrangement of the myelinated and nonmyelinated axons in the white matter and of the absence of junctional devices between the myelinated and unmyelinated axons was to produce expansion of the extracellular space in the white matter [1]. Swelling was not confined to the extracellular space, but was also evident in the astrocytes and ependymal cells in the acute stage. This phenomenon is essentially similar to the condition associated with hematogenous edema observed in other conditions [3].

There is a very good correlation between the present electron microscopic observations with serum infusion and the study of the tissue water content previously published [7]. The water content was similar immediately after and at 72 h after infusion. Wide extracellular spaces were also present to much the same extent immediately after and at 72 h after infusion. After 8 days the water content returned to normal in the previous study, and the extracellular spaces also returned to normal in our present fine structural study. The density of edema fluid in the distended extracellular space was lower 72 h after infusion than immediately after infusion. This implies that the electron-dense material was removed during this period. The presence of electron-dense material within the vacuoles of the reactive astrocytes as well as the macrophages indicates removal of the extracellular dense material. Uptake of extracellular material by astrocytes has been observed in other edematous conditions [5]. Another possible route of escape of the dense material is through the vascular wall into the bloodstream or through the ependymal lining into the CSF. Density of extracellular fluid is also influenced by contact with fixative and dehydrating agents during preparation. Total replacement by these solutions is common in ventricular and subarachnoid fluid. Partial replacement also occurred in the markedly widened extracellular space in the severely edematous white matter, especially in the peripheral zone of the tissue block. In spite of this important consideration, the difference in the density of the extracellular fluid immediately after and 72 h after infusion is striking in most cases and indicates that removal of the electron-dense material precedes clearance of the water content. Klatzo et al. [5] suggested that the presence of proteinaceous macromolecules in the hematogenous extracellular fluid plays a key role in producing and maintaining an increase in the water content, and removal of such substances leads to a decline in the water content. The previous investigation by Marmarou et al. [6] supported this theory, and our present study confirms their conclusion on morphological grounds.

Summary

Electron microscopic studies were performed immediately after and 72 h and 8 days after infusion of serum directly into brain tissue using the infusion model of brain edema. Electron-dense edema fluid was observed in the expanded extracellular spaces of the white matter immediately after serum infusion. Similarly expanded extracellular spaces were observed at 72 h, but the density of the fluid was considerably decreased. The extracellular space had returned to normal 8 days after serum infusion. Active phagocytosis of the electron-dense material was observed in the macrophages and astrocytes in the involved area. Swelling of the astrocytes was followed by extensive fibrillary gliosis of the astrocytes. These observations are consistent with the measurements of water content previously studied, and provide further support for the concept introduced by Klatzo, that loss of water from edematous tissue is closely allied to the dynamics of protein clearance.

References

1. Hirano A (1969) The fine structure of brain edema. In: Bourne G (ed) The structure of function of nervous tissue. Academic, New York, p 69
2. Hirano A (1981) A guide to neuropathology. Igaku-Shoin, New York
3. Hirano A, Llena JF (1983) Morphological aspects of brain edema. In: Federoff S, Hertz L (eds) Advances in cellular neurobiology, vol 4. Academic, New York, p 223
4. Hirano A, Zimmerman HM, Levine S (1964) The fine structure of cerebral fluid accumulation. III: Extracellular spread of cryptococcal polysaccharide in acute stage. Am J Pathol 45:1–19
5. Klatzo I, Chui E, Fujiwara K, Spatz M (1980) Resolution of vasogenic brain edema. In: Cervos-Navarro J, Ferszt R (eds) Advances in neurology. Brain edema. Raven, New York, p 359
6. Marmarou A, Tanaka K, Shulman K (1982) The brain response to infusion edema: Dynamics of fluid resolution. In: Brock M, Hartman A (eds) Treatment of cerebral edema. Springer, Berlin Heidelberg New York, p 11

Vascular Permeability and Cerebral Oedema in Experimental Brain Tumours *

P. L. LANTOS [1], P. J. LUTHERT, and B. R. DEANE

Key words: Transplantable rat gliomas, angiogenesis, vascular permeability, blood-brain barrier, cerebral oedema

Introduction

Blood vessels play a crucial role in the development of tumours: they provide all the necessary nutrients essential for progressive growth. The process of angiogenesis, the formation of vascular abnormalities and the complex relationship which exists between blood vessels and the tumour tissue are of paramount importance for the understanding of tumour development, the delivery of therapeutic agents and the design of imaging techniques. Vascular pathophysiology is more ominous in tumours of the brain than in neoplasms of any other organ: the developing cerebral oedema is a life-threatening event which poses a considerable challenge to both neurosurgeons and neurologists. Therefore, investigations which may elucidate the mechanisms underlying the formation of cerebral oedema have not only theoretical importance, but also practical value.

Structural and functional abnormalities of the vasculature in both human and experimental brain tumours have been well documented [4, 12, 15, 16], but there has been no comprehensive and sequential study of the pathophysiology of the vasculature in a reliable and well-characterised experimental brain tumour model. This paper will review some of the results obtained in a transplantable rat glioma system. The aim of this work was to follow the process of vascularisation, to describe morphological abnormalities of blood vessels relevant to oedema formation, to quantify these changes in different areas of the tumour and adjacent brain and in tumours of different sizes, to evaluate the permeability of blood vessels, and to assess possible transport pathways in the formation and resolution of cerebral oedema.

Materials and Methods

Cerebral tumours were produced in BD-IX rats by intracerebral injection of 3×10^5 cultured glial cells. The cell line, A15A5, was cloned at the 28th passage from the culture of a primary mixed glioma induced by transplacental administration of

---

* The work reported in this paper was supported by the Wellcome Trust.

[1] Department of Neuropathology, Institute of Psychiatry, London SE5 8AF, Great Britain

N-ethyl-*N*-nitrosourea to a syngeneic rat [13]. The cells were suspended in phosphate-buffered saline (PBS) at a concentration of 2×10^7 ml^{-1}, and 15 µl of this suspension was injected to each experimental animal.

Control rats each received injections of 15 µl PBS alone. The technique of transplantation and the procedures for light and electron microscopy have been previously described [8, 9]. General features of the vasculature (vessel density, endothelial hyperplasia and endothelial cytology) were assessed according to the microscopical angiogenesis grading system [2], while three features of the endothelial cells which may be particularly relevant to cellular transport, i.e., cytoplasmic vesicle content, fenestrations and intercellular junctions, were also quantified [9]. In the permeability studies, the protein tracer horseradish peroxidase (HRP) was used with or without Evans blue: HRP was administered either IV into the femoral vein or into the lateral cerebral ventricles. Details of the preparation of the tracers and methods of injection have been published elsewhere [10]. The in vitro features of this cell line were studied by Roscoe and her group [3], who demonstrated that A15A5 was highly malignant and glial. It was not shown until more recently, by immunocytochemistry, however, that these cells contain both glial fibrillary acidic protein and glutamine synthetase, two antigens present in astrocytes [13b]. The morphology of brain tumours produced by the intracerebral injection of these cells has already been reported [5, 6].

Results and Discussion

A sequential light and electron microscope study of angiogenesis revealed that on the basis of tumour vasculature three consecutive stages of tumour growth could be distinguished: avascular, early vascular and late vascular. These stages were related to the size of the tumours: the neoplasms grew to a diameter of about 1 mm during the avascular stage, after which capillary sprouts began to penetrate the tumours. The early vascular stage, during which the neoplasms reached 4 mm in diameter, was characterised by the appearance of an homogeneous vasculature of small immature capillaries up to 5 µm in diameter. These blood vessels appeared to be similar to those seen in normal embryonic vascularisation of the brain. The capillary buds were composed of one or more poorly differentiated endothelial cells, enclosing one or more slit-like or irregular lumina. The number of intercellular tight junctions frequently exceeded that of endothelial cells in each capillary bud (Fig. 1). Central zones of the tumours remained avascular and occasionally suffered necrosis. In the late vascular stage of growth, continued endothelial proliferation resulted in the formation of large, irregular blood vessels, up to 50 µm in diameter. The blood vessels varied in shape and size, and developed structural abnormalities associated with malignant gliomas. As the tumours increased in size, three zones could be distinguished on the basis of vascularisation: the avascular, often necrotic centre, the periphery, containing an homogeneous population of capillaries, and an intermediate zone supplied by pleomorphic, frequently abnormal blood vessels.

In these transplanted gliomas the blood vessels were classified into four groups according to size and ultrastructure. Type I included capillary buds and sprouts with immature endothelial cells surrounding slit-like or irregular lumina less than 3 µm

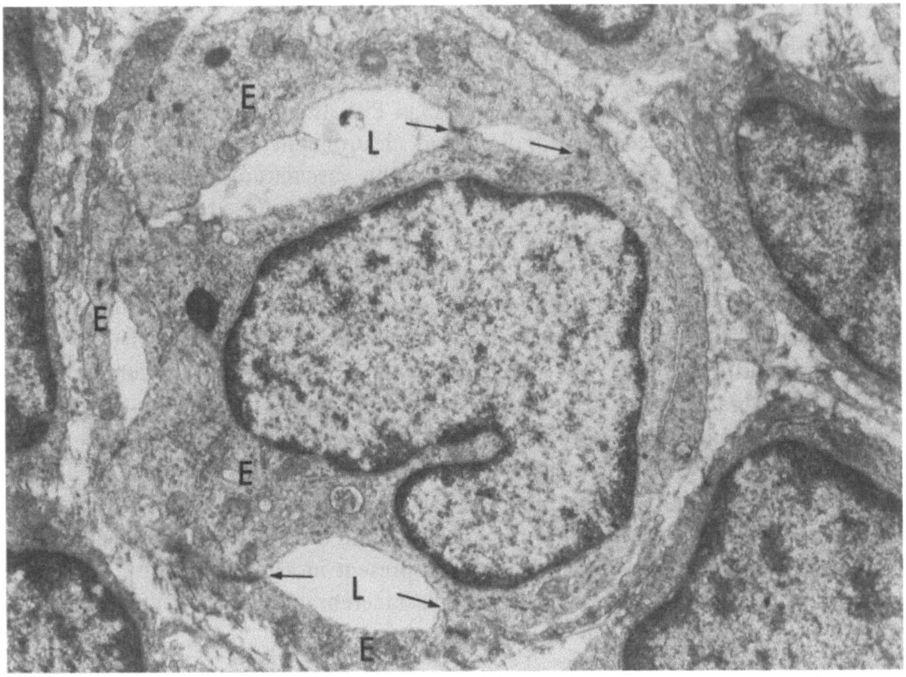

Fig. 1. Four endothelial cells (*E*) surrounding irregular lumina (*L*) to form seven intercellular junctions (*arrows*) in a complex capillary sprout. ×14 100 (Courtesy of Elsevier/North-Holland)

in diameter. Type II vessels were small, rounded immature capillaries with luminal diameters up to 5 μm. Types III and IV were both abnormal vessels which differed only in size: type III vessels were surrounded by up to six endothelial cells, while type IV comprised sinusoidal vessels lined by up to 15 endothelial cells [8].

A comprehensive quantitative assessment of morphological abnormalities [9] has been carried out. Blood vessel density, endothelial hyperplasia and endothelial cytology were assessed according to the microscopic angiogenesis grading system (MAGS) [2]. This system not only gives information on the vascular supply of tumours, but also provides a reliable index of malignancy. The values obtained indicated that the transplantable rat astrocytomas were gliomas of a high grade of malignancy. The score for areas of cerebral cortex around tumours exceeded that for control cortex, but was lower than that for the gliomas. This finding suggested that angiogenesis arose from host vessels around the tumour, resulting in a new population of small capillaries, initially outside the tumour. Endothelial structural alterations, which were thought to represent possible mechanisms of increased endothelial transport, were assessed: cytoplasmic vesicle content, fenestrations and abnormal intercellular junctions were evaluated. Cytoplasmic vesicle content was 3–6 times greater in tumour blood vessels (Fig. 2) than in capillaries from normal brain, but fenestrations and abnormal endothelial junctions were infrequently seen and were unevenly distributed [9].

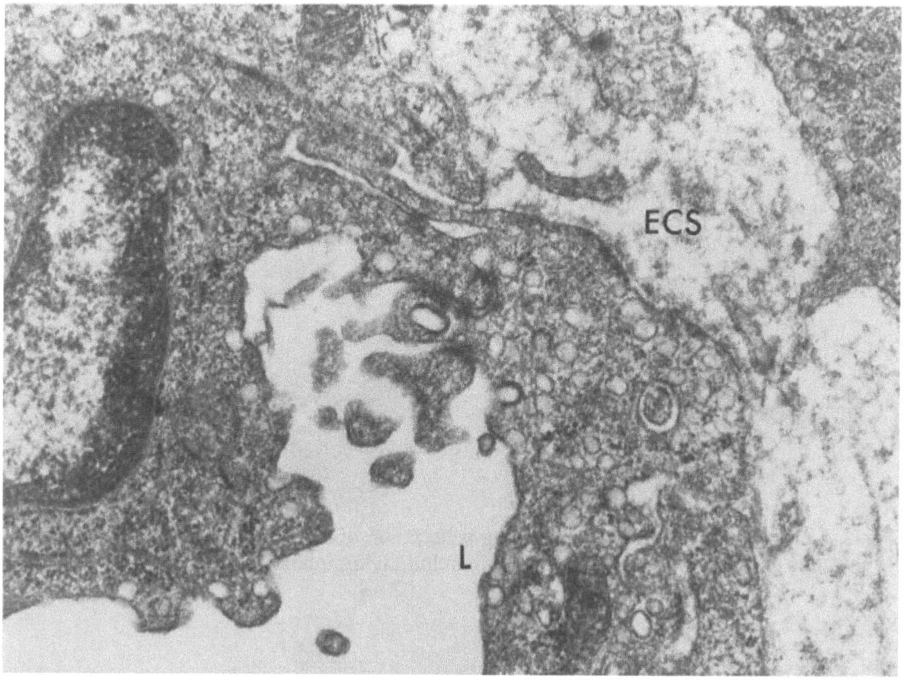

Fig. 2. Endothelial lining of a blood vessel within a tumour, showing many cytoplasmic vesicles. *L*, lumen; *ECS*, extracellular space. ×27 400 (Courtesy of Elsevier/North-Holland)

A morphometric study of the microvasculature of these tumours was subsequently carried out [13 a]. Sections containing the entire tumour and the surrounding brain were analysed using a digitising tablet. Blood vessel boundary (circumference), diameter and frequency, sample area and fractions occupied by viable tumour, necrosis and brain tissue were measured. In the centre of tumours vascular density decreased to 20% of the value for normal cortex, but vessel size more than doubled. The vascular surface area fraction reached a maximum at the tumour edge.

To elucidate the direction and time-course of transport processes which may affect the formation of oedema, the protein tracer horseradish peroxidase (HRP) was given with or without Evans blue to tumour-bearing rats, either IV or into the lateral ventricles of the brain. The movement of HRP into tumours and surrounding brain either from blood or from the ventricular cerebrospinal fluid was studied by light and electron microscopy at various intervals after injection of the tracer. The time-course of subsequent clearance of the HRP from the tumours and adjacent brain was also investigated. The IV-injected HRP rapidly penetrated all vascularised tumours and became evenly distributed within 10–20 min (Fig. 3). The HRP persisted in sufficient quantity within the tumours for several hours, after which it gradually disappeared, showing no reaction product after 12 h. Intraventricularly injected HRP penetrated periventricular brain tissue only to a distance of 1–2 mm within

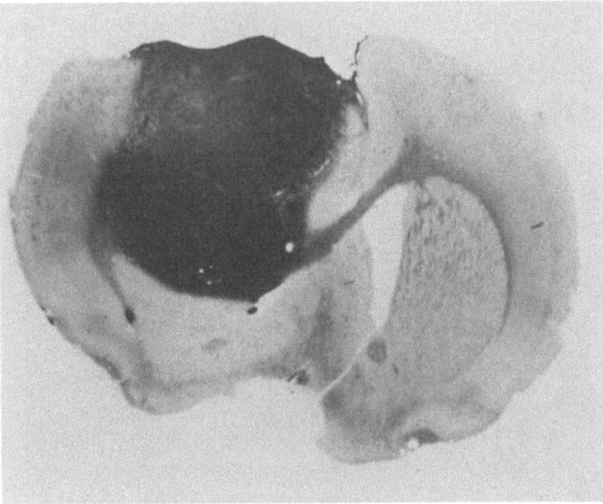

Fig. 3. Coronal slice of a rat brain showing penetration of HRP into the tumour 20 min after IV injection of the tracer. ×3 (Courtesy of Churchill Livingstone)

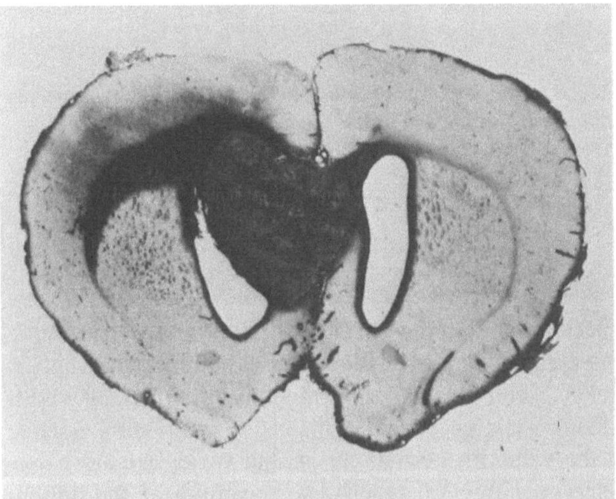

Fig. 4. Coronal slice, 100 μm thick, from a rat brain perfused 20 min after intraventricular injection of HRP. The tracer spread less than 1 mm from both the subarachnoid space and ventricular cavity, but penetrated the tumour and the ipsilateral corpus callosum. ×5 (Courtesy of Elsevier/North-Holland)

2 min, and the reaction product remained visible in this region for at least 20 min. In tumour-bearing animals, however, HRP penetrated further into periventricular tumours (Fig. 4) than into the adjacent brain [10].

These results confirm that IV-injected tracers penetrate the endothelial lining of tumour blood vessels, while the blood-brain barrier apparently remains intact in the brain tissue distant from the tumour. This finding suggests that the morphological abnormalities are indicative of, and probably responsible for, the abnormal permeability. Following IV or intraventricular administration (Figs. 5 and 6), the tracer

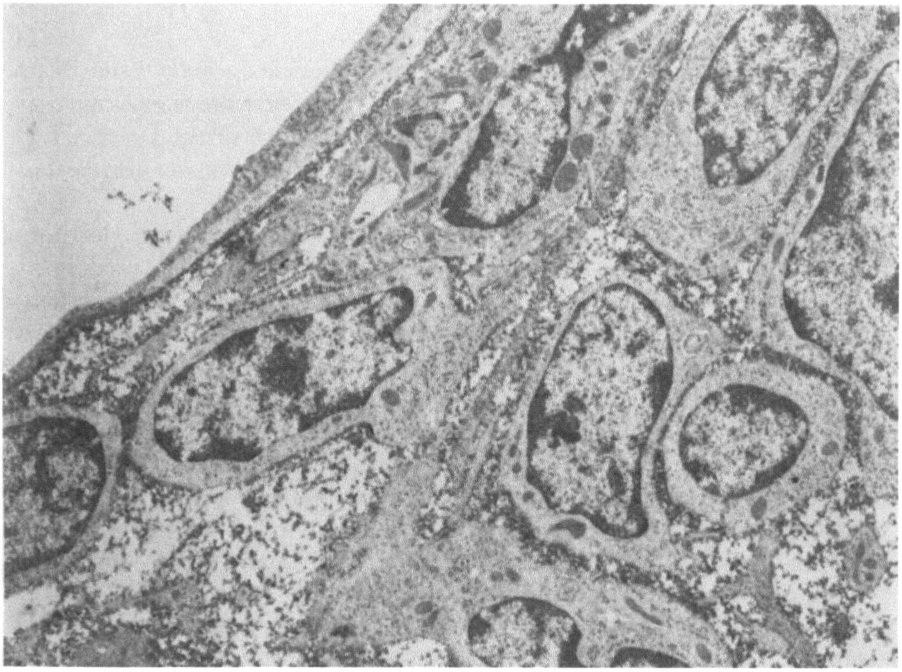

Fig. 5. Electron micrograph of perivascular area of a tumour showing dense reaction product in the widened extracellular space 10 min after intraventricular injection of HRP. ×11 100 (Courtesy of Elsevier/North-Holland)

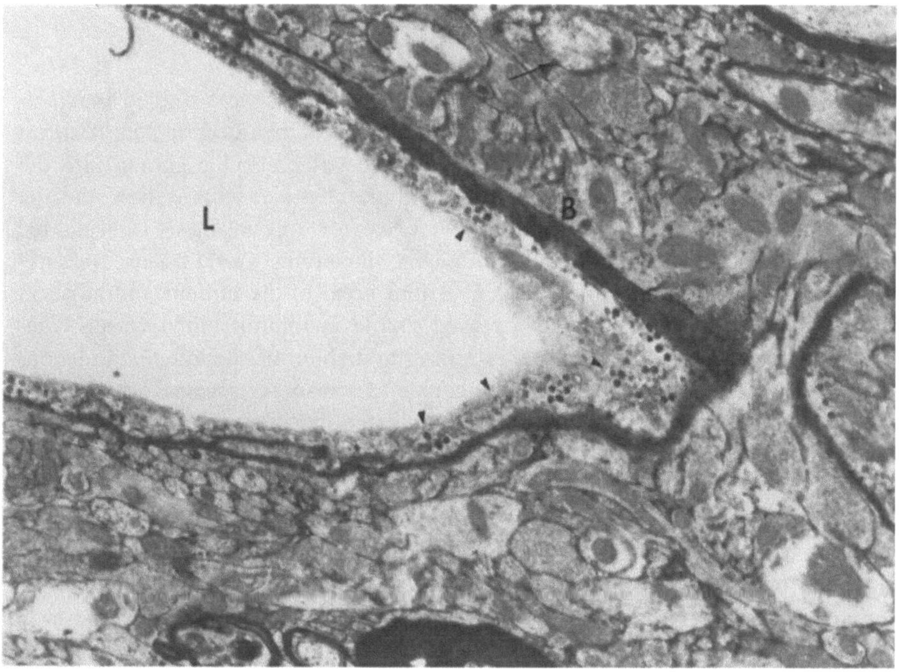

Fig. 6. Electron micrograph showing reaction product in endothelial vesicles (*arrow heads*), basement membrane (*B*) and extracellular space (*arrow*) 15 min after intraventricular injection of HRP. *L*, lumen. ×16 300 (Courtesy of Elsevier/North-Holland)

spreads throughout the largest tumours but fails to penetrate the brain tissue distant from the gliomas, or in the case of intraventricular injection, more than 2 mm away from the ependymal lining. This failure of tracer to spread away from the lesion suggests that an effective clearance mechanism may remain operational in the surrounding brain.

In addition to the sink effect of the CSF [7] and the drainage into cervical lymphatic vessels [1], clearance directly back into the cerebral vessels may occur in response to exogenous protein or oedema, perhaps by "retrograde" vesicular transport. Consequently, vesicular transport may play a role not only in the formation, but also in the resolution of cerebral oedema [10].

To quantify increased vascular permeability, the flux of mannitol from the blood into the normal brain or tumour tissue was measured [11] using a specially devised technique by which a steady level of radioactively labelled mannitol can be achieved rapidly and maintained in the bloodstream [14]. The apparent transfer constant for the movement of mannitol across the blood-brain barrier was increased more than 100-fold in the region of the tumour compared with values obtained for the brains of control rats or for brain tissue distant from the tumours [11].

These investigations have contributed to the knowledge of morphological and physiological abnormalities of the blood vessels in transplantable malignant brain tumours, and the information obtained is of potential value in the treatment of cerebral tumours and in the control of brain oedema.

Summary

Angiogenesis, vascular pathology and permeability changes were studied in experimental brain tumours. Malignant gliomas were produced by injecting neoplastic rat astrocytes cloned from an ethylnitrosourea-induced pleomorphic glioma into the brain of syngeneic animals. A sequential analysis of the vascularisation and the development of vascular abnormalities were carried out in these transplanted tumours. Standard morphometric parameters, including vessel-tissue measurements, revealed significant differences in various areas of the tumour and adjacent brain. Endothelial vesicle content increased sixfold in tumour blood vessels compared with normal capillaries, but fenestrations and abnormal endothelial junctions were infrequent. The direction and time-course of transport processes which could affect the accumulation of oedema were investigated in different tumour areas and in tumours of various sizes by injecting horseradish peroxidase IV or into the lateral cerebral ventricles. The findings revealed that blood vessels lacked an effective blood-brain barrier and this increased permeability was consequently confirmed by quantitative assessment of the flux of radioactively labelled mannitol across the endothelium from the blood into tumour or normal brain. The findings with electron-dense tracers strongly suggested that failure of an effective clearance mechanism in tumour blood vessels could also contribute to the formation of oedema. These studies, having established a reliable experimental system, provide a basis for further investigations of the pathophysiology of the blood-brain barrier and are of clinical importance in relation to drug delivery and imaging techniques.

Acknowledgements. The authors are indebted to Dr. M. Swash and Churchill Livingstone, Edinburgh, for permission to reproduce Fig. 14 from the chapter entitled "Tumours of the Nervous System" in "*The Scientific Basis of Clinical Neurology*" and to Elsevier/North-Holland Biomedical Press B.V. and the Editor of the *Journal of the Neurological Sciences* to reproduce the following figures from this journal: vol. 49 (1981), pp. 55–66: Fig. 3; vol. 49 (1981), pp. 67–77: Figs. 5, 7, 9, 10; vol. 65 (1984), pp. 47–58: Fig. 8; vol. 65 (1985), pp 59–68: Fig. 4.

References

1. Bradbury MWB (1979) The concept of a blood-brain barrier. Wiley, Chichester
2. Brem S, Cotran R, Folkman J (1972) Tumor angiogenesis: a quantitative method for histologic grading. J Natl Cancer Inst 48:347–356
3. Claisse PJ, Roscoe JP, Lantos PL (1979) Cellular heterogeneity in an ethylnitrosourea-induced glioma: malignancy, karyology and other properties of tumour cell types. Br J Exp Pathol 60:209–224
4. Cox DJ, Pilkington GJ, Lantos PL (1976) The fine structure of blood vessels in ethylnitrosourea-induced tumours of the rat nervous system. Br J Exp Pathol 57:419–430
5. Davaki P, Lantos PL (1980) Morphological analysis of malignancy: a comparative study of brain tumours. Br J Exp Pathol 61:655–660
6. Davaki P, Lantos PL (1981) The development of brain tumours produced in rats by the intracerebral injection of neoplastic glial cells: a fine structural study. Neuropathol Appl Neurobiol 7:49–61
7. Davson H (1976) The blood-brain barrier. J Physiol 255:1–28
8. Deane BR, Lantos PL (1981a) The vasculature of experimental brain tumours. 1: A sequential light and electron microscope study of angiogenesis. J Neurol Sci 49:55–66
9. Deane BR, Lantos PL (1981b) The vasculature of experimental brain tumours. 2: A quantitative assessment of morphological abnormalities. J Neurol Sci 49:67–77
10. Deane BR, Papp MI, Lantos PL (1984a) The vasculature of experimental brain tumours. 3: Permeability studies. J Neurol Sci 65:47–58
11. Deane BR, Greenwood J, Lantos PL, Pratt OE (1984b) The vasculature of experimental brain tumours. 4: The quantification of vascular permeability. J Neurol Sci 65:59–68
12. Hirano A, Matsui T (1975) Vascular structures in brain tumors. Hum Pathol 6:611–621
13. Lantos PL, Roscoe JP, Skidmore CJ (1976) Studies of the morphology and tumorigenicity of experimental brain tumours in tissue culture. Br J Exp Pathol 57:95–104

13a. Luthert PJ, Lantos PL (1985) A morphometric study of the microvasculature of a rat glioma. Neuropathol Appl Neurobiol (in press)

13b. Pilkington GJ, Martin TM, Lantos PL (1985) Cloned neoplastic cells from a chemically induced rat glioma: immunocytochemical characterization. Br J Exp Pathol (in press)

14. Pratt OE (1974) An electronically controlled syringe drive for giving an injection at a variable rate according to a present programme. J Physiol 237:5P–6P
15. Waggener JD, Beggs JL (1976) Vasculature of neural neoplasms. Adv Neurol 15:27–49
16. Weller RO, Griffin RL (1978) Transmission and scanning electron microscopy of the microcirculation of gliomas. Adv Neurol 20:569–575

Electron Microscopic and Behavioral Studies in Experimental Lead Encephalopathy *

R. A. CLASEN [1], T. J. HOEPPNER, J. F. HARTMANN, S. PANDOLFI, and J. R. CLASEN

Key words: Lead encephalopathy, cerebral edema, electron microscopy, visual discrimination

Review

There is much concern that even at the relatively low levels of lead which do not result in acute toxicity, alterations in cognitive function may occur [10]. Impairments in learning following early lead exposure have been reported in a number of species. Ewes were exposed to lead before breeding and throughout gestation [4]. At 4 months of age, the lambs born to them had a mean blood lead level of 14 μg% (control 4.7 μg%). At 5 months, the lambs were taught to discriminate between a circle and a triangle and then among circles of different sizes. The prenatally exposed lambs took significantly longer than controls to learn the size discrimination. This may be interpreted as a defect in reversal learning.

Newly born rhesus monkeys were placed with a surrogate mother having a lead base [1]. In 2 months the blood lead ranged from 160 to 400 μg% and the monkeys developed convulsions and had decreased physical activity. One animal developed visual impairment. Following removal of the surrogate mother the convulsions subsided, but the animals continued to show reduced social interaction and abnormal behavior patterns. In a second set of experiments infant monkeys were given lead in their diet. They developed a blood lead level of 60–100 μg% in 4 weeks, accompanied by anemia and hyperactivity. When the blood levels approached 300 μg% the animals developed intermittent convulsions, diminished social interaction, and increased vocalization. When the lead was discontinued the convulsions disappeared, but the abnormal behavioral patterns persisted. These same workers were not able to produce clinical symptoms by administering lead to juvenile rhesus monkeys. It has also been reported that the oral administration of lead to adult rhesus monkeys produced no changes in behavioral tests [8].

There have also been several reports of behavioral changes in the absence of gross cerebral changes, in lead-poisoned rodents. In one of these, the dose was adjusted so that no changes in body weight occurred in either dams or pups [2]. Diminished

* This work was supported by Research Grant ES-00775 from the U.S. Public Health Service and the Otho S.A. Sprague Memorial Institute.
[1] Rush-Presbyterian-St. Luke's Medical Center, 1753 West Congress Parkway, Chicago, Illinois, 60612, USA

learning in a T maze was seen with blood levels as low as 46 μg%. The animals were not hyperactive, but this has been reported in both rats [11] and mice [12] exposed to lead in the neonatal period. In both cases this was associated with growth retardation.

The effect of chronic lead exposure on learning in monkeys is less clear. Defects in reversal learning have been reported [3] but others found no significant defects in visual discrimination learning [14].

The present study examines acquisition and retention of color and pattern discriminations. Color discrimination is a simple task, and its retention at a high level would be expected for prolonged periods. Pattern discrimination is more difficult for young monkeys and its acquisition extends over a long period of time. For a given task acquisition is generally more sensitive to disruption than retention.

Materials and Methods

The methods for administering lead and vitamin D, the dosage schedule, the chemical analysis of blood, and the preparation of brain for light and electron microscopy have been described elsewhere [5, 6]. The present report is based on studies in ten lead-poisoned animals and four controls. Three controls received neither lead nor vitamin D, and one received vitamin D only. The animal that received vitamin D had slightly higher blood lead levels than other controls, but otherwise did not differ from them.

Motor activity was measured by placing the animal in a special cage equipped with a device which recorded movement. The animals were placed in this cage overnight for a 12-h period.

Form and color discrimination was tested using a device modeled after the Wisconsin General Testing Apparatus and designed so that it could be readily attached to the home cage of each animal. Essentially, it consisted of two food wells over which the plexiglas discriminanda were placed. A shield prevented the animal from seeing where the food was placed. Initially, the animals were trained to take food from the wells. Then they were trained to slide the plexiglas cover from over the food wells to obtain the food. All animals learned to do this in 2 or 3 days. Each subsequent session consisted of 20 trials in which red and green food well covers were located on the left and right, respectively, in random order. The food pellet was located under the red cover. Animals were given at least four sessions per week until they reached a criterion of 90% correct on 2 successive days. After this, red-green discrimination was tested at irregular intervals to assess retention.

After animals reached criterion on the red-green discrimination, a pattern discrimination was begun. A white circle on a black background was matched in area to a white square on a black background. The discrimination was between a square and a circle, the square being correct. The position of the discriminanda was randomly ordered within the 20 trial sessions. In this period, animals generally received two to four sessions of pattern discrimination per week.

Results

Morphologic Changes

Six rhesus monkeys developed neurologic symptoms and were successfully perfused for electron microscopic studies. In the acute stage of the disease, all animals showed gross evidence of cerebral swelling as previously described [10]. The major histological basis of this was the formation of areas of edema scattered throughout the white matter. The edema fluid was rich in protein according to light microscopy, and on electron microscopy was found to consist of granular material deposited in an expanded extracellular space (Fig. 1). Astrocytic processes in these areas were swollen but necrotizing changes were not seen. The gray matter occasionally also showed small focal areas of such edema with more prominent swelling of glia. These gray matter areas were not seen by light microscopy.

Collections of edema fluid were also found in the perivascular space of some of the larger blood vessels (Fig. 2). This was not associated with evidence of damage to the vessel wall. Some of the smaller blood vessels, on the other hand, showed evidence of severe damage. This consisted in swelling of the endoplasmic reticulum and the formation of lamellar bodies within endothelial cytoplasm (Fig. 3). In other vessels large portions of the vessel wall were denuded of endothelial cytoplasm.

Perivascular globules were found in both gray and white matter of lead-poisoned animals (Fig. 3). They were identical with the structures previously described in the rat and in humans [6].

Two rhesus monkeys died during the course of the experiment from causes other than lead poisoning. Two monkeys proved to be resistant to development of the encephalopathy. These were sacrificed after 8 months. The brains of both groups of animals were normal according to light microscopy.

In one animal the lead dosage was doubled after 4 months of exposure. After 1 week this animal developed convulsions and ataxia followed by weakness and lethargy. This animal was fed by stomach tube for 4 days, after which he appeared to have completely recovered. The animal was sacrificed 7 months after the onset of neurologic symptoms and the brain was studied by light microscopy. The cerebellum showed a few minor vascular changes, but no cerebral lesions were found.

One animal (Bruce) developed convulsions and ataxia after 3 months. This animal was not sacrificed and apparently completely recovered. At 4 months after the apparent recovery the lead dosage was increased, and 3 weeks after this the animal developed convulsions and blindness. On the following day, the animal was found dead. The brain was fixed by immersion and studied by means of light microscopy. The primary visual and visual association areas had a spongy appearance. These areas showed marked loss of neurons, numerous plump astrocytes, and marked capillary proliferation. The underlying white matter was edematous (Fig. 4). The overt blindness which the animal developed just prior to death was probably the result of this edema, which is also viewed as the immediate cause of death.

Fig. 1. Electron photomicrographs of white matter vessels. *Above* control animals. ×15 060. *Below* lead-poisoned animals. ×12 530

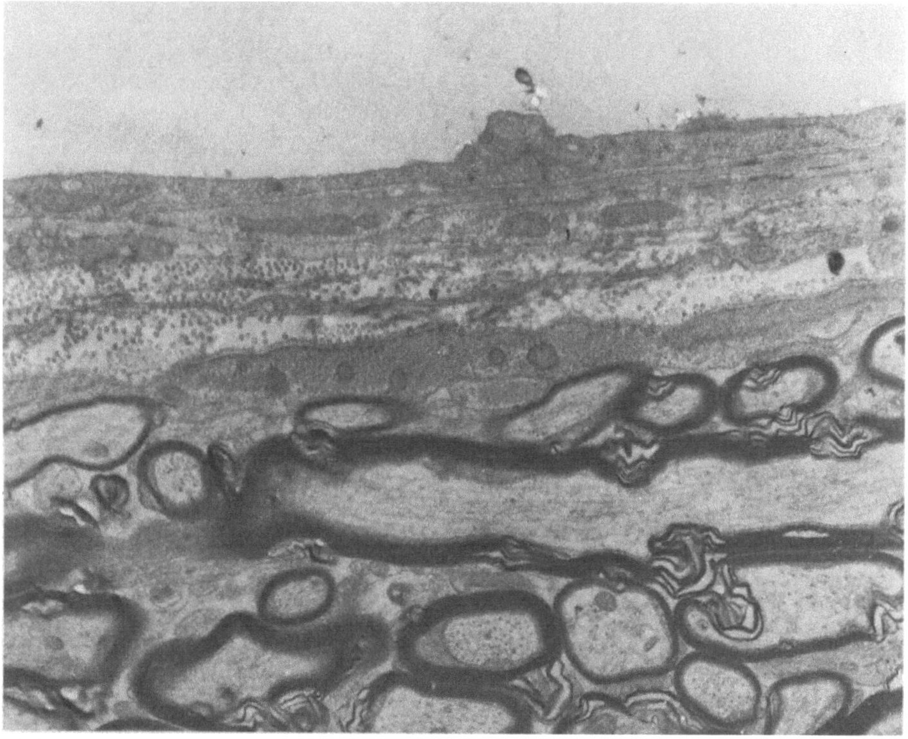

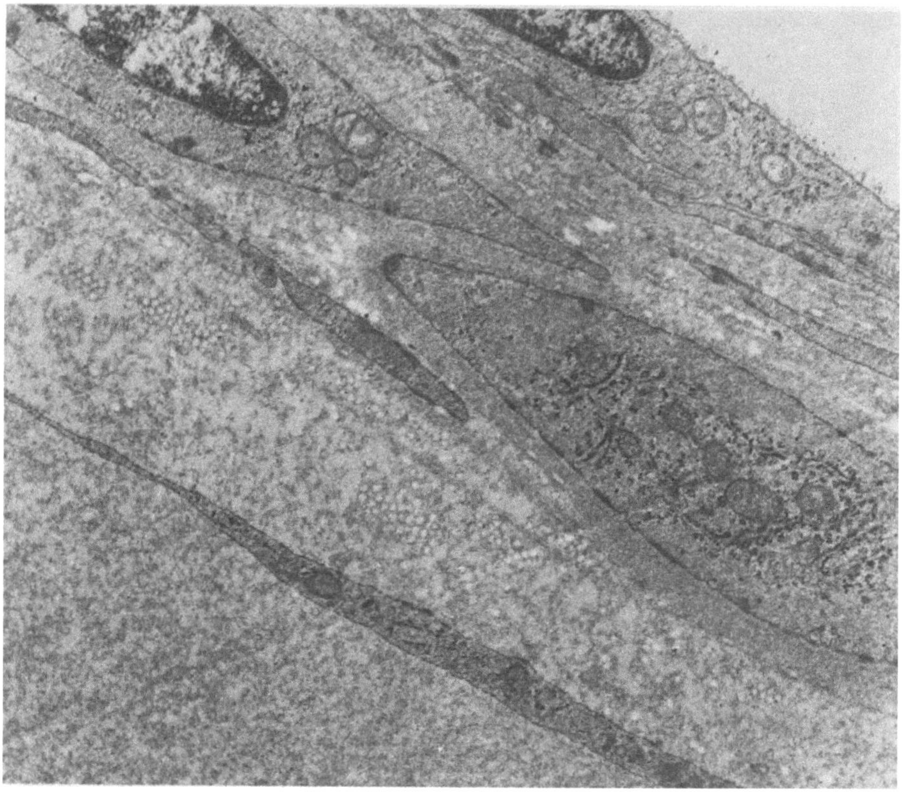

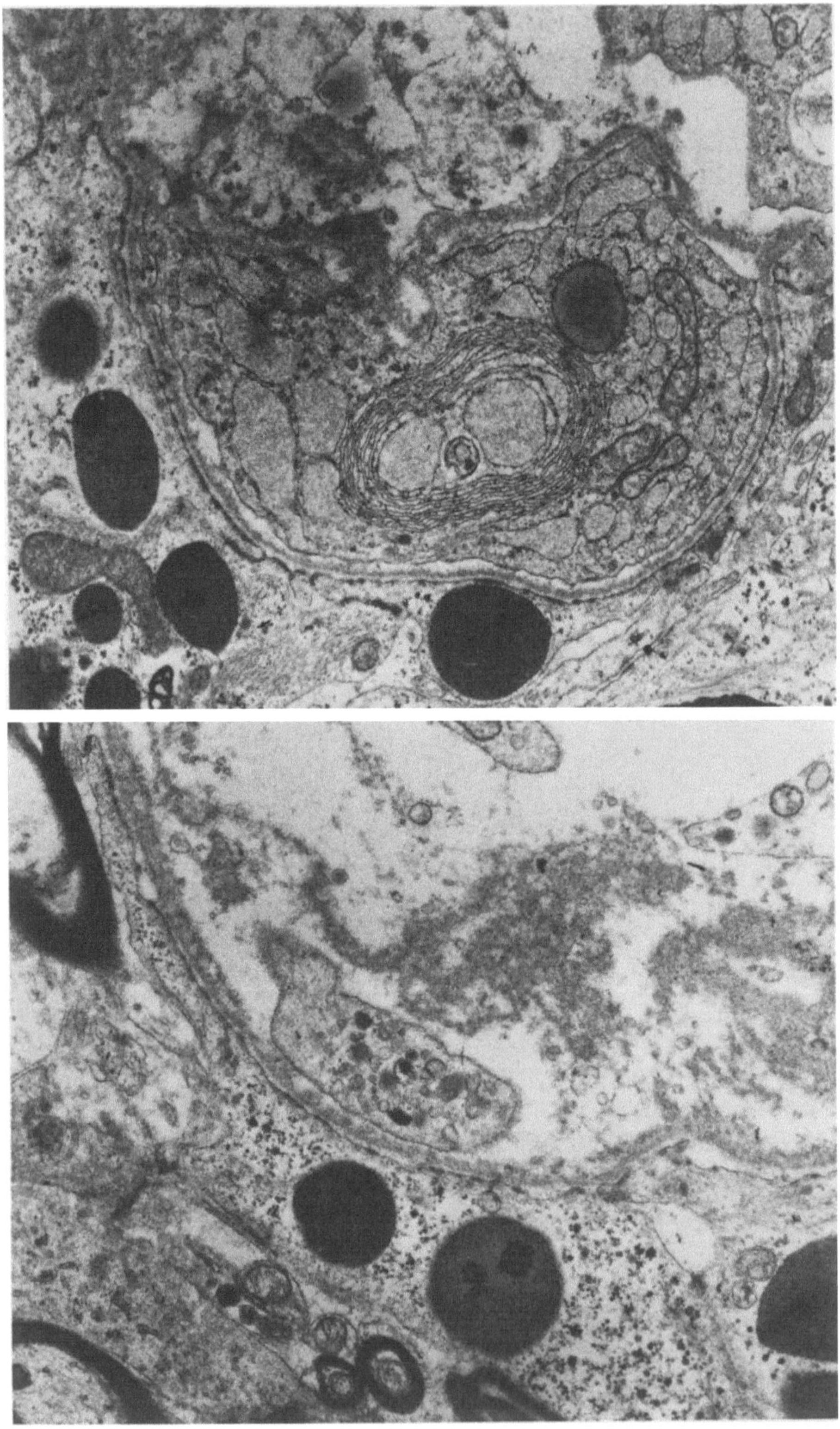

Behavioral Studies

There was no difference in monitored motor activity between controls and lead-poisoned animals.

Experimental and control groups required the same number of sessions to learn the red-green discrimination to a criterion of 90% correct 2 days in succession: 9.2 ± 0.4 (standard error) $n=6$, for those receiving lead, and 9.3 ± 1.1 sessions, $n=4$, for controls. In subsequent months the discrimination was retained equally well in both groups (Fig. 5).

The square/circle discrimination proved to be more difficult for both groups (Fig. 5). Only three of four controls and three of six lead-treated animals reached a criterion of at least 90% correct on 2 days in succession in the time over which they were tested. The lead-treated animals required 35.6 ± 7.4 sessions to reach criterion and the control animals, 23.3 ± 5.7 sessions. This is not a statistically significant difference. The discrimination was retained equally well in both groups. Of the lead-treated animals that did not reach criterion one became lethargic, collapsed, and died after 12 sessions, one showed a gum lead line but no abnormal behavior and was sacrificed after 25 sessions, and the third became lethargic, then comatose and was sacrificed before starting this discrimination training. One control monkey was sacrified after 19 sessions without reaching criterion.

The animals receiving lead who developed the encephalopathy showed symptoms of lethargy, generalized weakness, ataxia, and convulsions. Surprisingly, performance on the learning tasks generally showed little or no indication of impending distress. On the final day of testing the mean performance was 95.0% ± 1.2% for red-green discrimination and 85.0 ± 4.2% for square-circle discrimination. These scores are not significantly different from those reached by these animals in the preceding weeks, nor are they different from those of control animals at comparable times before sacrifice (92.5% ± 0.7% and 82.5% ± 4.6%, respectively on the red-green and square-circle discimination).

Thus, these group data show no evidence of impairment on the acquisition or retention of color or pattern discrimination in lead-poisoned juvenile rhesus monkeys.

In contrast to the group data, one monkey (Bruce) showed an apparent effect of the lead well before the appearance of acute toxicity. The learning pattern for Bruce is shown in Fig. 6. In this individual animal, there is loss of the recently learned red-green discrimination during the early period when the blood lead level measured was 1207 μg%. Following the onset of symptoms and recovery, both discrimination skills were learned to criterion and accurate performance was maintained even in the period just before clinical onset of the terminal disease. Since chronic lesions were found in both the striate and parastriate cortex (Fig. 4), it can be assumed that the disease process occurred in these areas before the first onset of clinical symptoms.

Fig. 2. Electron photomicrographs of damaged blood vessels. × 16 520

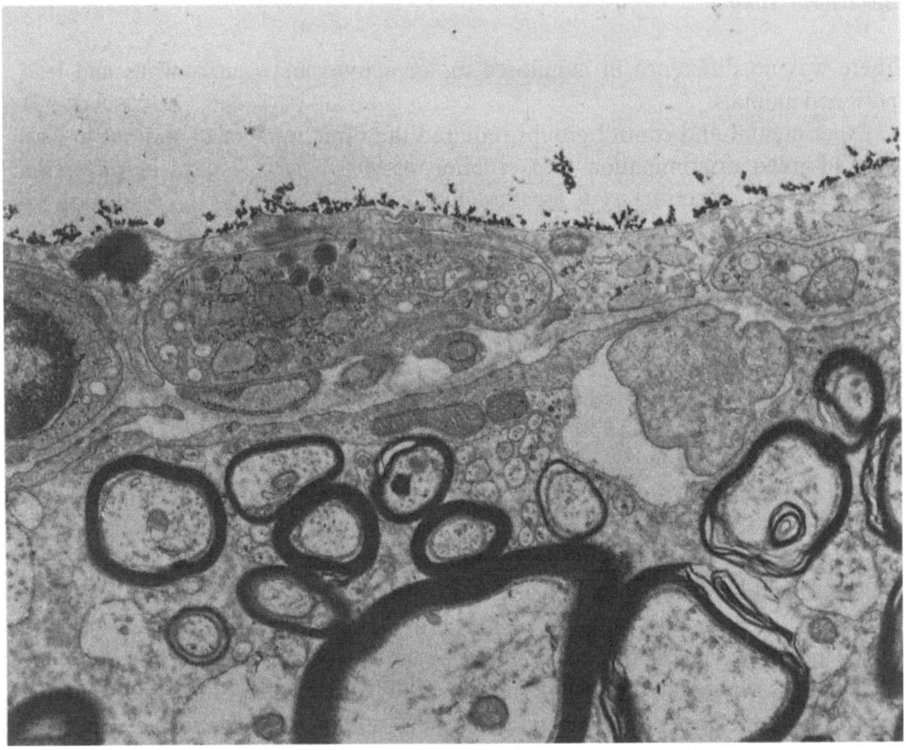

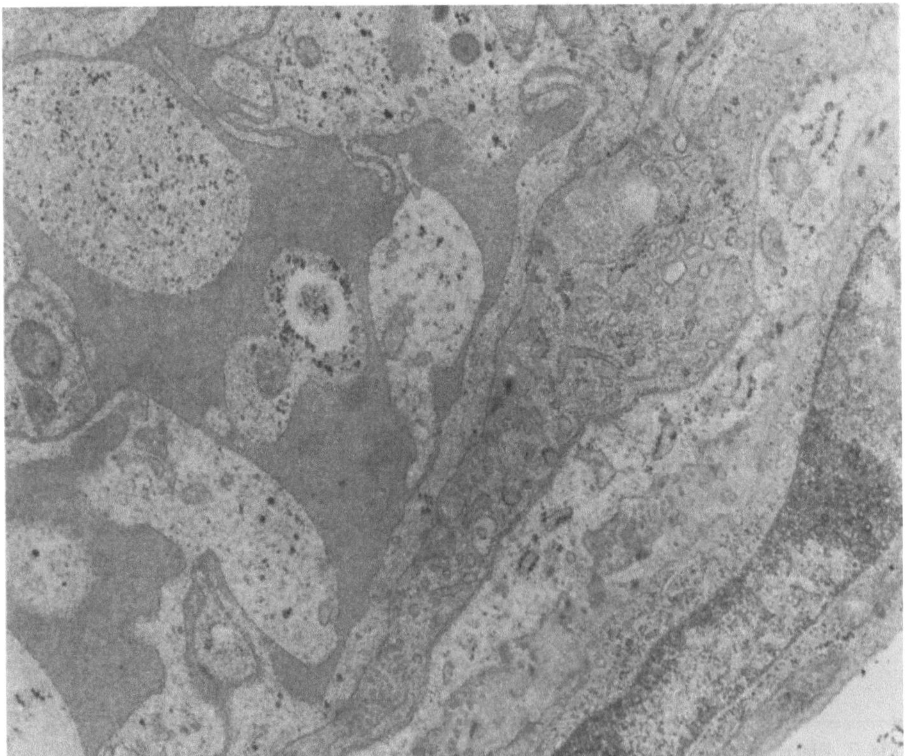

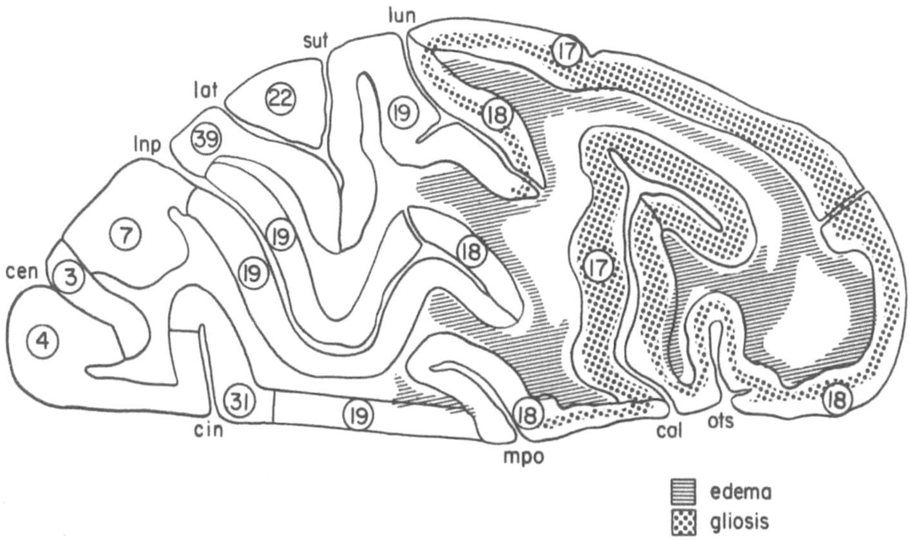

Fig. 4. Diagram of the extent and location of morphological changes seen in the brain of Bruce, based on a coronal section through the occipital lobes, with labeled sulci and cortical areas identified

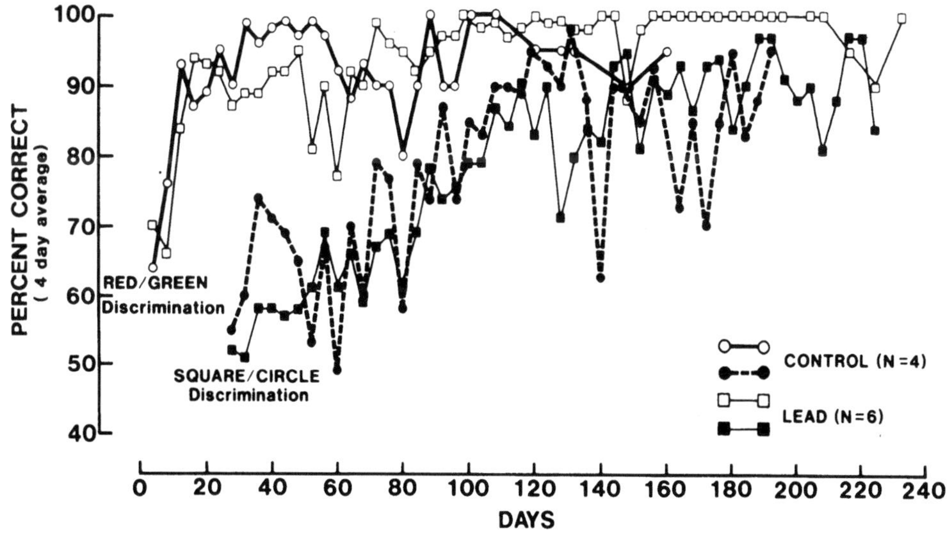

Fig. 5. Learning curves for control and lead-poisoned animals

Fig. 3. Electron photomicrographs of edematous white matter (*above* × 12 180) and edematous gray matter (*below* × 17 860)

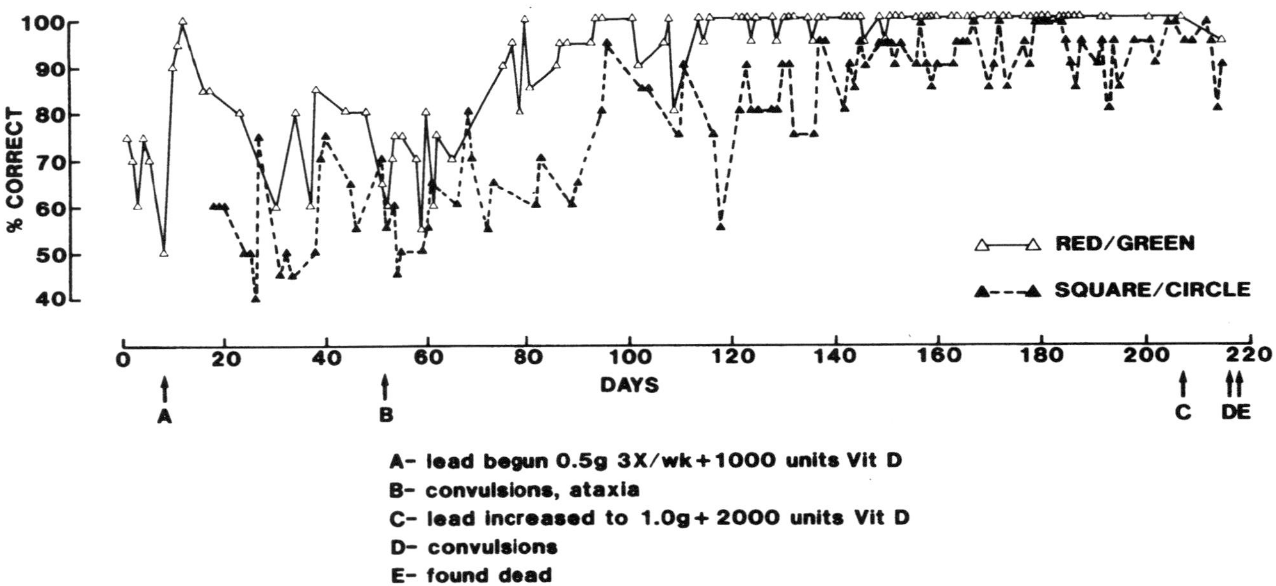

Fig. 6. Learning curve for Bruce, a lead-treated animal

Discussion

In this experimental model of vasogenic edema, the edema fluid is found in the perivascular space of larger bloods vessels (Fig. 1). This is not accompanied by any marked morphological evidence of damage to the vessel wall, while the capillaries show extensive damage (Fig. 2). In the lead-poisoned rat the toxin is concentrated in damaged capillaries [13]. It is most likely that these damaged capillaries are the source of the extracellular edema fluid associated with the disease and that the edema fluid in the perivascular spaces is a secondary phenomenon. In the dog with cryogenic edema leakage of plasma is confined to the vessels adjacent to the lesion, and larger, more distant vessels with perivascular edema fluid show no evidence of increased permeability [9].

Chemical studies in the lead-poisoned rat have shown that the cerebral swelling is equally distributed between the vasogenic extracellular component and a cytotoxic component of intracellular glial edema [7]. In the monkey, this intracellular component as judged morphologically (Fig. 1), is less prominent than in the rat. In the monkey, however, axonal edema is also seen [5].

The group behavior data show no evidence of lead-induced impairment in visual learning during either acquisition or retention of color and pattern discrimination (Fig. 5). One monkey receiving lead did show a loss of the recently learned red-green discrimination and needed slightly longer than average for acquisition of the square-circle discrimination. Both of these were eventually learned to criterion despite the extensive damage to the visual cortex subsequently observed. This is most probably attributable to progressive compensation by the remaining cerebral cortex during the gradual destruction of the visual cortex. The extensive neural damage in the animal is most probably attributable to the very high levels of lead achieved in the blood, which were three times those in any other animal.

Summary

One-half gram of lead subacetate and 1000 units of vitamin D were given three times a week by gastric gavage to newly weaned rhesus monkeys. During the period of toxification the animals were trained to discriminate forms and colors. There was no clear difference in the rate of learning or retention for lead-poisoned animals and controls. At about 3 months most animals developed ataxia, convulsions and, in some cases, blindness. In the period immediately preceding the development of symptoms the performance of the group of lead-treated animals on both color and form discrimination was normal. Only in one animal was there a deterioration in performance preceding the appearance of symptoms. This animal was found to have histologically chronic lesions in both the primary visual and visual association cortex. Some animals were sacrificed by perfusion fixation. Electron microscopic examination of these animals showed protein-rich extracellular edema involving primarily white matter, but also found in gray matter. The perivascular space of many larger intrinsic vessels was distended by edema fluid but the endothelium of these vessels appeared normal. Vessels of capillary size showed severe damage. It was concluded that the source of the edema fluid is damaged capillaries and that the fluid migrates to the perivascular space of the larger vessels as a secondary phenomenon.

References

1. Allen JR, McWey PJ, Suomi SJ (1974) Pathological and behavioral effects of lead intoxication in the infant rhesus monkey. Environ Health Perspect 7:239–246
2. Brown DR (1975) Neonatal lead exposure in the rat: Decreased learning as a function of age and blood lead concentrations. Toxicol Appl Pharmacol 32:628–637
3. Bushnell PJ, Bowman RE (1979) Reversal learning defects in young monkeys exposed to lead. Pharmacol Biochem Behav 10:733–742
4. Carson TL, VanGelder GA, Karas GC, Buck WB (1974) Slowed learning in lambs prenatally exposed to lead. Arch Environ Health 29:154–156
5. Clasen RA, Hartmann JF, Coogan PD, Pandolfi S, Laing I, Becker RA (1974) Experimental acute lead encephalopathy in the juvenile rhesus monkey. Environ Health Perspect 7:175–185
6. Clasen RA, Hartmann JF, Starr AJ, Coogan PS, Pandolfi S, Laing I, Becker R, Hass GM (1974) Electron microscopic and chemical studies of the vascular changes and edema of lead encephalopathy: A comparative study of the human and experimental disease. Am J Pathol 74:215–238
7. Clasen RA, Pandolfi S, Hoeppner TJ, Clasen JR (1984) Treatment of acute lead encephalopathy. In: Go KG, Baethmann A (eds) Recent progress in the study and therapy of brain edema. Plenum, New York, pp 633–642
8. Goode JW, Johnson S, Calandra JC (1973) Evaluation of chronic oral administration of lead acetate to rhesus monkeys. Toxicol Appl Pharmacol 25:465–466
9. Hindo WA, Clasen RA, Rayudu GVS, Pandolfi S (1972) Technetium in cryogenic cerebral injury and edema. Arch Neurol 27:526–534
10. LaPort RE, Talbott EE (1978) Effects of low levels of lead exposure on cognitive function. Arch Environ Health 33:236–239
11. Michaelson JA, Sauerhoff MW (1974) An improved model of lead-induced brain dysfunction in the suckling rat. Toxicol Appl Pharmacol 28:88–96
12. Silbergold EK, Goldberg AM (1974) Hyperactivity: A lead-induced behavior disorder. Environ Health Perspect 7:227–232
13. Toews AD, Kolber A, Hayward J, Krigman MR, Morell P (1978) Experimental lead encephalopathy in the suckling rat: Concentration of lead in cellular fractions enriched in brain capillaries. Brain Res 147:131–138
14. Zook BC, London WT (1980) Experimental lead paint poisoning in nonhuman primates. II: Clinical pathologic findings and behavioral effects. J Med Primatol 9:286–303

A Model for Brain Edema

S. I. RAPOPORT [1]

Key words: Brain edema, blood-brain barrier, compliance, hydraulic conductivity

Introduction

Brain edema associated with dilatation of the brain extracellular space has a number of causes, but it is termed "vasogenic" if the major cause is damage to the blood-brain barrier (BBB). Vasogenic edema occurs in tumors, trauma, vasculitis, a cold lesion, acute hypertension, infarction, radiation, and osmotic BBB opening. Extracellular edema which is not clearly vasogenic arises in association with increased CSF pressure and hydrocephalus [21], can be induced locally by intracerebral injection of fluid [8], and may accompany brain edema initiated by decreasing plasma tonicity (osmotic edema) or by metabolic inhibition (cytotoxic edema).

In 1978, I presented a model [12] which identified and interrelated major factors which characterize water movements between the intracranial compartments in the intact and edematous brain: cerebrovascular permeability and hydraulic conductivity, tissue hydraulic conductivity, and tissue elastic compliance. This model provides a frame of reference for designing critical experiments and for interpreting the significance of clinical and experimental observations, and will be discussed in this paper.

The Model

Figure 1 is a simplified diagram of the intracranial compartments. The brain is represented as a hollow cylinder with an outer region of gray matter, region a, and an inner region of white matter, region b. The model places capillaries only in gray matter, as the capillary surface area in gray matter is about five times greater than that in white matter. Fluid that leaks from capillaries in region a accumulates in region a, or flows centrifugally through region a into subarachnoidal cerebrospinal fluid (CSF), or centripetally through subcortical white matter into ventricular CSF. Flow from gray matter to subarachnoidal CSF is frequently ignored in edema studies [16], but clearly occurs [3]. CSF leaves the cranium through the valvular arachnoid villi or by lymphatic drainage [3].

---

[1] Laboratory of Neurosciences, National Institute on Aging, National Institutes of Health, Bethesda, Maryland, 20205, USA

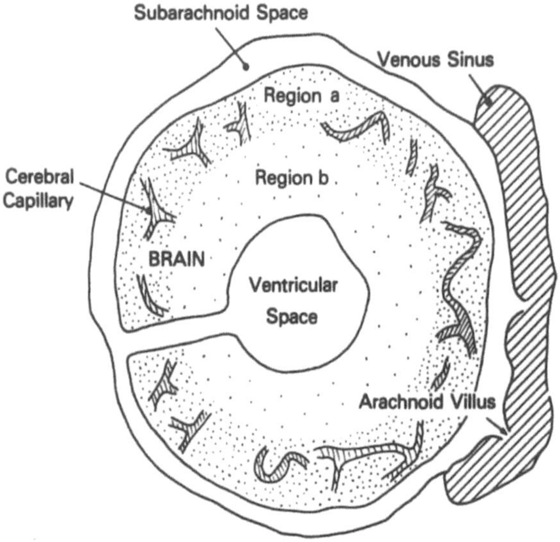

Fig. 1. Representation of intracranial compartments. The brain is a hollow cylinder with ventricular and subarachnoidal spaces that communicate via a conduit. It is composed of an outer region of gray matter (region a), which contains capillaries, and an inner region of white matter (region b), which is avascular. [12, 13]

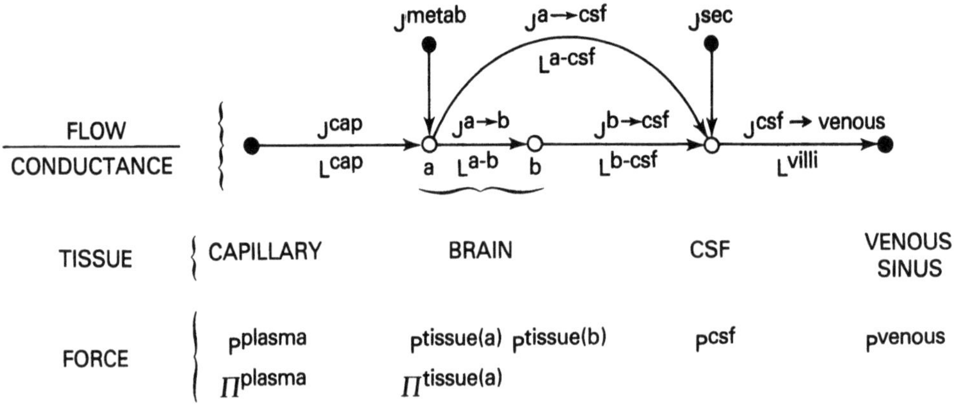

Fig. 2. Equivalent circuit for brain. Positive direction of fluid flow is from capillary to venous sinus blood. *J* designates a flow, *L* a hydraulic conductivity. *P* and *Π* are hydrostatic and osmotic pressures that contribute to driving forces for flow. Sources of fluid are marked as *filled circles*, and junctions of flow, as *open circles*. [12]

Figure 2 is a linear representation of the model in Fig. 1, where individual forces, flows, and conductivities are identified. Each circle represents a relevant intracranial compartment (capillary, brain regions a and b, CSF, venous sinus blood, metabolic compartment, choroid plexus). The filled circles are sources or sinks for fluid flow. Thus, if BBB damage occurs in region a, sources are the capillary bed and metabolic water production in region a.

The general equation that relates fluid flow between any two compartments (arrows in Fig. 2 represent positive flows) to the driving force is

$$\text{Flow (J)} = \text{Hydraulic conductivity (L)} \times \text{Driving force } (\Delta P, \Delta \Pi). \quad (1)$$

Flows are volume flows J (in units of $cm^3\ s^{-1}$), forces are hydrostatic pressure differences P between the compartments (P, mmHg or dyn cm^{-2}), or osmotic pressure differences (Π, mmHg or dyn cm^{-2}); conductances are ratios between flows and driving forces (L $cm^3\ s^{-1}\ mmHg^{-1}$). For volume flow between region a and CSF, for example,

$$J^{a\text{-}csf} = L^{a\text{-}csf}(P^a - P^{csf}). \quad (2)$$

From Fig. 2, it is possible to write eight linear equations with the same form as Eq. 1 (e.g., Eq. 2). In these equations, interstitial hydrostatic pressure contributes to the driving force for fluid movements across the capillary wall and between individual intracranial regions. Interstitial hydrostatic pressure also sets regional tissue volume, by virtue of the compliance relation. For an increment in tissue hydrostatic pressure, ΔP^{brain}, the increment in volume is given as ΔV^{tissue} (fractional increment per g brain), where k = tissue compliance [12, 13]:

$$k = \Delta V^{tissue} / \Delta P^{tissue}\ mmHg^{-1}. \quad (3)$$

When equations of the form of Eq. 1, are combined with Eq. 3, a complete description of the system results.

Table 1 gives best estimates of individual parameters illustrated in Fig. 2 for the intact human brain [12]. Net CSF production is 0.35 $cm^3\ min^{-1}$, of which 70% is formed at the choroid plexus and 30% is extrachoroidal [10, 12]. The nonchoroidal contribution is water derived from cerebral capillaries (18%) and from the metabolism of glucose (12%), which is oxidized at a rate of 0.156 μmol $g^{-1}\ min^{-1}$ in the human brain [12]. White matter compliance k_b is derived from observed relations between increments in white matter volume and increments in intracerebral hydrostatic pressure [15] (Fig. 3), and is equal to gray matter compliance k_a in the intact brain. White matter hydraulic conductivity is estimated according to Marmarou (personal communication, cited in [12]). Hydraulic conductivity of gray matter (region a) is probably about the same, as rates of loss of intracerebrally injected macromolecules are equivalent in the caudate nucleus and internal capsule of the intact rat brain [3].

The driving force for water flow at intact cerebral capillaries is the sum of osmotic and hydrostatic pressure differences across the capillary wall. Plasma protein oncotic pressure can be taken as 25 mmHg. Due to the impermeability of the BBB to proteins, interstitial oncotic pressure is approximately 0. Total osmolality of both plasma and interstitial fluid due to salts and nonprotein solutes is approximately 0.3 osmol, or 5100 mmHg. Plasma hydrostatic pressure can vary between 25 mmHg and 32 mmHg, whereas interstitial hydrostatic pressure can be taken as 0 [6, 12, 15, 20].

Net pressure differences across the cerebral capillary wall result in fluid efflux from plasma to brain, given as follows:

$$\begin{aligned} J^{cap} = L^{cap}\{ & P^{plasma} - P^{tissue(a)} \\ & - \sigma_{oncotic}(\Pi^{oncotic,\ plasma}\quad \Pi^{oncotic,\ tissue(a)}) \\ & - \sigma_i (RTC_i^{plasma} - RTC_i^{tissue(a)})\} \end{aligned} \quad (4)$$

Table 1. Estimated values for various parameters in model for water movement through a normal and through an edematous brain. Data from Rapoport [11–13]

Parameter	Units	Normal brain	Edematous brain
CSF secretion, J^{sec}	$cm^3\ s^{-1}$	4×10^{-3}	Same
Metabolic water prod., J^{metab}	$cm^3\ s^{-1}$	2.8×10^{-5}	Reduced
Capillary volume flow, J^{cap}	$cm^3\ s^{-1}$	1.1×10^{-3}	11×10^{-3}
Villus conductivity, L^{villi}	$cm^3\ mmHg^{-1}\ s^{-1}$	0.001	Same
Capillary conductivity, L^{cap}	$cm^3\ mmHg^{-1}\ s^{-1}$	1.5×10^{-4}	1.5×10^{-2}
Brain conductivity, L^{brain}	$cm^3\ mmHg^{-1}\ s^{-1}$	2.5×10^{-4}	6.6×10^{-3}
Conductivity, $L^{a\text{-}b}$	$cm^3\ mmHg^{-1}\ s^{-1}$	9.4×10^{-5}	5.6×10^{-4}
Conductivity, $L^{a\text{-}csf}$	$cm^3\ mmHg^{-1}\ s^{-1}$	1.9×10^{-4}	2.8×10^{-4}
Conductivity, $L^{b\text{-}csf}$	$cm^3\ mmHg^{-1}\ s^{-1}$	1.9×10^{-4}	1.1×10^{-3}
Region a compliance, k_a	$mmHg^{-1}$	0.001	0.003
Region b compliance, k_b	$mmHg^{-1}$	0.001	0.1
α	mmHg	1000	0
Region a volume, $V^{brain(a)}$	cm^3	1000	1029
Region b volume, $V^{brain(b)}$	cm^3	500	660
$\sigma_{oncotic}$	–	1.0	0.93
σ_i for salts	–	1.0	0
$\Pi^{salts,\ plasma}$	mmHg	5100	Same
$\Pi^{salts(a)}$ or $\Pi^{salts(b)}$	mmHg	5100	Same
$\Pi^{oncotic,\ plasma}$	mmHg	25	Same
$\Pi^{oncotic,\ (a)\ or\ (b)}$	mmHg	0	<25
p^{plasma}	mmHg	32	32
p^{brain}	mmHg	0	Variable
p^{csf}	mmHg	0	0
$t_{½(i)}$	min	16.4	2.2
$t_{½(ii)}$	min	26.3	346

where C_i and σ_i are the concentration and osmotic reflection coefficient, respectively, of a salt or small solute i. Because of the approximate impermeability of the BBB to salts as well as to proteins, plasma and tissue salts (e.g., Na^+ or Cl^+) exert effective osmotic pressures across the capillary wall and contribute to the net driving force for water flow across these walls (Eq. 4). The osmotic reflection coefficients for salts at the intact cerebral capillary, σ_i, approximate 1 [5, 11], as does the osmotic reflection coefficient for proteins, $\sigma_{oncotic}$. At non-neural capillaries without interendothelial tight junctions (zonulae occludens) $\sigma_i \ll 0.1$, and salts do not contribute significantly to osmotic driving forces across the capillary walls [7].

Table 1 also provides estimates for many of the variables in an injured, edematous brain (see below).

Steady State

In the intact brain, linear equations in the form of Eq. 1 can be written to describe flows between compartments. A steady state occurs when compartmental volumes and intercompartmental flows do not change with time. Then, net compartmental

Fig. 3. Relation between changes in brain volume and in interstitial hydrostatic pressure in white matter of cat brain, calculated from data of Reulen et al. [15]. Lines are chord compliances (Eq. 3), $k = \Delta V^{tissue}/\Delta P^{tissue}$ (in $mmHg^{-1}$) at different interstitial pressures. [12, 13]

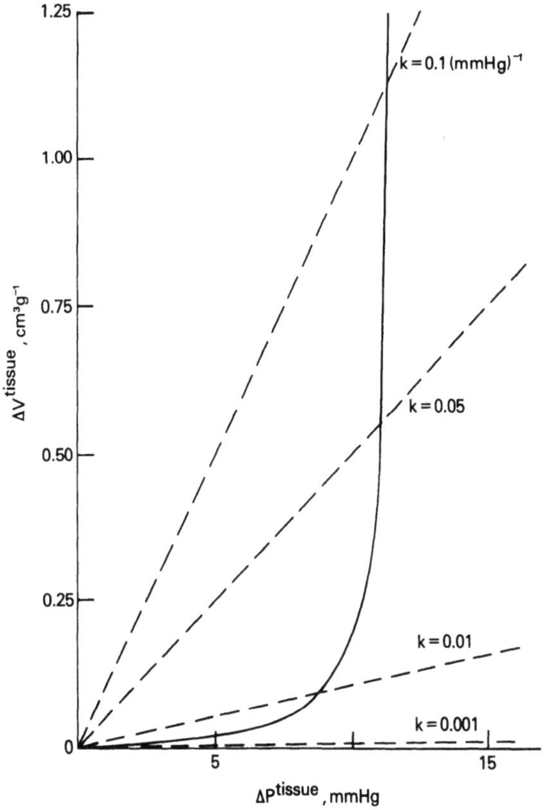

influx plus production from a source (filled circle) equals net efflux, and the following relations obtain among flows [12]:

$$J^{metab} + J^{cap} = J^{a\text{-}b} + J^{a\text{-}csf} = J^{brain\text{-}csf} \quad (5)$$

$$J^{a\text{-}b} = J^{b\text{-}csf} \quad (6)$$

$$J^{brain\text{-}csf} + J^{sec} = J^{csf\text{-}venous}. \quad (7)$$

For fluid movement from brain to CSF, two conductivities in series ($L^{a\text{-}b}$ and $L^{b\text{-}csf}$) are in parallel with a third ($L^{a\text{-}csf}$) (Figs. 1 and 2). These three conductivities are represented by an overall brain hydraulic conductivity, L^{brain},

$$L^{brain} = L^{a\text{-}csf} + (L^{a\text{-}b} \cdot L^{b\text{-}csf})/(L^{a\text{-}b} + L^{b\text{-}csf}). \quad (8)$$

Flow from brain to CSF at the steady state is given in terms of the tissue pressure around gray matter capillaries and the overall brain hydraulic conductivity (Eq. 8),

$$J^{brain\text{-}csf} = L^{brain}\,(P^{tissue(a)} - P^{csf}). \quad (9)$$

Note that the hydrostatic pressure in white matter does not come into play; $J^{brain\text{-}csf}$ is, of course, fluid that is produced by metabolism as well as by capillary

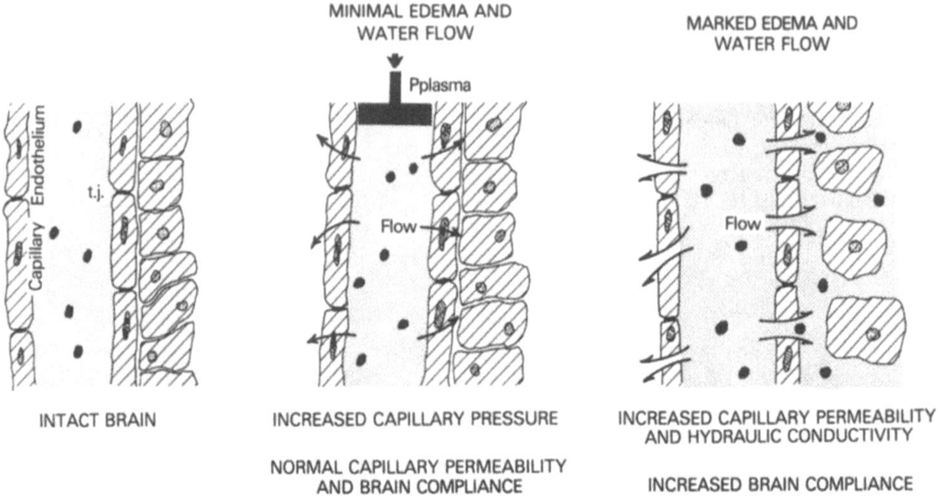

Fig. 4. Diagrams of capillary and surrounding tissue of intact brain (*left*), brain with normal capillary but with increased capillary hydrostatic pressure, leading to flow of ultrafiltrate into parenchyma (*center*), and swollen brain with damaged capillary and extravasated plasma protein and salts (*right*). *Stippling* represents plasma salts, and *large dots*, plasma protein

filtration into region a. The driving force for fluid movement out of the brain is the hydrostatic pressure in gray matter, vis-à-vis the CSF hydrostatic pressure. If CSF pressure is reduced, then fluid movement from the brain is accelerated even in the normal brain [15]. If CSF pressure is elevated, as in hydrocephalus, then fluid movement out of the brain is retarded, and water may accumulate intracerebrally [21].

Why is Edema Insignificant in the Intact Brain?

As illustrated in Fig. 4 (left and center), cerebral capillaries are assumed to be impermeable to salts as well as to proteins, so that plasma fluid that enters the brain is a salt- and protein-free ultrafiltrate. Solute flux from the capillaries due to filtration approximates zero, as $\sigma_i = 1$ for salts and proteins:

$$\text{Solute flux (i)} = (1 - \sigma_i) \times C_i \times J^{cap}. \qquad (10)$$

Dilution of interstitial osmolality by salt-free ultrafiltrate which is forced into the brain reduces the driving force for further fluid flow (Eq. 4). A coefficient α, aproximately equal to 1000 mmHg, has been derived [12, 13] to relate the net change in tissue osmotic pressure to the net change in tissue volume caused by water movement from capillaries to region a:

$$\alpha = -\Delta\Pi^{\text{tissue(a)}} / \Delta V^{\text{tissue(a)}}. \qquad (11)$$

For a reduction in tissue osmotic pressure by 1 mmHg, tissue volume will rise by only 0.001 cm^3 per g.

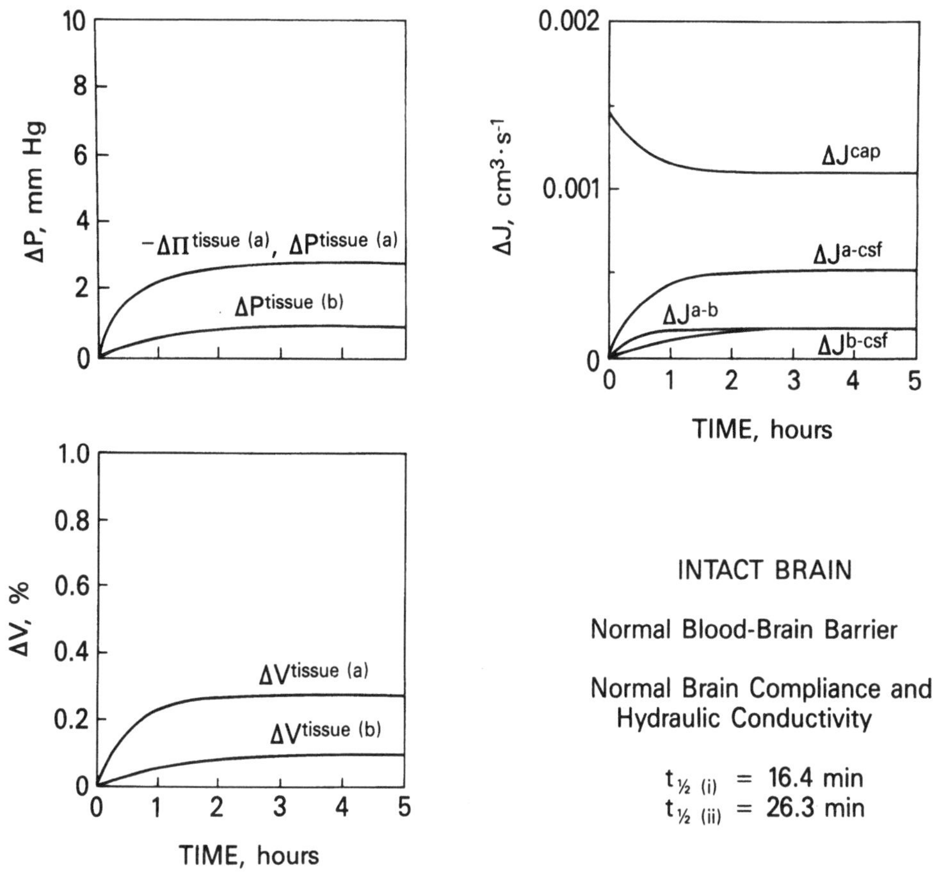

Fig. 5. Changes in pressures, volumes and flows following a 10-mmHg increment in driving force across capillaries of the intact brain. Parameters used are given for normal brain in Table 1. $t_{1/2(i)} = 16.4$ min, $t_{1/2(ii)} = 26.3$ min

Equations of the following form have been derived to describe time-dependent changes in gray and white matter tissue volumes following a step increment in driving force across the capillary wall:

$$\Delta V^{tissue} = \Delta V^{tissue(inf)} + A' \exp\{-0.693\ t/t_{1/2(i)}\} + B' \exp\{-0.693\ t/t_{1/2(ii)}\} \qquad (12)$$

where $\Delta V^{tissue(inf)}$ is the change in tissue volume at infinite time after the increment in driving force (i.e., at the new steady state), A′ and B′ are constants defined from the parameters in Table 1, and $t_{1/2(i)}$ and $t_{1/2(ii)}$ are the two half-times which describe the process [12]. Time-dependent changes in tissue hydrostatic pressure, ΔP^{tissue}, are derived from Eq. 12 by the compliance relation (Eq. 3), and flows are derived by equations of the form of Eq. 1 (e.g., Eqs. 2 and 4).

Fig. 4 (center) indicates that capillary ultrafiltrate free of salts or proteins will be forced into the brain following a one-step change in hydrostatic pressure, without marked swelling of the tissue. Figure 5 illustrates time-courses of regional volumes and pressures, and of intercompartmental flows, calculated with Eq. 12 and with the parameters for the normal brain (Table 1), following a 10-mmHg increment in driving force across the capillaries. This increment can be induced by elevating capillary hydrostatic pressure by 10 mmHg or by reducing capillary plasma osmotic pressure by 10 mmHg. $\Delta P^{tissue(a)}$ reaches 2.72 mmHg and $\Delta P^{tissue(b)}$, 0.91 mmHg after several hours, and $\Delta \Pi^{tissue(a)}$ falls by 2.72 mmHg (cf. Eq. 11). Corresponding to time changes in hydrostatic pressure are changes in regional volumes. As k_a and k_b are both equal to 0.001 $mmHg^{-1}$ (Table 1), gray matter volume rises only by 0.27% of the initial value at the steady state, and white matter volume only by 0.09%.

Immediately after the 10-mm elevation in capillary driving force, ΔJ^{cap} is equal to 1.5×10^{-3} cm^3 s^{-1}; it declines to $1 \times 10^{-3} cm^3$ s^{-1} after several hours. Incremental flow at first is greater between region a and region b than between region b and CSF, due to fluid accumulation within region b. At the steady state, however, both flow terms are equal, and their sum equals ΔJ^{cap} (Eqs. 5–7).

The calculated half-times for the changes in regional volumes and pressures are $t_{1/2(i)} = 16.4$ min and $t_{1/2(ii)} = 26.3$ min (Eq. 12). $t_{1/2(i)}$ is related mainly to the inverse of capillary hydraulic conductivity, and corresponds to an experimental value of 15 min in animal studies [4, 5]. $t_{1/2(ii)}$ is related mainly to the inverse of brain hydraulic conductivity, which retards fluid movement from region a to b, and directly to compliance of region b, k_b. The low compliances of regions a and b, each 0.001 mmHg in the intact brain, limit brain swelling to 0.27% or less in response to the 10-mmHg pressure increment.

In summary, the impermeability of intact capillaries to salts as well as to proteins limits the increment in tissue hydrostatic pressure for a given increment in driving force across the capillaries (Fig. 4, center), because extracellular fluid is diluted by capillary ultrafiltrate. Sequentially, a low brain compliance limits brain swelling in response to any increment in tissue hydrostatic pressure.

Effect of Damage to the Blood-Brain Barrier

With the model, it is possible to examine the effect on brain parameters of BBB damage without concomitant changes in brain compliance or conductivity. With BBB damage, capillary hydraulic conductivity L^{cap} is assumed to be increased 100-fold above normal, and the capillary is assumed to become permeable to salts to the extent that $\alpha = 0$ (Table 1) [12, 13]. σ_i for salts approximates 0 in Eqs. 4 and 10, as it does in leaky non-neural capillaries, and $\sigma_{oncotic}$ falls to 0.93 [1, 19]. The net result is that Eq. 4 reduces to

$$J^{cap} = L^{cap\text{-}a} \left\{ (P^{plasma} - P^{tissue} - \sigma_{oncotic} (\Pi^{plasma} - \Pi^{tissue(a)} \right\}. \quad (13)$$

Damage to the BBB also allows plasma protein into the extracellular space of region a, so that $\Pi^{tissue(a)}$ may rise by up to 25 mmHg. Comparison of Eq. 13 with Eq. 4 shows that the net effect of BBB opening on the driving force for fluid flow across the capillary wall, assuming P^{plasma} constant and $C_i^{plasma} = C_i^{tissue}$, is to augment the driving force by the term, $\sigma_{oncotic} \times \Delta \Pi^{oncotic, tissue(a)}$. By letting this increment equal 10 mmHg, we can compare time-dependent changes in tissue parameters after BBB opening, calculated with the aid of Eq. 12 and illustrated in Fig. 6, to

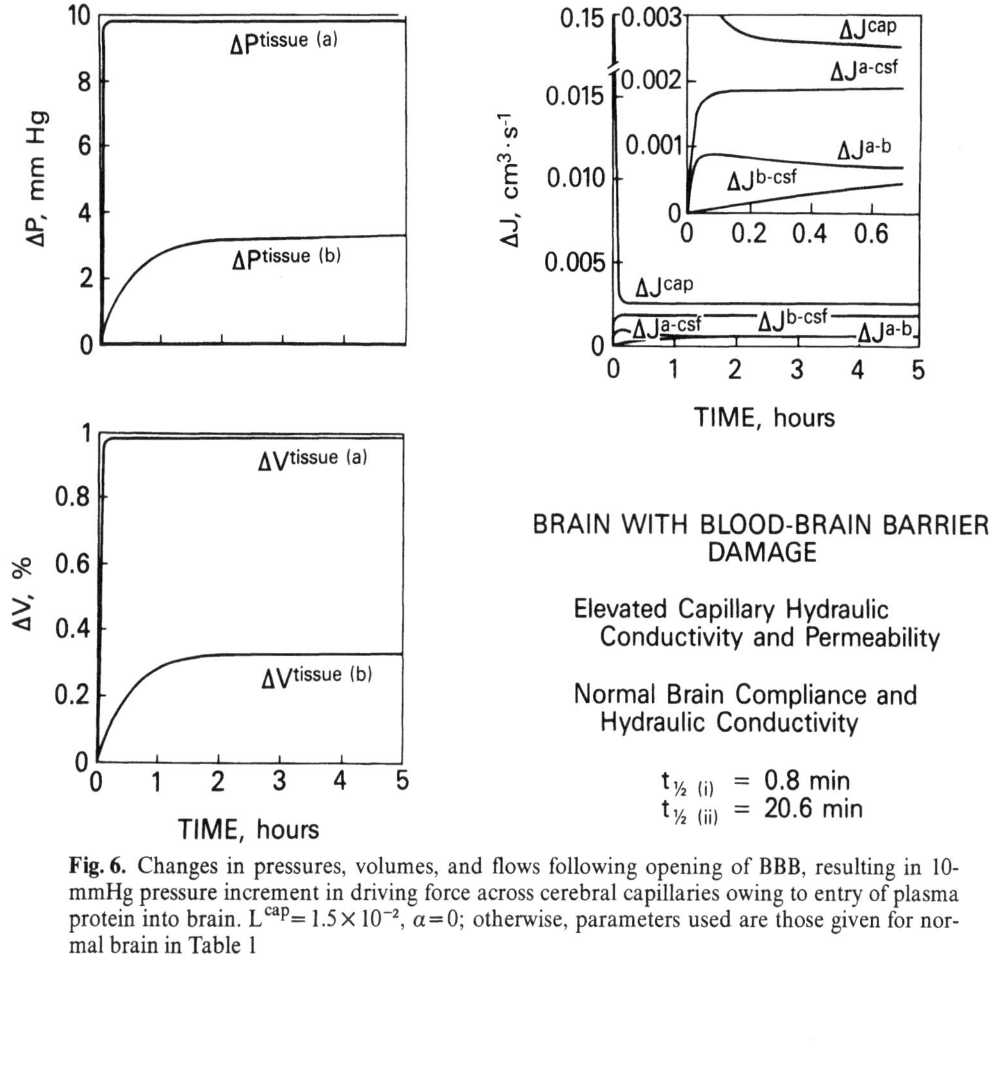

Fig. 6. Changes in pressures, volumes, and flows following opening of BBB, resulting in 10-mmHg pressure increment in driving force across cerebral capillaries owing to entry of plasma protein into brain. $L^{cap} = 1.5 \times 10^{-2}$, $\alpha = 0$; otherwise, parameters used are those given for normal brain in Table 1

calculated changes in the normal brain following an equivalent increment in driving force across the capillaries (Fig. 5).

Figure 6 illustrates that BBB damage (1) accelerates accumulation of capillary fluid in region a, (2) makes the steady-state hydrostatic pressure of region a approximate the increment in driving force, and (3) allows protein into region a. $t_{1/2(i)} = 0.76$ min, as against 16.4 min for the intact brain, and $t_{1/2(ii)} = 20.6$ min, as against 26.3 min for the intact brain. $\Delta P^{tissue(a)}$ at the steady state equals 9.84 mmHg following the 10-mmHg increment in driving force at the capillaries, as compared with 2.7 mmHg in the intact brain. Because a low compliance is retained, tissue volumes do not rise above 1% of initial values. As $\alpha = 0$, dilution of the region a extracellular space due to ultrafiltration of salts does not occur, and $\Delta P^{tissue(a)}$ rises to slightly less than 10 mmHg, to counteract the imposed increment in driving force due to protein accumulation.

Blood-Brain Barrier Opening and Increased Tissue Compliance

If cerebrovascular permeability remains elevated for many hours, capillary filtrate continues to enter the gray matter. Driven by the hydrostatic pressure difference between gray and white matter, fluid dissects its way through white matter at a rate of 2.5 mm h^{-1} [14, 15]. The pressure head causes brain compliance and hydraulic conductivity to rise with time, as illustrated for white matter in Table 2 and Fig. 3 [6, 8, 12, 14, 17]. k_b of white matter attains 0.1 mmHg (Fig. 3), as myelin fibers separate and tissue adhesion weakens [2]. At 1 or 2 days after barrier opening by a cold lesion, net brain water is increased by 8% and plasma protein has infiltrated the brain intercellular space [9, 11–13] (Fig. 4, right).

The compliance and hydraulic conductivity of gray matter do not increase substantially, as they do in white matter, even with continued interstitial hypertension. Gray matter water does not increase by more than 1.5% in cerebral edema, as against increases of 8% or more in white matter [9, 12]. Assuming that $\Delta P^{tissue(a)} = 25$ mmHg following BBB [15, 17, 20], k_a approximates 0.003 $mmHg^{-1}$ in the edematous brain [12].

Table 1 provides best estimates of model parameters for the edematous brain, with prolonged BBB opening associated with elevated brain compliance and conductivity. The data were derived from animal experiments with cold injury edema [6, 9, 12, 14, 15]. k_a is assumed to equal 0.003 $mmHg^{-1}$ and k_b to equal 0.1 $mmHg^{-1}$ (see above). Hydraulic conductivities $L^{a\text{-}b}$ and $L^{b\text{-}csf}$, arising primarily in white matter, are assumed to be sixfold above normal, whereas $L^{a\text{-}csf}$ is assumed to be elevated twofold in less distorted gray matter. As after BBB opening alone (section: "Effect of Damage to the Blood-Brain Barrier"), L^{cap} is elevated 100-fold, $\alpha = 0$, σ_i for salts $= 0$ and $\sigma_{oncotic} = 0.93$.

The parameters for the edematous brain in Table 1 were inserted into Eq. 12 and equations derived from it to calculate times courses and steady-state values of volumes, pressures and flows following BBB opening associated with instantaneous elevations in brain compliance and hydraulic conductivity. The results are illustrated in Fig. 7 for an increment $\sigma_{oncotic} \times \Delta\Pi^{tissue(a)} = 10$ mmHg.

Following transition from normal to edematous parameters (Table 1), $\Delta P^{tissue(a)}$ rapidly approaches the initial 10-mmHg increment in tissue osmotic pressure, $\Delta\Pi^{tissue(a)}$, caused by protein entry into the brain through the damaged capillaries. Capillary hydraulic conductivity is increased 100-fold and $\alpha = 0$. $t_{1/2(i)}$, which governs the rate of rise of $\Delta P^{tissue(a)}$, is equal to 2.2 min. The steady-state volume elevation of $\Delta V^{tissue(a)}$ is about threefold that in Fig. 5, because of the threefold difference in compliance between the two conditions. ΔJ^{cap} is initially equal to 0.15 cm^3 s^{-1}, then falls to 0.008 cm^3 s^{-1}, about twice the steady-state value in the less conductive brain with isolated BBB damage (Fig. 7).

The effects of increasing brain compliance and conductivity in association with BBB opening are recorded mainly in white matter (cf. Figs. 6 and 7). $t_{1/2(ii)}$, which governs the rate of swelling of region b, is prolonged to 346 min, as against 26.3 min in the intact brain and 20.6 min in the brain with isolated BBB modification. The rate of rise of $\Delta V^{tissue(b)}$ approximates that found with experimental cold-injury edema [9].

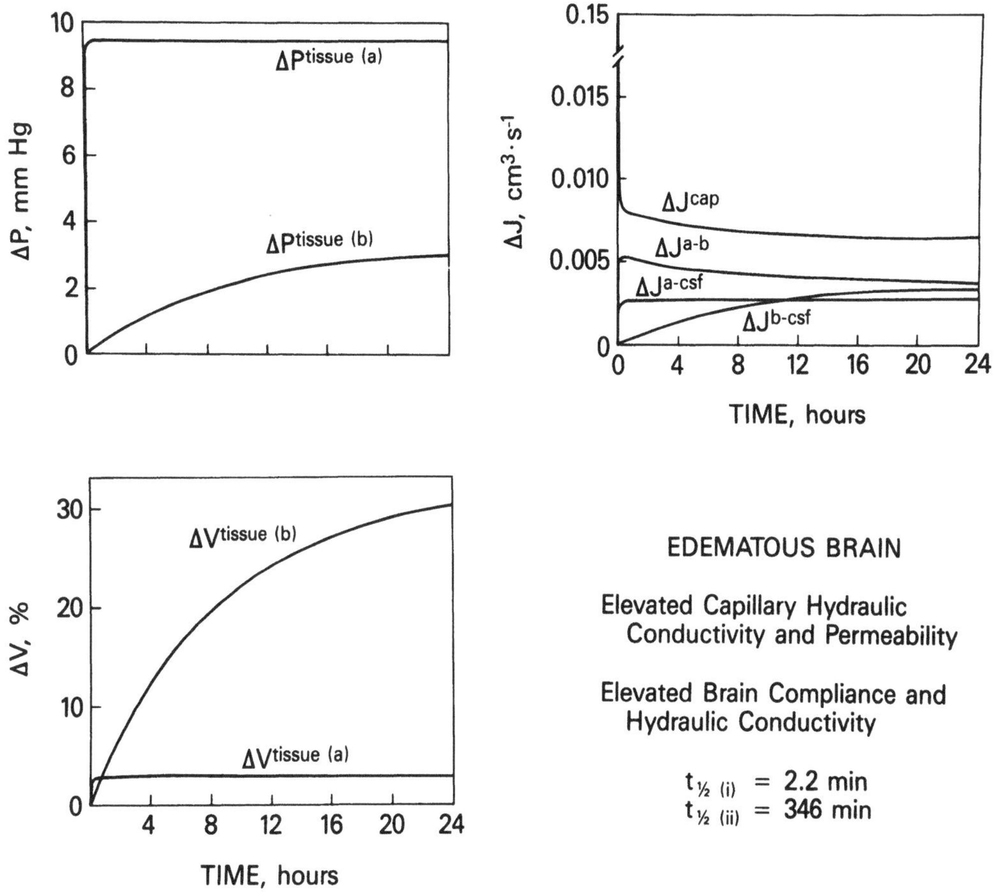

Fig. 7. Changes in pressures, volumes, and flows following opening of BBB and 10-mmHg increment in capillary driving force due to entry of plasma protein into brain. Brain compliance and hydraulic conductivity are increased, as given for edematous brain in Table 1. $t_{1/2(i)} = 2.2$ min and $t_{1/2(ii)} = 346$ min

Table 2. Resistance and compliance of brain during infusion of fluid via a micropipette

Volume (ml)	Resistance (mmHg ml^{-1} min^{-1} × 10^3)	Compliance (ml mmHg^{-1} × 10^5)	Pressure (mmHg)
0 –0.05	6.4±2.5	5.3± 4.0	29
0.1–0.19	2.2±0.7	10.6±10.1	10
0.2–0.29	1.6±1.0	22.9±19	10
0.3–0.39	1.4±1.0	30.5±25	17
0.4–0.49	0.8±0.2	32.7±13	18

Fluid was infused into white matter of the cat brain through a micropipette at a fixed rate. Line pressure was measured. Tissue resistance decreases as compliance increases. Data from Marmarou et al. [8]

After about 24 h, $\Delta P^{tissue(b)}$ reaches the same steady-state level as after isolated BBB opening. Due to a higher tissue compliance, however, $\Delta V^{tissue(b)}$ is elevated to 30% of the initial tissue volume, as against 3.5% following isolated BBB opening (cf. Figs. 6 and 7). The time courses of the individual intercompartmental volume flows, following BBB opening plus elevations of brain compliance and conductivity, reflect the rapid filling of region a (ΔJ^{cap} falls 20-fold within 30 min), and the slower filling of region b ($\Delta J^{a\text{-}b} \gg \Delta J^{b\text{-}csf}$ immediately after BBB opening, but both become equal eventually at the steady state).

Conclusions

We have discussed three conditions in which brain edema might develop: (1) when the driving force increases across the intact capillary wall, (2) when the driving force increases because capillary permeability and hydraulic conductivity rise, and (3) when the driving force increases because capillary permeability and hydraulic conductivity rise and plasma protein enters the brain, and brain compliance and hydraulic conductivity also are elevated.

With intact capillaries, brain swelling is not more than 0.27% of the initial volume per 10-mmHg increment in driving force (case 1). Furthermore, ΔV^{tissue} is not more than 1% of the initial volume if the BBB is altered but brain compliance is unaffected, per 10-mmHg increment in force (case 2). In case 3, $\Delta V^{tissue(b)}$ rises to about 30% of its initial value per 10 mmHg by 24 h, and marked edema and distortion of brain tissue develop. This case represents potentially lethal vasogenic edema.

Several factors are not taken into account in the model of vasogenic brain edema. These include the exact time dependence of compliance and conductance changes in individual regions, in relation to interstitial hydrostatic pressure. The role of capillaries in white matter is ignored, although capillary transport of solutes such as chloride [18] may help to resolve the edema process. Brain metabolism also is ignored, but may help to regulate intercellular adhesion, metabolic water production and the resorption or degradation of extravasated proteins.

Summary

A hydrodynamic-elastic model is used to examine water movement and accumulation in the intact brain, and in the brain in which the blood-brain barrier is damaged and brain compliance is elevated. In the intact brain, cerebral capillaries are impermeant to salts and proteins, and capillary hydraulic conductivity is very low. Salt- and protein-free plasma water that might be forced slowly into the brain will immediately dilute perivascular osmolality and thereby reduce the driving force across the capillary for further fluid accumulation. If cerebrovascular permeability and hydraulic conductivity are increased, and plasma protein enters the brain, this protection is lost and interstitial hydrostatic pressure rises rapidly. If the defect remains for some time, brain compliance and hydraulic conductivity are elevated markedly, particularly in white matter, leading to profound swelling and maximal edema by 1 and 2 days. Plasma filtrate containing salt and protein moves from less compliant gray matter into compliant white matter because of the interstitial hydrostatic pressure difference.

References

1. Aukland K (1973) Autoregulation of interstitial fluid volume. Edema-preventing mechanisms. Scand J Clin Lab Invest 31:247–254
2. Clasen RA, Cooke PM, Pandolfi S, Carnecki G (1963) The effects of focal freezing on the central nervous system. Presbyterian St Luke's Hosp Med Bull 2:36–46
3. Cserr HF (1983) Flow of brain interstitial fluid and drainage into cerebrospinal fluid and lymph. In: Ishii S, Nagai H, Brock M (eds) Intracranial pressure V. Springer, Berlin Heidelberg New York, pp 618–621
4. Fenstermacher JD (1984) Volume regulation of the central nervous system. In: Staub NC, Taylor AE (eds) Edema. Raven, New York, pp 383–404
5. Fenstermacher JD, Johnson J (1966) Filtration and reflection coefficients of the rabbit blood-brain barrier. Am J Physiol 211:341–346
6. Go KG, Patberg WR, Teelken AW, Gazendam J (1976) The Starling hypothesis of capillary fluid exchange in relation to brain edema. In: Pappius HM, Feindel W (eds) Dynamics of brain edema. Springer, Berlin Heidelberg New York, pp 63–67
7. Granger DN, Perry MA (1983) Permeability characteristics of the microcirculation. In: Mortillaro NA (ed) The physiology and pharmacology of the microcirculation, vol 1. Academic, New York, pp 157–208
8. Marmarou A, Takagi H, Shulman K (1980) Biomechanics of brain edema and effects on local cerebral blood flow. In: Cervos-Navarro J, Ferszt R (eds) Brain edema. Pathology, diagnosis and therapy. Adv Neurol 28:345–358
9. Pappius HM, McCann WP (1969) Effects of steroids on cerebral edema in cats. Arch Neurol 20:207–216
10. Pollay M, Curl F (1967) Secretion of cerebrospinal fluid by the ventricular ependyma of the rabbit. Am J Physiol 213:1031–1038
11. Rapoport SI (1976) Blood-brain barrier in physiology and medicine. Raven, New York, pp 1–316
12. Rapoport SI (1978) A mathematical model for vasogenic brain edema. J Theor Biol 74:439–467
13. Rapoport SI (1979) Roles of cerebrovascular permeability, brain compliance, and brain hydraulic conductivity in vasogenic brain edema. In: Popp AJ, Bourke RS, Nelson LR, Kimelberg HK (eds) Neural trauma. Raven, New York, pp 51–62
14. Reulen HJ, Graham R, Fenske A, Tsuyumu M, Klatzo I (1976) The role of tissue pressure and bulk flow in the formation and resolution of cold-induced edema. In: Pappius HM, Feindel W (eds) Dynamics of brain edema. Springer, Berlin Heidelberg New York, pp 103–112
15. Reulen HJ, Graham R, Spatz M, Klatzo I (1977) Role of pressure gradients and bulk flow in dynamics of vasogenic brain edema. J Neurosurg 46:24–35
16. Reulen HJ, Tsuyumu M, Prioleau G (1980) Further results concerning the resolution of vasogenic brain edema. In: Cervos-Navarro J, Ferszt R (eds) Brain edema. Pathology, diagnosis and therapy. Adv Neurol 28:375–381
17. Shulman K, Marmarou A, Weitz S (1975) Gradients of brain interstitial fluid pressure in experimental brain infusion and compression. In: Lundberg N, Ponten U, Brock M (eds) Intracranial pressure II. Springer, Berlin Heidelberg New York, pp 221–223
18. Smith QR, Rapoport SI (1984) Carried-mediated transport of chloride across the blood-brain barrier. J Neurochem 42:754–763
19. Starling EH (1896) On the absorption of fluids from the connective tissue spaces. J Physiol (Lond) 19:312–326
20. Staub NC (1974) Pulmonary edema. Physiol Rev 54:678–811
21. Weller RO, Mitchell J (1980) Cerebrospinal fluid edema and its sequelae in hydrocephalus. In: Cervos-Navarro J, Ferszt R (eds) Brain edema. Pathology, diagnosis and therapy. Adv Neurol 28:111–123

Colloid Osmotic Pressure of Cat Brain Homogenate Relative to Autogenous Cerebrospinal Fluid, Measured by Means of an Electronic Osmometer with a Rigid Semipermeable Copper Ferrocyanide Membrane

M. KOBARI[1], F. GOTOH, M. TOMITA, T. SHINOHARA, Y. TERAYAMA, and B. MIHARA

Key words: Brain swelling, cerebral ischemia, colloid osmotic pressure, electronic osmometer, staverman's reflection coefficient

Introduction

The physicochemical mechanisms of brain swelling in pathologic conditions, e.g., during cerebral ischemia, remain obscure. Using excised cat brain tissue in Ringer's solutions containing various amounts of polyethylene glycol (PEG) 6000 as an osmometer, we demonstrated previously that an ambient osmotic pressure of 578 mmHg was required to suppress the swelling of the brain tissue [4]. Although the observed osmotic pressure was thought to be equal to the colloid osmotic pressure of the intracellular fluid in the brain tissue (π_{ICF}), the value might have been overestimated due to the "PEG space" in the tissue sample, which was represented by the extracellular space accessible to PEG molecules. We therefore attempted to reestimate the value of π_{ICF} using an electronic osmometer with a rigid semipermeable membrane devised by ourselves [3].

Methods

Figure 1 gives a schematic illustration of the electronic osmometer. The theoretical background, detailed description, and basic characteristics of the device have been reported previously [3]. In short, the apparatus comprised a rigid semipermeable membrane made of a baked clay disk impregnated with copper ferrocyanide, a stainless steel mount, and a semiconductor strain-gauge pressure transducer. The sample substance was placed on the rigid semipermeable membrane. The negative pressure inside the hermetic chamber filled with reference fluid was measured by the pressure transducer and was recorded on a DC recorder.

Experiments were carried out in five cats anesthetized with α-chloralose and urethane. A small amount of cerebrospinal fluid was aspirated by puncture of the cisterna magna. After craniectomy the cerebral hemispheres were quickly removed. The cortical tissue was carefully sliced off and immediately homogenized. Measurements of the colloid osmotic pressure of the brain homogenate (π_{BH}) relative to the

---

[1] Department of Neurology, School of Medicine, Keio University, 35 Shinanomachi, Shinjuku-ku, Tokyo 160, Japan

Fig. 1. Cross-sectional diagram of the electronic osmometer. *A*, sample receptacle; *B*, rigid semipermeable membrane comprising a baked clay disk impregnated with copper ferrocyanide; *C*, stainless steel mount; *D*, pressure chamber; *E*, needle for drainage of reference fluid; *F*, rubber stopper; *G*, semiconductor strain-gauge transducer. [3]

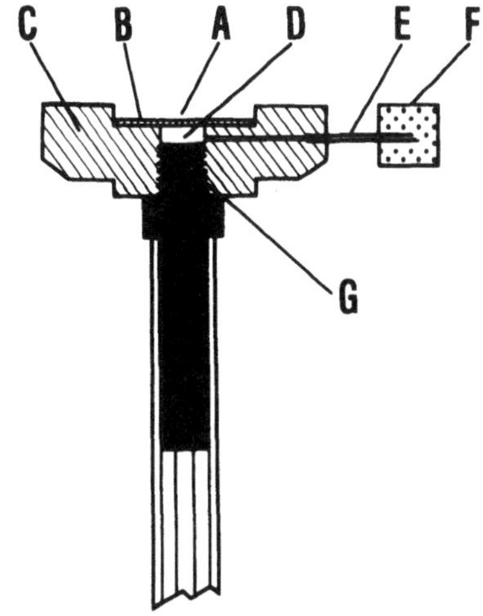

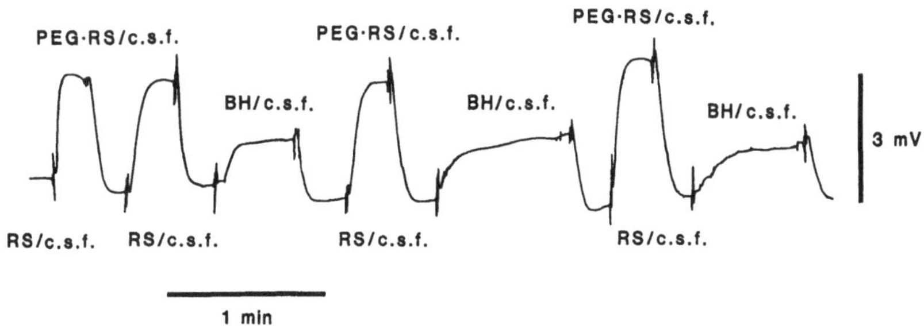

Fig. 2. Example of a recording of pressure changes in the pressure chamber in response to Ringer's solution (*RS/c.s.f.*), a calibrating solution of 72 g/l PEG 6000 in Ringer's solution (*PEG · RS/c.s.f.*) and brain homogenate (*BH/c.s.f.*). For details see text

autogenous cerebrospinal fluid were first made within 5 min and thereafter at arbitrary intervals up to 2 h after excision of the brain tissue. A 72 g/liter solution of PEG 6000 in Ringer's solution was used for calibration. All measurements were performed at room temperature.

Results

An example of a recording of the colloid osmotic pressure of the PEG solution and brain homogenate is shown in Fig. 2. The osmotic pressure of the Ringer's solution (RS/CSF) was regarded as the base level. The four large upward deflections (PEG · RS/CSF) are estimates of the osmotic pressure of the solution of PEG 6000 in Ringer's solution at 72 g/liter. This solution has been reported to have an osmotic pressure of 578 mmHg [4]. The three small wide upward deflections (BH/CSF) are the measures of π_{BH}. It is clear from the recording that reproducibility of the measurements was fairly good for both the PEG solution and brain homogenate.

The absolute value of π_{BH} was calculated by comparing the heights of the two curves. The values of π_{BH} were plotted against time after removal of the brain tissue, and a regression line was calculated for each animal. The values of the slope of the regression line for the five animals were −0.42, −1.31, +0.28, −0.41, and −0.02 mmHg/min. The overall average slope was −0.38±0.27 mmHg/min (mean±SEM). The values of π_{BH} for the five cases were 302±10, 317±11, 292±13, 344±23, and 333±24 mmHg. The total average of π_{BH} for all experiments was 317±10 mmHg (mean±SEM).

Discussion

The validity of the present electronic osmometer has been discussed in a previous communication [3]. The semipermeability of the membrane (Staverman's reflection coefficient, σ) is known to be determined by the characteristics of the membrane itself and the solute in the solution. In the case of the osmometer used in the present experiments, the value of σ for PEG solutions containing high-molecular-weight PEG (above 6000) was almost constant. Although the precise molecular weight of the proteins constituting cytosol is not known, they are assumed to be mostly higher than 6000. It seemed appropriate therefore to use 72 g PEG 6000 solution per liter dissolved in Ringer's solution, with its osmotic pressure of 578 mmHg, for calibration of π_{BH}.

The change in π_{BH} with time after removal of the brain tissue was −0.38 mmHg/min. This relatively small value implies a minimal effect of autolysis of proteins during the measurements. Cat brain homogenate was demonstrated to have a high colloid osmotic pressure of 317 mmHg. It is well accepted that mild homogenization of tissue destroys the cell membrane, while leaving the subcellular organelles and probably protein molecules intact [2]. We therefore assumed that π_{BH} would represent the colloid osmotic pressure of the intracellular fluid in the brain tissue (π_{ICF}). However, since the protein concentration in the cytosol could be diluted by the extracellular fluid during homogenization there was a possibility of underestimating the actual π_{ICF} with the present method. Using excised brain tissue in Ringer's solutions containing various concentrations of PEG 6000 as an osmometer, we previously found that an ambient osmotic pressure of 578 mmHg was required to suppress the swelling of brain tissue [4]. The observed osmotic pressure was thought to be equal to the π_{ICF}, although the value might have been overestimated because of the "PEG space" in the tissue sample, which was represented by the extracellular space accessible to PEG molecules.

A definitive value of π_{ICF} cannot therefore be offered at present, because of methodological limitations. However, the level of colloid osmotic pressure of the intracellular fluid in cat brain tissue, which is far in excess of the systemic arterial blood pressure, should be emphasized. We speculate that under physiological conditions such high colloid osmotic pressure is counterbalanced by the osmotic effect exerted by active ion transport across the cell membrane. The process is supported by the cellular metabolism, and is frequently accompanied by passive water outflow [1]. The ion transport mechanism, however, may be disturbed in pathologic conditions, e.g., cerebral ischemia, and both ions and water may thus accumulate inside the cell, giving rise to brain cell swelling.

In conclusion, the colloid osmotic pressure of the intracellular fluid of cat brain tissue can be said to lie between 317 and 578 mmHg. This high colloid osmotic pressure may represent the intrinsic potential for brain cell swelling under pathologic conditions.

Summary

Using an electronic osmometer with a rigid semipermeable copper ferrocyanide membrane, we measured the colloid osmotic pressure of cat brain homogenate (π_{BH}). Samples of cerebrospinal fluid and fresh cerebro-cortical tissue were obtained from the animals, and the tissue was immediately homogenized. Measurements were first made within 5 min and thereafter at arbitrary intervals up to 2 h after excision of the brain tissue. The values of π_{BH} were plotted against time, and a regression line was calculated for each animal. The mean value of the slope of the regression lines was -0.38 ± 0.27 mmHg/min (mean $\pm$ SEM). This relatively small value implies a minimal effect of autolysis of intracellular protein during the measurements. The mean value of π_{BH} for all measurements was 317 ± 10 mmHg. π_{BH} was thought to represent the colloid osmotic pressure of the intracellular fluid of the brain tissue. The value was lower than the previously presented figure of 578 mmHg, which was obtained by using excised brain tissue in Ringer's solutions containing various concentrations of polyethylene glycol 6000 as an osmometer. Some of the methodological problems inherent in both methods are discussed. It is concluded that the colloid osmotic pressure of the intracellular fluid of cat brain tissue can be considered to lie between 317 and 578 mmHg.

References

1. Macknight ADC, Leaf A (1977) Regulation of cellular volume. Physiol Rev 57:510–573
2. Newsholme EA, Leech AR (1983) Biochemistry for the medical sciences. Wiley, Chichester, pp 2–4
3. Tomita M, Gotoh F (1970) Electronic osmometer with rigid membrane of copper ferrocyanide. Keio J Med 19:163–175
4. Tomita M, Gotoh F, Sato T, Yamamoto M, Amano T, Tanahashi N, Tanaka K (1979) Determination of the osmotic potential for swelling of cat brain in vitro. Exp Neurol 65:66–77

Exudation of Plasma Protein Fractions in Vasogenic Brain Edema*

K. G. Go[1], H.J. Houthoff, J. Hartsuiker, D. van der Molen-Woldendorp, F. Zuiderveen, and A. W. Teelken

Key words: Blood-brain barrier, brain edema, plasma protein fractions

Introduction

The passage of plasma proteins into the brain is pertinent to the question of resolution of vasogenic brain edema, as the proteins give rise to the colloidosmotic pressure of brain interstitial fluid, one of the parameters in the Starling relation of transcapillary fluid exchange [6].

Other important aspects of the entrance of plasma proteins into the brain concern the penetration of antibodies in inflammatory and autoimmune diseases. Furthermore, knowledge of the differential passage of the various plasma protein fractions may contribute to the interpretation of cerebrospinal fluid (CSF) protein spectra in pathologic conditions.

For human CSF, a relation has been found between the rate of passage of various plasma proteins into the brain and their molecular sizes [2], while influences of changes in barrier permeability have also been noted. In a study using anionic and cationic horseradish peroxidase (HRP), the significance of electric charge was demonstrated in determining the rate of migration of the tracer in the brain [9].

This study was undertaken to assess whether in various models of barrier injury, as used in our previous studies on the exudation of HRP and anti-HRP antibody, the exudation of various endogenous plasma proteins was differential (for some data see Table 1), that is, susceptible to the factors mentioned, or entirely non-

Table 1. Some characteristics of the plasma proteins studied

	AAT	Alb	IgG	AMG	IgM
Molecular weight ($\times 10^3$)	54	65	156	820	900
Molecular charge (isoelectric point)	4.5	4.7	5.5–8.6	5.2	7.0–7.4
Serum concentration (mg/ml)	2.9	31	16.5	2.4	0.5

* The investigation reported in this paper was supported by the Netherlands Organization for the Advancement of Pure Research.

[1] Departments of Neurosurgery, Pathology and Neurology, University of Groningen, The Netherlands

selective. Two approaches were chosen, one based on visualization of the various fractions by immunoelectron microscopy and the other on the analysis of edema fluid acquired following cold injury in cats.

Materials and Methods

Morphological Studies

Protein Purification

The endogenous serum protein tracers used included α_1-antitrypsin (AAT), albumin (Alb), immunoglobulin G (IgG), α_1-macroglobulin (AMG), and immunoglobulin M (IgM). All proteins were purified from whole rat serum, starting with separation by gel electrophoresis over a DEAE 52 column, with successive preparative methods for the fractions containing each of the proteins. The AAT-containing fraction was further purified over a G150 S Sephadex column and a Con A-Sepharose column. For AMG purification, the α_1-protein-containing fraction was separated over a G200 S Sephadex column. The final protein fractions were tested in polyacrylamide gel electrophoresis, with only one band for each AAT and AMG. The purified proteins were used for raising antibodies (AAT and AMG) in rabbits, for testing the specificity of the antisera and for finding the optimal antibody dilutions.

Antisera: Raising and Specificity Testing

Commercially purchased rabbit antisera to rat albumin (Nordic, Tilburg, The Netherlands), rat IgG, and rat IgM (Miles, Elkhart, Ind, USA) were used. Rabbit antisera to AAT and AMG were raised by immunization of rabbits with 1–2 mg antigen in complete Freund's adjuvant. Following two boosters, a high-titer antiserum was obtained. The specificity of the antisera was tested in Ouchterlony immunodiffusion and immunoelectrophoresis. Following absorption of the commercial antisera, the resulting monospecific antisera were used in optimal dilutions for detection of the endogenous tracers.

Models of Damage to the Blood-Brain Barrier

Rats with an average body weight of 200 g were anesthesized with urethan (1.5 g/kg body weight) and subjected to the following injuries.

Hyperosmolar Perfusion. Injections of 0.6 ml 4 *M* urea solution were given into the left internal carotid artery over 15 s through a cannula in the left external carotid artery. The animals were killed by perfusion with fixative through a cannula within the thoracic aorta 10 s or 60 min later.

Cold Injury. A rod of dry ice was applied to the dura of the left parietal cortex for 1 min through a 5-mm trephine hole in the skull. The animals were killed by perfusion with fixative 10 s or 60 min later.

Hypertension. Mean arterial pressure, recorded through a cannula in the femoral artery, was raised to 180 mmHg by means of a metaraminol infusion into the tail vein. The animals were killed 30 min later.

Ischemia. A vertical incision was made between the left orbit and the left auditory canal; through this the temporalis muscle was retracted, and the left zygoma and the coronoid process of the mandibula were removed, exposing the inferotemporal fossa and the skull base. Through a craniectomy in the area in front of the foramen ovale the left middle cerebral artery was visualized as it crossed the olfactory tract [11] and clipped with a Scoville clip. The clip was removed after 3 h, and the animal was killed by perfusion 4 days later.

Intraventricular Collagenase Injection. The left lateral cerebral ventricle was punctured at a depth of 5 mm with a 25-mm needle, through a burr hole in the coronal suture and 1.2 mm lateral of the sagittal suture; 0.25 mg collagenase (Calbiochem) in 0.2 ml saline was injected into the ventricle at a rate of 0.2 ml/16 min. The animals were killed 3 h later by perfusion fixation [4].

Tissue Preparation and Tracer Detection

The rats were killed by perfusion fixation through the cannulated abdominal aorta. After perfusion with Ringer-lactate for 30 s, freshly prepared Na-cacodylate-buffered 1% paraformaldehyde (650 mosmol) was perfused for 30 s, followed by 2% paraformaldehyde and 0.1% glutaraldehyde in the same buffer for 4 min. Following removal and coronal sectioning of the brain, fixation was continued by immersion in the same fixative at 4 °C for 24 h. For light microscopy (LM), 4-µm paraffin sections were used. For electron microscopy (EM), 30-µm Vibratome sections were used. The Vibratome sections were pretreated with 10% v/v DMSO in phosphate-buffered saline (PBS), but otherwise the tracer detection methods in LM and EM were comparable. Following preincubation with methanol-H_2O_2 for 30 min and with 5% normal porcine serum, the sections were incubated for 45 min at room temperature or for 10 h at 4 °C with one of the rabbit antisera in its optimal dilution (1 : 160 to 1 : 400). In the next step, the sections were incubated with peroxidase-conjugated porcine anti-rabbit Ig antibodies (Dako, Copenhagen, Denmark) diluted 1 : 50 for 30 min at room temperature or 12 h at 4 °C. For visualization of the peroxidase label, the diaminobenzidine reaction was performed for 5–10 min at room temperature. Dilution and rinsing between the steps were performed with PBS. For EM, the Vibratome sections were then postfixed in 2% glutaraldehyde and 1% OsO_4, dehydrated, and flat-embedded in epoxy resin. Unstained 1-µm epoxy sections were used for LM and unstained ultrathin sections, for EM.

Analysis of Edema Fluid

In cats of 3 kg body weight, anesthesia was induced with phenobarbitone and pentobarbitone and maintained with nitrous oxide-oxygen. A freezing injury was inflicted by application of a freezing probe at –30 °C to the dura for 5 min. A platform holding 25-g needles 4–13 mm in length was stereotactically aimed at the freezing lesion until all the needles had been inserted into the brain [3]. The needles were connected to polyethylene tubes containing a fluid gasoline seal, which prevented evaporation and concentration of the edema fluid that subsequently collected within the tubes. The tubes were removed every hour, plugged with metal wires at either end, and stored at -20 °C. Plasma samples were also collected hourly from an arterial cannula. Colloid osmotic pressure was measured using a colloid osmometer constructed in the laboratory according to Aukland and Johnsen [1].

The total protein content of plasma and edema fluid was determined by mixing 0.025 ml of the 1:100 diluted sample with 1 ml of a (500 m*M*) NAOH/(33 m*M*) EDTA solution and adding 0.25 ml of a (4.5 m*M*) hyamine solution, with photometric reading at a wavelength of 439 nm. IgG and albumin were assayed in plasma and edema fluid by Laurell's electroimmunoassay [10]. The (1:20 for IgG and 1:400 for albumin) diluted 1-μl samples were placed in 2.5-mm wells punched out in an agarose gel layer of 1.50 mm thickness. The agarose gel was composed of 1% agarose-litex (Glastrup, Denmark) and 1% polyethylene glycol 6000 (Merck) dissolved in 0.02 *M* barbital buffer pH 8.6; it contained the antiserum against cat IgG (Cappel Labs) (300 μl antiserum/30 ml agarose solution) or the antiserum against cat albumin (Cappel Labs) (100 μl antiserum/30 ml agarose solution). Electrophoresis was performed at a field strength of 2–3 V/cm for 16–22 h. Subsequently the gel was pressed lightly between layers of filter paper, rinsed in saline, and dried. The gel plates were then stained for 10 min with Coomassie Brilliant Blue R-250 (5 g in 450 ml ethanol, 100 ml acetic acid, 450 ml distilled water) and destained twice in the same solvent the following day. The reference cat IgG was purchased from Cappel Labs and the reference cat albumin was extracted from cat serum by ammonium sulfate precipitation and subsequent dialysis against distilled water.

Results

Morphological Studies

The results obtained in the model with hyperosmolar urea perfusion are presented in detail. For the other experimental models only data differing from this first model in the exudation pattern of the proteins are given.

Hyperosmolar Urea Perfusion

Light Microscopy. The observations recorded in LM are displayed in Table 2. At 10 s survival exudation spreading into the surrounding brain was only obvious for Alb and, to a lesser extent, for IgM. In addition, Alb was also prominently present in pericytes. However, in the lining of capillaries and larger vessels, IgG, AMG, and IgM were the proteins most conspicuously present.

At 60 min survival spreading into the surrounding brain of Alb and IgM was no longer discernible, but both these proteins were still obviously present in pericytes.

Table 2. Hyperosmolar urea perfusion (detection of protein tracer exudation in light microscopy)

	AAT	Alb	IgG	AMG	IgM
Survival 10 s					
Capillary lining cells	±	±	++	++	++
Pericytic uptake	–	++	–	–	–
Extravascular spreading	–	+	–	–	+
Survival 60 min					
Capillary lining cells	±	±	++	++	++
Pericytic uptake	–	++	–	–	+
Extravascular spreading	–	–	+	+	–

The exudation and spreading of IgG and AMG into the surrounding brain had become considerable by 60 min survival. The presence of the other proteins in the lining of capillaries and larger vessels at 60 min survival was similar to that at 10 s survival, although to a lesser extent. As in each animal the presence of all protein tracers could be studied and as the variability in results between the animals was minimal, the differences in protein tracer exudation were interpreted as reflecting the type of barrier damage inflicted by this experimental model.

Electron Microscopy. The results in EM (Fig. 1) showed similar differences in exudation of the various plasma proteins as were observed in LM. Alb was rarely visualized in the endothelial lining, but it was conspicuously present in the perivascular spaces, the extracellular space of the brain, and vesicles of pericytes. AAT also was nearly lacking from the endothelial cells but it was prominent in the extracellular space; moreover, sometimes AAT was found in the cytoplasm of perivascular astrocytes. The presence of IgG, AMG, and IgM at 10 s survival remained confined to the cytoplasm of endothelial cells, with only incidentally some perivascular localization of tracers, especially of AMG. The morphology of the endothelial cells with cytoplasmic tracer localization regularly showed indications of regressive changes with the formation of large and irregular vesicles. With none of the tracers was a localization in the usual cytoplasmic vesicles observed.

Fig. 1a–f. Hyperosmolar urea perfusion at 10 s survival in one animal. *Bar*, 1 μm in each case. **a** Endogenous albumin as tracer. A small amount of tracer is present in the endothelial cytoplasm (→). There is some perivascular edema (*). **b** Endogenous albumin as tracer. A large amount of tracer is present in the perivascular spaces. **c** Endogenous AAT as tracer. A large amount of tracer is present in the extracellular spaces and in the swollen cytoplasm of an astrocytic endfoot. **d** Endogenous IgM as tracer. Tracer is prominent in the endothelial cytoplasm, in the abluminal side of the basement membrane (→), and in swollen cytoplasmic processes (*). **e** Endogenous IgG as tracer. Tracer is prominent in the endothelial cytoplasm, with sparing of cytoplasmic vesicles and organelles. **f** Endogenous AMG as tracer. Tracer is conspicuous in the endothelial cytoplasm and the abluminal side of the basement membrane (→). Note the regressive changes with large and irregular empty vesicles in the endothelial cell containing tracer

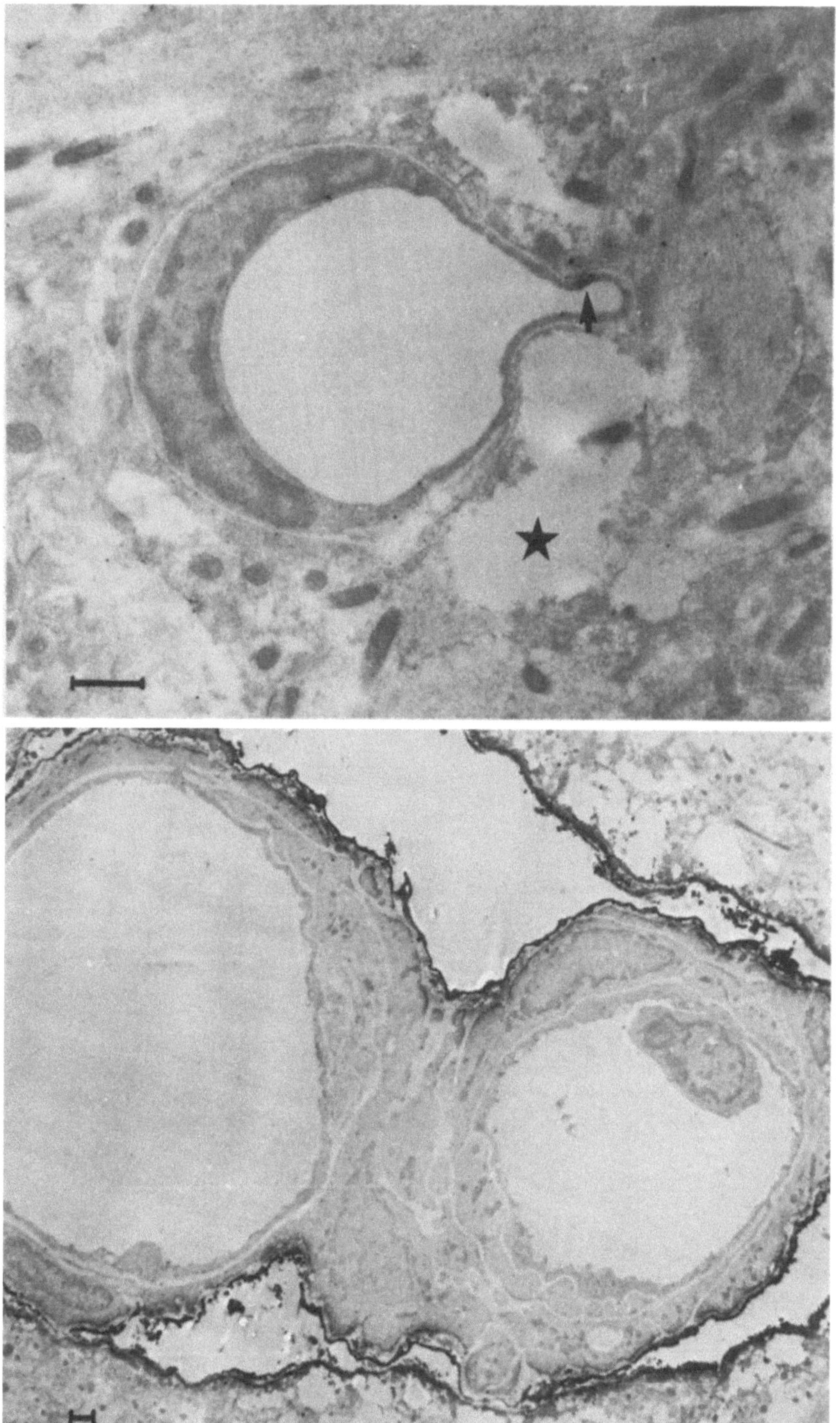

a

b

Fig. 1 a, b

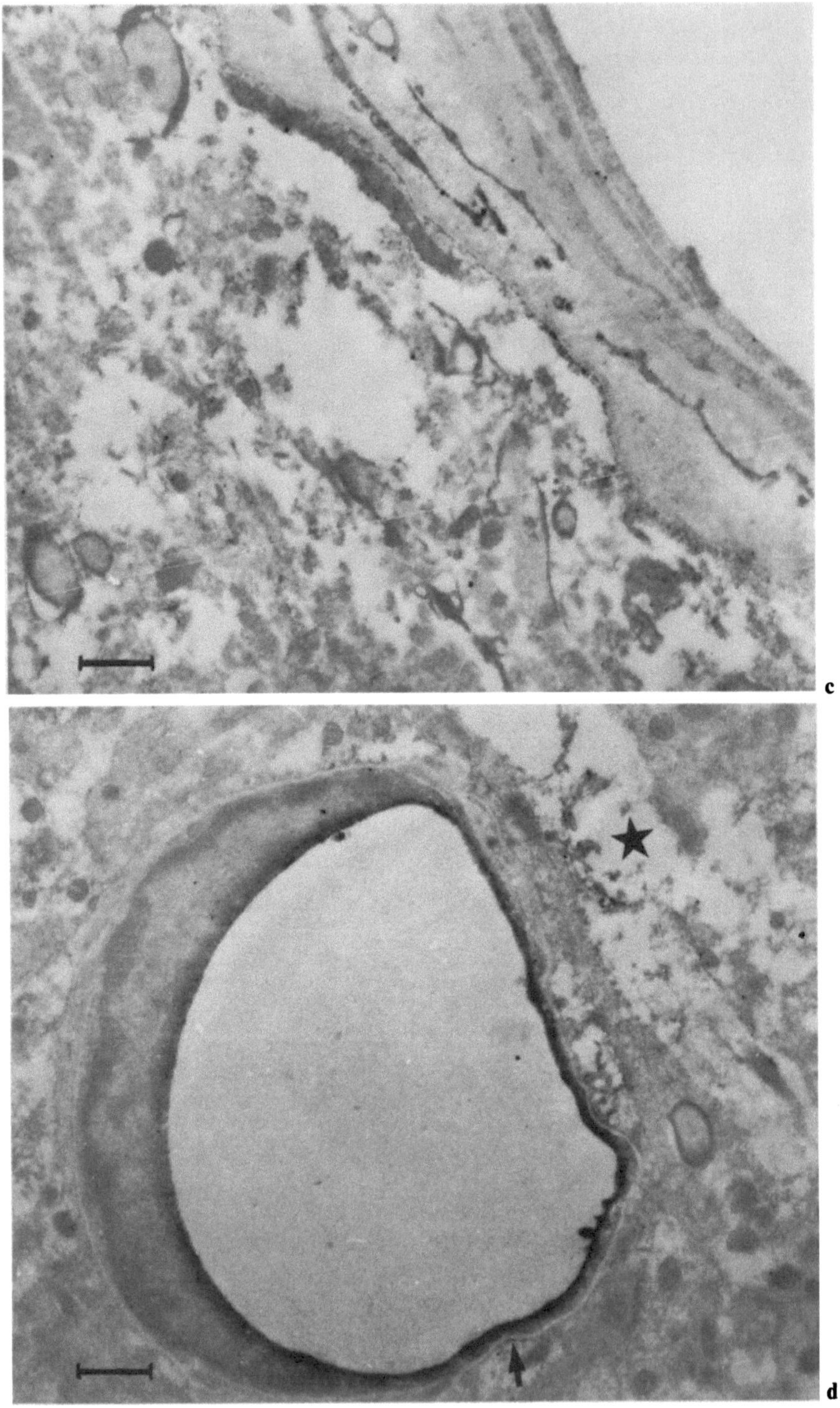

Fig. 1 c, d

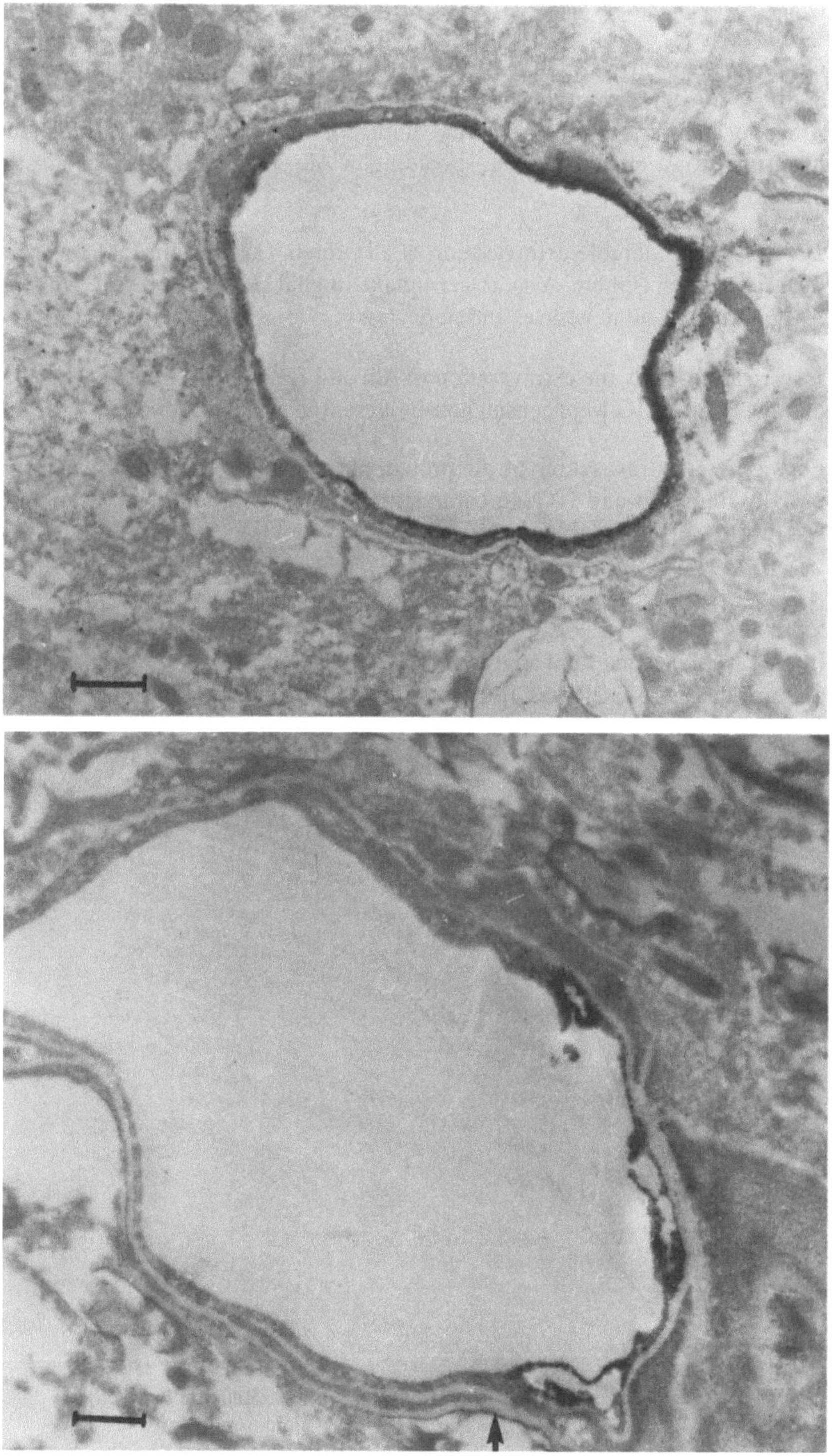

e

f

Fig. 1 e, f

Other Experimental Models

Cold Injury. As early as 1 min after injury the exudation and spreading of Alb, IgG, and IgM into the brain areas surrounding the lesion site was already conspicuous. Alb appeared to be present in the lining of many capillaries throughout both hemispheres. At 60 min survival spreading of Alb, IgG, and AAT was most prominent, in that order.

Ischemia. Considerable extravasation of all proteins apart from IgM was present in the affected hemisphere. Also, tracer uptake in glial cells was present. Only Alb and AMG were present in vesicles and pericytes.

Hypertension. Only the extravasation of Alb and IgG was prominent. These proteins and AAT and AMG were conspicuously present in pericytic vesicles.

Collagenase. Extravasation of all protein tracers apart from IgM was noted, especially from Alb and IgG. In contrast, the lining of capillaries and larger vessels was mostly devoid of protein tracers.

Analysis of Edema Fluid

In the cats the edema fluid analyzed (Table 3) had a lower total protein content than plasma; therefore COP was also lower in edema fluid. In contrast to the Alb con-

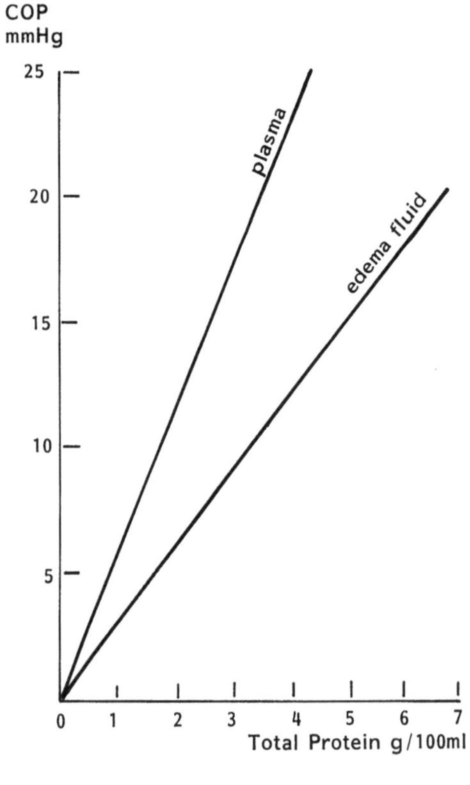

Fig. 2. Relation between colloid osmotic pressure (*COP*) and total protein content for plasma and edema fluid

Table 3. Mean contents (g/100 ml) of total protein, albumin (Alb) and immunoglobulin G (IgG) in plasma and edema fluid, mean colloid osmotic pressure (COP, mmHg) of plasma and edema fluid, and mean edema fluid plasma ratios for total protein, albumin and IgG contents, and COP

	COP	Total protein	Alb	IgG
Plasma	36.1 ± 9.5	6.61±1.30	2.80±0.36	2.23±1.08
Edema fluid (EF)	23.1 ±10.7	3.98±1.09	2.41±0.53	2.95±1.80
EF/plasma ratio	0.65± 0.29	0.64±0.16	0.82±0.10	1.37±0.70

tent, which also seemed lower in edema fluid than in plasma, the IgG content was higher in edema fluid. Assuming that a down-gradient passage of IgG from plasma to brain through the impaired blood-brain barrier is usual, this indicates that IgG must have accumulated in edema fluid. Accordingly, in edema fluid the proportion of IgG is elevated, and that of Alb reduced. As albumin constitutes the protein fraction mainly contributing to COP, this is reflected by the lower COP exerted by the proteins in edema fluid (3.05 mmHg per g protein) than in plasma (5.76 mmHg per g protein).

Discussion

The results of both the morphological studies and the analysis of edema fluid indicate that the presence of any protein fraction at a particular site in the tissue is obviously the result of transfer through the disrupted blood-brain barrier and of removal by migration or by cellular uptake. The factors that determine the passage through the barrier are molecular size, plasma concentration, and electrical charge of the protein, while the last factor also determines mobility during migration. Particularly Alb was remarkable by its great mobility as visualized in the morphological studies. Even by 10 s after the injury it has migrated from the extracellular spaces as far as the perivascular spaces, while the presence of IgG and IgM is still largely confined to the endothelium. AAT, another small-molecular protein, like Alb, had reached the extracellular spaces by 10 s according to EM.

The passage of AMG, which even advances into the perivascular spaces to some degree within 10 s as shown by LM, is highly remarkable considering that its molecular weight is one of the highest of all fractions and that it is not very abundant in plasma, which is probably due to its negative charge. As visualized in LM, it takes 60 min for IgG and AMG to reach the extracellular spaces. It is possible that earlier spreading of AMG has eluded LM. Cellular uptake into pericytes as a mechanism of removal was particularly conspicuous with Alb.

In the study of protein passage through the disrupted blood-brain barrier horseradish peroxidase (HRP) has always been used as the standard tracer.

Our previous studies using anti-HRP antibody (of the IgG class) as a tracer have indicated the prevalence of diffuse cytoplasmic imbibition as the mechanism of passage through the endothelium; the prominence of vesicles with the use of HRP may be due to the exogenous nature of the protein [8].

In the present study pertaining to endogenous protein fractions, cytoplasmic imbibition was again observed as the relevant mechanism of passage through the endothelium. The different behavior of the various fractions, moreover, demonstrates the inadequacy of HRP as a standard tracer.

The analysis of edema fluid in the cat model has indicated the accumulation of IgG with respect to Alb. It may reflect concentration of IgG, with removal of Alb and fluid migration or cellular uptake, whereas IgG is retained.

With reference to the Starling relation governing transcapillary fluid exchange, in contrast to other tissues, in brain tissue the movement of fluid (water and Na^+) between blood and brain is greatly restricted by the blood-brain barrier. Nevertheless the blood-to-brain passage of Na^+ has been found to be dependent on blood pressure, in accordance with the Starling relation [5, 7].

The COP is the other parameter determining fluid exchange in the Starling relation [6]. Following microinfusion of fluid into cerebral white matter of cats, the retention of fluid within the tissue seemed to depend on the presence of protein in the fluid, as saline was retained for a shorter time than a protein solution (A. Marmarou, personal communication). The lower level of COP per gram of protein in brain edema fluid with respect to plasma (on account of the lower proportion of Alb in the edema fluid) is compatible with reabsorption.

Furthermore, the protein content of edema fluid may determine the proton NMR (nuclear magnetic resonance) parameters of brain edema relevant to NMR imaging of edematous cerebral lesions.

Summary

In rats the exudation of endogenous α_1-antitrypsin, albumin, IgG, α_1-macroglobulin, and IgM (with mol. wt. 45, 65, 156, 820, and 900 000, respectively) was evaluated by light- and electron microscopy using an immunoperoxidase method with specific antibodies, after BBB disruption caused by freezing injury, hyperosmolar carotid perfusion, acute hypertension, intraventricular collagenase injection, or ischemia following middle cerebral artery occlusion. The exudation of the respective protein fractions varied widely and seemed dependent on other factors than molecular weight alone. Passage through the endothelium occurred neither through junctions nor by vesicular transport, but only by diffuse cytoplasmic imbibition.

In cats with a freezing lesion, edema fluid was collected in polyethylene tubes connected to needles inserted into the edematous brain. In samples of plasma and edema fluid, total protein, albumin, and colloid osmotic pressure were determined. The results suggested a relative increase in IgG in the extracellular edema fluid with respect to albumin, suggesting uptake of the latter into cellular elements or removal into the circulation.

References

1. Aukland K, Johnsen HM (1974) A colloid osmometer for small fluid samples. Acta Physiol Scand 90:485–490

2. Felgenhauer K, Schliep G, Rapic N (1976) Evaluation of the blood-CSF barrier by protein gradients and the humoral immune response within the central nervous system. J Neurol Sci 30:113–128
3. Gazendam J, Go KG, Van Zanten AK (1979) Composition of isolated edema fluid in cold-induced edema. J Neurosurg 51:70–77
4. Gazendam J, Houthoff HJ, Huitema S, Go KG (1984) Cerebral edema formation and blood-brain barrier impairment by intraventricular collagenase infusion. In: Go KG, Baethmann A (eds) Recent progress in the study and therapy of brain edema. Plenum, New York, p 159
5. Go KG, Pratt JJ (1975) The dependence of the blood to brain passage of radioactive sodium on blood pressure and temperature. Brain Res 93:329–336
6. Go KG, Patberg WR, Teelken AW, Gazendam J (1976) The Starling hypothesis of capillary fluid exchange in relation to brain edema. In: Pappius HM, Feindel W (ed) Dynamics of brain edema. Springer, Berlin Heidelberg New York, p 63
7. Go KG, Koster-Otte L, Pratt JJ (1979) Brain sodium uptake after choroid plexectomy. Brain Res 170:325–331
8. Houthoff HJ, Go KG, Gerrits PO (1982) The mechanisms of blood-brain barrier impairment by hyperosmolar perfusion. An electron cytochemical study comparing exogenous HRP and endogenous antibody to HRP as tracers. Acta Neuropathol 56:99–112
9. Houthoff HJ, Moretz RC, Rennke HG, Wisniewski HM (1984) The role of molecular charge in the extravasation and clearance of protein tracers in blood brain barrier impairment and cerebral edema. In: Go KG, Baethmann A (ed) Recent progress in the study and therapy of brain edema. Plenum, New York, p 67
10. Laurell CB (1972) Electro immuno assay. Scand J Clin Lab Invest [Suppl 124] 29:21
11. Tamura A, Graham DJ, Mc Cullouch J, Teasdale GM (1981) Focal cerebral ischemia in the rat. 1. Description of technique and early neuropathological consequences following middle cerebral artery occlusion. J Cereb Blood Flow Metab 1:53–60

Development of Brain Edema Following Fluid Percussion Injury

A. MARMAROU[1], T. NAKAMURA, H. SAKAMOTO, L. JENKINS, and D. P. BECKER

Key words: Brain edema, fluid percussion injury, gravimetric method

Introduction

The progressive increase in brain volume following severe mechanical injury ultimately leads to intracranial ischemia and hypertension. The severity of the problem is in part reflected in the statistic that 50% of patients who succumb to head injury die of excessively high intracranial pressure [1, 2]. The objective of the present research is to identify the role that brain edema plays in this swelling process and to determine in a well-defined model of brain injury how edema affects cerebral blood flow.

Experimental models of closed head injury produced by mechanical impact have been studied extensively, but relatively few studies have quantified the amount of edema developed by direct tissue water measurement. Tornheim et al. measured tissue density following mechanical impact to the closed skull of cats [3–5]. In animals sacrificed 48 h after trauma findings of unilateral fracture of the frontal bone, subarachnoid hemorrhage, and significant edema of the contused hemisphere were recorded [3]. Although this model continues to yield valuable data, Tornheim views the lack of morphological reproducibility introduced by the thickness and contour of the cranial bones as a primary weakness of it [3]. The studies described in this report utilized the fluid percussion model which obviates the variability introduced by the container properties of bone. Our first goal was to establish the amount of edema developed following fluid percussion impact and to document the concomitant change in intracranial pressure and volume status.

Methodology

The fluid percussion model has been described in detail in other reports [6]. In brief, adult cats (2.5–3.5 kg) were anesthetized with IV Brevital titrated to absence of the lid reflex. The animals were intubated, paralyzed with pancuronium bromide (0.05–0.1 mg/kg), and kept normocapnic by means of mechanical ventilatory support. Arterial blood samples were obtained to confirm normal pH and normal levels of carbon and oxygen.

[1] Division of Neurosurgery, Medical College of Virginia, Richmond, VA, USA

Following reflection of the scalp and associated musculature, a large burr hole 11 mm in diameter was made over the midline of the parieto-occipital region (central injury site) or 90° laterally over the temporo-parietal region (TP injury site), and a hollow metal screw was inserted tightly into the cranium over the intact dura. The fluid percussion device described by Sullivan [6] was attached securely to the injury screw. Brain trauma was produced by the release of a weighted pendulum which struck a fluid-filled plexiglas column attached to the injury screw.

Following injury, the animals were kept unconscious by means of a mixture of nitrous oxide (70%) and oxygen (30%) and maintained in a special ICU (intensive care unit), specifically designed and staffed to provide continuous care and support for 24 h. During this period, ventricular and cisternal fluid pressure, arterial pressure, pressure volume index (PVI), somatosensory evoked potentials, and resting EEG were recorded and followed on stripcharts. Upon sacrifice of the animals at 24 h the brains were removed and the spatial distribution of water was determined gravimetrically [7, 8].

Results

Control levels of tissue water content compared favorably with normal levels for the adult cat (68.8% in white matter, 80.9% in gray matter) [8]. All animals studied 24 h after fluid percussion injury developed significant brain edema. The distribution of water content typical of central injury is shown in Fig. 1, where the dashed lines cor-

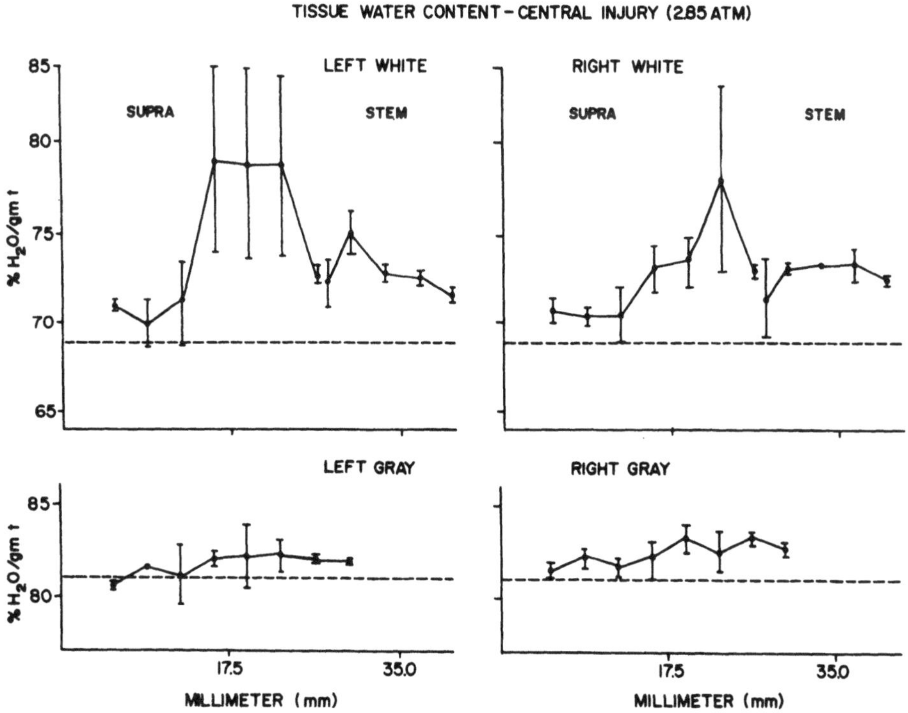

Fig. 1. Typical distribution of water content in the brain affected by central injury

respond to normal control level. White matter water content was elevated throughout the hemisphere. The edema was most pronounced in the brain stem. The water content of the gray matter was essentially normal, with a slight increase to 83% in the region directly under the percussion injury. In the group as a whole ($n = 3$), central injury produced a maximum tissue water content in the brain stem of 76.75% + 3.8% (SD) by weight. The finding that edema of cortex is normal and increase of water content confined to white matter suggests the edema fluid is of vasogenic origin. The characteristic distribution for central impact is that edema is most pronounced in the brain stem, with less water above the tentorium, and it is symmetrically distributed within the white matter.

With TP injury ($n = 3$) maximum edema is developed in the injured hemisphere, with a water content of 83.3% + 8.08% (SD) by weight in the white matter along the axis of impact. The water content of gray matter following TP impact was not significantly elevated [81.74% + 0.89% (SD) by weight]. Spatially, brain stem water was increased symmetrically with temporal parietal impact, but the increase in brain stem water was less marked than that seen with central injury.

Discussion

A severe fluid percussion injury is immediately followed by a rapid rise in arterial and intracranial pressure. The intracranial pressure rise averaged 32.4 mmHg in previous studies, and pressure returned to normal levels approximately 1 h after central percussion impact. These findings prompted a study of tissue water content by Corales et al. [9] to determine whether the rise in ICP following traumatic injury was caused by brain edema. Studies performed 5 and 30 min after central injury indicated no increase in water content in any area of the brain, either during the elevation or after the transient rise in pressure subsided. This was not the case in animals sacrificed 24 h after injury. All animals developed significant brain edema. With central injury the edema is symmetrically distributed, with a high brain stem component. With lateral injury, edema is most severe in the injured hemisphere with less edema found in the brain stem. In the current central impact studies ventricular and cisternal fluid pressure averaged 6.8 ± 1.6 mmHg (mean + SD) at 2 h after injury and gradually increased to a mean level of 15.5 mmHg at 24 h after impact. The pressure volume index decreased from a control value of 1.035 ml to one of 0.6 ml at 24 h. With lateral injury, the PVI decreased to an average of 0.48 (± 0.2) ml by 10 h after the impact. This exhaustion of buffering capacity was followed by dissociation of ventricular and cisternal pressure by 18 h after impact, suggesting tentorial impaction.

Summary

Brain edema does indeed develop following mechanical fluid percussion injury. With a central impact, edema is most pronounced in the brain stem. Lateral impact produces greater supratentorial involvement and leads to tentorial impaction within 18 h. The development of brain edema and eventual exhaustion of buffering capacity appears to be the major factor in the subsequent rise of ICP and neurologic deterioration seen in this model.

References

1. Becker DP, Miller JD, Ward JD, Greenberg RP, Young HF, Sakalas R (1977) The outcome from severe head injury with early diagnosis and intensive management. J Neurosurg 47:491–502
2. Marshall LF, Smith RW, Shapiro HM (1979) The outcome with aggressive treatment in severe head injuries. I. The significance of intracranial pressure monitoring. J Neurosurg 50:20–25
3. Tornheim PA, McLaurin RL, Thorpe JF (1976) The edema of cerebral contusion. Surg Neurol 5:171–175
4. Tornheim PA, McLaurin RL (1978) Effect of dexamethasone on cerebral edema from cranial impact in the cat. J Neurosurg 48:220–227
5. Tornheim PA, McLaurin RL, Sawaya R (1979) Effect of furosemide on experimental traumatic cerebral edema. Neurosurgery 4:48–52
6. Sullivan HG, Martinez J, Becker DP, Miller JD, Griffith R, Wist AO (1976) Fluid percussion model of mechanical brain injury in the cat. J Neurosurg 45: 520
7. Marmarou A, Poll W, Shulman K, Bhagavan H (1978) A simple gravimetric technique for measurement of cerebral edema. J Neurosurg 49: 530–537
8. Marmarou A, Tanaka K, Shulman K (1982) An improved gravimetric measure of cerebral edema. J Neurosurg 56:246–253
9. Corales RL, Miller JD, Becker DP (1980) Intracranial pressure and brain water content in acute graded experimental cerebral trauma. In: Shulman K, Marmarou A, Miller JD, Hochwald G, Becker DP, Brock M (eds) Intracranial pressure IV. Springer, Berlin Heidelberg New York, pp 280–283

Biomechanics of Vasogenic Brain Edema Application of Biot's Consolidation Theory and the Finite Element Method

T. NAGASHIMA[1], N. TAMAKI, T. SHIRAKUNI, S. MATSUMOTO, Y. SEGUCHI, and T. TAMURA

Key words: Brain edema, extracellular fluid, biomechanics, computer simulation, finite element method

Introduction

Although many factors are known to modify the process of the brain edema, little is known about the mechanism of the progression and resolution of vasogenic brain edema. In 1978, Rapoport [6] first elaborated a mathematical model of vasogenic brain edema. He adequately defined many factors with a hydraulic compartment model and proposed a theoretical basis of the research of vasogenic brain edema. We have tried to extend this model to give a more comprehensive one. The model was based on the well-established concept that the edema fluid propagates as bulk flow through extracellular space depending on hydrostatic pressure gradient. We applied Biot's theory of consolidation, which describes the behavior under loading of porous deformable material containing viscous fluid. The finite element method (FEM) was introduced to evaluate the theoretical model [12]. We can visualize the complex mathematical model by application of the FEM using advanced computer techniques. The result of the simulation was compared with results obtained in animal experiments.

Materials and Methods

Animal Experiments

Twenty adult cats were used for the study. After production of a cortical cold lesion at the right parietal lobe, Evans blue (2% solution, 1 ml/kg) was injected IV. The cats were sacrificed 3, 6, 12, 48 h after the procedure. The extension of Evans blue was recorded and the specific gravity of the brain was measured. Five cats were studied with NMR-CT scan to observe the edema progression.

Computer Simulation by the FEM

The linear consolidation theory (Biot) [2] was introduced to analyze the time-dependent phenomenon of vasogenic brain edema. Consolidation is a quasi-static

[1] Department of Neurosurgery, Kobe University School of Medicine, 7-5-1 Kusunoki-cho, Chuo-ku, Kobe, Hyogo 650, Japan

transient phenomenon in which the equilibrium of the stress and flow of interstitial fluid are closely coupled. The following principles were assumed: (a) fluid flow throughout the brain tissue according to Darcy's law; (b) conservation of mass of the interstitial fluid; (c) equilibrium of the whole body; (e) validity of Hooke's law of deformation; and (e) Terzaghi's concept of effective stress [11].

The basic finite element program used in this study was developed by Verruijt [11]. Parameters varying over time: interstitial pressure, effective stress, and brain deformation, were plotted with an X-Y plotter after a 32-step calculation. The brain slice equivalent to that used in animal experiments was selected for a two-dimensional finite element model; it corresponds to a slice 9.5 mm forward of the interaural line on the cat stereotaxic map (Fig. 1, left). The finite element mesh is constructed with 198 nodes and 336 triangular elements (Fig. 1, center). The interstitial pressure of the nodes corresponding to the cold injury was set at a higher level than the intraventricular pressure, which was assumed to be stable during the process. Material properties are reported as follows: Young's modulus (3.9×10^{-2} kgf/cm^2) [1], bulk modulus (3.84×10^5 dyn/cm^2) [10], compressibility of the fluid (5.0×10^{-10} m^2/N) [11], hydraulic conductivity (5.0×10^{-8}m/s) [9], extracellular space (15%) [3], and Poisson's ratio (0.5) [1]. Poisson's ratio was assumed to be 0.499 instead of 0.5. The Young's modulus of the gray matter was assumed to be 10 times that of the white matter. The hydraulic conductivity of the white matter was assumed to be 100 that of the gray matter (Fig. 1, right). These values were applied for the simulation.

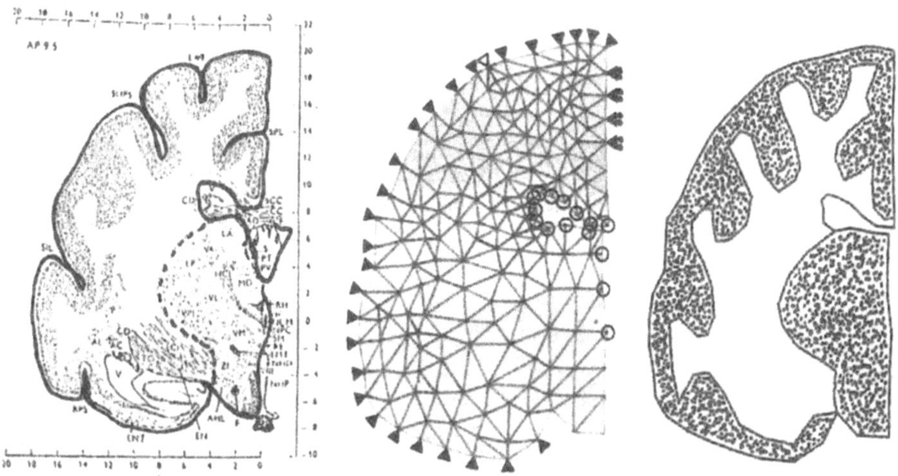

CORONAL SECTION of CAT BRAIN (9.5 mm forward of interaural line) | MESH and BOUNDARY CONDITION | MATERIAL PROPERTIES

Fig. 1. The finite element model. *Open circles,* unfixed nodes that can absorb fluid; *open triangle,* fixed node supplying fluid; *closed triangles,* fixed nodes; *closed triangle* with *two small circles,* nodes restricted to vertical movement. Other nodes are unfixed, and water supply is impossible

Results

Animal Experiments

There were decreasing gradients of the specific gravity from the cortical lesion to the ventricle (Fig. 2). The gradient of the specific gravity became less steep when the process reached the maximum. The edema extended to the neighboring gyrus and the ventricular wall by 24 h after the injury. NMR images of the experimental edema caused by cold injury (Fig. 3) demonstrated the same distribution as Evans blue staining.

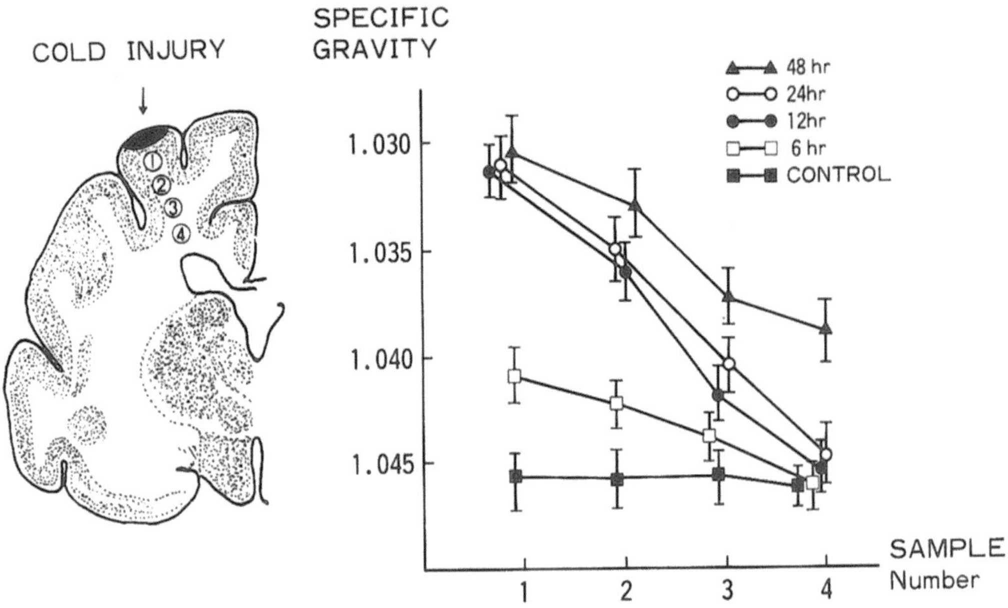

Fig. 2. The gradients of specific gravity of the brain in the animal experiments

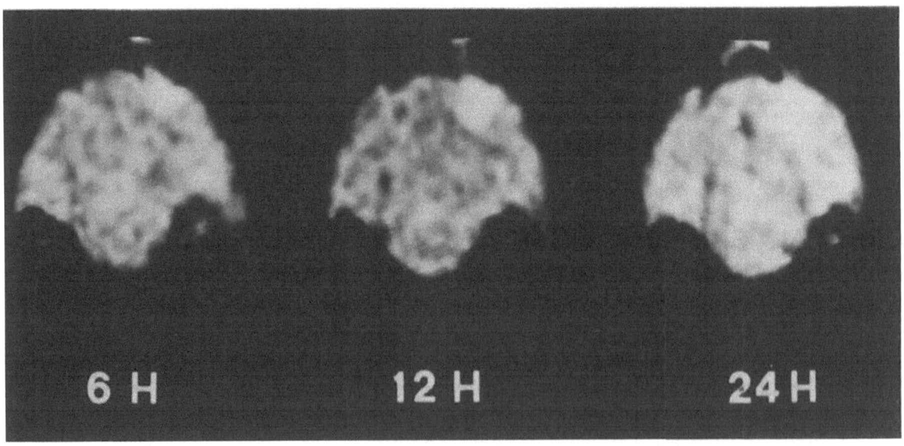

Fig. 3. NMR images demonstrating progression of cold-induced brain edema in the cat

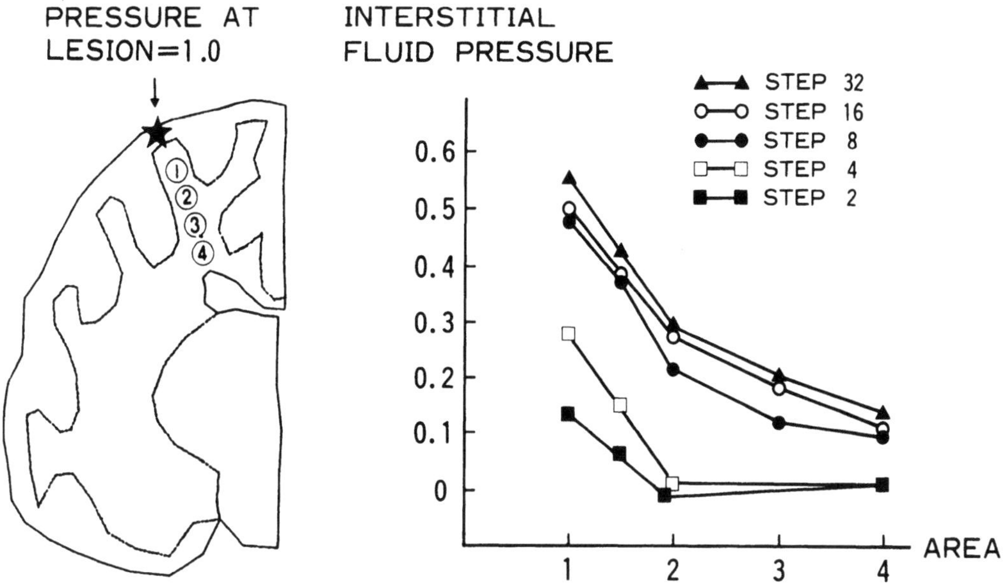

Fig. 4. Gradients of the simulated interstitial pressure

Computer Simulation

The gradient of interstitial pressure was represented in the same fashion as the study of specific gravity in the animal experiments (Fig. 4). The process reached the plateau phase at step 24. The two-dimensional analysis showed the progression of edema through the white matter, which has high hydraulic conductivity (Fig. 5, center). The elevation of interstitial pressure was not remarkable in the gray matter, which has low hydraulic conductivity. The effective stress was also propagated in the white matter (Fig. 5, right). The deformation of the brain under the given conditions was not significant.

When the smaller value of bulk modulus was used for the simulation, adequate deformation of the brain was observed. If the process reached the plateau at 48 h after the procedure the hydraulic conductivity of the brain was computed to be 0.6×10^{-3} cm/s. This value is much higher than the reported one [9]. The result of computer simulation gave a good representation of the actual progression of vasogenic brain edema observed in the animal experiments.

Discussion

In the present study, we attempted to model the progression of vasogenic brain edema mathematically. Rapoport [6] defined intraparenchymal fluid movement with a simple equation in his mathematical model. The equation, however, was not adequate for description of the spatial and time-dependent progression of the vasogenic brain edema. On the other hand, Hakim [4] defined intracerebral stress and

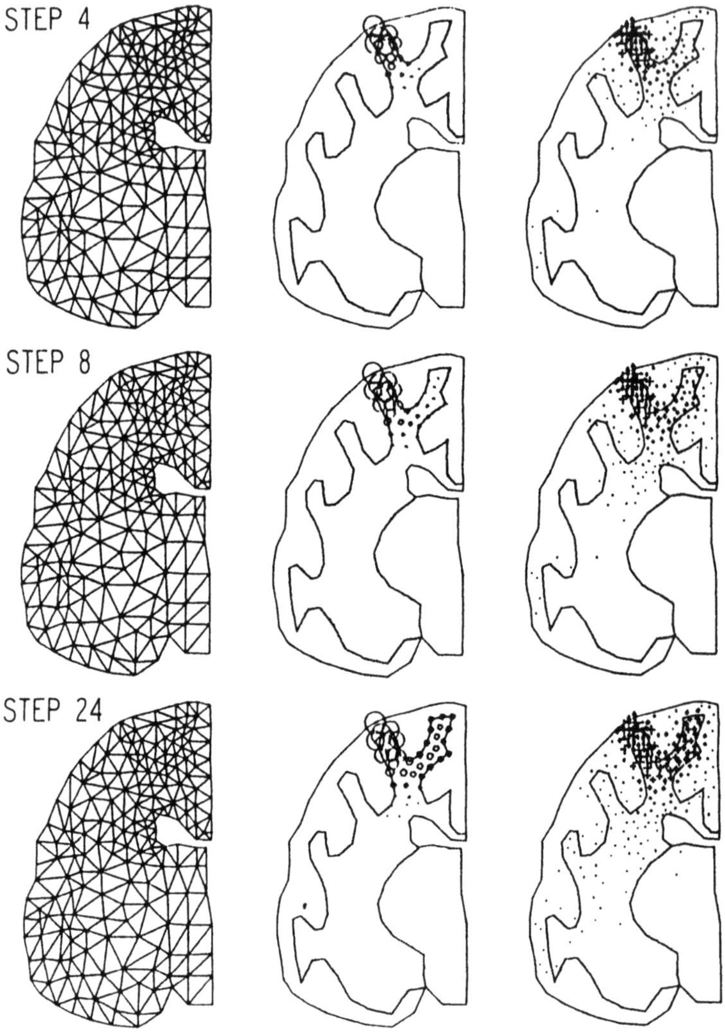

Fig. 5. Two-dimensional progression of the vasogenic brain edema represented by the computer simulation. *Left,* finite element meshes and deformation; *center,* interstitial pressure; *right,* effective stress

called the brain a "visco-elastic sponge." The mechanical factors that modify the progression of edema were defined as follows in the present study: (a) interstitial pressure, (b) hydraulic conductivity of the brain, (c) bulk modulus of the brain, (d) Young's modulus of the brain, (e) Poisson's ratio of the brain, (f) viscosity of the interstitial fluid, (g) compressibility of the interstitial fluid, (h) deformation of the brain, (i) intracerebral stress, (j) cerebrospinal fluid pressure. Since these factors are clinically important, we proposed a comprehensive model to integrate them.

Biot's theory of consolidation can be used to predict the time course of stress and strain in a porous deformable solid in which fluid seepage occurs. It is well known in clinical practice that the brain, when stressed, shows not instantaneous but gradual deformation. It is also known that extracellular fluid moves by bulk flow depending on the hydrostatic pressure gradient [7, 8]. A simple mechanism to explain such a complex phenomenon was well described by Biot's theory. The details of the theory are not within the scope of this paper and can be found elsewhere [2].

The FEM has been introduced to solid, fluid, gas, and thermodynamics, and its value is well established in the various fields. The FEM is based on continuum mechanics. The basic concept of the method is that any continuum can be adequately modeled into an aggregate of subdivisions (finite element), in each of which the behavior is described by a separate set of assumed functions. The time-dependent process can also be described by the step-by-step technique.

The result of the computer simulation showed that the progression of vasogenic brain edema was adequately modeled by Biot's theory of consolidation. The quality of the simulation of time-dependent changes in interstitial pressure, intracerebral stress, and brain deformation was very good.

The hydraulic conductivity of the brain computed from the simulation was much higher than the reported one [9]. This is because the hydraulic conductivity of the brain increases significantly when the extracellular space increases in size [5]. The bulk modulus reported by Sahai [10] seems to be too large.

The bulk modulus of the brain was predicted to be smaller than the value reported by Sahar according to the result of the simulation. A quantitative study is now needed to determine adequate values for bulk modulus and the hydraulic conductivity of the brain. Comparative studies with clinical and animal experiments seem promising as a means of determining the unknown material properties of the brain. As the next step of the study, time-dependent changes in cerebrospinal fluid pressure and Starling's equation will be incorporated in the model. In considering the future of the FEM in biomechanical research on brain edema, this new method will provide a completely novel approach to analysis of the complex behavior of vasogenic brain edema.

Summary

Biot's theory of consolidation was applied to describe the progression of vasogenic brain edema. The finite element method (FEM) was introduced to evaluate the model and to analyze the pathomechanics of the vasogenic brain edema. A finite element model was constructed with 336 triangular elements and 198 nodes. The progression of edema was simulated by the model. The result of the simulation was compared with the progression of cold-induced brain edema in cats. The progression of vasogenic brain edema was adequately modeled by Biot's theory of consolidation. The FEM will provide a completely innovative approach to biomechanical research on brain edema.

References

1. Aoyagi N, Masuzawa H, Sano K, Kihira M, Kobayashi S (1980) Compliance of the brain. Brain Nerve 32:47–56
2. Biot MA (1955) Theory of elasticity and consolidation for a porous anisotropic solid. J Appl Physiol 26:182–185

3. Fenske A, Samii H, Reuren J, Hey O (1973) Extracellular space and electrolyte distribution in cortex and white matter of dog brain in cold induced oedema. Acta Neurochir 28:81–94
4. Hakim S, Venegas JG, Burton JD (1976) The physics of the cranial cavity, hydrocephalus and normal pressure hydrocephalus: Mechanical interpretation and mathematical model. Surg Neurol 5:187–210
5. Marmarou A, Takagi H, Shulman K (1980) Biomechanics of brain edema and effects on local cerebral blood flow. Adv Neurol 28
6. Rapoport SI (1978) A mathematical model for vasogenic brain edema. J Theor Biol 74:439–467
7. Reulen HJ, Graham R, Spatz M, Klazo I (1977) Role of pressure gradients and bulk flow in dynamics of vasogenic brain edema. J Neurosurg 46:24–35
8. Reulen HJ, Matsudaira T, Tack A, Fenske A, Prioleau R (1978) Clearance of edema fluid into cerebrospinal fluid. J Neurosurg 48:754–764
9. Rosenberg GA, Kyner WT, Estralda E (1980) Bulk flow of brain interstitial fluid under normal and hyperosmolar conditions. Am J Physiol 238:F42–F49
10. Sahar A, Hochwald GM, Ransohoff J (1970) Experimental hydrocephalus: Cerebrospinal fluid formation and ventricular size as a function of intraventricular pressure. J Neurol Sci 11:81–91
11. Verruijt A (1977) Generation and dissipation of pore water pressure. In: Gudenhus G (ed) Finite elements in geomechanics. Wiley, Chichester
12. Zienkiewicz OC (1977) The finite element method, 3rd edn. McGraw-Hill, London

Dynamics of Fluid Movement Through Brain Parenchyma and into the CSF in Vasogenic Brain Edema

M. TSUYUMU[1], H.-J. REULEN, and Y. INABA

Key words: Vasogenic brain edema, normal pressure hydrocephalus (NPH), edema resolution, tissue compliance

List of Abrreviations

C20 and C45	– control groups
CSF	– cerebrospinal fluid
L20 and L45	– lesion groups
NPH	– normal-pressure hydrocephalus
PVL	– periventricular low-density area
TIP	– tissue infusion pressure
TP	– tissue pressure

Introduction

Previous studies have shown that vasogenic edema spreads in the white matter by bulk flow and not by diffusion [1, 6, 8–12]. On the basis of the pressure-volume curve of the brain extracellular space in edema [2, 7, 9] it was concluded that fluid mobility must be significantly greater in the edematous than in the normal brain.

The present study was an attempt at further investigation of the biomechanics of fluid movement through the white matter in vasogenic brain edema and PVL. For this purpose, an artificial CSF labeled with Evans blue and ^{35}S-thiosulfate was infused into the white matter at a known infusion rate.

Materials and Methods

The 21 cats used in these experiments were divided into four groups (L20, L45, C20, C45). In the groups of animals subjected to cold lesion (L20, L45) a small craniotomy was performed over the right frontal pole. Cold injury edema was produced 24 h prior to the experiment by applying a metal plate (4 × 10 mm in area) previously cooled to –65 °C to the exposed dura for 45 s. Groups C20 and C45 were control animals.

[1] Department of Neurosurgery, Tokyo Medical and Dental University, School of Medicine, 1-5-45, Yushima, Bunkyo-ku, Tokyo 113, Japan

During the experiment the femoral vessels were unilaterally catheterized and arterial blood pressure was monitored with a pressure transducer. All animals were tracheotomized, treated with muscle relaxants, and mechanically ventilated at a normal rate with a conventional Starling pump. The acid-base status and blood gases in the arterial blood were intermittently checked by the Astrup micromethod and kept within normal ranges. End-tidal CO_2 was measured continuously. Each animal's head was fixed in a stereotaxic holder.

Four burr holes corresponding to the coordinates were made with a dental drill for insertion of the probes. For positioning of the four needles in the brain the following coordinates were used, according to the Horsley-Clark method and the atlas of Reinoso-Suarez [5]. TIP (tissue infusion pressure in the right hemisphere); AP +22.0, lateral 3.5, vertical 15.5. In animals with cold lesion, corrections (AP +20.5, lateral 3.0) were made for the mass shift caused by edema. This location corresponds to a point approximately 3.0 mm forward of the frontal apex of the right lateral ventricle. The point for TP (tissue pressure in the right hemisphere) was placed 5.0 mm away from the point TIP. For the ventricular fluid pressure measurement in the left lateral ventricle and a ventriculocisternal perfusion through the right lateral ventricle the following stereotaxic coordinates were used; VPP (ventricular perfusion pressure, right); AP +12.0, lateral 4.5, vertical 17.0 (Fig. 1a and b).

(^{35}S)-Sodium thiosulfate was prepared with a radioactivity level of approximately 20 000 counts/ml, mixed with synthetic CSF, and stained with Evans blue for visualization of the extent of its distribution. This solution was infused into the tissue at the point TIP at a rate of 0.20 ml/h in groups C20 and L20 and 0.45 ml/h in groups C45 and L45.

Tissue pressure was measured using the cotton-wick technique described previously [7], at the point described above and, at the end of the experiment, at the exact site of the tissue infusion.

Both lateral ventricles and the cisterna magna were cannulated, and a ventriculocisternal perfusion with synthetic CSF was established through the right lateral ventricle with a perfusor. The perfusion rate was 2.25 ml/h. The cisternal outflow was collected during every 15 min for measurement of volume and activity.

Tissue infusion and ventriculocisternal perfusion lasted for 90 min in all experiments. At the end of the experiment the animals were sacrificed by exsanguination, and the brains were removed and quickly frozen with a mixture of acetone and liquid nitrogen. Then a 4- to 5-mm horizontal slice was cut from each brain to include the edematous and blue-stained area where the fluid containing ^{35}S activity and Evans blue had been infused (Fig. 1a and b). Consecutive 1-mm tissue blocks were then cut from the cortex to the caudate nucleus for determination of tissue water content and ^{35}S activity (Fig. 1a and b).

Tissue water content was determined by weighing both fresh samples and samples dried at 105 °C for 48 h. The ^{35}S radioactivity of tissue samples and cisternal outflow was determined by liquid scintillation.

The thiosulfate space was computed from the following equation:

$$\text{Space\%} = \frac{\text{cpm/g tissue (wet weight)}}{\text{cpm/g infusion solution}} \times 100 . \tag{a}$$

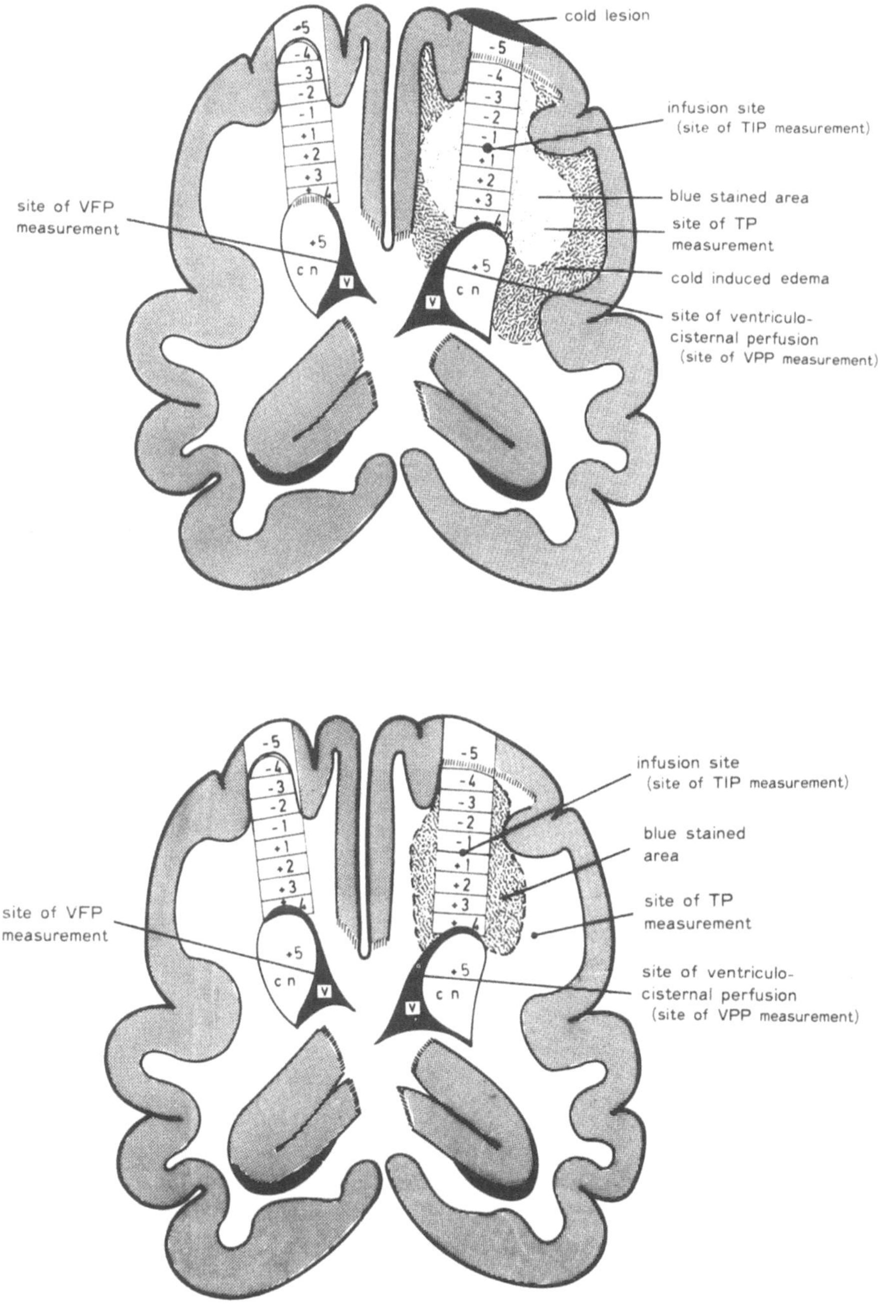

Fig. 1.a Schematic of horizontal tissue slices used for edema study in lesion groups (L20, L45). Infusion site where TIP was measured and the site for TP measurement are shown. Consecutive tissue blocks for water content and ^{35}S radioactivity analysis are numbered +*5* to –*5*. *Blue-stained area* signifies the extension of infused fluid in edematous white matter after 90 min tissue infusion. *Na-Fluorescein-stained* area shows extent of the cold-induced edema. Block, –5 = cortex; block +5 (*cn*) = caudate nucleus; blocks –4 to +4 = white matter; *V*, ventricle **b** Same schematic used in control groups (C20, C45). *Blue-stained area* was smaller than in lesion groups (see Table 1)

The drainage into the ventricular CSF of the infused solution in the tissue was calculated based on the principle of dilution method as follows;

$$\text{Drainage into the ventricle} = \frac{\text{cpm/g in cisternal outflow}}{\text{cpm/g infusion solution}} \times (\text{V}-\text{C perfusion rate} + 22.0) \quad \text{(b)}$$

in which 22.0 is the CSF production rate in the cat [14].

Results

Tissue Infusion Pressure (TIP)

In the control groups the initial rise in TIP was much steeper and the initial peaks were higher than in the corresponding two groups with cold-induced edema. Then the TIP in cold lesion animals subsided earlier than in control groups. However, 30 min after the beginning, TIP was nearly the same in all groups and decreased slowly until the end of the experiment (Fig. 2).

Water Content

In Fig. 3, the increase in water content of the consecutive tissue blocks is given in relation to the distance from the infusion site to each tissue block.

In both groups of cold lesion animals the increase in water content was always higher than in animals with infusion only. This may be explained by the cold-induced edema already present before the tissue infusion. As shown previously, cold lesion edema is most pronounced close to the lesion and slowly declines towards the deep white matter. Animals with a tissue infusion rate of 0.45 ml (L45, C45) had a higher increase in water content than those in groups C20 and L20. The increase in water content in block 4 exceeded 5% in all groups, but it was markedly greater in the groups with the high infusion rate.

Thiosulfate Space

The thiosulfate space (Fig. 4) was computed on the assumption that thiosulfate is distributed within the extracellular space at the same concentration as in the infusion solution. In cold lesion animals the extracellular space is already enlarged by the edema fluid and it can be assumed that the fluid infused becomes diluted by the edema fluid. This would lead to an underestimation of the thiosulfate space in cold lesion animals. The actual extracellular space in the brains of these animals, especially in the blocks adjacent to the lesion, would thus be greater.

Drainage of Infused Solution into CSF

The drainage into the CSF (Fig. 5) was practically zero during the first 15 min, after which it increased rapidly until end of the experiment, reaching about 1 μl/min at 90 min. In the groups with the fast infusion rate the labeled fluid arrives earlier in

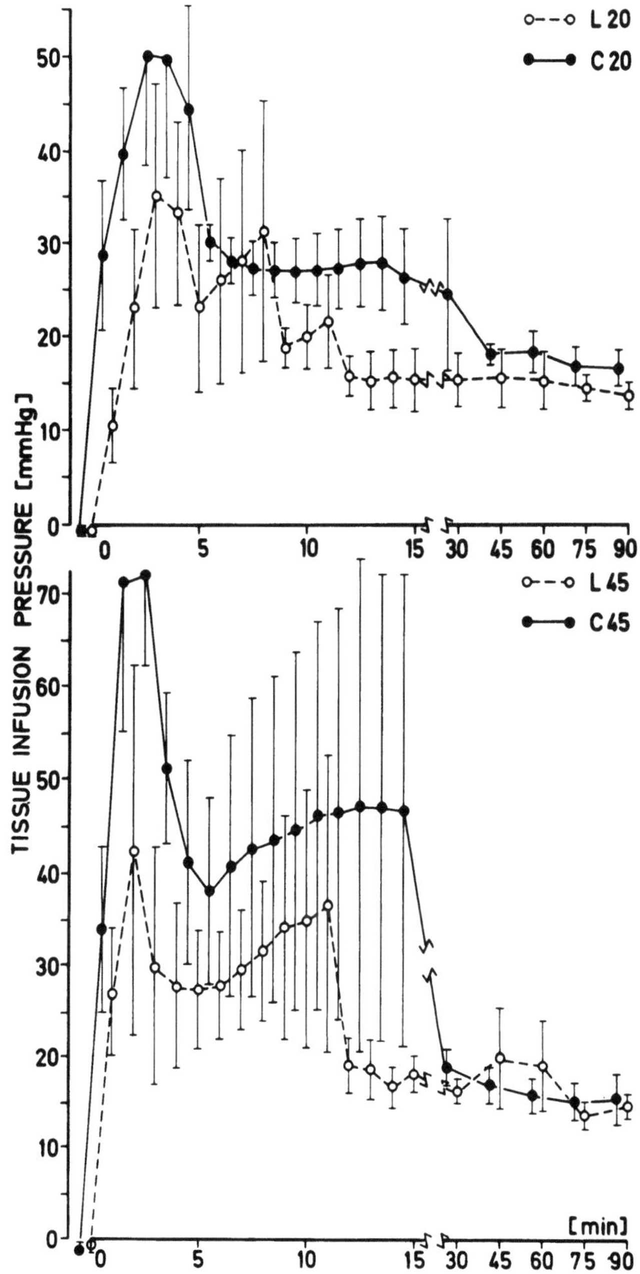

Fig. 2. Time-course of tissue infusion pressure during the experiment in each group. *L 20,* lesion group with infusion rate of 0.20 ml/h; *C20,* control group, 0.20 ml/h, *L 45,* lesion group, 0.45 ml/h; *C45,* control group, 0.45 ml/h

the ventricle (about 30 min after the beginning of the experiment) than in the groups with low infusion rate.

Morphological Observation of Edema and Evans Blue Spreading

The extension of the staining with Evans blue was measured (Table 1). It is obvious that the longitudinal extension is greater in cold lesion animals than in control ani-

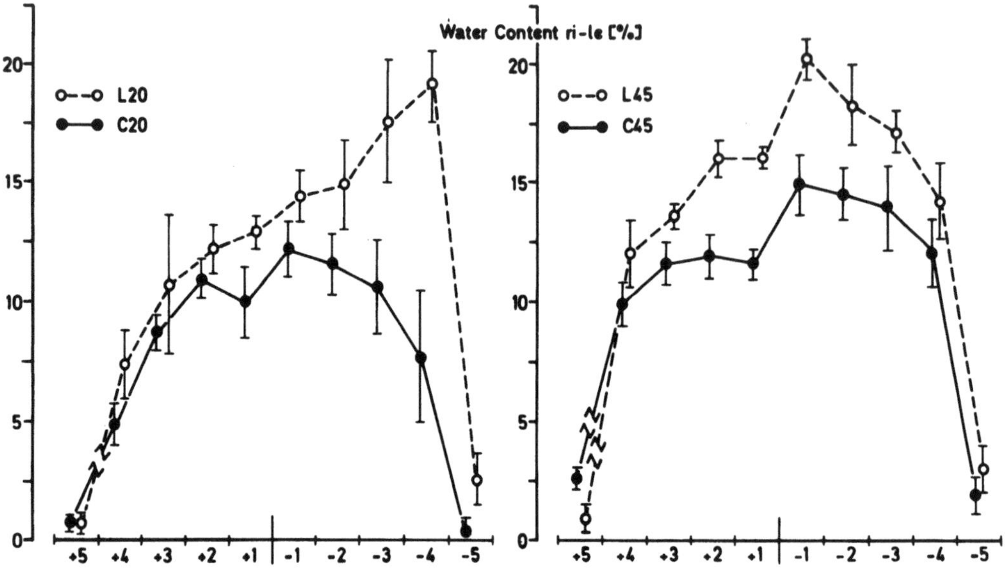

Fig. 3. Distribution of tissue water content in the control groups (C20, C45) and lesion groups (L20, L45). The *solid lines* correspond to animals without cold lesion and the *dotted lines,* to animals with cold lesion. Tissue water content is given as a difference between respective tissue blocks of experimental (*right*) hemisphere and control (*left*) hemisphere. Block +5 = caudate nucleus; blocks +4 to –4 = white matter; block –5 = cortex (see Fig. 1a, b)

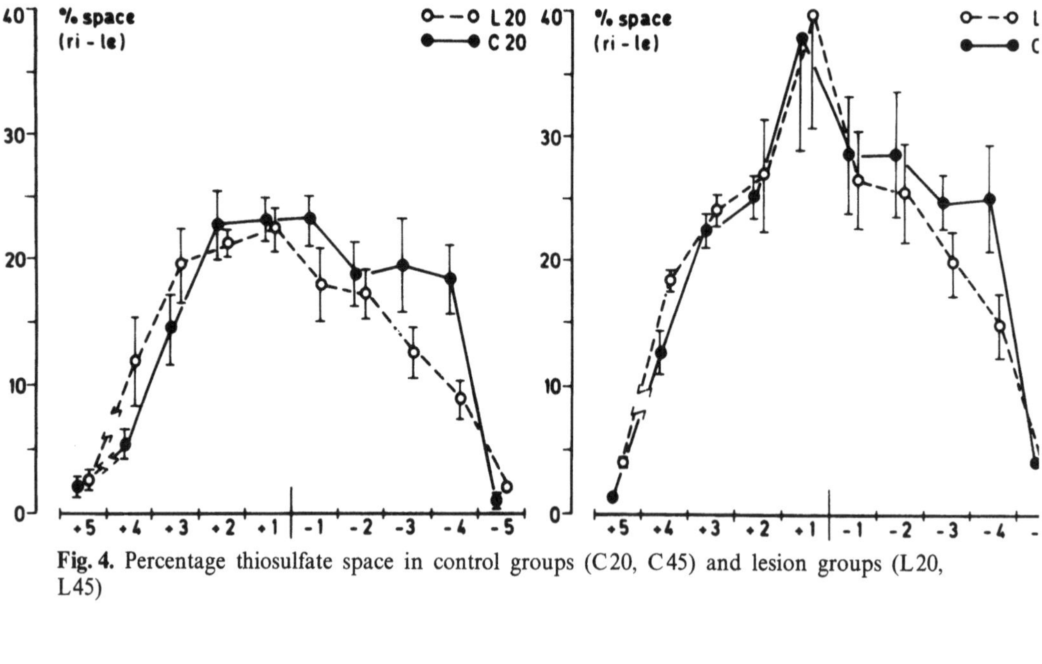

Fig. 4. Percentage thiosulfate space in control groups (C20, C45) and lesion groups (L20, L45)

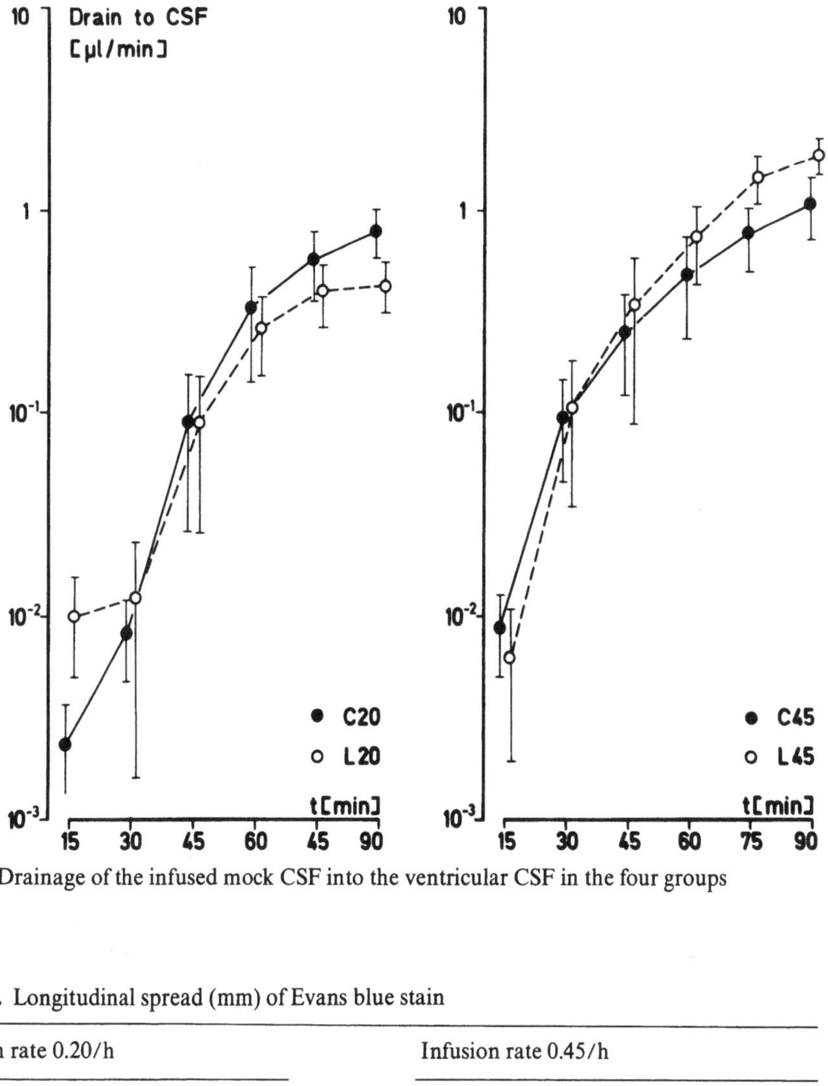

Fig. 5. Drainage of the infused mock CSF into the ventricular CSF in the four groups

Table 1. Longitudinal spread (mm) of Evans blue stain

Infusion rate 0.20/h		Infusion rate 0.45/h	
Control (C20)	Cold lesion (L20)	Control (C45)	Cold lesion (L45)
6.50±0.56	8.64±1.33	7.20±0.06	10.30±0.56

mals. This means that the fluid infused spreads more extensively in edematous tissue than in control tissue.

The edema fluid was labeled with Na fluorescein. Under ultraviolet light it was possible to distinguish the border to the cold-induced edema and the extent of infused solution. The extension of Na fluorescein staining exceeded the Evans blue staining in both the longitudinal and the lateral directions in all experiments. This is schematically shown in Fig. 1a. Thus, the spreading of the infused solution in the cold lesion groups always remained within the edema territory.

Discussion

In this study, small amounts of labeled mock CSF, 0.20 and 0.45 ml/h, were infused into the white matter to simulate extravasation of edema fluid from leaky vessels [3].

Since the tissue infusion pressure reflects the resistance of the tissue to infusion and extracellular volume expansion, this pressure probably gives a raw measure of the tissue resistance (R = pressure/flow). It is obvious from Fig. 2 that initially a much lower pressure is needed in edematous brains than in normal brains to overcome the tissue resistance (in both infusion groups). This may be explained by the fact that in edema the extracellular space is already widely distended [12] and the compliance (C = dV/dP) of the extracellular space is increased. This has been predicted previously on the basis of the pressure volume curve of the brain extracellular space in edema [2, 7, 9].

The infused and Evans-blue-stained mock CSF spreads further in brains that are already edematous before the infusion. Since the duration of the infusion is equal in all groups this means that spread through the enlarged extracellular spaces in edema is faster, i.e., fluid moves at higher speed, although the infusion pressure is slightly lower in these animals. It can be concluded that the impedance to fluid movement is significantly reduced if the brain has become edematous and the extracellular spaces are distended.

This explains why in a lesion involving long-term impairment of the blood-brain barrier (e.g., a tumor) only very small pressure gradients through the tissue are necessary to sustain edema. The same reasoning can also be applied to the biomechanics of normal-pressure hydrocephalus with PVL, where following a history of high ventricular pressure with periventricular edema even small increases of ventricular pressure (within a normal range) can maintain the edema propagation, i.e., PVL.

The amount of infused fluid draining into the ventricular CSF was determined in these experiments. The fluid labeled with ^{35}S-thiosulfate can be detected in the ventricular CSF after as little as 30 min of infusion. After about 90 min the drainage seems to reach a plateau, which is nearly the same in all groups. (If we assume that the infused fluid is diluted to some extent by edema fluid then the actual clearance of brain extracellular fluid into the ventricular CSF could be slightly underestimated in animals with cold injury edema.) In contrast to these relatively uniform clearance rates in the various groups, the amount of edema and the size of extracellular space in the white matter bordering the ventricle (block 4) vary greatly. This means that edema drainage can vary within a certain range, as shown in this and our previous experiments [13], but is eventually limited by some as yet unknown factors. A similar limitation of edema fluid entry into the ventricle has recently been described by Marmarou et al. [4].

One possible explanation for this limitation of CSF clearance is that the ventricular ependyma functions as a hindrance or a bottleneck [8], i.e., the impedance of the ependymal lining may become higher than that of fluid migration through the tissue [4]. Marmarou et al. [4] assume that in this case fluid would continue to migrate through the white matter, thus causing further expansion of the edema volume. This may become important in all forms of acute and severe impairments of the BBB, and lead ultimately to a rapid increase in tissue volume and uncontrollable intracranial pressure.

Summary

Mock CSF with ^{35}S-sodium thiosulfate was infused into the normal cat brain, and the results were compared with those recorded in an edematous brain 24 h after a cold lesion was made at the right frontal pole. Using the ventriculocisternal perfusion technique, the drainage of extracellular fluid was quantitatively measured.

High pressure is needed to overcome the high resistance of the tissue against fluid propagation initially when tissue compliance is low. Once the extracellular space is distended, i.e., when compliance is high, even a small increase in perfusion pressure can cause edema propagation.

When there is a history of high-pressure hydrocephalus, a small increase in ventricular pressure can initiate and maintain periventricular low density area (PVL), the location of which may be related to the large tissue compliance of the white matter adjacent to the frontal pole of the lateral ventricle.

The drainage of edema fluid into ventricular CSF seems to reach a plateau at about 90 min with either infusion rate. The ventricular ependyma might act as a hindrance or a bottleneck for the drainage of edema into CSF.

References

1. Bruce DA, Weeme CT, Kaiser G, et al. (1976) The dynamics of small and large molecules in the extracellular space and cerebrospinal fluid following local cold injury of the cortex. In: Pappius HM, Feindel W (eds) Dynamics of brain edema. Springer, Berlin Heidelberg New York, pp 122–128
2. Guyton AC, Granger HJ, Taylor AE (1971) Interstitial fluid pressure. Physiol Rev 51:527–563
3. Marmarou A, Shapiro K, Poll W, et al. (1976) Studies of kinetics of fluid movements within brain tissue. In: Beks JWF, Bosh DA, Brock M (eds) Intracranial pressure III. Springer, Berlin Heidelberg New York, pp 1–4
4. Marmarou A, Nakamura T, Tanaka K, Hochwald GM (1984) The time course and distribution of water in the resolution phase of infusion edema. In: Go KG, Baethmann A (eds) Brain edema. Plenum, New York, pp 37–44
5. Reinoso-Suarez F (1961) Topographischer Hirnatlas der Katze. Merck, Darmstadt
6. Reulen HJ (1976) Vasogenic brain edema. New aspects in its formation, resolution and therapy. Br J Anaesth 48:741–752
7. Reulen HJ, Kreysch H (1973) Measurement of brain tissue pressure in cold induced cerebral edema. Acta Neurochir 29:29–40
8. Reulen HJ, Tsuyumu M (1981) Pathophysiology of formation and natural resolution of vasogenic brain edema. In: de Vlieger M, de Lange SA, Beks JWF (eds) Brain edema. Wiley, New York, pp 31–48
9. Reulen HJ, Graham R, Spatz M, et al. (1977) Role of pressure gradients and bulk flow in dynamics of vasogenic brain edema. J Neurosurg 46:24–35
10. Reulen HJ, Tsuyumu M, Tack A, et al. (1978) Clearance of edema fluid into cerebrospinal fluid: A mechanism for resolution of vasogenic brain edema. J Neurosurg 48:754–764
11. Reulen HJ, Tsuyumu M, Prioleau G (1980) Further results concerning the resolution of vasogenic brain edema. Adv Neurol 28:375–389
12. Shulman K, Marmarou A, Weitz S (1975) Gradients of brain interstitial fluid pressure in experimental infusion and compression. In: Lundberg N, Ponten U, Brock M (eds) Intracranial Pressure II. Springer, Berlin Heidelberg New York, pp 211–214
13. Tsuyumu M, Reulen HJ, Prioleau RG (1981) Movement of edema fluid through the brain tissue into CSF. Part I. Edema fluid clearance rate. Acta Neurochir 57:2–13
14. Vates TS Jr, Bonting SL, Oppelt W (1964) Na-K activated adenosine triphosphate formation of cerebrospinal fluid in the cat. Am J Physiol 206:1165–1172

The Effect of Lymphatic Blockage on Resolution of Vasogenic Brain Edema

E. CSANDA[1], S. KOMOLY, and O. MAJOR

Key words: Vasogenic brain edema, ^{90}Y implantation, cold injury, lymphatic blockage, brain edema resolution, protein clearance, water content

Introduction

Between 1961 and 1974 the research group in Szeged established the relation of brain and extracranial lymphatics in animal experiments [4, 7]. The cervical lymph nodes and vessels were ligated in dog, cat, rabbit, and rat, and the animals were examined by means of neuropathological, neurochemical, neurophysiological methods. Learning disturbances, behavior changes, and slowing down of the EEG were observed, whereas the CSF pressure was elevated; in the brain edema of the white matter and semilunar gaps opening in the vessel walls were found. In 1975 the research group in Budapest performed experiments designed to examine lymphatic drainage of substances in the brain, implanting yttrium-90 (^{90}Y) rods into the deep white matter or applying it to the cortical surface in the same animal species. The Virchow-Robin spaces (VRS) were found to play the same role as the lymph vessels in the body outside the cranial cavity. The sudanophilic myelin breakdown substances moved in the VRS between the vessel walls toward the brain surfaces, entering the CSF space. After some hours the Sudan-positive material was detected in the upper third of the cervical lymph nodes which are known to communicate with the CSF space [5].

Reulen et al. [9] demonstrated in cold injury (CI)-induced brain edema (BE) that the vasogenic edema fluid moved toward the ventricles, the CSF playing an important role in the resolution of the brain edema. In our previous experiments we confirmed the communication of CSF space and lymphatics by injecting markers (stains or the subjects' own blood) into the CSF [5]. The proteins in the body outside of the brain are related to lymphatic pathways. Our recent work has been concerned with the transport of protein in vasogenic BE. Therefore we repeated the lymphatic blockage experiments and carried out tests in CI and ^{90}Y-induced BE combined with simultaneous blockage of extracranial lymph nodes and vessels in cat and rat.

---

[1] Institute of Neurology, Semmelweis Medical University, Budapest, Hungary

Material and Methods

The test animals were 105 rats of both sexes, with an average weight of 200 g, used in pentobarbitone general anesthesia. Cold injury (CI) was inflicted with a tube containing liquid nitrogen after removal of the right parietal bone. The exposure time was 30 s and the injured surface was 12.56 mm^2. The lymphatic blockage was achieved by cauterization of the superficial and deep, paracarotid lymph nodes. All other anatomical structures were carefully preserved. Sham-operated animals were used as controls. Both their sternoclavicular muscles were cauterized. Animals were sacrificed after 6, 12, 24, 48, and 72 h. The water content was determined by measurement of tissue weights. To study protein-rich BE quantitatively, 4 mg/100 g body weight Evans blue was given 4 h before sacrifice. The content of Evans blue was determined photometrically at 613 nm after germanin extraction. The original germanin method of Jancsó was adapted for brain investigations [8]. Before extraction the stain containing blood was washed out from the cerebral vessels by a short saline perfusion. Three cats underwent lymphatic blockage (LB), and three sham-operated cats were used as controls. Five cats had LB combined with CI- or ^{90}Y-induced BE.

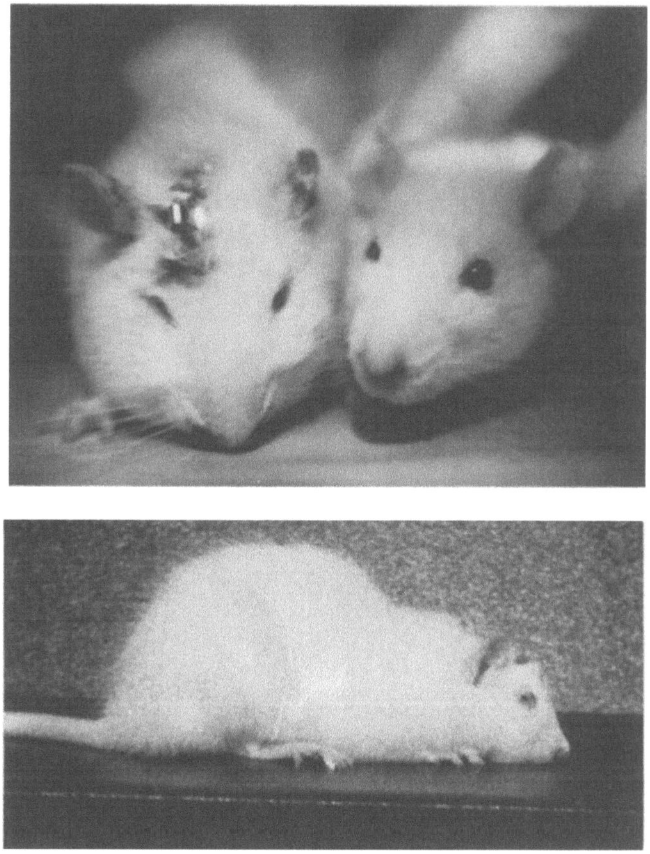

Fig. 1. Rat after cervical lymphatic blockage

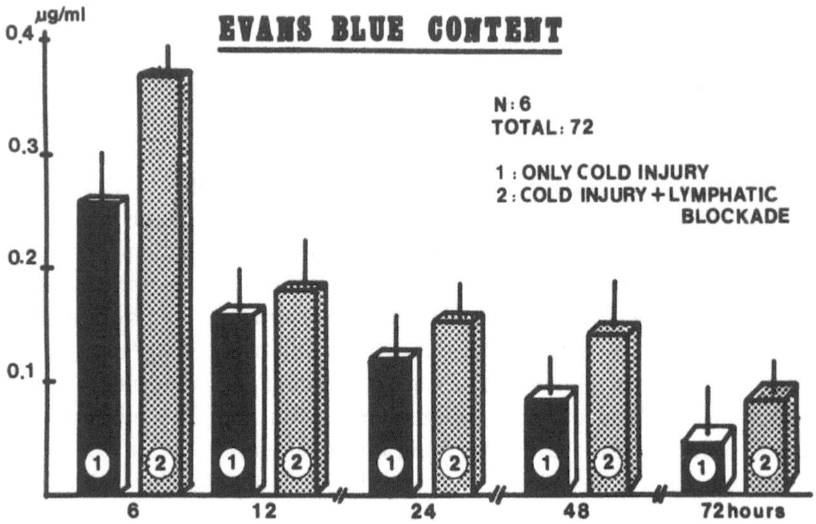

Fig. 2. Changes in Evans blue content of rat brain 6–72 h after cold injury, with and without cervical lymphatic blockage

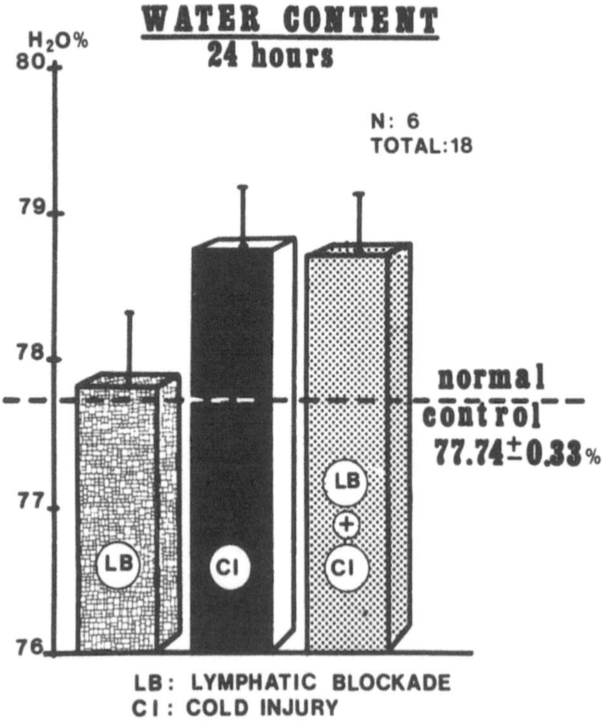

Fig. 3. Water content of rat brain 24 h after cervical lymphatic blockage (*LB*), cold injury (*CI*) and a combination of these two procedures (*LB + CI*)

Results

The animals with LB had swollen heads 24 h after the operation. They were apathetic and had a decreased tendency to move. The fur of rats was matted. The animals with CI combined with LB were conspicuously more apathetic and somnolent. The rats held themselves strangely (Fig. 1).

Light and electron microscopic study of the brain of cats showed opening of the Virchow-Robin spaces, which were filled with vacuolated macrophages, and accumulation of PAS-positive substances. The peak of BE (studied by means of the macroscopical Evans blue method) was prolonged in the CI+LB group. Light-microscopical evidence of a loss of white matter, especially from the corpus callosum, reflected brain edema in the CI, ^{90}Y plus LB, and LB alone groups; we never observed this in sham-operated animals.

Quantitative measurements of Evans blue in rat brain showed the Evans blue content (EBCO) was highest after 6 h in both the CI and the CI+LB groups (Fig. 2). This was the time at which the difference in EBCO in different groups was most pronounced: the CI+LB animals had significantly higher amounts than the CI animals. At later stages the differences between the CI and CI+LB groups were less significant, but in all CI+LB animals the EBCO was higher than in CI group.

Changes in the water content of the brain were different. In the brains of LB animals there was no increase in water content. The increase in water content in the CI and CI+LB groups is shown in Fig. 3. There was no remarkable difference between these two groups.

Discussion

There are two main possibilities for resolution of BE: one is movement of the edema fluid to the ventricles by bulk flow, and the second is the so-called sink effect of the brain capillaries. The latter – in the form of contraluminal transport of water from the perivascular spaces into the vascular lumen – seems to function efficiently in the LB animals. In the brains of these animals the appearance of VR spaces with vacuolated cellular elements and PAS-positive substances can lead to the conclusion that LB upsets the clearance of brain protein metabolites.

Cserr et al. [6] and Bradbury [1] demonstrated a direct communication of CNS and extracranial lymphatics by injecting ^{131}I albumin into the caudate nucleus. They found a higher proportion of this marker in the cervical lymph than in the CSF in the cisterna magna. These experiments prove the role of the extracranial lymphatic system in the clearance of proteins from the extracellular spaces in the brain. These observations are in keeping with our previous findings in ^{90}Y-induced demyelinization: the clearance of myelin break-down products are lymph dependent. While Cserr et al. [6], Bradbury [1], and Casley-Smith et al. [2] assume a direct communication between brain substance and cervical lymph (via vessel wall?), we believe that the CSF is an important link between brain substance and the extracranial lymphatic system. The strictly unilateral hemispheric processes lead to the accumulation of decomposed myelin substances in the cervical lymph nodes on both sides.

In our LB experiments we tried to block all lymph nodes and vessels in the neck, being aware of the high revascularization capacity of the lymphatic system. Therefore, we performed the LB at the same time as CI was inflicted, and the measurements were carried out not later than 72 h later. The comparative study with LB, CI, and LB + CI groups showed that protein clearance was slowed down by LB, whereas LB seems not to influence the water content of normal or edematous brain tissue.

Summary

The effect of lymphatic blockage on resolution of vasogenic brain edema caused by ^{90}Y implantation or cold injury was examined in animal experiments. The lymphatic blockage was performed by ligation of cervical lymph nodes and vessels. Brain edema was measured by photometric determination of Evans blue content of the brain. The water content was determined by tissue weight measurement. Light and electron microscopical studies were also carried out. The experiments confirmed the importance of the connection between the brain tissue and extracranial lymphatics in the resolution of brain edema. Lymphatic blockage slows down protein clearance while it does not substantially influence the water content of normal or edematous brain tissue.

Acknowledgement. We very much appreciate the work of Gábor Jancsó Jr in adapting the original germanin extraction method for brain edema analysis. Furthermore we wish to express our thanks to Mesdames Rita Vértessy and Clara Dóczi for their skillful technical assistance.

References

1. Bradbury M (1981) Lymphatics and the central nervous system. Trends Neurosci 4: 100–101
2. Casley-Smith JR, Földi-Börcsök E, Földi M (1976) The prelymphatic pathways of the brain as revealed by cervical lymphatic obstruction and the passage of particles. Br J Exp Pathol 57:179
3. Csanda E (1980) Radiation brain edema. Adv Neurol 28:
4. Csanda E, Földi M, Obál F, Zoltán ÖT (1968) Cerebral edema as a consequence of experimental cervical lymphatic blockage. Angiologica 5:55
5. Csanda E, Obál F, Obál F Jr (1983) Central nervous system and lymphatic system. In: Földi M, Casley-Smith JR (1983) Lymphangiology. Schattauer, Stuttgart, pp 475–508
6. Cserr HF, Cooper DN, Milhorat TH (1977) Flow of cerebral interstitial fluid as indicated by the removal of extracellular markers from rat caudate nucleus. Exp Eye Res [Suppl] 25:461–473
7. Földi M, Csanda E, Obál F, Madarász I, Szeghy G, Zoltán ÖT (1963) Über Wirkung der Unterbindung der Lymphgefäße und Lymphknoten des Halses auf das Zentralnervensystem im Tierversuch. I. Z gesamte exp Med 137:483
8. Jancsó GA, Szolcsányi J, Jancsó M (1967) A simple method for measuring the amount of Azovan-Blue exuded into the skin in response to an inflammatory stimulus. J Pharm Pharmacol 19:486–487
9. Reulen HJ, Graham R, Fenske A, Tsuyumu M, Klatzo I (1976) The role of pressure and bulk flow in the formation and resolution of cold-induced edema. In: Pappius HM, Feindel W (eds) Dynamics of brain edema. Springer, Berlin Heidelberg New York, pp 103–112

Brain Edema Model Induced with Typhoid Endotoxin in Rabbits

Y. PEI-LAN [1], Z. PEI-FANG, Y. YU-JIA, P. LONG-XING, and F. BEN-CHENG

Key words: Brain edema, endotoxin animal model

Introduction

This paper describes an animal model of brain edema. Preliminary experiments were performed to screen several kinds of animals and bacteria. A model for brain edema induced with olive oil [1] has been developed further. The purpose of the research is to produce an animal model of acute brain edema with typhoid endotoxin. The model is similar to the acute brain edema caused in children by bacterial infection.

The study was divided into three parts.

First Part

Method

Comparisons were made of 40 rabbits in pairs, which were randomly divided into experimental and control groups. Typhoid endotoxin and sterile normal saline were injected into the right side of the internal carotid artery in the experimental and control groups. Evans blue in normal saline solution (2.5%, 1 ml/kg) was injected into the right ear vein of animals in both groups. The animals were then kept under observation for 6 h. All animals that survived longer than 6 h were killed with pentobarbital IV. After death, the brains were removed from the skulls, and four samples $3 \times 10 \times 10$ (mm) were taken from corresponding points on both sides of each. The water content of each sample was determined by wet-dry weight measurement. The amount of sodium and potassium in the dry samples were also determined.

Results

The average water content of samples from the right hemispheres of the experimental animals was much higher than that of control samples (right anterior 81.98 ± 0.41

[1] Department of Pediatrics. The First Affiliated Hospital, Laboratory of Electron Microscopy and Department of Pathology, Hunan Medical College, Changsha, Hunan, China

vs 78.79 ± 0.13, $P < 0.001$; right posterior 81.95 ± 0.50 vs. 78.16±0.13, $P < 0.001$). The average sodium contents of samples on the right side in the experimental group were slightly higher than the control values. There was no significant change in the potassium level. Bluish discoloration occurred in 20/20 of the experimental rabbits' brains, but only 1/20 (a small area of 3 × 4 mm) of the control brains. Unequal pupil size was observed in 18/20 of the experimental group, but in none of the animals in the control group. Some (6/20) of the experimental rabbits showed protrusion of the eyeballs (4 of both and 2 on the right) but this was not seen in any of the controls. More evident fall in body temperature and reduction in heart rate were seen in the experimental rabbits than in the controls.

Second Part

Method

Light microscopic investigations were performed in 17 rabbits.

Results

Diffuse or focal edematous regions were common findings in cerebrum, cerebellum, and hippocampus, in the area around the ventricle; and the perivascular spaces and the spaces around nerve cells and glia cells were widened in these regions. In staining processes with Cajal's stain the astrocytes were swollen and closely attached to the walls of the blood vessels (Fig. 1). PAS-positive substances increased in amount in the edematous region. ATPase of capillaries of the edematous region decreased or disappeared.

Third Part

Method

Kinetic studies with electron microscopy were performed in eight rabbits. They were killed by perfusion fixation at 10 min, 2 h, and 6 h after the injection of endotoxin. As the vascular endotheliopathy progressed and capillary permeability increased (Fig. 2), electron microscopy revealed swelling of the astrocytes initially (Fig. 3), and then necrosis of nerve cells. It indicated that the thyphoid endotoxin induced both vasogenic and cytotoxic brain edema [2]. No pathologic changes were observed in the control group.

Except for a few cases of brain edema produced by bacterial exotoxin [3] or bacteria injected into the brain causing a local brain edema [4], there have been no reports of brain edema models produced by bacterial endotoxin. The pathologic findings in our brain edema model are mixed in type (i.e., vasogenic and cytotoxic). They are quite similar to those seen in the acute brain edema caused by bacterial infection in children [5].

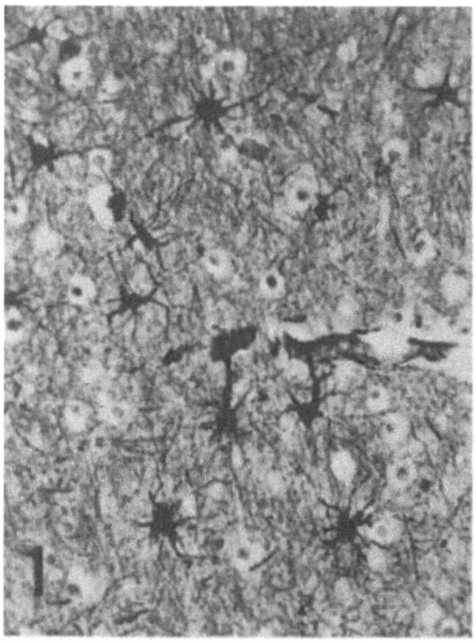

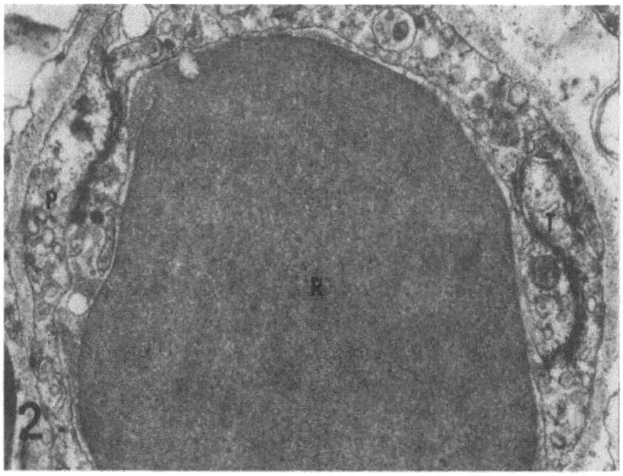

Fig. 1. Processes of astrocytes of perivascular region, swollen in edematous area. Cajal, ×139

Fig. 2. Capillary of experimental rabbit killed 10 min after injection of endotoxin. Pinocytotic vesicles (*P*) increased in number. Tight junction (*T*) remained unchanged. Red cell ×20 900

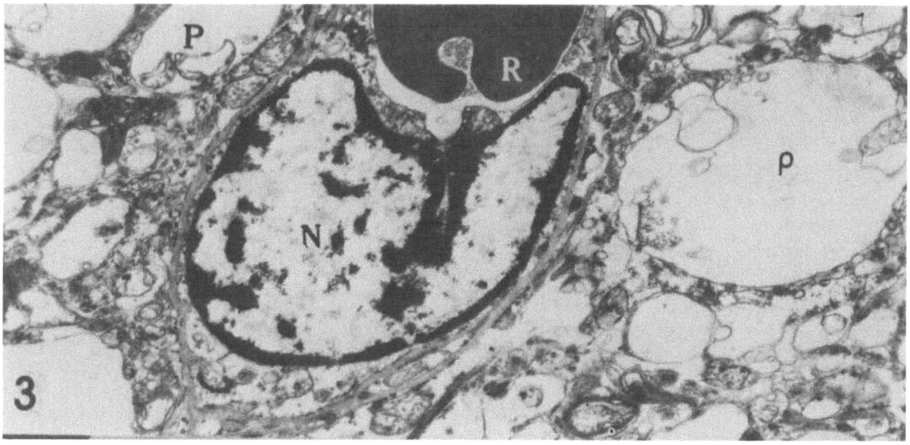

Fig. 3. Capillary of experimental rabbit killed 2 h after injection of endotoxin. There were swelling processes (*P*) of neuroglia cells (*N*) around the capillary. Tight junction remained unchanged. *R*, red cell. ×6960

Summary

Brain edema was induced by injecting typhoid endotoxin into the right internal carotid artery of experimental rabbits. Injection of normal saline was used as control. Altogether 65 rabbits were used for the investigation.

Evan's blue discoloration was demonstrated on the toxin injected on the same side of the brain of all the rabbits. In the control group only one rabbit's brain showed slight bluish discoloration. The average water content in brain samples of experimental rabbits was much higher than that in controls ($P < 0.001$).

As the vascular endotheliopathy progressed and capillary permeability increased, the brain tissue began to show swelling of the astrocytes and then necrosis of the nerve cells on light and electron microscopy.

References

1. Yang Yu-jia, Yu Pei-lan, Zhao Xiang-wen (1983) Experimental acute brain edema in rabbits. Bull Hunan Med Coll 8:171
2. Klatzo I (1967) Neuropathological aspects of brain edema. J Neuropathol Exp Neurol 26:1
3. Gardner DE (1974) Brain edema, an experimental model. Br J Exp Pathol 55:453
4. Hirano A, et al. (1964) The fine structure of cerebral fluid accumulation. III: Extracellular spread of cryptococcal polysaccharides in the acute stage. Am J Pathol 45:1
5. Department of Pediatrics. The First Affiliated Hospital, Hunan Medical College (1976) Septic shock in children. The People's Press, Hunan, pp 123–134

The Mucopolysaccharides of the Ground Substance in Ischemic Edema

I. FEIGIN [1]

Key words: Mucopolysaccharides, brain edema, ischemia

Ischemic edema is authoritatively viewed as a unique entity, which should be distinguished, for example, from vasogenic, cytotoxic, and hydrocephalic cerebral edema. The mucopolysaccharides (MPSS) of the ground substance of the human brain in hypoxia and ischemia were studied histochemically, since these greatly influence the water content of normal and edematous tissues. The neutral MPS were disclosed by periodic acid-Schiff staining, and the acidic MPS (glycosaminoglycans) by the metachromatic staining with toluidine blue after saponification.

All observations described in this report pertain to the human brain. The neutral mucopolysaccharides (MPSS) of the ground substance are stained by the periodic acid-Schiff (PAS) technique. The cortex is more deeply stained than the arcuate white matter (w.m.), and this in turn is more deeply stained than the deep w.m. Microdensitometer readings for these tissues in three instances were: (a) 0.215, 0.180, 0.162; (b) 0.227, 0.207, 0.187; and (c) 0.189, 0.147, 0.101, respectively, confirming this relationship.

The MPS are present as an interstitial, i.e., extracellular, ground substance. This is demonstrated by simultaneously staining these and the variously formed elements of the neural tissues, i.e., astrocytes, myelin, axons etc., and noting the distinction.

The acidic MPSs (glycosaminoglycans) are demonstrated by their metachromatic violet staining with toluidine blue at about pH 4. The violet color is evident on viewing in an aqueous medium. When the section is dehydrated in alcohol and mounted permanently, the color becomes blue. In brain, this staining with toluidine blue is evident only after saponification of the tissues with KOH, presumably because this frees the reactive acid groups [1]. The acid MPSs of cortex, arcuate w.m., and deep w.m. are present in the same proportions as the neutral MPSs. The same proportions hold for the water content of these tissues in normal brains (85%, 79%, 71%), reflecting the functional effects of the MPSs. This also accounts for the high resistance of the cerebral cortex and the moderate resistance of the arcuate w.m. to edema.

The MPSs strongly influence the physiologic properties of tissues in normal and edematous states. Their large molecules influence a large volume of tissue, their "domains." They increase viscosity and osmotic pressure. They tend to bind water and some cations. In a static sense, i.e., at equilibrium, their "exclusion effect" tends to bar the presence of some large solutes such as albumin. In a dynamic sense they

---

[1] New York University Medical Center, New York, N.Y. 10016, USA

act as a “molecular sieve,” restricting the movement of water and solutes into their domain and thus impeding the spread of edema.

In the brain, they appear to maintain the integrity of the tissues in the presence of a water content (edema) which causes injury when the MPS content is not as great. It is the balance betwen MPS and water that determines tissue injury in edema.

The MPS are not significantly changed in hypoxic tissues in which neurons show ischemic necrosis but no other tissue element is altered. There is a decrease in the histochemical staining of MPSs early in ischemic infarction involving neurons together with other tissue elements. Later, as microglia and macrophages proliferate and vessels become hyperplastic, the MPSs increase beyond normal values. The MPSs are also increased when lakes of fluid appear with severe edema, these apparently derived from plasma proteins. As an infarct becomes old the MPSs are again decreased to below normal levels. The changes in neutral and acidic MPSs are parallel.

Cerebral edema is authoritatively viewed as being divided into four basic types: vasogenic, cytotoxic, hydrocephalic, and ischemic. Our studies in humans suggest that cerebral edema assumes a single basic pattern recognized in all clinical circumstances studied, i.e., hemorrhage, tumors (both primary and secondary), inflammation, hypoxia and acidosis, trauma, hypertension, hydrocephalus, and diffuse sclerosis. This edema involves mostly the deep w.m., tends to spare the arcuate w.m., is rare in gray matter, and almost always spares the cerebral cortex unless it is necrotic. These differences reflect the differing MPS content of these tissues.

The edema is extracellular, this being most obvious when it is severe and lakes of serum protein components, which stain like MPSs, are found in the tissue interstices. Most w.m. astrocytes degenerate very early in edema, as can be demonstrated with gold sublimate stains, while a minority are preserved and may hypertrophy. This astrocytic degeneration is the most sensitive histological indicator of edema, and is permanent, remaining recognizable for an indefinite period. Late in edema the myelin sheaths tend to degenerate while the axons tend to be preserved. The preservation of the astrocytes and myelin of the arcuate w.m. when these degenerate and are lost in the deep w.m. is a highly significant histological indication of edema.

Edema may be the essential pathogenetic mechanism in the demyelinating diseases. The arcuate preservation characteristic of edema is noted in diffuse sclerosis of both the leukodystrophy and the Schilder types. In metachromatic leukodystrophy the metachromatic bodies (sulfatides) indicative of the metabolic defect may be present in both the demyelinated w.m. and the preserved arcuate w.m. Being evident in both, the metabolic defect does not account for the difference in the two sites. The plaques of multiple sclerosis may be the result of focal edema injury to myelin rather than immune cell-mediated injury, the explanation generally favored. Focal edema is possible when the role of the MPS is considered.

Summary

Hypoxia limited to neurons is associated with no change in MPS. Hypoxia affecting other elements as well (infarction) is associated first with a decrease in MPS, but as microglia proliferate and macrophages are mobilized, the MPS are increased above normal. When lakes of fluid accumulate with very severe edema and necrosis, the glycolipid plasma components stain as do MPS. Finally, as the infarct becomes obsolete, the MPS are decreased below normal. In non-hypoxic circumstances, edematous tissues show no change in MPS early and when of moderate intensity, increased MPS when severe with lakes of fluid, and finally decreased MPS in tissues with residual injury after edema had subsided.

These patterns of changes do nothing to alter the concept offered in earlier studies, that the edema noted with ischemia does not differ fundamentally from that in other clinical circumstances, and is extracellular in all.

Reference

1. Feigin I (1981) The effect of saponification on the mucopolysaccharides of the ground substance of the human brain: The relation to focal edema and multiple sclerosis. J Neuropathol Exp Neurol 40:102–111

Distribution of Lectin Receptors on Cerebral Endothelium*

S. NAG [1]

Key words: Lectin, cationized ferritin, cerebrovascular, endothelium

Introduction

The finding that increased cerebrovascular permeability in acute hypertension is associated with reduction of endothelial surface charge [3] suggests the occurrence of alterations in factors contributing to charge. About 50% of the net negative charge on endothelium is thought to be due to sialyl residues [2]. Since no published reports are available of the distribution of sialyl and other monosaccharide residues on cerebral endothelium this ultrastructural study was undertaken.

Monosaccharide residues on the endothelial luminal plasma membrane of intracerebral cortical vessels of rats were localised using biotinylated lectins. In addition, the distribution of certain lectins and anionic groups following pretreatment of brain slices with neuraminidase was also studied.

Materials and Methods

Following anesthesia the brains of female Wistar-Furth rats (180–200 g) were fixed in situ by perfusion of 500 ml 2% glutaraldehyde in 0.1 *M* cacodylate buffer (pH 7.2) containing 4.35% sucrose and 0.05% $CaCl_2$. Brains were then fixed for an additional 2–4 h and sliced with a tissue chopper, after which the slices were further cut into rectangular blocks each containing one or two penetrating arterioles. The superficial molecular layer of these blocks was excised to allow incubating solutions to enter vascular lumina.

Blocks were washed in phosphate-buffered saline (PBS) and placed in PBS containing 0.01 *M* glycine and 1% bovine serum albumin for 30 min, after which they were incubated in biotinylated lectin solutions (Vector Laboratories, Burlingame, Calif) for 90 min at 37 °C with constant gentle agitation. The concentration of concanavalin A (Con A), peanut agglutinin (PNA), *Ricinus communis* I agglutinin (RCA I), *Dolichos biflorus* (DBA), soybean agglutinin (SBA) and *Ulex europeus* I (UEA I) was 0.750–1 mg/ml Dulbecco's PBS, while the wheatgerm agglutinin (WGA) concentration was 0.050 mg/ml.

---

* This work was supported by the Heart and Stroke Foundation of Ontario.

[1] Department of Pathology (Neuropathology), Queens' University and Kingston General Hospital, Kingston, Ontario K7L 3N6, Canada

Blocks were washed with PBS and incubated with avidin D-horseradish peroxidase (HRP), 15 μg/ml, for 30 min at room temperature, followed by several rinses in PBS and incubation in Tris-HCl buffer (pH 8.0) containing 3,3′-diaminobenzidine (0.048%) and hydrogen peroxide for 20 min to demonstrate conjugates of biotinylated lectin and avidin D-HRP reaction product.

Specificity of lectin binding was demonstrated by competitive inhibition in which blocks were incubated with biotinylated lectins along with 0.1 *M* of the appropriate monosaccharides as described previously [8]. In addition, control blocks were incubated with avidin D-HRP and substrate medium without lectin.

Anionic groups on cerebral endothelium were demonstrated using cationized ferritin (CF), as described previously [3].

Some brain blocks were incubated with 4 units/ml of type X neuraminidase (Sigma Chemical Co., St. Louis, Mo) for 1 h before incubation with biotinylated WGA, SBA and PNA, or cationized ferritin.

Brain blocks were processed for electron microscopy as described previously [3].

Results

Lectin Distribution on Endothelium

The structure of intracerebral cortical vessels was as reported previously [4]. Controls incubated with avidin D-HRP only and with biotinylated lectins and their corresponding competing sugars did not demonstrate lectin binding on endothelium (Fig. 1 a). An exception was WGA binding, which was only partially blocked by incubation with 0.5 *M* *N*-acetylglucosamine or 0.25 *M* of each of *N*-acetylglucosamine and *N*-acetylneuraminic acid.

The pattern of Con A, RCA I, and WGA binding to endothelium of intracerebral arterioles and capillaries was similar. Conjugates of lectin and avidin D-HRP formed a uniform linear deposit on the luminal plasma membrane of endothelium (Fig. 1 b). Pinocytotic vesicles which opened onto the vascular lumen showed lectin binding on the plasma membrane within vesicles. Lectin binding was observed on the plasma membranes at the luminal end of interendothelial spaces, but not on membranes within the space. Although a similar pattern of lectin binding was observed with SBA, DBA and UEA I, the intensity of staining was less pronounced than that observed with the other lectins (Fig. 1 c). Binding of PNA to endothelium was not observed.

Neuraminidase Pretreatment

The SBA and avidin D-HRP conjugates on endothelium were present in larger amounts than in vessels not pretreated with neuraminidase (Fig. 1 d). No alteration of WGA binding was observed.

After pretreatment of blocks with neuraminidase PNA-binding sites were demonstrated on endothelium. The pattern of binding on the endothelial luminal plasma membrane of intracerebral vessels was the same as observed using the other lectins (Fig. 1 e and f).

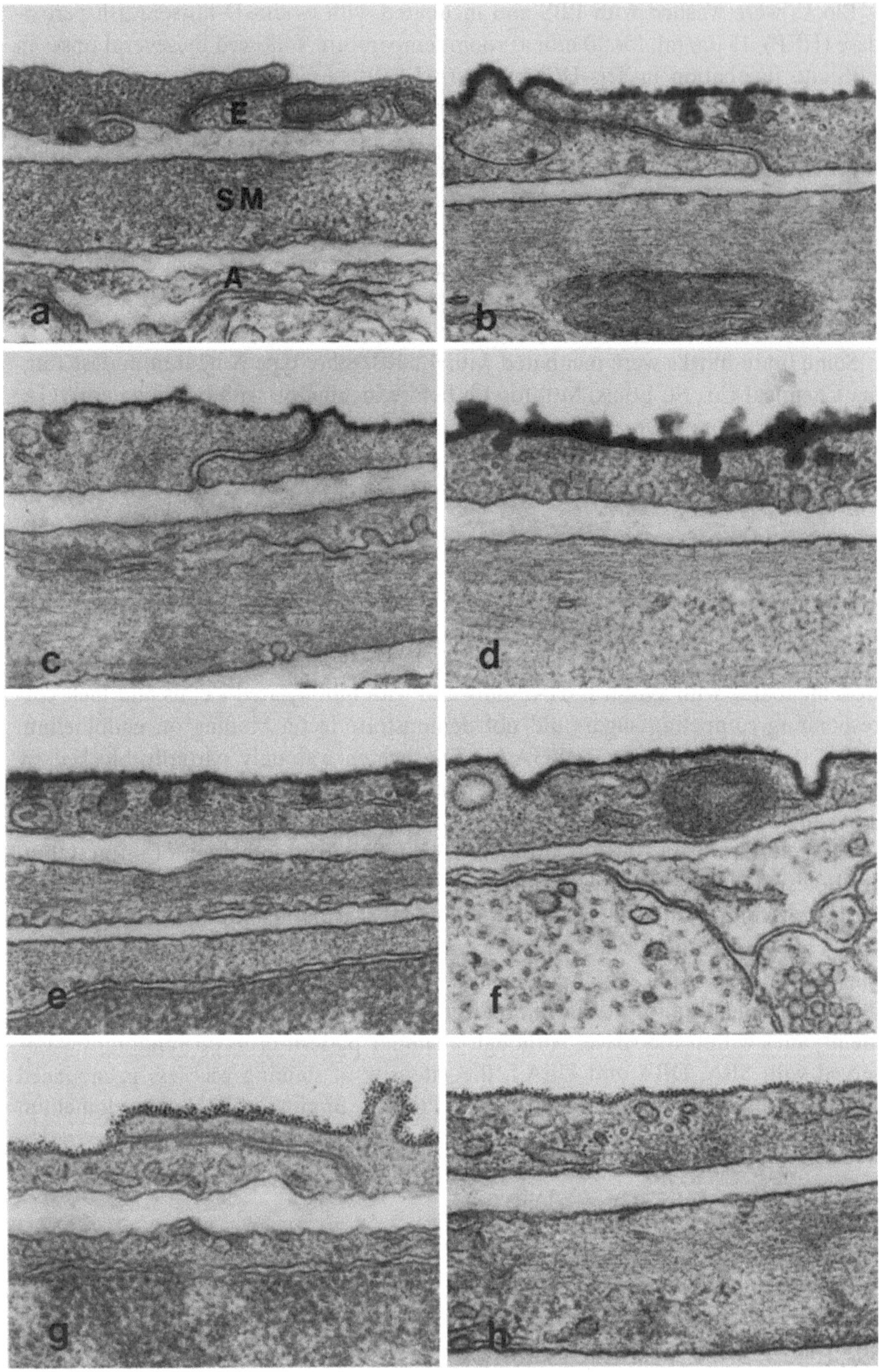
E
SM
A
a
b
c
d
e
f
g
h

Anionic Groups on Endothelium

Linear continuous deposits of CF (Fig. 1 g) were observed on the endothelial luminal plasma membrane of arterioles, venules, and capillaries, as reported previously [3]. No CF binding was observed on plasma membranes within interendothelial spaces or within pinocytotic vesicles which opened onto the vascular lumen.

Following neuraminidase pretreatment there was a reduction in the number of CF particles on the endothelial luminal plasma membrane of intracerebral vessels.

Discussion

The distribution of specific oligosaccharide residues on the endothelial luminal plasma membrane of intracerebral vessels has been documented in this study with biotinylated lectins following prior fixation.

This study demonstrates binding of Con A, RCA I, WGA, and SBA to cerebral endothelium, indicating the presence of α-D-mannosyl, α-D-glucosyl, B-D-galactosyl, β-N-acetylglucosaminyl, N-acetylneuraminic (sialic) acid and α-N-acetylgalactosaminyl groups on the luminal plasma membrane. These groups have been demonstrated on noncerebral endothelium by light [5] and electron microscopy [6, 8]. Simionescu et al. (1982) found the same pattern of lectin binding regardless of whether live or fixed endothelium was used.

There was some uncertainty as to whether α-L-fucosyl groups were present on rat noncerebral endothelium, since they could not be demonstrated by light microscopy [5, 7]. However, an electron microscopic study [8] and the present study have demonstrated these groups on endothelium of murine capillaries and on cerebral endothelium.

The major difference between cerebral and noncerebral endothelium appears to be in the binding of PNA. This lectin has been reported to bind to noncerebral endothelium, but it did not bind to cerebral endothelium in this study. However, following neuraminidase pretreatment of brain blocks there was exposure of β-D-gal-(1-3)-D-gal-N-acetyl residues, to which PNA binds. Similar findings have been reported in choroid plexus endothelium [9]. These authors observed PNA binding to endothelium only after tissues had been pretreated with neuraminidase.

Fig. 1. a Arteriolar segment from a control brain block incubated in avidin D-HRP only. The vessel wall consists of endothelium (*E*) resting on basement membrane, a single layer of smooth muscle (*SM*), and adventitia (*A*). Nonspecific binding of avidin D-HRP conjugates on endothelium is not present. Conjugates of lectin and avidin D-HRP are present on the endothelium luminal plasma membrane of arterioles with WGA (**b**) and SBA (**c**). Lectin binding is present on plasma membranes within pinocytotic vesicles which are open to the vascular lumen but not on membranes within interendothelial spaces. Following neuraminidase pretreatment the SBA and avidin D-HRP conjugates are increased (**d**) and PNA binding is demonstrable on arteriolar (**e**) and capillary endothelium (**f**). Arteriolar segments show CF binding on the endothelial luminal plasma membrane prior to incubation with neuraminidase (**g**) and following neuraminidase pretreatment (**h**), when fewer CF particles are present on the endothelium. ×39 400

Following neuraminidase pretreatment the SBA and avidin D-HRP conjugates on endothelium were increased over those in vessels not pretreated with neuraminidase. Removal of sialic acid is known to expose more *N*-acetyl galactosaminyl residues, resulting in the accentuated staining observed [1, 5]. Binding of WGA was not altered following pretreatment of brain blocks with neuraminidase. Possibly, the number of sialic acid groups removed was not sufficient to produce reduced staining or more *N*-acetyl glucosaminyl groups were exposed so that the overall staining was not altered.

The distribution of anionic groups on endothelium corresponded to the distribution of sialyl groups. Fewer anionic groups were demonstrated on cerebral endothelium following neuraminidase pretreatment of tissues. Since only 50% of the charge is due to sialyl groups [2] it is not surprising that there is reduction but not loss of the anionic groups.

Summary

The distribution of saccharide residues on the endothelial luminal plasma membrane of intracerebral cortical vessels of rats was determined at the ultrastructural level with biotinylated lectins. In addition, the effect of neuraminidase pretreatment on binding of lectins and cationized ferritin was studied.

Binding of concanavalin A, *Ricinus communis* I and wheatgerm agglutinin was observed on the luminal plasma membrane of intracerebral capillary, venular and arteriolar endothelium. Lectin-avidin D-horseradish peroxidase conjugates were present in smaller quantities when biotinylated *Dolichos biflorus*, soybean and *Ulex europeus* I agglutinins were used. All these lectins have been observed to bind to noncerebral endothelium.

Binding of peanut agglutinin was only observed following pretreatment of brain slices with neuraminidase. In this respect cerebral endothelium differs from noncerebral endothelium, in which peanut agglutinin binding is demonstrable without prior neuraminidase treatment.

The distribution of anionic groups corresponded to the distribution of sialyl groups on endothelium. Reduction of anionic groups was observed following neuraminidase pretreatment of brain blocks.

The role of plasma membrane oligosaccharides in cerebrovascular permeability alterations and the genesis of cerebral edema remains to be determined.

Acknowledgements. The author would like to thank Dr. D. M. Robertson for valuable suggestions and Mrs. V. Norkum for skilled technical assistance.

References

1. Butters TD, Hughes RC (1978) Lectin binding to mosquito Aedes aegyptii and human KB cells: structural comparisons of membrane oligosaccharides. Carbohyd Res 61:159–168
2. Danon D, Skutelsky E (1976) Endothelial surface charge and its possible relationship to thrombogenesis. Ann NY Acad Sci 275:47–63
3. Nag S (1984) Cerebral endothelial surface charge in hypertension. Acta Nauropathol (Berl) 63:276–281

4. Nag S, Robertson DM, Dinsdale HB (1979) Quantitative estimate of pinocytosis in experimental acute hypertension. Acta Neuropathol (Berl) 46:107–116
5. Pena SDJ, Gordon BB, Karpati G, Carpenter S (1981) Lectin histochemistry of human skeletal muscle. J Histochem Cytochem 29:542–546
6. Pino RM (1984) Ultrastructural localization of lectin receptors on the bone marrow sinusoidal endothelium of the rat. Am J Anat 169:259–272
7. Schulte BA, Spicer SS (1983) Histochemical evaluation of mouse and rat kidneys with lectin-horseradish peroxidase conjugates. Am J Anat 168:345–362
8. Simionescu M, Simionescu N, Palade GE (1982) Differentiated microdomains on the luminal surface of capillary endothelium: distribution of lectin receptors. J Cell Biol 94:406–413
9. Vierbuchen M, Klein PJ (1983) Histochemical demonstration of neuraminidase effects in pneumococcal meningitis. Lab Invest 48:181–186

Semiquantitative Evaluation of Interendothelial Cleft Changes in Water Intoxication

J. CERVOS-NAVARRO[1], J. ARTIGAS, Y. NAKAGAWA, and R. FERSZT

Key words: Hypo-osmolar edema, interendothelial cleft, tight junction, blood-brain barrier, paracellular pathway

Introduction

It is generally held that the processes responsible for the selective permeability of the blood-brain barrier occur in the endothelium of brain microvasculature [1, 5, 11]. The precise mechanisms involved remain somewhat unclear; a variety of transendothelial transport mechanisms have been proposed [12, 13].

The existence of a paracellular pathway for water, ions, and small solutes has been postulated, and it is highly plausible that under some experimental conditions such a pathway does indeed exist [4–6, 10].

The physiological relevance of such a transport pathway, however, remains unclear. This is due in part to the lack of quantitative studies in this field. The aim of this report is to present a morphometric evaluation of changes in the interendothelial clefts of hypo-osmolar edema.

Materials and Methods

The experiments were performed in Wistar rats. The experimental animals received IV injections of distilled water in amounts equal to 10%, 15%, 20%, and 25% of their body weight. Distilled water was injected over a period of 120 min into the femoral vein while the arterial blood pressure was monitored. After water injection, the animals were immediately killed and perfused with Karnovsky solution. Tissue blocks from cortex, basal ganglia, corpus callosum, and brain stem were processed for electron microscopy.

A total of 365 capillaries and small cerebral venules were examined. The number of dehiscences and blisters and their width were calculated from electromicrographs. The morphological data subjected to statistical analysis were: the number of dehiscences, the width of dehiscences and blisters, and their mean value. The data were analyzed statistically.

[1] Institute of Neuropathology, Klinikum Steglitz, Free University Berlin, Hindenburgdamm 30, D-1000 Berlin 45

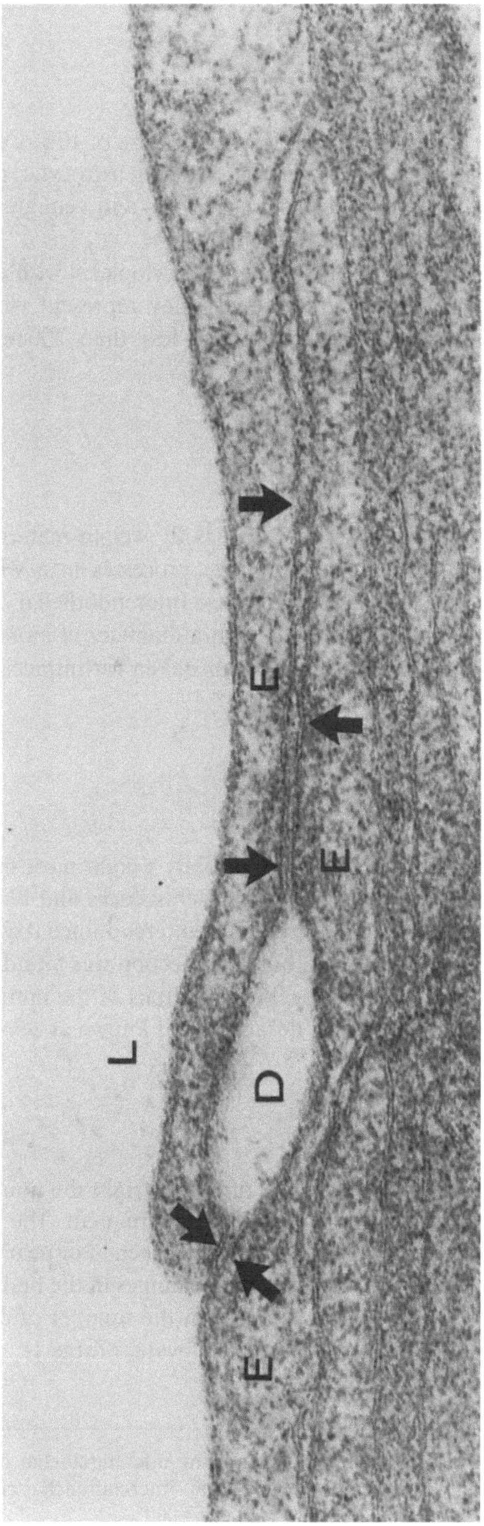

Fig. 1. Wall of a capillary showing interendothelial dehiscence. Water dosage 15% of body weight. Width of the dehiscences is 140 nm. Interendothelial clefts are indicated by *arrows*. *L*, lumen; *E*, endothelial cell; *D*, dehiscence. ×88 000

Results

Group 1

After IV administration of water at a dose of 10% of body weight, in areas of edema formation in the gray matter swollen astrocytic processes are most prominent around blood vessels, mostly arterioles and venules. The interfascicular glia is also swollen, but to a lesser degree.

The endothelial cells show a light cytoplasm with intact cyto-organelles. Some interendothelial clefts are evident; they represent widening of the interendothelial space between tight junctions by less than 200 nm (Fig. 1); we term them interendothelial dehiscences.

Group 2

After water at a dose of 15% of body weight material of very low electron density was found outside the astrocytic processes in a wide extracellular space around venules, arterioles, and capillaries. Interendothelial dehiscences are found quite frequently; some of them large with a diameter of more than 200 nm (Fig. 2); we term these structures, which can be mistaken for intracellular vacuoles, interendothelial blisters.

Group 3

After water at a dose of 20% of body weight most interendothelial spaces were enlarged, forming interendothelial dehiscences and blisters. In some sections no connection was apparent between the interendothelial clefts and the blisters, because of the large size of the cleft, but a connection was found when additional serial sections were cut. In addition, focal evaginations of the luminal endothelial cell membrane were found at this water dosage: this is known as zeiosis [3].

Group 4

After water at a dose of 25% of body weight the number of dehiscences and blisters increased strikingly. Zeiosis was also frequent. The microvillus-like structures produced by zeiosis were very frequently seen at or near the interendothelial clefts.

The control animals showed no changes in the brain endothelial cells.

A correlation was made between the number of dehiscences and blisters seen in electromicrographs and the dose of water (Table 1).

Fig. 2. Wall of a small venule, showing interendothelial blisters. Water dosage 25% of body weight. Width of the blisters is 600 nm. Interendothelial clefts are indicated by *arrows*. *L*, lumen; *E*, endothelial cell; *B*, blister. × 63 000

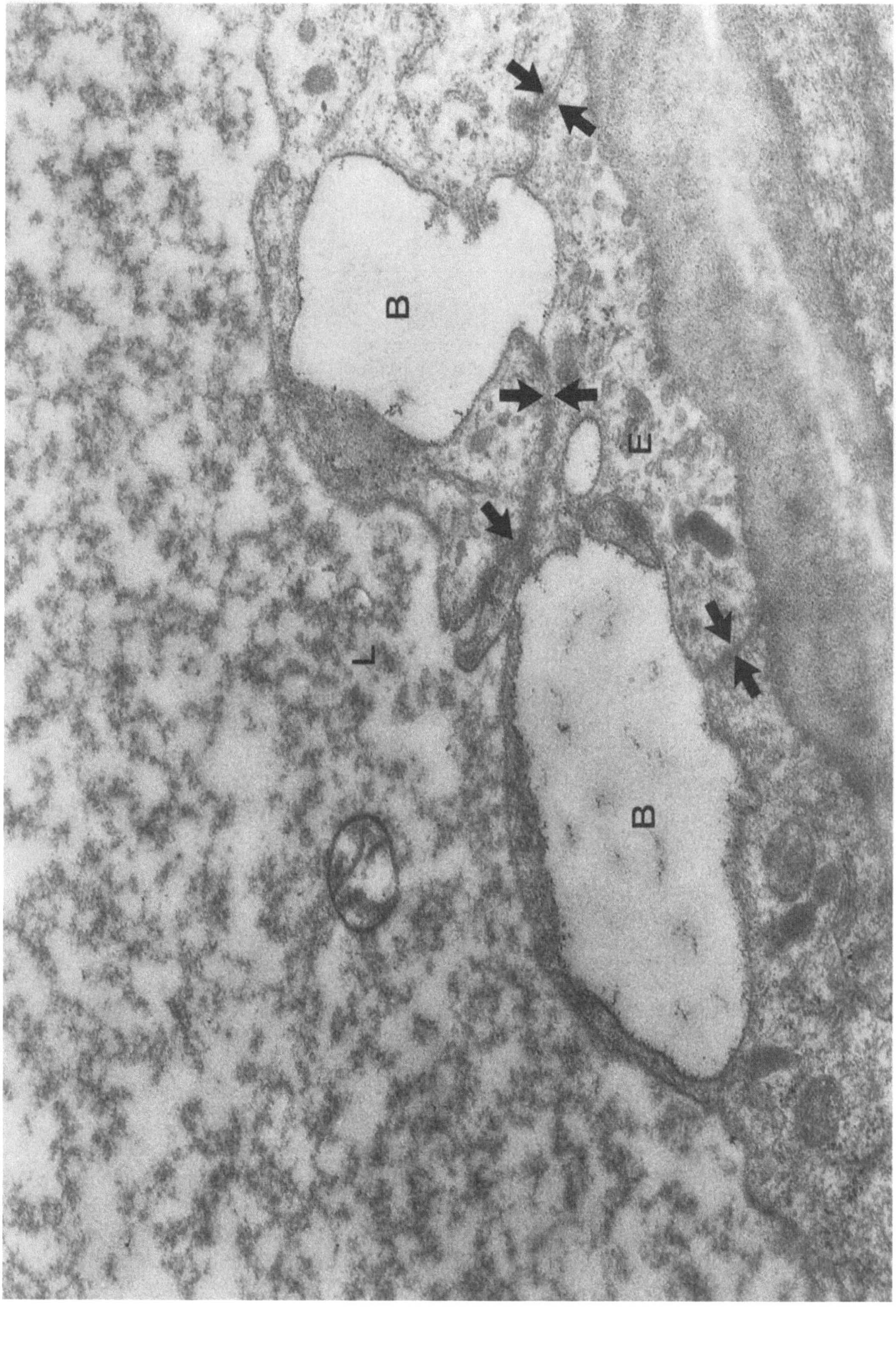
B
E
L
B

Table 1. Correlation between number of dehiscences or blisters and dose of water

Water dosage	Control	Water toxification			
		10%	15%	20%	25%
	(*n*=5)	(*n*=5)	(*n*=5)	(*n*=5)	(*n*=5)
Cerebral cortex	0/20	4/21	7/19	15/21	17/20
Basal ganglia	0/16	2/13	3/15	5/18	8/15
Corpus callosum	0/12	1/14	2/13	3/13	6/20
Brain stem	0/22	6/18	8/25	18/25	20/25
Total	0/70 (0%)	13/66 (19.7%)	20/72 (27.7%)	31/77 (40.2%)	51/80 (63.7%)

No. of vessels in which interendothelial dehiscences or blisters/no. of vessels examined in this study

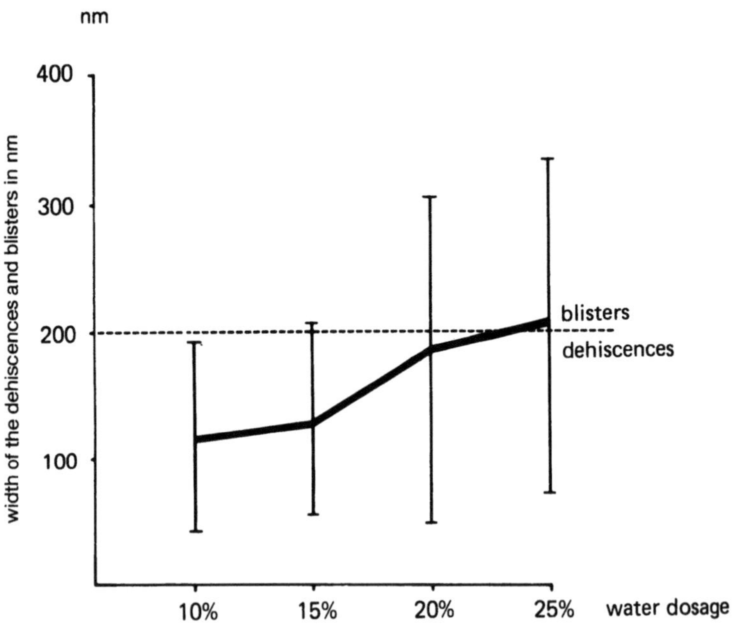

Fig. 3. Relationship between the width of the dehiscences or the diameter of blisters and the water dosage. Statistically, there are significant differences between groups 1 (10%) and 2 (15%) (low water dosage) compared with groups 3 (20%) and 4 (25%) (high water dosage)

There is a topographic pattern of these changes; the cerebral cortex and the brain stem show evidence of widening of endothelial clefts at a water dosage of 20% of body weight, followed by the cerebral cortex, the basal ganglia, and the brain stem at the slightly higher dosage of 25% of body weight.

There is a clear statistical correlation between the width of the dehiscences and the diameter of the blister and the water dosage (Fig. 3). At a water dosage of 10%, hardly any blisters are seen but only dehiscences, their mean width being 110 ± 60 nm. At a water dosage of 15% there are many more dehiscences and some blisters, the mean maximal width of these being 124 ± 59 nm. At a water dosage of 20% of body weight many dehiscences and blisters are found, with a mean diameter of 194 ± 130 nm. There is a further increase in the number and the size of blisters when the water dose is increased to 25% of body weight. In this case they have a mean width of 205 ± 129 nm.

Discussion

It has been suggested that the interendothelial clefts may constitute a paracellular pathway for the passage of water, ions, and small solutes in brain vessels [4–6, 10]. It seems that this pathway would be permeable in both directions, depending on the driving osmotic or pressure gradient [5, 9, 10].

Establishment of an osmotic or pressure gradient between both sides of the endothelial layer causes a widening of interendothelial clefts and, at a higher gradient, the formation of blisters between tight junctions [4, 8, 10]. The results of this quantitative study clearly show that the number and the size of blisters and the dehiscences found after water toxification are larger and are found at lower doses of water in areas shown by a gravimetric method to be prone to edema [8]. This regional variability of hypo-osmolar edema cannot be explained by differences in microvascular density alone.

Our results indicate that widening of dehiscences and formation of blisters between endothelial cells under the influence of an osmotic gradient correlate with the water dosage as well as with the degree and the location at which hypo-osmolar edema is formed.

In our opinion, this is consistent with the notion that tight junctions are permeable to ionic flows and water.

There is little doubt that the interendothelial changes we report are causally related to water toxification and correlate with the intensity of brain edema. The cytoplasmic mechanism for regulation of tight-junctional permeability is as yet ill defined. The interendothelial cleft represents a part of the environment of the endothelial cell, and its functional status may well be regulated by the endothelium. The endothelial cell might respond to physiologic or pathologic stimuli by increasing or decreasing the permeability of the tight junctions. Bentzel et al. and Duffey et al. [2, 7] showed that the permeability of tight junctions is apparently regulated by the formation of microfilaments in the cytoplasm adjacent to the tight junctions. In toad bladder studies they postulated that the control of the paracellular route of ions involves this specific interaction between microfilaments and specialized junctional domains of the plasma membrane.

It is not clear how the molecular biology and the function of tight junctions are influenced by water toxification. One additional feature associated with the formation of dehiscences and blisters is the evagination of the luminal cell membrane, particularly at high water dosage. This phenomenon is termed zeiosis and was observed in cells treated with cytochalasin B, probably due to disruption of microfilament attachment to the cell membrane [3].

We suggest that the formation of dehiscences and blisters is due to solute movement into the interendothelial clefts and the subsequent movement of water producing focal discontinuities in junctional protein fibrils with disruption of microfilaments and, according to the freeze-fracture technique, with reorientation and a disorder of tight-junctional elements.

Summary

The microvasculature in cortex, basal ganglia, corpus callosum and brain stem was studied by electron microscopy in rats with hypo-osmolar edema. Intravenous injection of water at 10%, 15%, 20%, and 25% of body weight for a period of 120 min leads to the formation of interendothelial clefts, the number being clearly related to the degree of water toxification. Blisters and dehiscences are most pronounced in cortex and brain stem. We assume that in hypo-osmolar edema a paracellular pathway for water, ions and small solutes from blood stream to the brain is visualized.

References

1. Brightman MW (1977) Morphology of blood-brain interfaces. Exp Eye Res [Suppl] 1–25
2. Bentzel CJ, Hainau B, Edelman A, Anagnostopoulos T, Benedetti EL (1976) Effect of plant cytokinins on microfilaments and tight junction permeability. Nature 264:666–668
3. Burgess DR, Grey RD (1974) Alterations in morphology of developing microvilli elicited by cytochalazin B. J Cell Biol 62:566–574
4. Cervós-Navarro J, Artigas J (1984) Ultrastructural of cerebral vessels in hypoosmolar edema. In: Go KG, Baethmann A (eds) Recent progress in the study and therapy of brain edema. Plenum, New York, pp 117–126
5. Cervós-Navarro J, Artigas J, Mrsulja B (1982) Morphofunctional aspects of the normal and pathological blood-brain barrier. Acta Neuropathol [Suppl] (Berl) VIII: 1–19
6. Cervós-Navarro J, Artigas J, Nakagawa Y, Sasaki S (1983) Morphological evidence of transjunctional fluxes of ions and water in the blood-brain barrier. J Cereb Blood Flow Metabol [Suppl 1] 3:415–416
7. Duffey ME, Hainau B, Ho S, Bentzel CJ (1981) Regulation of epithelial tight junction permeability by cyclic AMP. Nature 294:451–453
8. Hahm H, Ferszt R, Mueller J, Cervós-Navarro J (1980) Topography of diffuse brain edema. Adv Neurol 28:299–315
9. Luse SA, Harris B (1960) Electron microscopy of the brain in experimental edema. J Neurosurg 17:439–446
10. Nakagawa Y, Cervós-Navarro J, Artigas J (1984) A possible paracellular route for the resolution of hydrocephalic edema. Acta Neuropathol (Berl) 64:122–128
11. Spatz M, Mrsulja BB (1982) Progress in cerebral microvascular studies related to the function of the blood-brain barrier. Adv Cell Neurobiol 3:311–337
12. Van Deurs B (1977) Vesicular transport of horseradish peroxidase from brain to blood in segments of the cerebral microvasculature in adult mice. Brain Res 124:1–8
13. Westergaard E (1977) The blood-brain barrier to horseradish peroxidase under normal and experimental conditions. Acta Neuropathol (Berl) 39:181–187

Differences in Response of Large-Vessel Endothelium and Capillary Endothelium Following Intracarotid Mannitol

J. C. GODERSKY[1], T. SASAKI, and N. F. KASSELL

Key words: BBB, hyperosmolar solution, HRP, cerebral vascular endothelium

Introduction

Transient osmotic disruption of the BBB has been advocated by Neuwelt et al. [3] as a vehicle for increased drug delivery into the brain for treatment of central nervous system (CNS) malignancies. However, a number of drugs administered in this manner have been shown to be neurotoxic [4]. This study was designed to investigate the effects of hyperosmolar solutions on the endothelium of the major extracranial and intracranial arteries and to contrast this with the effects on the cerebral capillary endothelium. A potential risk of injury to the vessels exists if antineoplastic drugs are able to penetrate the vessel wall following the administration of mannitol.

Methods

Adult dogs were anesthetized with sodium pentobarbital and the end-tidal CO_2 adjusted to 36–40 torr. The left common carotid artery was exposed and cannulated with a 20-gauge catheter positioned at the origin of the ICA. The external carotid was then ligated. Evans blue dye (2.5 ml/kg of a 2% solution) was injected via the femoral vein, as was HRP (Sigma type II, 200 mg/kg). Mannitol (45 ml 25% solution) was infused into the left internal carotid artery over an interval of 30–35 s. The animals were sacrificed 10–20 min later by intracardiac perfusion with aldehydes. The cervical ICA, cavernous ICA, and major cerebral vessels were removed and further fixed by immersion. Peroxidase activity was demonstrated by means of the method of Reese and Karnovsky [5]. Macroscopic areas of HRP reaction product were recorded, and selected areas of the vessels and brain were processed for TEM. A total of nine dogs were studied, but two were excluded from the final analysis because of a rise of more than 50 mmHg in systolic blood pressure following mannitol injection. The vessels at the opposite side to where the mannitol injection was given were used as controls for this study.

[1] University of Iowa, Iowa City, Iowa 52242, USA

Results

The macroscopic distribution of HRP reaction product is demonstrated in Fig. 1. Dense staining was evident in the left cervical ICA (ipsilateral to the mannitol injection) and in the cavernous segment of the ICA bilaterally. The right cervical ICA was densely stained in the region corresponding to the carotid body, but lightly stained distal to this. As the ICA passed through the dura mater on the right side, a transition zone was noted over which the staining gradually diminished. Distal to this transition zone, reaction product was only seen at arterial bifurcations.

In contrast, staining was more pronounced and more widely distributed on the side of the mannitol injection. Major branch points and the origins of small vessels were the most consistently stained. Variable staining was evident along the remainder of the vessel. BBB breakdown predictably occurred in the vascular territory supplied by the stained arteries.

The accompanying ultrastructural changes are shown in Fig. 2. In the cervical ICA, HRP readily penetrated the endothelium and was evident within the muscular layers. Endothelial swelling was seen ipsilateral to the mannitol injection in two of seven cervical ICAs. In the cavernous ICA segment, reaction product was seen to enter the vessel from both the luminal and the abluminal (sinus side) surfaces; entry from the abluminal side was more pronounced. These extracranial segments of the ICA do not possess a significant barrier to protein transport. After the ICA enters the subarachnoid space, reaction product remains identifiable but its presence is less pronounced than in the more proximal portions of the artery. Vesicles and channels, frequently seen in the cervical and cavernous ICA, are reduced in number in the intracranial vessels. The intracranial arteries restrict protein (HRP) transport, but mannitol alters their ability to do so.

HRP was transported through the endothelium of both the extracranial and intracranial arterial segments, primarily by way of vesicles and/or channels. Occasion-

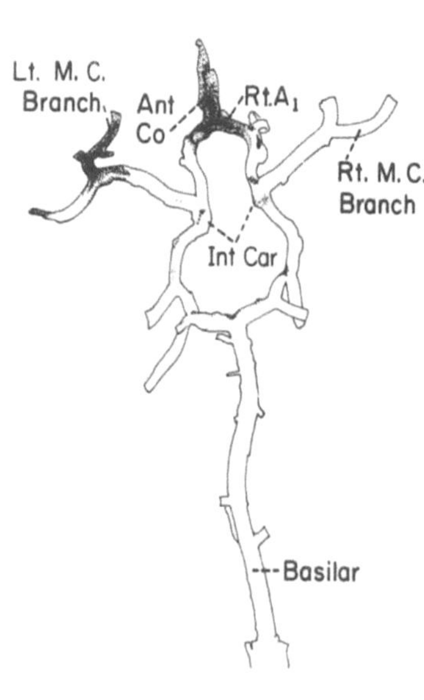

Fig. 1. Macroscopical distribution of HRP (*shaded areas*) is represented in the sketch. Mannitol was injected into the left internal carotid. (*Int Car*). Areas of dense staining are seen in left middle cerebral artery (*Lt. M. C.*) and in the region of the anterior communicating artery (*Ant Co*). Minimal staining is present on the right side and none is evident in the basilar artery (*Basilar*)

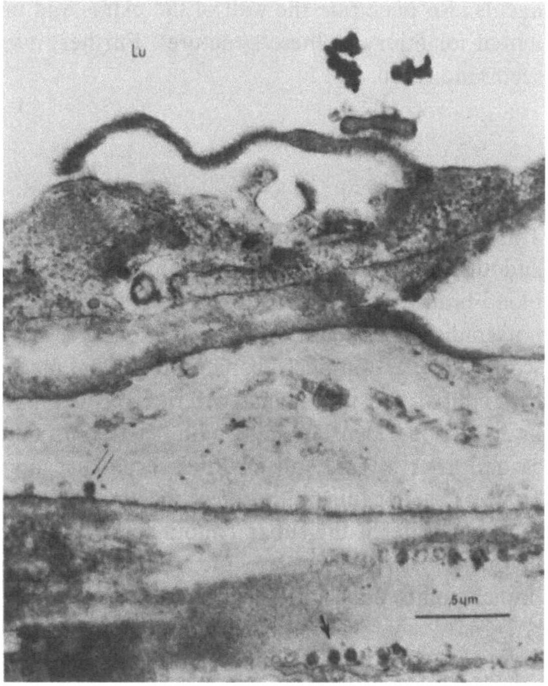

Fig. 2. Electron micrograph of a left middle cerebral artery branch, showing a small amount of HRP reaction product within the endothelial cell. A large amount of reaction product is evident in the deeper layers of the arterial wall (*arrows*) 15 min after mannitol injection

ally, dark staining of the endothelial junctions was noted, but disruption of these junctions was not seen.

Discussion

The site of the functional BBB has been localized to the tight junction of the capillary endothelium [1]. Studies of BBB breakdown concentrated on the alterations at the capillary level, and little attention has been paid to the function of the major intracranial arteries. Westergaard and Brightman [7] and Westergaard [6] have shown that under normal conditions, insignificant amounts of HRP reaction products do pass through the endothelium of cerebral arterioles (15–30 μm in diameter). Our study confirms and extends this observation to include the major intracranial vessels. When the BBB is disrupted by intracarotid mannitol infusion, the barrier function of the major cerebral vessels is also disturbed. Brightman et al. [2] demonstrated that hyperosmolar urea caused patchy areas of the vessels penetrating the brain substance to leak HRP. In our study this leak was most pronounced at sites of arterial branching, but also occurred with an irregular distribution along the main trunk of the arteries. The transition from endothelium without barrier function to endothelium with barrier function occurs as the ICA penetrates the dura.

Recently, BBB disruption has been proposed as a means of increasing delivery of antineoplastic drugs to CNS tumors. It is evident from our study that these cytotoxic agents also penetrate the wall of the extra- and intracranial arteries, creating a potential for injury to these structures. Further investigation of this potential hazard seems indicated.

Summary

This study was designed to investigate the effect of a hyperosmolar solution on the endothelium of the major extracranial and intracranial arteries in dogs. Transient blood-brain barrier (BBB) disruption was accomplished by mannitol infusion and horseradish peroxidase (HRP) was used as a marker for protein transport. Macroscopic and electron microscopic studies were made of the distribution of HRP in the extracranial and intracranial arteries and compared with the HRP distribution in brain sections. Dense staining with reaction product was seen in the cervical internal carotid artery (ICA) and in the cavernous segment of the ICA, suggesting an absence of barrier function in these locations. However, after the ICA penetrated the dura and entered the subarachnoid space, HRP reaction product was evident only in the vessels ipsilateral to the mannitol injection, most prominently at arterial branch points and small vessel origins.

Transmission electron microscopy (TEM) of the cervical and cavernous ICA segments consistently revealed numerous vesicles and tubules containing HRP both within the endothelial cell cytoplasm and penetrating into the muscular layers of the artery. In contrast, the endothelial cells of the major intracranial arteries contained fewer vesicles. Vesicles containing HRP reaction products were less prominent both within the endothelial cell and the muscle layers of the arterial wall; although dense staining was occasionally seen in the muscular layers. No evidence of tight junction disruption, by mannitol, was found. From these observations it is apparent that the endothelial cells of the major intracranial arteries do form a barrier to HRP penetration. Furthermore, this barrier can be altered by mannitol infusion.

References

1. Brightman JW, Reese TS (1969) Junctions between intimately apposed cell membranes in the vertebrate brain. J Cell Biol 40:648–675
2. Brightman MW, Hori M, Rapoport SI, Reese TS, Westergaard E (1973) Osmotic opening of tight junctions in cerebral endothelium. J Comp Neurol 152:317–326
3. Neuwelt EA, Frenkel EP, Diehl J, Vu LH, Rapoport SI, Hill S (1980) Reversible osmotic blood-brain barrier disruption in humans: implications for the chemotherapy of malignant brain tumors. Neurosurgery 7:44–52
4. Neuwelt EA, Barnett PA, Glasberg M, Frenkel EP (1983) Pharmacology and neurotoxicity of *cis*-diamminedichloroplatinum, bleomycin, 5-fluorouracil, and cyclophosphamide administration following osmotic blood-brain barrier modification. Cancer Res 43:5278–5285
5. Reese TS, Karnovsky MJ (1967) Fine structural localization of a blood-brain barrier to exogenous peroxidase. J Cell Biol 34:207–217
6. Westergaard E (1980) Ultrastructural permeability properties of cerebral microvasculature under normal and experimental conditions after application of tracers. In: Cervós-Navarro J, Ferszt R (eds) Adv Neurol 28:55–74
7. Westergaard E, Brightman MW (1973) Transport of proteins across normal cerebral arterioles. J Comp Neurol 152:17–44

Ultrastructure of Capillary Permeability in Human Brain Tumors – Gliomas Associated with Cerebral Edema (Low-Density Area)

S. SHIBATA[1], M. FUKUSHIMA, M. INOUE, and K. MORI

Key words: Glioma, vascular ultrastructure, cerebral edema, low density area

Introduction

Computed tomography (CT) reveals that intracerebral glioblastomas cause severe surrounding cerebral edema (low-density area), and astrocytomas may be accompanied by slight cerebral edema.

We recently observed five patients with glioblastomas who were developing severe cerebral edema and three patients with astrocytoma who also had slight cerebral edema. The CT and electron-microscopic findings of tumor vessels in these patients are discussed.

Materials and Methods

In five cases of glioblastoma and three of astrocytoma, the test material was obtained from surgically removed specimens. Following fixation for 10 min in 3% glutaraldehyde, 1% paraformaldehyde, and 0.1 *M* cacodylate buffer (pH 7.4) at 0° C, a block section of 1×1×3 mm was made of each under the stereoscopic microscope and reimmersed in the same fixing solution for 24 h. Then the section was frozen in Freon 22, which was cooled with liquid nitrogen in the EE-FED B frozen section apparatus (Nippon Denshi) and fractured at −130° C and 1×10^{-6} torr. The cut surface was shadowed with evaporated platinum-palladium and carbon in vacuo, and the tissues were dissolved in sodium hypochlorite solution for 1 h. After a rinse with distilled water, the replica membranes were submitted to the electron microscope study (100 B, Nippon Denshi).

A part of each block section was also used for conventional electron-microscopic examination.

[1] Department of Neurosurgery, Nagasaki University School of Medicine, 7-I Sakamoto-machi, Nagasaki 852, Japan

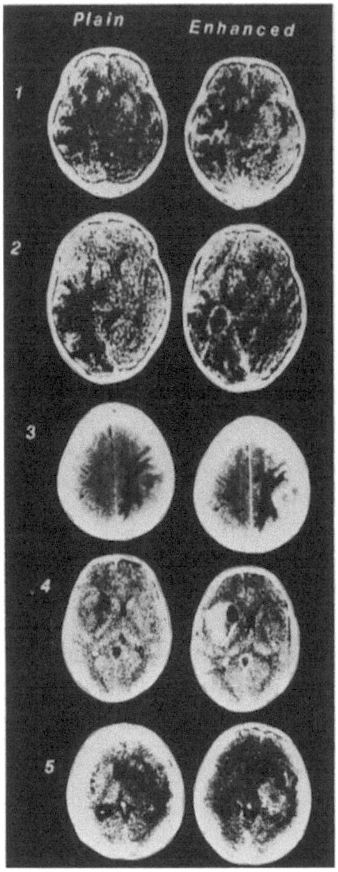

Fig. 1. CT of cases 1–5 (glioblastoma multiforme), showing large low-density area and peripheral ring, and nodular enhancement with effect in each case

▼ **Fig. 2.** Electron micrograph of an ultrathin section from a glioblastoma, showing surface infolding, endothelial hyperplasia, and enlarged perivascular space. ×3940

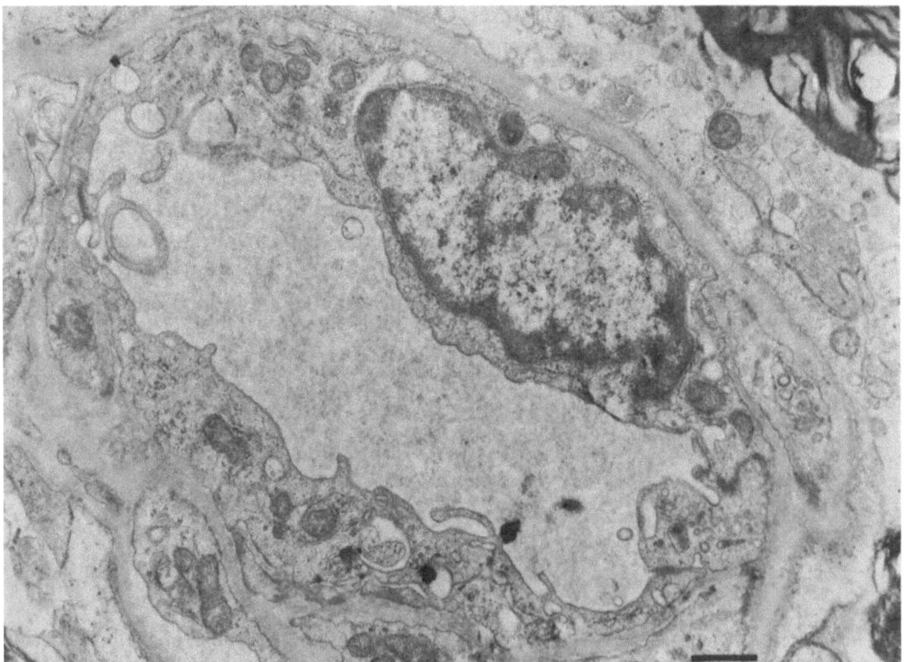

Results

Glioblastoma Multiforme

CT Scan

All cases were examined by CT scan. Patient 1 (75-year-old man) proved to have a large low-density area and irregular ring enhancement with a mass effect in the left temporal region. In case 2 (68-year-old woman) a large low-density area and thin ring enhancement were found, with a shift to the right of the midline structures in the left temporo-occipital region. In case 3 (58-year-old man) a slightly high-density ring that enhanced with contrast infusion was revealed in the right parietal region. There was marked ipsilateral cerebral edema. Patient 4 (36-year-old woman) showed a large mixed iso- and low-density mass with nodular enhancement in the left frontotemporal region. In case 5 (59-year-old man) CT showed a large low-density mass and irregular ring enhancement in the right temporal region.

Electromicrographs of Ultrathin Sections

Endothelial cells of the tumor capillaries tended to have marginal infoldings and hyperplasia. The basal lamina was swollen, and the perivascular space was enlarged (Fig. 2). Some of these cell junctions were shorter or longer than normal, or even open (Figs. 3 and 4). Increased pinocytotic vesicles of endothelial cells were found in the tumor capillaries.

Findings in Freeze-Fracture Replicas

Figure 5 shows a capillary replica of the glioblastoma. Pinocytotic vesicles appeared concave in the protoplasmic face (PF) and elevated in the extracellular face (EF). The density of pinocytotic vesicles increased markedly, amounting to 25 per μm^2 on average.

The tight junction in one area was seen as a network of six strands composed of particles measuring about 100 Å, but in the other area as one or two strands. These tight junctions had an irregular lining of intramembranous particles (Figs. 6 and 7).

Astrocytoma

CT Scan

The astrocytomas were also examined by CT scan (Fig. 8) and in case 6 (42-year-old woman with astrocytoma grade III) a right frontal, small, nonenhancing, low-density lesion was found. Patient 7 (34-year-old man with grade II astrocytoma) proved to have a left frontal, small, nonenhancing, low-density lesion. In case 8 (42-year-old man with cystic astrocytoma grade II) CT revealed a small low-density lesion with

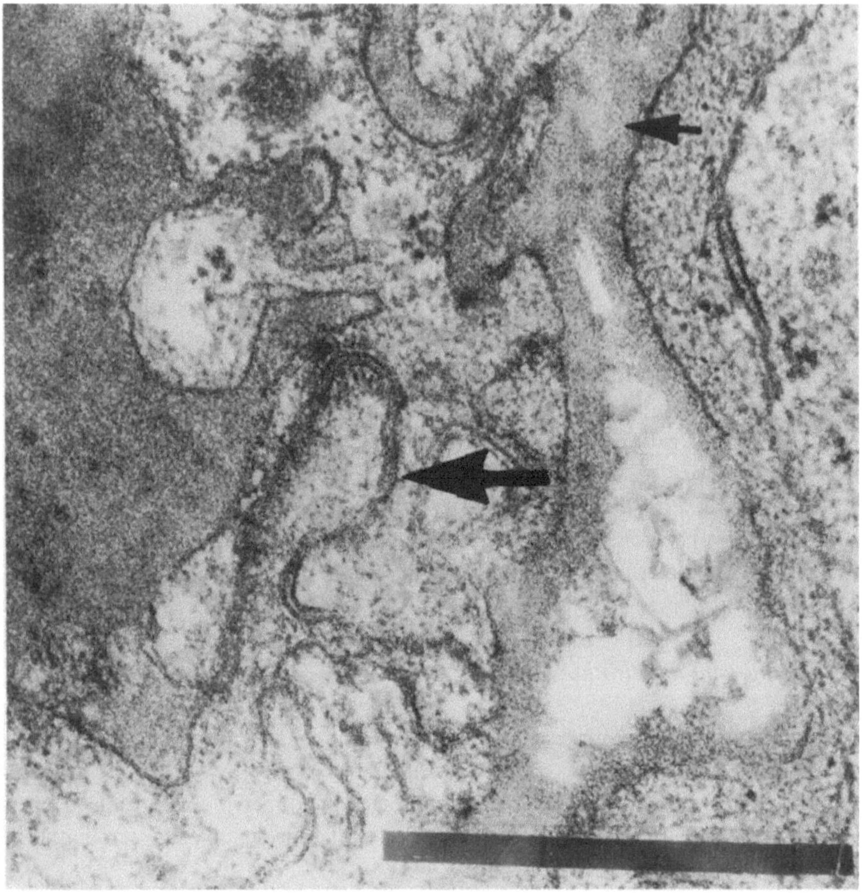

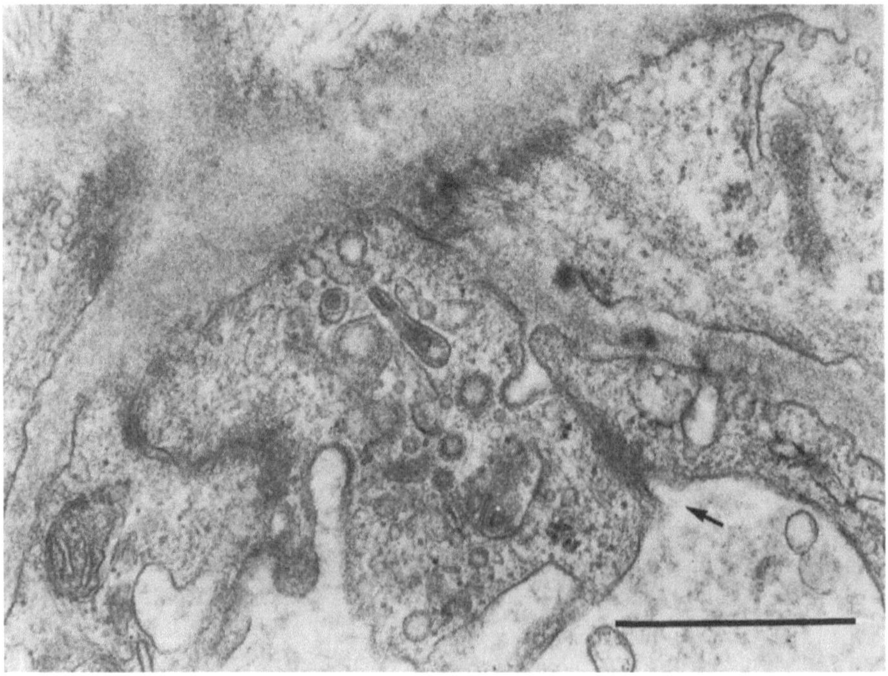

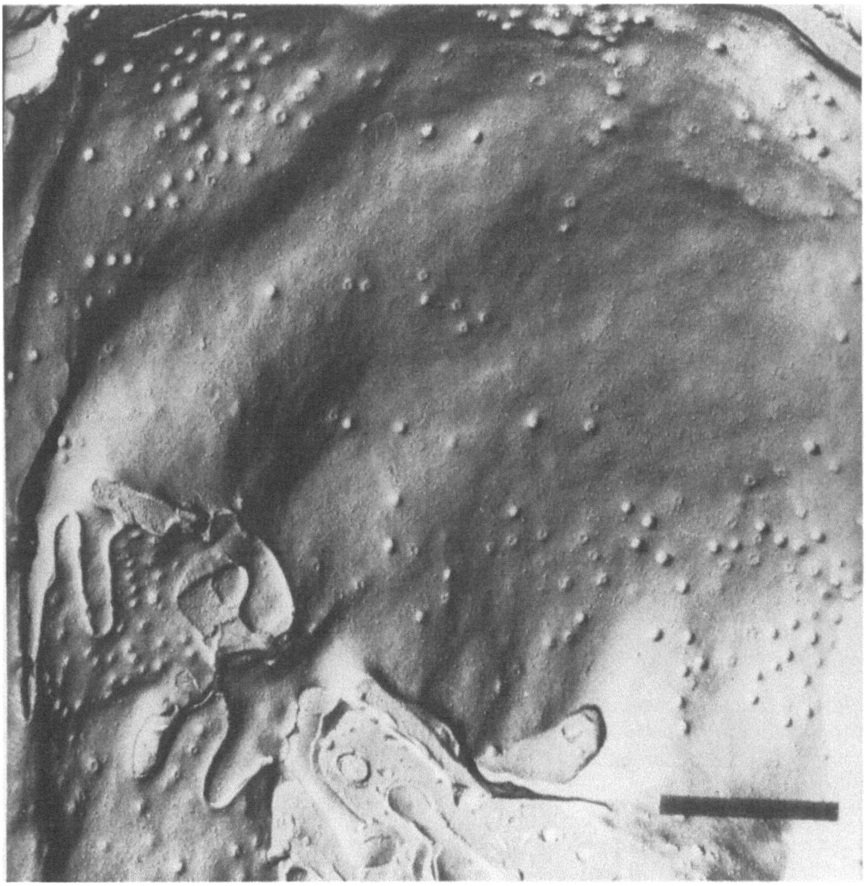

Fig. 5. Electron micrograph of the replica of the tumor capillary endothelium plasma membrane of glioblastoma, showing increased density of pinocytotic vesicles. ×6700

◄

Fig. 3. Ultrathin section from a glioblastoma, showing a tortuous, elongated junction between two capillary endothelial cells (*large arrow*) and a thick, irregular basal lamina (*small arrow*). ×20 000

Fig. 4. Ultrathin section of glioblastoma, showing a short tight junction. ×17 000

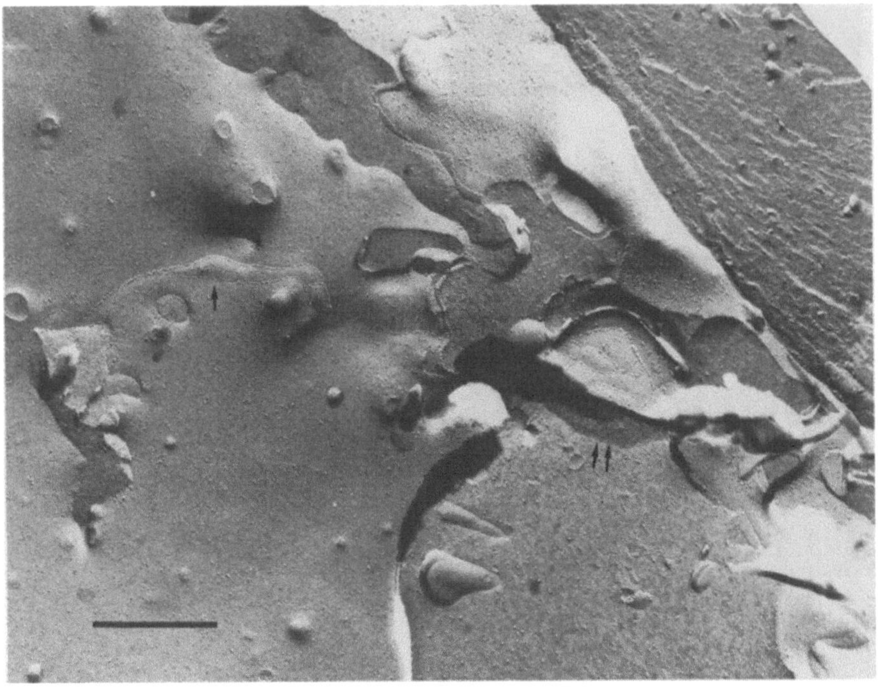

Fig. 6. P face of an endothelial membrane of glioblastoma with six strands (*double arrow*) and two strands (*single arrow*) of tight junction. This tight-junctional element appears as a discontinuous array of particles. × 12 280

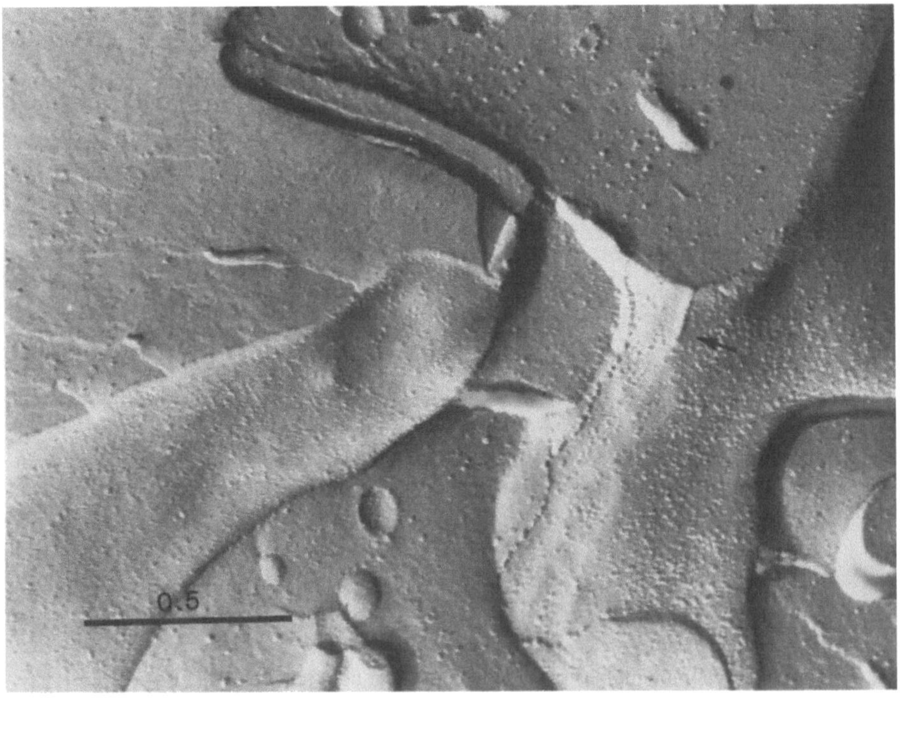

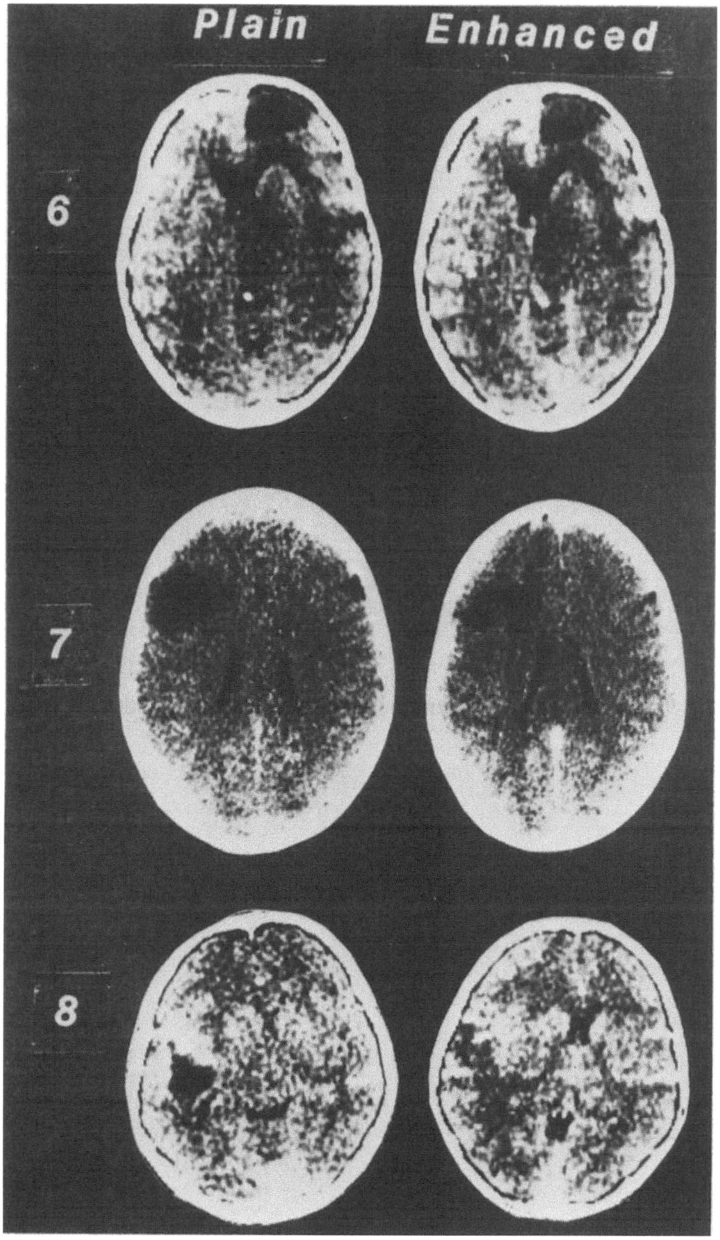

Fig. 8. CT of cases 6–8 (astrocytomas grade III and II), showing nonenhancing low-density lesions

Fig. 7. Tight junction of glioblastoma, showing two strands and appearing as a discontinuous array of particles. ×25 800

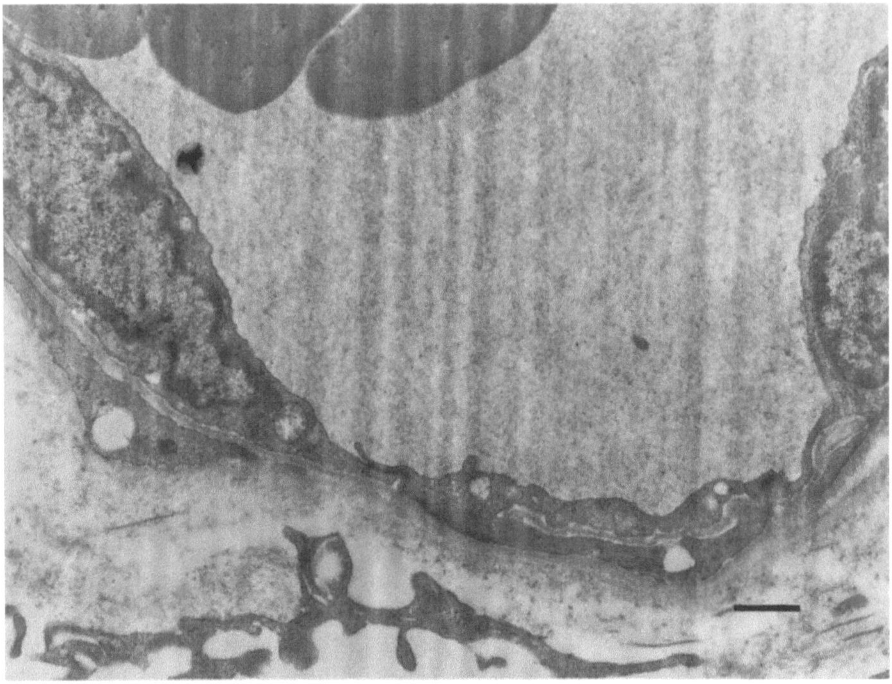

Fig. 9. Ultrathin section of astrocytoma showing smooth endothelial surface. ×3910

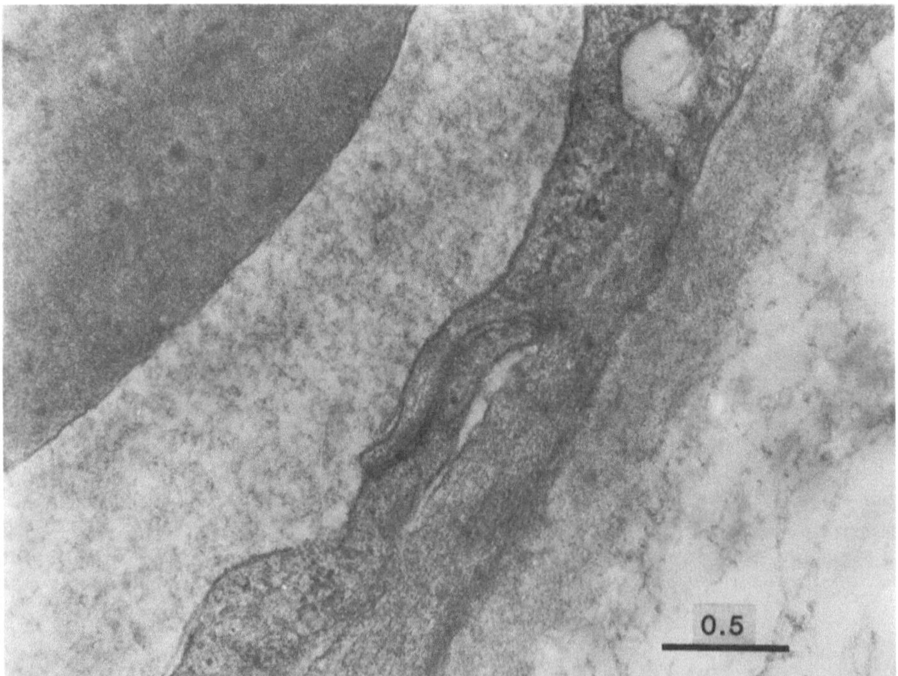

Fig. 10. Ultrathin section of astrocytoma showing a tight junction and a thin basal lamina. ×14 800

peripheral ring, nodular enhancement, and a slight mass effect in the left temporal region.

Electromicrographs of Ultrathin Sections

Endothelial cells of the tumor capillaries showed a smooth endothelial surface and regular tight junctions although the blood vessels appeared relatively normal (Figs. 9 and 10).

Findings in Freeze-Fracture Replicas

Figure 11 shows a capillary replica of the astrocytoma. The density of pinocytotic vesicles increased markedly, reaching 34 per μm^2 on average.

Tight junctions in the replica membrane appeared as six strands of particles about 100 Å in size, arranged in a network in the protoplasmic membrane of each endothelial cell. The particle lines were not disrupted (Fig. 12).

Discussion

According to the fluid mosaic model proposed by Singer and Nicolson in 1972 [5], protein particles float between the two layers of phospholipid membrane with their hydrophobic surface facing inward and its hydrophilic surface toward the outside of the membrane. In the freeze-fracture replica method, dissociation occurs in the central part of the hydrophobic part, which is the weakest in intermolecular condition. Accordingly, extensive three-dimensional observation of intramembranous structures becomes possible [3, 4]. In replica preparations, the inner surface of the membrane viewed from outside is called the protoplasmic face (PF) and the outer face looked from inside is called the extracellular face (EF).

A few reports are based on studies using the freeze-fracture replica method, which is considered more reliable than conventional ultrathin section specimens for quantitative study of pinocytotic vesicles developing from the endothelial cell membrane of cerebral tumor vessels [6]. In our present study the freeze-fracture replica method revealed a marked increase in the density of pinocytotic vesicles in both glioblastoma and astrocytoma compared with normal brain vessels, although the number of vesicles did not differ significantly between the two tumors (Table 1).

With the freeze-fracture replica method it is possible to observe a network composed of five or more strands of protein particles in the tight junction, and it was found that the zonula occludens of a very leaky epithelium consists in most places of only one or two junctional strands [1, 2, 7]. Significant differences have been found in the number of strands making up the tight junction. In glioblastomas they are composed of one or two strands, as against six or more in astrocytomas (Table 1). We conclude that the smaller number of strands in the tight junctions plays an important role in the increased permeability in the vessels of glioblastomas with severe perifocal edema, in addition to the increase in the density of pinocytotic vesicles.

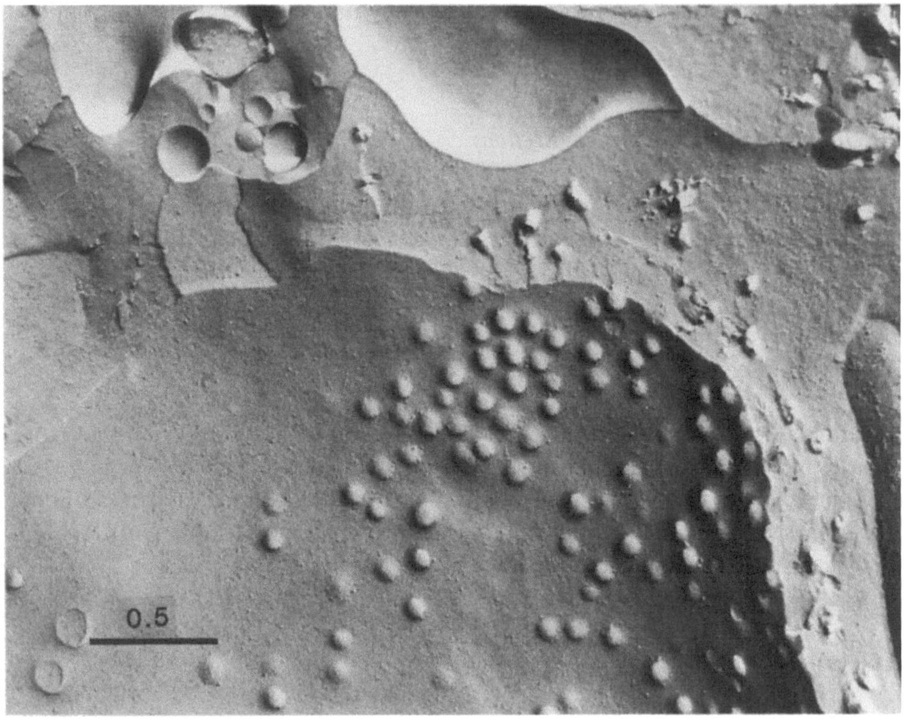

Fig. 11. Replica of astrocytoma, showing increased density of pinocytotic vesicles. ×14 800

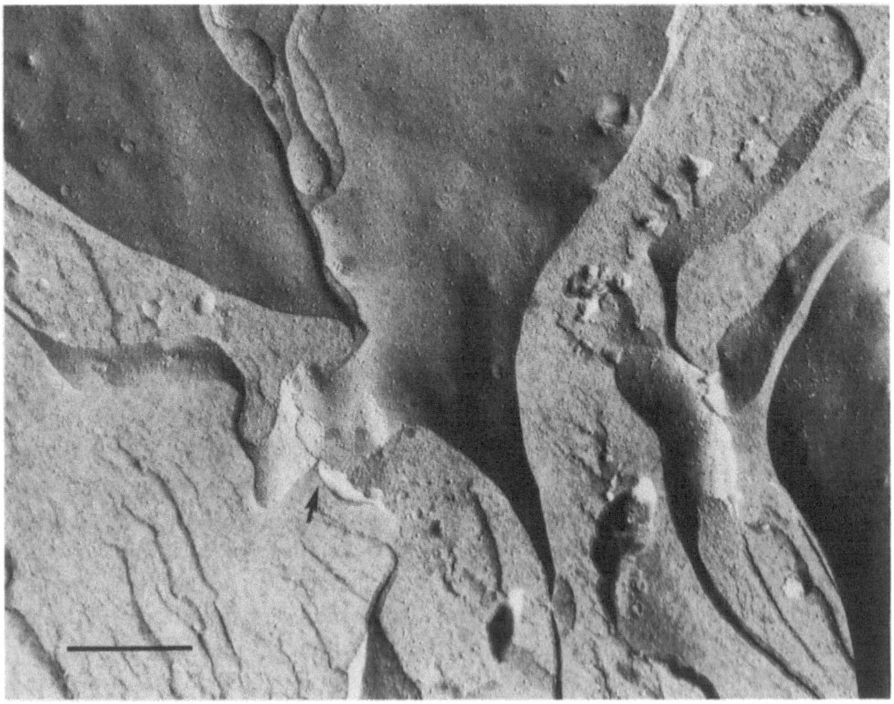

Fig. 12. Replica of astrocytoma showing seven sealing strands in a tight junction. ×20 600

Table 1. Composite values for capillaries from five glioblastomas and three astrocytomas

Case	Diagnosis	CT findings		Ultrathin section				Replica	
		Edema	CE	SI	TJ	BL	PS	PV (No./μm²)	TJ (strands)
1. TT 75M	Glioblastoma	+ + +	+ +	Marked	Short and elongated	Irregular	Large	35	2–6
2. UM 68F	Glioblastoma	+ + +	+	Marked	Short and elongated	Irregular	Large	15	?
3. KH 58M	Glioblastoma	+ + +	+ +	Marked	Short and elongated	Irregular	Large	19	?
4. KI 36M	Glioblastoma	+ + +	+ +	Marked	Short and elongated	Irregular	Large	20	2
5. YY 59M	Glioblastoma	+ + +	+	Marked	Short and elongated	Irregular	Large	24	3–4
6. KM 42F	Astrocytoma GIII	+	–	Moderate	Regular	Regular	Normal	37	?
7. TM 34M	Astrocytoma GII	+	–	Moderate	Regular	Regular	Normal	31	?
8. MS 47M	Astrocytoma GII	+	–	Moderate	Regular	Regular	Normal	?	7

M, male; F, female; CE, contrast enhancement; SI, surface infolding; TJ, tight junction; BL, basal lamina; PS, perivascular space; PV, pinocytotic vesicles

Summary

To elucidate the pathogenesis of perifocal edema in human brain tumors, we have observed the alteration of capillary permeability between the glioblastoma with pronounced edema (5 cases) and astrocytomas with slight edema (3 cases). Specimens were studied in conventional ultrathin sections and by the freeze-fracture replica technique.

In ultrathin sections of capillaries in glioblastomas, some of these cell junctions were tortuous and elongated, in fact, open. Other capillary abnormalities included endothelial hyperplasia with extensive vesicular formation, surface infolding of endothelial cells, irregularity of the basal lamina and the presence of a large collagen-filled extracellular space. In freeze-fracture replicas of capillary endothelium, the density of pinocytotic vesicles was markedly increased, reaching 25 per μm^2 on average. The tight junction in one area resembled a network of six strands, composed of about 100-Å particles, but in another area it looked like one or two strands.

The blood vessels appeared relatively normal in ultrathin sections of astrocytoma. In freeze-fracture replicas, pinocytotic vesicles increased markedly in density, to 34 per μm^2 on average. The tight junction was seen as a network of seven strands.

We conclude that the fact that there are fewer strands in the tight junction plays an important role in the increased permeability in the vessels of glioblastomas with severe perifocal edema, in addition to the increase in density of pinocytotic vesicles.

References

1. Bar-Sella P, Front D, Peyser E, Talmon A, Israel O, Nir I (1981) Correlation between radionuclides uptake and ultrastructural features of tight junctions in the capillary wall of meningiomas. J Neurol Neurosurg Psychiatry 44:1024–1028
2. Claude P, Goodenough DA (1973) Fracture faces of zonulae occludentes from "tight" and "leaky" epithelia. J Cell Biol 58:390–400
3. Simonescu M, Simonescu N, Palade GE (1974) Morphometric data on the endothelium of brain capillaries. J Cell Biol 60:128–152
4. Simonescu M, Simonescu N, Palade GE (1975) Segmental differentiations of cell junction in the vascular endothelium. The microvasculature. J Cell Biol 67:863–885
5. Singer SJ, Nicolson GL (1972) The fluid mosaic model of the structure of cell membranes. Cell membranes are viewed as two-dimensional solutions of oriented globular proteins and lipids. Science 175:720–731
6. Tani E, Ikeda K, Kudo S, Yamagata S, Higashi N, Fujihara E (1974) Fenestrated vessels in human hemangioblastoma. J Neurosurg 40:696–705
7. Wade JB, Karnovsky MJ (1974) Fracture faces of osmotically disrupted zonulae occludentes. J Cell Biol 62:344–350

Early Permeability Change of Macromolecules After Transient Global Ischemia

H. ARAI[1], M. SUZUKI, J. SUZUKI, and Y. IWASAKI

Key words: Global ischemia, blood-brain barrier, macromolecular tracer, Evans blue, horseradish peroxidase

Introduction

Vascular permeability to macromolecular tracers is known to increase in various types of brain damage [1, 3, 4]. In transient ischemia with hypoxia, extravasation of Evans blue–albumin complex (EB) and horseradish peroxidase (HRP) may take place by different mechanisms [1]. The early changes in vascular permeability to HRP and EB were studied by electron and fluorescence microscopy in rats subjected to three-vessel occlusion.

Materials and Methods

In male Wistar rats weighing 200–250 g anesthesia was induced with ether and, after tracheotomy, maintained with halothane with the aid of a Harvard rodent respirator 680. The basilar artery was exposed by a cervicoclival approach and dissected after electrocoagulation under an operating microscope. The bilateral common carotid arteries were temporarily occluded with Scoville's clips for 10 or 30 min. The rats with 10-min occlusion survived for 10, 30 and 60 min after the release of bilateral common carotid arteries, and those with 30-min occlusion survived for 10 and 30 min after the restoration of flow. At 5 min before sacrifice, the animals were given horseradish peroxidase (Type II, Sigma) 100 000 units/kg and 2% Evans blue 1 ml/kg via the femoral vein. Physiological variables such as blood pressure and electroencephalogram (EEG) were monitored continuously during the experiment. At the end of the experiment each animal was intracardially perfused with 200 ml heparinized normal saline and then with a mixture of 0.5% glutaraldehyde and 4% paraformaldehyde in Millonig's phosphate buffer at a pressure of 120 mmHg. Coronal sections were made with a cryostat from a brain slice through the optic chiasm and carefully examined for the presence of EB with a fluorescence microscope. The adjacent brain slice was cut into 50-μm sections with a vibratome and incubated for

[1] Divisions of Neurosurgery and Neuropathology, Institute of Brain Diseases, Tohoku University School of Medicine, 1-1 Seiryo-cho, Sendai City 980, Japan

peroxidase activity. HRP-positive areas of the brain were selected and processed for electron microscopy. The tissue for electron microscopy was post-fixed in osmium tetroxide, dehydrated through graded alcohols, and embedded in epoxy resin. Ultrathin sections were evaluated for HRP reaction products by a Hitachi H-600 electron microscope operating at 100 kV.

Results

In the control group, no extravascular leakage of either EB or HRP was detected with fluorescence and light microscopes. Even electron microscopic examination rarely revealed HRP, and any present was confined exclusively to the pinocytotic vesicles of the endothelium.

In the 10-min ischemia group (Fig. 1), as early as 10 min after release of the occlusion a few small foci of extravascular leakage of both EB and HRP were found in the cerebral cortex, hippocampus, and basal ganglia. The severity of extravasation of the tracers did not change after prolonged reflow.

In the 30-min ischemia group (Figs. 2–4) the leakage of HRP was more severe than that in rats subjected to 10-min ischemia. However, the number of EB-positive vessels and the intensity of fluorescence were similar to those in the 10-min ischemia group. Again, the severity of extravasation of EB and HRP was not different between animals with 10-min reflow and those with 30-min reflow.

In the electron microscopic examination (Figs. 5 and 6), the vessels in these lesions were seen to have increased numbers of pinocytotic vesicles with HRP re-

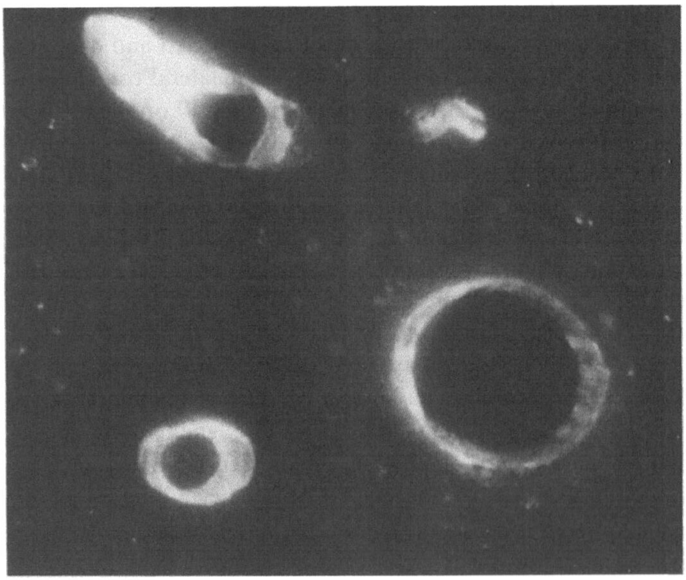

Fig. 1. Fluorescence photomicrograph of small vessels in the thalamus of the rat subjected to 10 min ischemia and 10 min reflow

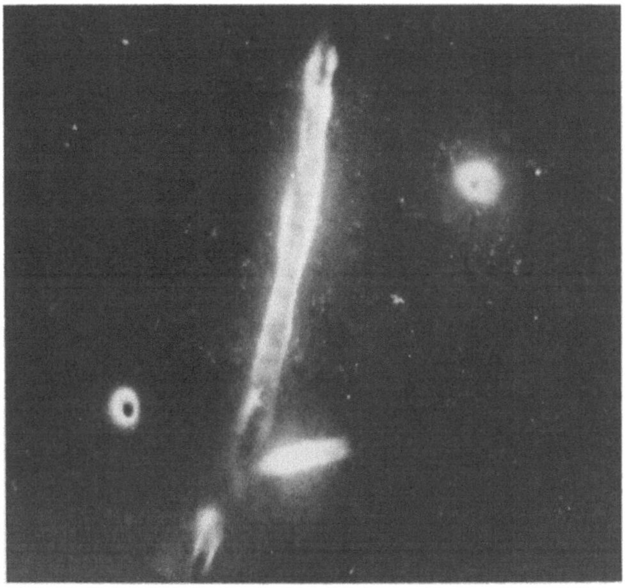

Fig. 2. Fluorescence photomicrograph showing the profile of the cerebral vessels with EB in the cortex of the rat subjected to 30 min ischemia and 10 min reflow

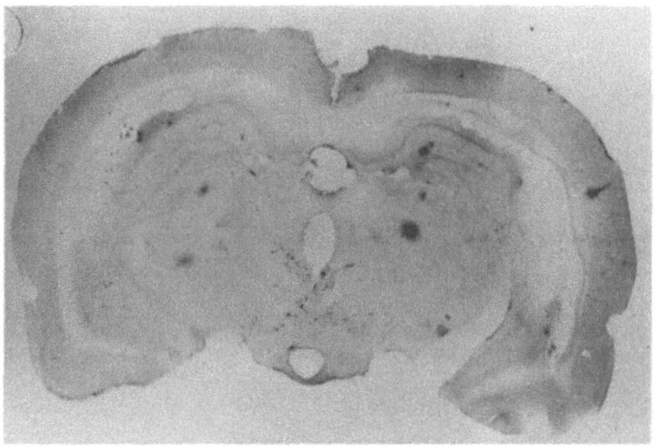

Fig. 3. Photomicrograph after 30 min ischemia and 10 min reflow. HRP reaction products are seen scattered through the cortex, hippocampus, and basal ganglia

action products, and the reaction products occasionally passed into the basement membrane and even into the intercellular spaces of the surrounding tissue. In the perivascular cerebral parenchyma, mild swelling of the perivascular astrocytic endfoot was occasionally seen. Between endothelial cells the tight junction did not seem to be disrupted. The HRP reaction products, however, often appeared to penetrate into the interjunctional spaces from the abluminal side of the vessel but not from the luminal side.

Discussion

The present study has clearly demonstrated that extravasation of both HRP and EB can occur within 10 min of reflow after transient global ischemia and the degree of the leakage does not depend on the duration of reflow time up to 1 h but it appar-

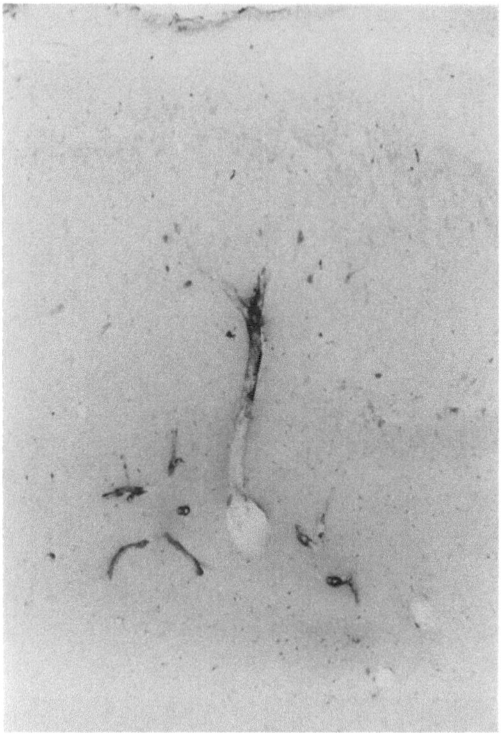

Fig. 4. Segments of large vessels 15–30 μm in diameter and containing HRP reaction products in their walls in the hippocampus

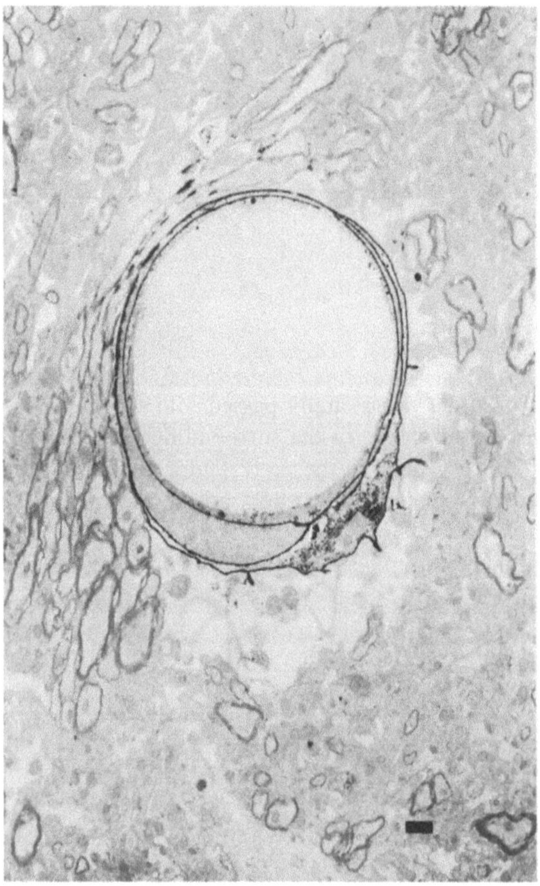

Fig. 5. Appearance after 30 min ischemia and 10 min reflow. HRP reaction products are seen in the basement membrane and even in the adjacent intercellular spaces. Swollen astrocytic processes are present adjacent to the vessel. (Bar = 1 μm)

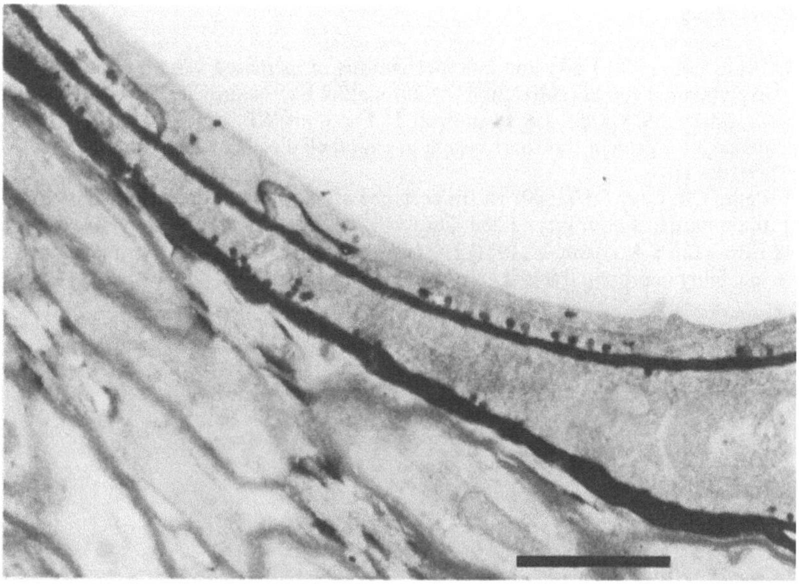

Fig. 6. Higher magnification of the same vessel as seen in Fig. 5 shows prominent pinocytosis of HRP and retrograde filling of HRP between the endothelium from the basement membrane. (Bar = 1 μm)

ently increases as a function of the duration of ischemia, at least in the case of HRP. At present, the leakage of HRP is thought to be due to the enhanced transendothelial vesiculocanalicular transport rather than to disruption or opening of tight junctions [1, 2], and in agreement with this hypothesis neither opening of the tight junction nor the passage of HRP through the intercellular space was verified in the present study. As the morphological studies suggest, if the transendothelial transport plays a major role in the leakage of HRP the increased vascular permeability during recirculation after ischemia could be an energy-dependent phenomenon. The mechanism of the leakage of EB is less clear than that of HRP, but diffuse staining of the vascular walls with EB seems to indicate that the leakage of EB may also reflect the increased transendothelial transport.

Summary

Transient global ischemia was induced in rats by occlusion of the basilar artery and temporary occlusion of the bilateral carotid arteries. Evans blue (EB) and horseradish peroxidase (HRP) were administrated 5 min before sacrifice to assess the permeability of the cerebral vessels to macromolecules following ischemic insult of 10, 30, or 60 min duration. There was an early change in permeability to EB and HRP within 10 min of reflow. There was no discrepancy in the vascular permeability to EB and HRP. Ultrastructural examination suggested that the change in permeability of the cerebral vessel to HRP was associated with the enhanced pinocytosis in the endothelial cells rather than with disruption or opening of the tight junction.

References

1. Petito CK (1979) Early and late mechanisms of increased vascular permeability following experimental cerebral infarction. J Neuropathol Exp Neurol 38:222–234
2. Lossinsky AS, Garcia JH, Iwanowski L, Lightfoot WE Jr. (1979) New ultrastructural evidence for a protein transport system in endothelial cells of gerbil brains. Acta Neuropathol 47:105–110
3. Petito CK, Levy DE (1980) The importance of cerebral arterioles in alterations of the blood-brain barrier. Lab Invest 43:262–268
4. Hossmann KA, Olsson Y (1971) The effect of transient cerebral ischemia on the vascular permeability to protein tracers. Acta Neuropathol 18:103–112

Disintegration of Orthogonal Arrays in Perivascular Astrocytic Processes as an Early Event in Acute Global Ischemia

M. SUZUKI[1], Y. IWASAKI, H. ARAI, T. YAMAMOTO, H. KONNO, T. YOSHIMOTO, and J. SUZUKI

Key words: Astrocyte, brain ischemia, orthogonal arrays, square assemblies, freeze-fracture

Introduction

Orthogonal arrays or square assemblies of intramembrane particles as revealed by a freeze-fracture technique are a distinctive specialization of the plasmalemma of certain types of cells [3]. In the mammalian central nervous system they have been observed in the astrocytes and ependymal cells. Although the function of membrane specialization has not yet been elucidated, a preponderance of the structure in the astrocytic processes facing small parenchymal vessels and subarachnoid spaces has led to the assumption that they might be involved in transport into and out of these compartments [1]. In addition, rapid disappearance of orthogonal arrays after circulatory arrest has recently been reported in the astrocytic membrane of the mouse brain [4].

In an effort to understand the role of this membrane specialization in the development of ischemic brain damage, we conducted sequential and quantitative observations of the freeze-fracture profiles of the astrocytic processes surrounding small cortical vessels of rats in acute global ischemia.

For a quantitative analysis of orthogonal arrays in astrocytic processes, three well-fixed rats were selected from each of the ischemic groups and five from the control group. In individual animals, 50 profiles of the astrocytic processes facing blood vessels were examined for the presence of either orthogonal arrays on the protoplasmic face or pits on the extracellular face of the plasma membrane.

Results

Histopathological examinations of paraffin sections revealed no abnormalities except for the presence of dark neurons occasionally encountered in animals subjected to ischemia for 30 and 60 min.

In thin sections, ultrastructural alterations of astrocytic processes became evident first in the animals of the 30-min ischemia group. Some perivascular astrocytic pro-

[1] Divisions of Neurosurgery and Neuropathology, Institute of Brain Diseases, Tohoku University School of Medicine, 1-1 Seiryo-cho, Sendai City 980, Japan

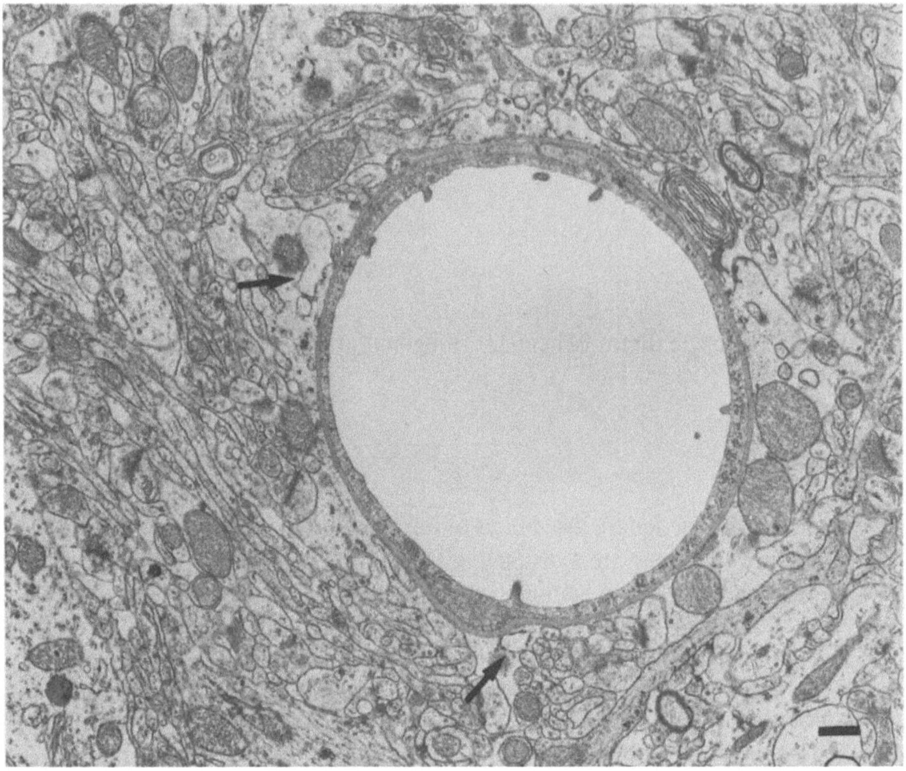

Fig. 1. Electron micrograph of a portion of deep cerebral cortex of a rat subjected to 30 min global ischemia. Note the swelling of the astrocytic processes with dilated rough endoplasmic reticulum (*arrows*). *Bar* = 1 μm

cesses appeared watery and swollen, while the rough endoplasmic reticula (rERs) were dilated and the ribosomes were detached from the rERs (Fig. 1). In the 60-min ischemia group astrocytic perikarya were also swollen. In contrast to obvious alterations in astrocytes, changes in neuronal cells were inconspicuous even in the sections from animals in the 60-min ischemia group.

In the deeper cortex of control animals, orthogonal arrays and pits (Fig. 2) were found only in the perivascular astrocytic processes. In controls they were encountered in approximately 70% of 50 profiles of perivascular astrocytic processes randomly examined (32.2 ± 5.4, mean ± SD). The tightly packed subunits seen in controls decreased in number as a function of the duration of ischemia, and in the ischemic groups, amorphous masses of large particles were more conspicuous in the plasma membrane of perivascular astrocytic processes. The number of the astrocytic processes with orthogonal arrays decreased even in the 5-min ischemia group (Fig. 3).

Fig. 3. Number of freeze-fracture profiles of perivascular astrocytic processes with orthogonal arrays or pits. Fifty profiles were examined for each animal. *Bar,* mean ± SD (From Suzuki [5])

Fig. 2. **A** Freeze-fracture profile of a perivascular astrocytic process in a 5-min ischemia rat. Note coexistence of orthogonal arrays (*asterisk*) and large disintegrated particles. *Bar*= 10 μm. **B** Pits in the astrocytic membrane of a 60-min ischemia rat. *Bar*= 10 μm

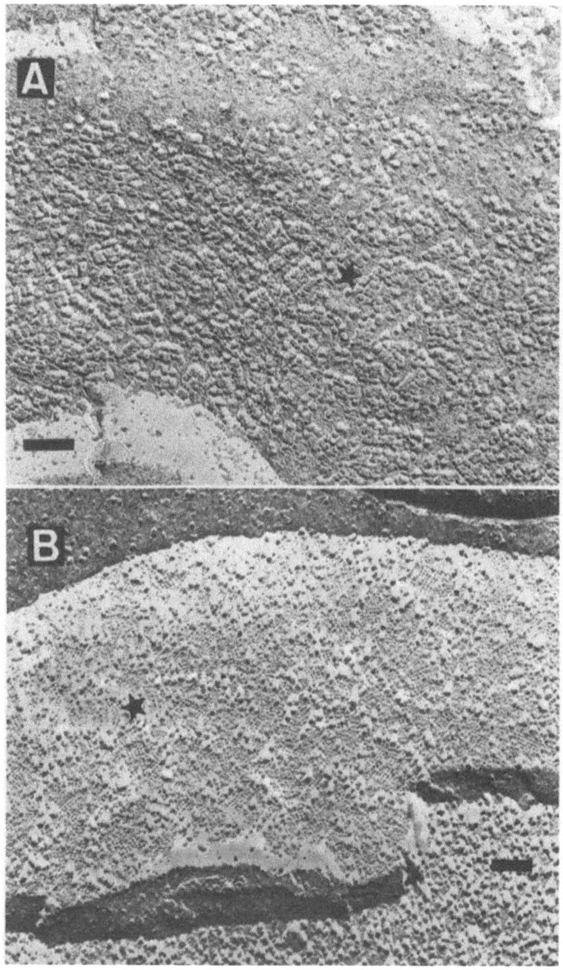

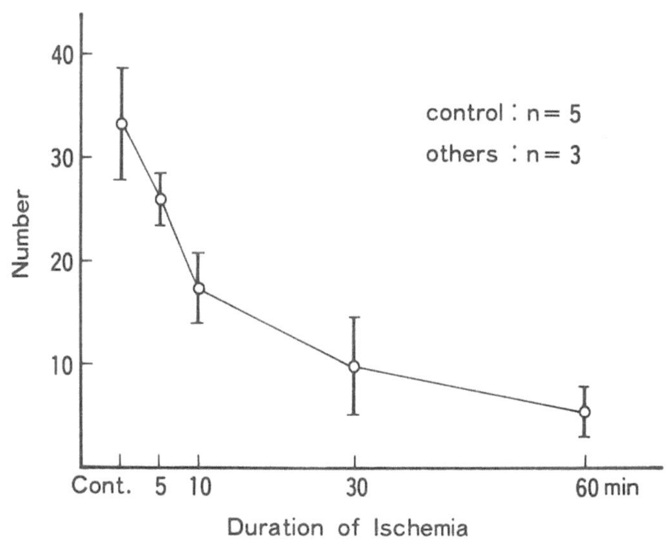

The number fell to half that in controls in the 10-min ischemia group, where swelling of the astrocytic process had not yet been detected by transverse electron microscopy. Apparently, disintegration of the orthogonal arrays preceded the swelling of the perivascular astrocytic processes.

Conclusion

At present, little is known about the factors regulating the assembly of the intramembrane particles, and the mechanism of astrocytic swelling appeared to be multifactorial [2]. Thus, the role of the particle assemblies in the development of astrocytic swelling has yet to be elucidated. It is now clear, however, that the orthogonal arrays in perivascular astrocytic processes, like those in the glial limitans [4], are labile under ischemic conditions and that disintegration of the structure apparently precedes the swelling of the astrocytic processes.

Summary

A quantitative freeze-fracture study of perivascular astrocytic processes in rat cerebral cortex disclosed rapid disintegration of orthogonal arrays of the intramembrane particles in acute global ischemia. The process apparently preceded the development of astrocytic swelling.

References

1. Anders JJ, Brightman MW (1970) Assemblies of particles in the cell membranes of developing, mature and reactive astrocytes. J Neurocytol 8:777–795
2. Hertz L (1981) Features of astrocytic function apparently involved in the response of central nervous tissue to ischemia-hypoxia. J Cereb Blood Flow Metab 1:143–153
3. Landis DMD, Reese TS (1974) Arrays of particles in freeze-fractured astrocytic membrane. J Cell Biol 60:316–320
4. Landis DMD, Reese TS (1981) Astrocytic membrane structure: Changes after circulatory arrest. J Cell Biol 88:660–663
5. Suzuki M (1984) Disintegration of orthogonal arrays in perivascular astrocytic processes as an early event in acute global ischemia. Brain Res 300:141–145

Arachidonic Acid Induces Opening of the Blood-Brain Barrier*

A. UNTERBERG [1], M. WAHL, and A. BAETHMANN

Key words: Arachidonic acid, free radicals, blood-brain barrier opening, cerebral arteries, cerebral veins

Introduction

A broad spectrum of cerebral insults causes a liberation of arachidonic acid in brain tissue. The membrane-bound arachidonic acid pool decreases markedly during hypoxia and a few minutes after the onset of cerebral ischemia [3, 7]. Moreover, recirculation after ischemia is associated with the appearance of metabolites of arachidonic acid, such as prostaglandins and leukotrienes [11]. Experimentally induced seizures also induce release of free unsaturated fatty acids [2]. Moreover, considerable amounts of arachidonic acid were detected in vasogenic edema fluid produced by a cortical freezing lesion [9]. In addition, this compound has been detected in CSF of patients with severe head injuries [10]. Arachidonic acid and its metabolites, prostaglandins, leukotrienes, and free radicals are regarded as potent mediators of secondary brain damage such as cytotoxic and vasogenic brain edema [1]. Exposure of brain slices to arachidonic acid induces cytotoxic cell swelling [5]. Inhibition of Na^+/K^+-ATPase and uncoupling of oxidative phosphorylation are thought to be the molecular cytotoxic mechanisms [6]. Moreover, arachidonic acid and free radicals were found to produce endothelial lesions, such as "dome-like protrusions" and "craters" in cerebral arterioles when extravascularly applied to pial vessels [8].

The aim of the present investigations was to clarify the effect of arachidonic acid and free radicals on blood-brain barrier function and the vasomotor effects on cerebral arteries and veins.

Materials and Methods

Mongrel cats of about 3 kg body weight were anesthetized with α-chloralose (50 mg/kg IV), and a cranial window was made above the parietal region. A fluid reservoir was formed around the opening with a quick-setting dental cement. The

* The study reported in this paper was supported by a grant from the Deutsche Forschungsgemeinschaft (Ba 452/6-5).

[1] Institute for Surgical Research, Klinikum Großhadern, and University of Munich, Marchioninistr. 15, D-8000 Munich 70

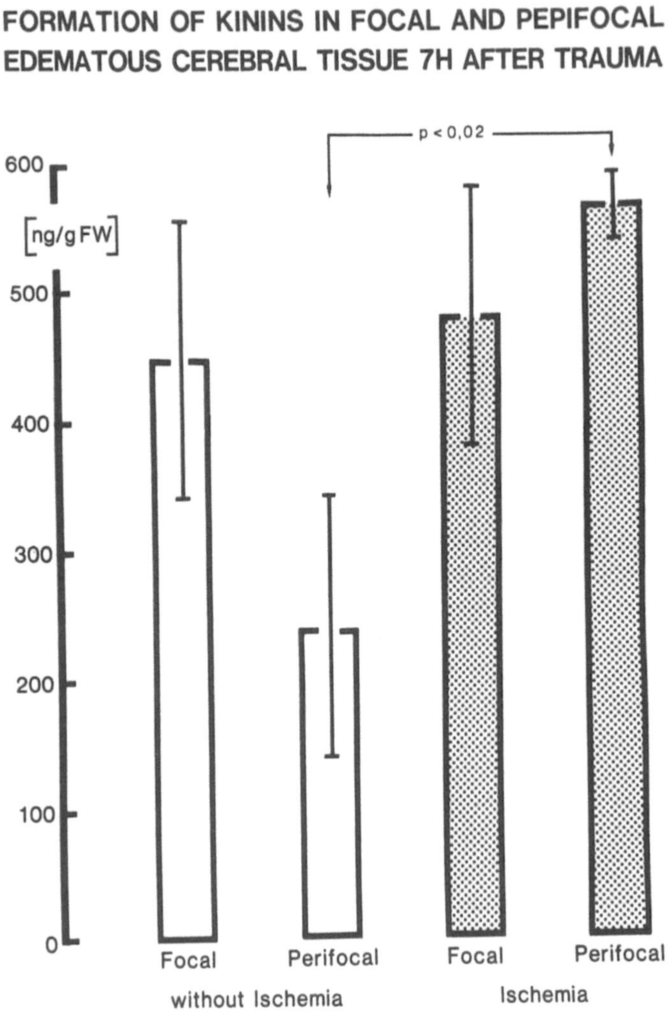

Fig. 1

dura was then covered with paraffin oil and slit. Na^+-fluorescein (mol. wt. 376), or fluorescein-labeled dextran (FITC-dextran, mol. wt. 19 400 or 62 000) was administered IV as a blood-brain barrier indicator. In a control period of 30 min, the exposed cerebral cortex was superfused with artificial CSF via plastic catheters perforating the wall of the reservoir. During this period, the indicators remained strictly confined within the intravascular space. Subsequently, Na^+-arachidonate (3×10^{-5} -3×10^{-3} *M*) dissolved in artificial CSF or xanthine-oxidase (0.25 units/ml) plus hypoxanthine (2 m*M)* was used for superfusion.

Changes in the blood-brain barrier permeability secondary to arachidonic acid or free radicals were intravitally observed by fluorescence microscopy [12, 13]. The vasomotor response of arteries and veins was determined from microphotographs.

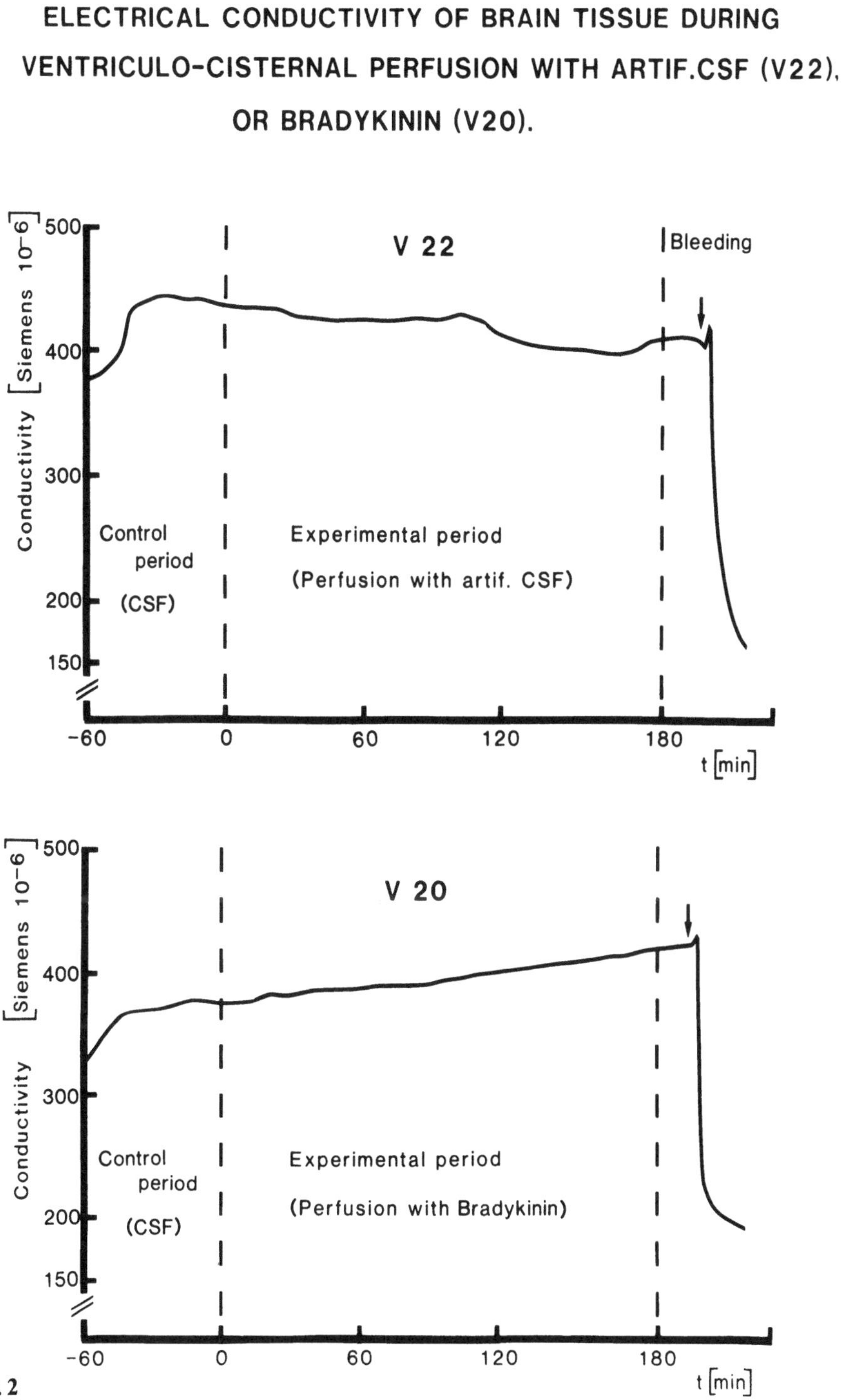
ELECTRICAL CONDUCTIVITY OF BRAIN TISSUE DURING
VENTRICULO-CISTERNAL PERFUSION WITH ARTIF.CSF (V22),
OR BRADYKININ (V20).
V 22
Bleeding
Conductivity [Siemens 10⁻⁶]
500
400
300
200
150
Control
period
(CSF)
Experimental period
(Perfusion with artif. CSF)
-60
0
60
120
180
t [min]
V 20
Conductivity [Siemens 10⁻⁶]
500
400
300
200
150
Control
period
(CSF)
Experimental period
(Perfusion with Bradykinin)
-60
0
60
120
180
t [min]

Fig. 2

Results and Discussion

Vasomotor Effects

The effect of arachidonic acid on the diameter of cerebral arteries is summarized in Table 1. Lower concentrations of arachidonic acid (3×10^{-5} and 3×10^{-4} *M*) induced a moderate constriction, whereas 3×10^{-3} *M* arachidonate revealed a slight dilatation. This is in disagreement with findings of other authors, who detected marked dilatations of feline pial arteries in response to arachidonic acid [4, 14].

Table 2 summarizes the effect of arachidonate on the diameter of pial veins. Significant changes of the diameters of veins could not be detected either after 1 or after 30 min of administration of arachidonic acid.

Superfusion of the free radical generating system (xanthine-oxidase plus hypoxanthine) induced a dramatic increase of the vascular diameter in arteries and veins, up to 200% and more of the initial resting diameter. The dilatating response

Table 1. Vascular diameter of pial arteries as percentage of control diameter 1 and 30 min after superfusion with Na^+ arachidonate

		Na^+ arachidonate (*M*)		
		3×10^{-5}	3×10^{-4}	3×10^{-3}
1 min	$\bar{x}$	91.95*	89.88*	101.05
	SEM	±1.65	±1.79	±3.88
	n	12	14	13
30 min	$\bar{x}$	87.78*	90.69*	109.42*
	SEM	±3.10	±2.24	±4.24
	n	9	14	13

* Significantly different from resting diameter ($P < 0.05$ or less)

Table 2. Vascular diameter of pial veins as percentage of control diameter 1 and 30 min after superfusion with Na^+ arachidonate

		Na^+ arachidonate (*M*)		
		3×10^{-5}	3×10^{-4}	3×10^{-3}
1 min	$\bar{x}$	102.18	99.65	98.38
	SEM	±1.72	±1.76	±3.41
	n	14	15	11
30 min	$\bar{x}$	97.66	96.23	97.18
	SEM	±2.22	±2.89	±2.92
	n	10	16	9

appeared immediately upon administration of the substances and was not attenuated as exposure continued.

Blood-Brain Barrier Permeability

When Na^+ fluorescein was used as barrier indicator it was seen that the minimum concentration of Na^+ arachidonate inducing extravasation was 3×10^{-5} *M* in two experiments. In three experiments a concentration of 3×10^{-4} *M* was required to open the barrier and in another two experiments as much as 3×10^{-3} *M* Na^+ arachidonate caused increased permeability of pial vessels. Superfusion with this concentration also induced barrier opening for larger indicators such as FITC-dextran (19 400 and 62 000 mol. wt.).

The variability of arachidonate concentrations causing barrier opening cannot be directly explained by findings recorded in our experiments. It may perhaps result from metabolism of the fatty acid to free radicals or other intermediates, since it was also demonstrated that superfusion of the cortex with the free radical-generating system caused barrier damage.

Superfusion of xanthine oxidase plus hypoxanthine induced leakage of Na^+ fluorescein and FITC dextran in distinct areas, preferentially around small venules. Superfusion with xanthine oxidase alone, however, did not induce any leakage. Further experiments should elucidate whether prostaglandins or leukotrienes also induce barrier disturbances and whether inhibition of arachidonate metabolism prevents barrier opening.

Taken together, extravascular administration of arachidonate and a free radical-generating system induces gross opening of the blood-brain barrier. Substantial structural damage to endothelial cells is the most likely cause of barrier opening. This damage might be attributable to arachidonic acid itself or to its intermediates, such as free radicals. The findings support the concept that release of arachidonic acid in injured brain enhances secondary damaging processes, such as blood-brain barrier dysfunction.

Acknowledgements. We highly appreciate the excellent technical and secretarial help of Angelika Konrad, Ulrike Goerke, and Ruth Demmer.

Summary

Arachidonic acid is released after various insults to the brain, e.g., seizures, ischemia, or head injury. The fatty acid and its metabolites are considered as mediators of secondary brain damage, such as brain edema. The purpose of the present investigations was to study the effect of arachidonic acid and free radicals on blood-brain barrier function and on the vasomotor response of cerebral vessels under physiological conditions.

In chloralose anesthesia feline pial vessels were studied by intravital fluorescence microscopy. Intravenously administered Na^+ fluorescein (mol. wt. 376) and FITC dextran (mol. wt. 19 400 or 62 000) were used as blood-brain barrier indicators. The vasomotor response of arteries and veins to artificial CSF, Na^+ arachidonate

(3×10^{-5} to 3×10^{-3} *M*), or a free-radical-generating system (xanthine-oxidase plus hypoxanthine) was microphotographically determined.

Cortical superfusion with arachidonate caused extravasation of fluorescein and FITC dextran from the pial vasculature. Effective concentrations varied between individual experiments from 3×10^{-5} to 3×10^{-3} *M*. Arachidonate 3×10^{-3} *M* was always required to open the blood-brain barrier for FITC dextran. Extravasation of fluorescein and FITC dextran was also induced by exposure of the cerebral cortex to free radicals generated by xanthine-oxidase (0.25 units/ml) plus hypoxanthine (2 m*M*).

The diameters of arteries and veins were only minimally affected by arachidonate, but were found to increase markedly upon administration of the free-radical-generating system.

These findings support the concept that arachidonic acid and free radicals enhance blood-brain barrier dysfunction under pathophysiological conditions.

References

1. Baethmann A, Oettinger W, Rothenfußer W, Geiger R (1979) Biochemical aspect of cerebral edema. In: Mrsulja BB, Rakic LM, Klatzo I, Spatz M (eds) Pathophysiology of cerebral energy metabolism. Plenum, New York, pp 189–209
2. Bazan NG (1971) Changes in free fatty acids of brain by drug-induced convulsions, electroshock, and anesthesia. J Neurochem 18:1379–1385
3. Bazan NG, Rodriguez de Turco EB (1980) Membrane lipids in the pathogenesis of brain edema. – Phospholipids and arachidonic acid, the earlier membrane components changed at the onset of ischemia. Adv Neurol 28:197–205
4. Busija DW, Heistad D (1983) Effects of indomethacin on cerebral blood flow during hypercapnea in cats. Am J Physiol 244:H519–H524
5. Chan PH, Fishman RA (1978) Brain edema: Induction in cortical slices by polyunsaturated fatty acids. Science 201:358–360
6. Chan PH, Fishman RA, Longar S, Chen S, Chew S (1983) The role of arachidonic acid in cellular brain edema. In: Sun GY, Bazan NG, Wu JY, Porcellati G, Sun AY (eds) Neural membranes. Humana, Clifton, pp 141–152
7. Gardiner M, Nilsson B, Rehncrona S, Siesjö BK (1981) Free fatty acids in the rat brain in moderate and severe hypoxia. J Neurochem 36:1500–1505
8. Kontos HA, Wei EP, Povlishock JT, Dietrich WD, Magiera CJ, Ellis EF (1980) Cerebral arteriolar damage by arachidonic acid and prostaglandin G_2. Science 209:1242–1245
9. Maier-Hauff K, Lange M, Schürer L, Guggenbichler C, Vogt W, Jacob K, Baethmann A (1984) Glutamate and free fatty acid concentrations in extracellular vasogenic edema fluid. In: Go KG, Baethmann A (eds) Recent progress in the study and therapy of brain edema. Plenum, New York, pp 183–192
10. Maier-Hauff K, Baethmann A, Vogt W, Jacob K, Marguth F (1984) Mediator compounds in CSF of neurosurgical patients with raised intracranial pressure. In: Piotrowski W, Brock M, Klinger M (eds) Advances in neurosurgery, vol 12. Springer, Berlin Heidelberg New York, pp 302–306
11. Moskowitz MA, Kiwak KJ, Hekimian K, Levin L (1984) Synthesis of compounds with properties of leukotrienes C_4 and D_4 in gerbil brains after ischemia and reperfusion. Science 224:886–889
12. Unterberg A, Wahl M, Baethmann A (1985) Effects of bradykinin on permeability and diameter of pial vessels in-vivo. J Cereb Blood Flow Metab (in press)
13. Wahl M, Unterberg A, Baethmann A (1985) Intravital fluorescence microscopy for the study of blood-brain barrier function. Int J Microcirc Clin Exp (in press)
14. Wei EP, Ellis EF, Kontos HA (1980) Role of prostaglandins in pial arteriolar response to CO_2 and hypoxia. Am J Physiol 238:H226–H230

Cell Volume Regulation of Glial Cells During Anoxia and Hyposmotic Exposure In Vitro *

O. KEMPSKI[1], M. ZIMMER, A. NEU, F. VON ROSEN, and A. BAETHMANN

Key words: Cytotoxic brain edema, anoxia, cell volume regulation, glia, membrane permeability

Introduction

The swelling of dendrites and glial cells is a morphologically significant feature of cytotoxic brain edema, which is regularly observed in cerebral ischemia. Cellular hydrops is usually explained by a disturbed double Donnan equilibrium [10], and it is thought to be an immediate result of failing ion pumps in the presence of a reduced supply of metabolic energy.

The rapid onset of cell swelling, however, together with the complete breakdown of ion gradients as soon as 3 min after the induction of ischemia, strongly suggests an involvement of other factors than shortage of energy for the ion pumps alone.

A cytotoxic insult causes many physiological parameters to change simultaneously in vivo, making it almost impossible to analyze the underlying molecular processes. Therefore, an in vitro model has been devised to allow the study of effects of tissue damage (which leads to cytotoxic cell swelling in vivo) in strictly controlled conditions [7]. C-6 glioma cells are used as model cells with glial characteristics. The system allows fast and detailed analysis of pathophysiologically relevant changes in cell volume, intracellular electrolytes, and ion fluxes, and of such extracellular parameters as pH, PO_2, and lactate.

This report focuses on the effects of anoxia, and of anoxia combined with inhibition of anaerobic glycolysis, on glial cell volume, intracellular electrolyte concentrations, and transmembranous ion fluxes. The results suggest that depletion of brain metabolic energy alone does not explain ischemic cell swelling in vivo.

Methods

C-6 glioma cells were grown at 37° C in Dulbecco's MEM (DMEM) supplemented with 10% FCS in a humidified atmosphere of 5% CO_2 and 95% room air in plastic

---

* The study reported in this paper was supported by grants from the Deutsche Forschungsgemeinschaft (Ba 452/6-3 and Ke 338/1-1).

[1] Institute for Surgical Research, Ludwig-Maximilians University, Munich, Klinikum Großhadern, Marchioninistr. 15, D-8000 Munich 70

petri dishes. For the experiments the cells were harvested and suspended in a test chamber as previously described.

The cells were initially kept under control conditions (pH = 7.35, PO_2 = 60 mmHg, t = 37° C) for 30–60 min. This was followed by interruption of the oxygen supply to the chamber, which led to a drop of the PO_2 to 0 mmHg within approximately 5 min. In some experiments, iodoacetate (2.5 m*M*) was added to block glycolysis in both the presence and the absence of oxygen. Samples of suspended cells were collected from the incubation chamber before and during anoxia for various analyses, including cell volume.

In a second set of experiments, anoxia was combined with reduction of the osmolality of the medium to test the volume-regulatory capacity of the cells [7, 8]. For this purpose, hypotonic fluid was added to the chamber to reach a final osmolality of 160 mosmol/liter. The concentrations of potassium, calcium, and magnesium were kept normal.

Cell volume was measured by flow cytometry (Metricell) as described by Kachel [5]. Intracellular electrolytes were determined by atomic absorption spectophotometry. The cells were briefly washed in $CaCl_2$ (identical osmolality) and centrifuged through phthalate oil [4] to remove extracellular sodium. The remaining extracellular contamination was assessed by the addition of tritiated inulin.

Transmembranous sodium and potassium fluxes were studied in nontrypsinized cultures using sodium-22 and potassium-42 in parallel experiments.

Results and Discussion

Glial cells in vitro maintain a constant cell volume for more than 2 h when exposed either to anoxia alone or to anoxia plus iodoacetate (Table 1). Cell swelling did not occur in either group, even with complete anoxia documented by the marked rise of extracellular lactate to almost double the concentration found in normoxic experiments. This was never observed when iodoacetate had been added, proving the effective inhibition of glycolysis.

On the other hand, in the anoxic group anaerobic glycolysis was obviously sufficient to maintain ion gradients, whereas anoxia plus iodoacetate led to a marked depletion of intracellular potassium ($P < 0.05$, Table 1). Conversely, intracellular sodium increased in these circumstances, though without attaining statistical significance.

As described before [7, 8], exposure of C-6 glial cells to hypotonicity led to immediate swelling, with volumes up to 150% of the control volume. Swelling was followed by a regulatory volume decrease (RVD) to normal cell size. Corresponding findings recorded in the current experiments are given in Table 2, where the approximate swelling maxima are calculated from best-fit regressions of the volume decay curves for only the first 15 min of hypotonic exposure. All four groups had an initial regulatory decrease in cell volume. However, when hypotonic exposure had been combined with anoxia and iodoacetate, secondary swelling developed. The volume of these cells after 60 min exposure was again 44% above normal.

These findings may have particular significance for the in vivo situation, since glial cells of the ischemic brain have to cope with sudden changes in the extracellu-

Table 1. Cell volumes and intracellular potassium and sodium concentrations of C-6 glioma cells and extracellular lactate before and after normoxia, anoxia, and anoxia+iodoacetate (2.5 m*M*)

	Preincubation (60 min)				Experimental Incubation (120 min)			
	Cell vol. (μm³)	K^+ i.c. (m*M*)	Na^+ i.c. (m*M*)	Lactate (m*M*)	Cell vol. (μm³)	K^+ i.c. (m*M*)	Na^+ i.c. (m*M*)	Lactate (m*M*)
Normoxia (*n*=7)	1007.9 ±20.0	167.1 ±26.8	22.4 ± 3.1	0.96 ±0.14	1032.4 ±38.9	166.6 ±43.0	26.0 ± 4.2	2.81 ±0.31
Anoxia (*n*=6)	1012.9 ±30.1	160.4 ±12.5	47.8 ±16.3	1.07 ±0.21	1087.0 ±26.9	155.4 ±14.6	40.3 ±11.3	4.19 ±0.38
Anoxia + iodoacetate (*n*=7)	1051.6 ±49.9	153.5 ±12.6	16.5 ± 3.7	1.30 ±0.17	1030.8 ±47.8	38.8 ± 7.8	50.2 ± 8.5	1.01 ±0.13

Electrolyte concentrations are expressed as micromoles per liter cell mass

Table 2. Cell volume and intracellular potassium and sodium concentrations of C-6 glioma cells before and after hyposmotic exposure

	Isotonic, 300 mosmol/liter			Hypotonic, 160 mosmol/liter					
	60 min preincubation			30 s, calculated data			60 min, measured data		
	Cell vol. (% control)	K^+ i.c. (m*M*)	Na^+ i.c. (m*M*)	Cell vol. (% control)	K^+ i.c. (m*M*)	Na^+ i.c. (m*M*)	Cell vol. (% control)	K^+ i.c. (m*M*)	Na^+ i.c. (m*M*)
Normoxia (*n*=6)	100	139.5 ±10.4	26.4 ±3.4	147.6	94.3	17.8	106.8 ±3.2	50.4 ± 6.4	19.1 ±3.5
Iodoacetate (*n*=6)	100	143.9 ±31.9	28.6 ±6.4	144.3	99.3	19.9	110.7 ±4.8	71.4 ±12.9	26.7 ±2.1
Anoxia (*n*=6)	100	120.6 ±10.8	13.7 ±2.5	144.2	83.8	9.5	116.2 ±8.9	62.1 ± 9.6	12.7 ±1.9
Anoxia + iodoacetate (*n*=6)	100	127.3 ±20.1	9.2 ±2.9	161.9	79.1	5.7	144.6 ±4.8	40.6 ± 9.4	48.7 ±5.9

The 30-s data are calculated from a regression analysis of cell volume changes during the first 15 min after osmotic swelling and from the isotonic electrolyte concentration

Table 3. Decrease in extracellular ^{42}K activity in C-6 glioma cells incubated in isotonic (300 mosmol/liter) and hypotonic (160 mosmol/liter) after a 2-h equilibration with ^{42}K

Time (min)	0.5	1	3	10	15	30	60
Isotonic exposure (^{42}K i.c., % of control)	94.7 ±2.2	93.1 ±3.5	90.8 ±1.4	82.9 ±2.9	74.6 ±1.5	60.3 ±3.9	44.8 ±5.3
Hypotonic exposure (^{42}K i.c., % of control)	90.3 ±0.8	88.9 ±0.8	59.8 ±7.1	46.3 ±6.8	38.6 ±3.4	27.7 ±4.1	8.1 ±1.4

Results are expressed as the percentage of ^{42}K found in the cells as against the ^{42}K activity after equilibration. Results from three identical experiments per group (± SD) are given

lar environment. The homeostatic maintenance of functions may involve volume regulatory mechanisms. Failure of homeostasis by glial cells would promote cytotoxic edema caused, for example, by an accumulation of "edema mediators" [3] such as neurotransmitters (especially glutamate [6]), free fatty acids, or potassium. This hypothesis is supported by findings of Ames et al. [1, 2] who studied the effects of anoxia in the isolated retina. Up to 40 min of anoxia and substrate deprivation were tolerated without significant swelling if retinas had been incubated in a large extracellular volume. On the other hand, retina did swell in response to anoxia if the extracellular volume was small or if the retinas were placed in medium previously conditioned by other anoxic retinas.

These findings underline the importance of cell volume regulation in anoxia. To attain further elucidation of the mechanisms involved in cell volume control, studies on membrane permeability for sodium and potassium were performed in C-6 glial cells during hyposmotic exposure. The data (Table 3) show that efflux of potassium from the cells was increased five times during the first 10 min of RVD. Influx of potassium was only slightly increased. Calculation of net fluxes showed a loss of potassium-42 from the cells, primarily during the first 5 min of volume regulation. Therefore, the initial phase of RVD can be attributed to an efflux of potassium accompanied by anions that have not yet been identified. However, a second mechanism seems to come into effect thereafter. Reestablishment of the membrane potential and extrusion of sodium ions may occur during this phase, as shown in cerebrovascular endothelium [9]. This secondary phase of RVD cannot be inhibited by ouabain [7] but is susceptible to metabolic deprivation, as shown in this study.

The fact that glial cells can maintain a normal volume in anoxia over a period of more than 2 h is still unexplained. MacKnight concedes, in a recent review on volume regulation [11], that if the loss of potassium from cells exceeds sodium entry, cells may initially even shrink. This was indeed observed in several experiments in this study. MacKnight concludes, however, that such shrinking should be transient and eventually followed by swelling. The present study demonstrates that glial cells can maintain cell volume much longer than observed in vivo after the complete stop of metabolic energy production. This suggests the involvement of other pathogenetic mechanisms during the formation of cytotoxic brain edema in vivo and not pump failure alone.

Hence, the in vitro results reported herewith support the hypothesis [3] that release or activation of mediator substances constitute the initial mechanisms of cell swelling during cerebral anoxia/ischemia. Only thereafter failure of energy supply supervenes as it interferes with the active processes providing maintenance of a normal cell volume.

These findings may obtain additional, clinical relevance, since they could open new pathways for the therapy of cytotoxic brain edema.

Summary

The experiments reviewed in this report demonstrate that anoxia of up to 2 h duration does not cause swelling of C-6 glioma cells in an in vitro system designed to study mechanisms of cytotoxic brain edema under controlled conditions. The cells do not even swell when anoxia is combined with iodoacetate to inhibit anaerobic glycolysis. On the other hand, complete shutdown of cellular energy production by anoxia plus iodoacetate abolishes the normalization of cell volume regulation after osmotic swelling in hypotonic medium, which is always found under normoxic conditions. It is concluded that depletion of brain metabolic energy, before causing so-called Donnan swelling, will primarily affect the capacity of cells to regulate cell volume. This is particularly relevant in conditions associated with the release or activation of extracellular edema mediators.

References

1. Ames A, Nesbett FB (1983) Pathophysiology of ischemic cell death. I: Time of onset of irreversible damage; importance of different components of the ischemic insult. Stroke 14:219
2. Ames A, Nesbett FB (1983) Pathophysiology of ischemic cell death. III: Role of extracellular factors. Stroke 14:233
3. Baethmann A, Oettinger W, Rothenfusser W, Kempski O, Unterberg A, Geiger R (1980) Brain edema factors. Current state with particular reference to plasma constituents and glutamate. Adv Neurol 28:171–195
4. Bui AH, Wiley JS (1981) Cation fluxes and volume regulation by human lymphocytes. J Cell Physiol 108:47–54
5. Kachel V (1976) Basic principles of electrical sizing of cells and particles and their realization in the new instrument 'Metrizell'. J Histochem Cytochem 24:211–230
6. Kempski O, Gross U, Baethmann A (1982) An in vitro model of cytotoxic brain edema: cell volume and metabolism of cultivated glial and nerve cells. In: Driesen W, Brock M, Klinger M (eds) Advances in Neurosurgery, vol 10. Springer, Berlin Heidelberg New York
7. Kempski O, Chaussy L, Gross U, Zimmer M, Baethmann A (1983) Volume regulation and metabolism of suspended C6 glioma cells: an in vitro model to study cytotoxic brain edema. Brain Res 279:217
8. Kempski O, Zimmer M, Chaussy L, Baethmann A (1984) Volume and metabolism of C6 glioma cells suspended in hypotonic medium: an in vitro model to study cytotoxic brain edema. In: Go KG, Baethmann A (eds) Recent progress in the study and therapy of brain edema. Plenum, New York
9. Kempski O, Spatz M, Valet G, Baethmann A (1985) Cell volume regulation of cerebrovascular endothelium in vitro. J Cell Physiol
10. MacKnight ADC, Leaf A (1977) Regulation of cellular volume. Physiol Rev 37:510
11. MacKnight ADC (1984) Cellular response to injury. In: Staub NC, Taylor AE (eds) Edema. Raven, New York

Cerebral Blood Flow, Energy Utilization, Serotonin Metabolism, (Na, K)ATPase Activity, and Postischemic Brain Swelling

B. B. MRŠULJA [1], B. M. DJURIČIĆ, Y. UEKI, R. CAHN, V. CVEJIĆ, H. MARTINEZ, D. V. MIĆIĆ, T. STOJANOVIĆ, and M. SPATZ

Key words: Brain, edema, factors

Introduction

Cerebral blood flow (CBF) is normally tightly controlled to match the level of oxidative metabolism in the brain. However, numerous studies have pointed out a lack of any association between blood flow and metabolism in various pathophysiologic conditions [3, 7]. Recently, the concept of "ischemic flow threshold(s)" has been developed; these thresholds refer to those critical low levels of blood flow, and consequently oxygen supply, at which energy-requiring cell functions fail [2]. An upper ischemic flow threshold (CBF 16–20 ml/min/100 g tissue) is associated with the failure of synaptic transmission and lower ischemic threshold (below 10 ml/min/100 g tissue) and with membrane failure, as indicated by net Na^+-K^+ leakage and tissue swelling with simultaneous ATP depletion [1].

Reintroduction of oxygen and glucose to an ischemic tissue triggers a series of events, some of which are unique to the postischemic period. It has been shown that reestablishment of CBF after 15 min of circulatory arrest in the gerbil markedly enhances the formation of brain edema [12]. Among the factors contributing to the development of brain edema the following have been considered: energy failure which leads to an equilibration of ion concentration gradients across the cell membrane [8]; brain hypoperfusion [17]; hypoactivity of (Na, K)ATPase [12]; and dysfunction of serotonin metabolism [4, 13].

The objective of this study was to correlate the levels of CBF, energy status and metabolism, serotonin level and turnover, and (Na, K)ATPase activity in the hippocampus of gerbils exposed to either 5 or 15 min of ischemia and 1 h of reflow with the degree of brain swelling. The hippocampus is likely to be the most sensitive structure with reference to the effects of ischemia [9]. Our preliminary study revealed that brain edema is different in degree 1 h after 5 and 15 min of ischemia.

Materials and Methods

Edematous changes in the gerbil hippocampus associated with bilateral occlusion of the common carotid arteries were studied in animals subjected to either 5 or 15 min

[1] CVD Research Group, Institute of Biochemistry, School of Medicine, Višegradska 26, 11000 Belgrade, Yugoslavia

of ischemia followed by 1 h of reflow. Animals were prepared as described by Kirino [9].

For the measurement of ATP, P-creatine, glucose, lactate, and serotonin contents, gerbils were sacrificed by microwave irradiation (1.25 kW to the head, 2.3 s). (Na, K)ATPase activity was measured in the preparation of synaptosomal membranes. Serotonin turnover was measured by a pharmacological approach according to which the monoamine oxidase inhibitor pargyline HCl (75 mg/kg body weight IP) was administered 60 min before sacrifice and amine levels were determined by the method of Laverty and Taylor [10]. Cerebral blood flow was measured by the hydrogen clearance technique [15], with a platinum electrode stereotaxically introduced into the hippocampus.

The utilization rate of immediate energy reserves (URIER) was estimated by the method of least-squares analysis of the decline in (ATP + P-creatine) during 60 s of ischemia and refers to the half-time (t/2). Glucose, lactate, ATP, and P-creatine levels were determined in neutralized perchloric acid extracts by enzymatic fluorimetric procedures [11]. The brain water content was obtained by the wet tissue/dry tissue procedure and the volume of brain swelling was calculated [6].

Results

Cerebral Blood Flow and Brain Swelling

The cerebral blood flow measured at the end of 5 and 15 min ischemia was 12.2 ± 2.3 ml/min/100 g tissue and 6.8 ± 1.0 ml/min/100 g tissue, respectively. Tissue swelling was 0.4% and 1.9%, respectively. Therefore, the CBF level of 12.2 ml/min/100 g tissue was above the assumed critical threshold for edema formation. After 1 h of reflow hypoperfusion was found in both groups (31.9 in the 5-min group and 23.3 ml/min/100 g tissue in the 15-min group), while brain swelling was markedly increased in the 15-min ischemia group only (Table 1). However, it should be

Table 1. Cerebral blood flow, water content, brain swelling, and (Na, K)ATPase activity in gerbil hippocampus 1 h after either 5 or 15 min of ischemia

Parameter	Control	1 h after ischemia for	
		5 min	15 min
Cerebral blood flow (ml/min/100 g)	136.0 ±0.7	31.9 ±5.9[a]	23.3 ±2.8[a]
Water content (ml/100 g wet weight)	78.29±0.04	78.483±0.051	78.99±0.04
Brain swelling (calculated; %)	–	0.9	3.9
(Na, K)ATPase activity (nMol Pi/min/mg protein)	106±10	97±2	31±3[a]

Numbers given are means ± SEM for 5–8 animals.

[a] Statistically significant difference ($P < 0.01$; Student's *t*-test) compared with control

pointed out that in the 5-min ischemia group the CBF level was higher, with 8.6 ml/min/100 g tissue, than in the 15-min ischemia group at 1 h after ischemia. In both animal groups the CBF levels during reflow were markedly above the assumed critical level for edema formation.

URIER and the Level of Energy Metabolites

During the period of hypoperfusion (1 h after either 5 or 15 min of ischemia) the hippocampal levels of glucose were significantly enhanced in both groups, while lactate was above normal only in the 15-min ischemia group (Table 2). ATP and P-creatine recovered normal levels in the 5-min ischemia group, but in the 15 min group these metabolites were not fully normalized (Table 2). These changes in lactate, ATP, and P-creatine content correspond to the more severe hypoperfusion recorded in the 15-min than in the 5-min ischemia group (Table 1). The half-time (t/2) for URIER at 1 h after 5 min ischemia was close to normal, while it was about three times the normal duration in the 15-min ischemia group (Fig. 1). These data suggest a diminished ability of edematous tissue to utilize immediate energy reserves.

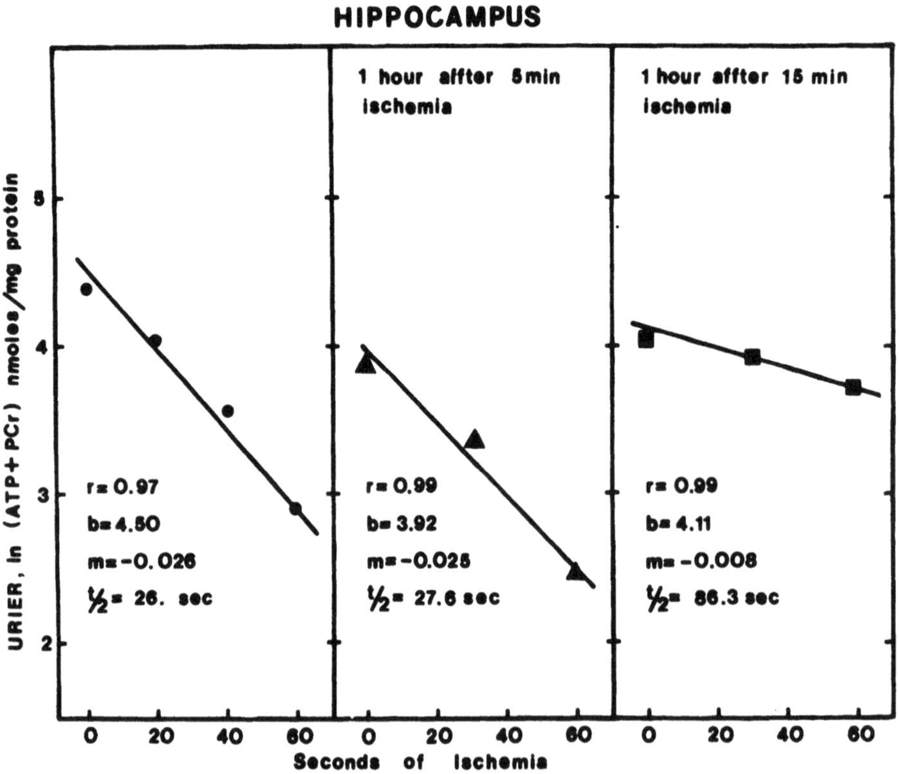

Fig. 1. Decline of immediate energy reserves (ATP + P-creatine) during 60 s of ischemia in gerbil hippocampus. Utilization rate of immediate energy reserves (*URIER*) refers to the half-time. Note that (ATP + P-creatine) concentrations are given as ln values

Table 2. ATP, P-creatine, glucose, and lactate in gerbil hippocampus 1 h after either 5 or 15 min of ischemia

Parameter (nMol/mg protein)	Control	1 h after ischemia for	
		5 min	15 min
ATP	28.9±1.6	25.3±0.8	18.6±1.3[a]
P-Creatine	50.9±3.7	48.0±1.6	38.4±2.8[b]
Glucose	13.7±0.6	24.4±1.0[b]	20.6±2.2[b]
Lactate	9.1±1.9	11.0±3.4	39.0±4.4

Numbers given are means ± SEM for 5–8 animals.
[a,b] Statistically significant difference (Student's *t*-test; [a] $P<0.01$, [b] $P<0.05$) compared with control

Table 3. Serotonin content and serotonin turnover rate in gerbil hippocampus 1 h after either 5 or 15 min of ischemia

Parameter	Control	1 h after ischemia for	
		5 min	15 min
Serotonin content (ng/g wet weight)	614±62	613±52	625±93
Serotonin turnover rate (μg/h/g wet weight)	0.542±0.031	0.536±0.042	0.842±0.034[a]

Numbers given are means ± SEM for 7 animals
[a] Statistically significant difference ($P<0.01$; Student's *t*-test) compared with control

Serotonin Levels and Turnover

The levels of serotonin (5-HT) were the same in both ischemic groups and in controls; however, in the 15-min ischemia group the 5-HT turnover rate was increased (Table 3). Therefore, brain swelling is coincident with the increased release of the monoamine.

(Na, K)ATPase and Its Kinetics

Reduced activity of (Na, K)ATPase was found after 1 h of reflow following 15 min of ischemia, but not following 5 min of ischemia (Table 1). The observed reduction in (Na, K)ATPase activity corresponds to the postischemic brain swelling.

Kinetic studies reveal that in the 15-min ischemia group affinity of the enzyme for the substrate decreased 2.5-fold (K_m in controls is 3.9 mMol, as against 10.0 mMol in the ischemic group; Figs. 2 and 3).

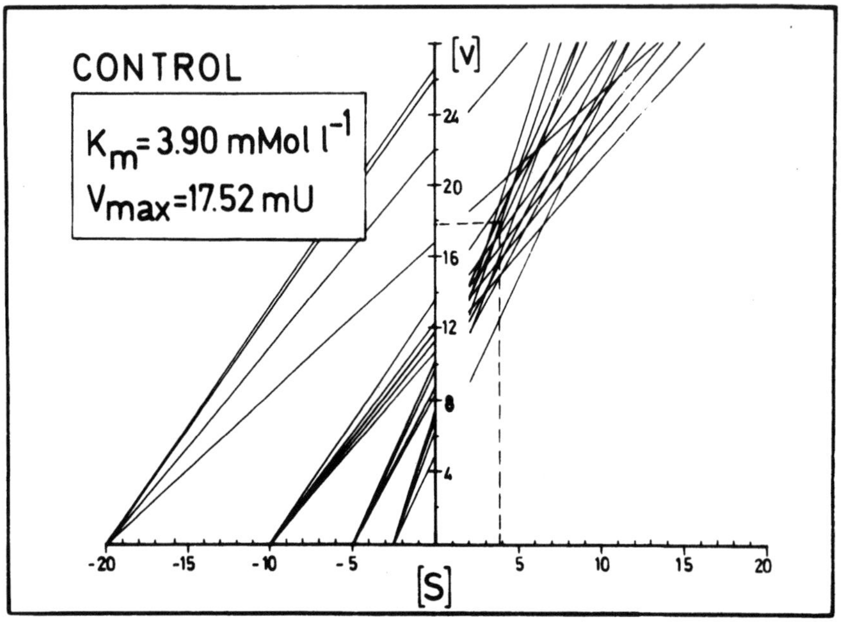

Fig. 2. Kinetic plot of (Na, K)ATPase activity in gerbil brain; rate of *p*-nitrophenyl phosphate hydrolysis (*V*) is plotted against substrate concentration (*S*). Method used for estimation of K_m and V_{max} is that of Eisenthal and Cornish-Bowden [5]

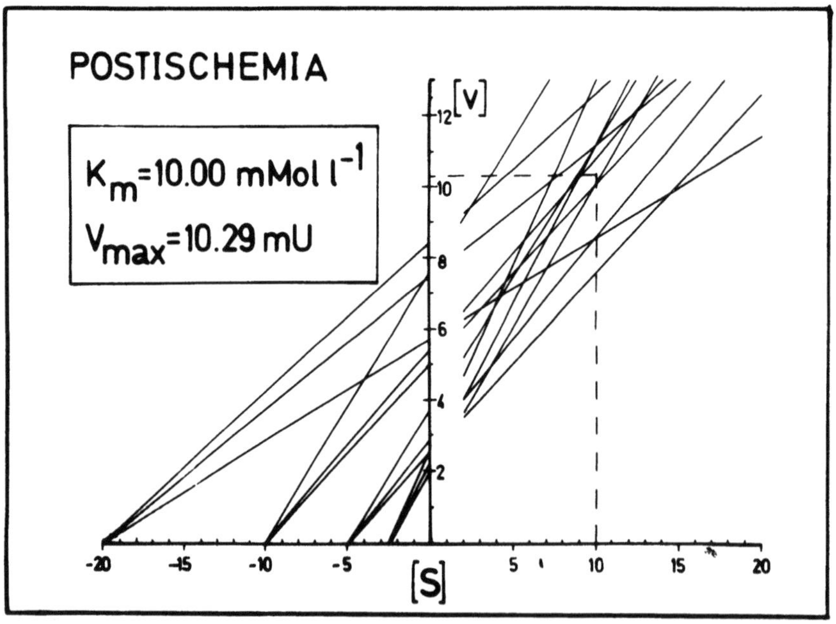

Fig. 3. Kinetic plot of (Na, K)ATPase activity in gerbil brain after 15 min of ischemia. Other conventions as in Fig. 2

Discussion

The accumulation of water in a tissue is common in ischemia and subsequent reflow. It appears that brain edema during ischemia is related to the degree of cerebral blood flow reduction and the duration of interruption of the blood supply. In this study, when CBF remained above 10 ml/min/100 g tissue (5 min of ischemia) brain swelling was insignificant (0.4%). When CBF was reduced below 10 ml/min/100 g tissue (15 min of ischemia) there was marked brain swelling by 1.9%.

The pathogenic mechanisms involved in the development of edema induced by ischemia are complex and the subject of some controversy. It might be expected that an increase in tissue water content would occur when the ionic pump breaks down as a consequence of the energy failure caused by the blood supply cessation. However, depletion of tissue energy reserves seems not to be a major mechanism of edema formation, because the time courses of the decrease in high-energy phosphates (ATP + P-creatine) and the development of ischemic brain edema do not appear to be interrelated. ATP and P-creatine are reduced to below 10% of the initial values within 90 s after the onset of ischemia [14], whereas brain swelling appears if CBF is below 10 ml/min/100 g tissue (ischemia for longer than 5 min); this CBF level is the ischemic threshold for edema formation. Yet this ischemic CBF threshold does not account for postischemic brain swelling: at 1 h after either 5 or 15 min of ischemia hypoperfusion was present, but the actual figures were far above the critical value (Table 1). Brain swelling, however, was enhanced in the 15-min ischemia group only (Table 1). On the other hand, ATP and P-creatine were almost fully restored after 1 h of reflow (Table 2), but more significantly, the rate of their utilization was considerably prolonged in the 15-min ischemia group (Fig. 1). Hence, edematous tissue has an altered capacity for utilization of available energy reserves.

Another striking finding was the hypoactivity of (Na, K)ATPase and the increased release of serotonin in the 15-min but not in the 5-min ischemia group (Tables 2 and 3).

(Na, K)ATPase activity and 5-HT content have been shown to correlate closely with the formation and resolution of ischemic brain edema [4, 12]. Drugs known to reduce 5-HT release also attenuate the degree of brain swelling after ischemia [13] and prevent or reduce ischemic damage to the spinal cord [18]. Indeed, brain swelling was observed when 5-HT release was enhanced (Table 2), even though CBF was far above the critical threshold (Table 1). Hypoactivity of (Na, K)ATPase coincided recognizably with both brain swelling and increased 5-HT release (Table 3). Reduced (Na, K)ATPase activity appears in spite of substrate (ATP) availability. Kinetic studies revealed changes induced in the enzyme molecule by ischemia (lower substrate affinity). Also, there is evidence that the activity of (Na, K)ATPase is inversely proportional to the degree of amine release [16].

In conclusion, ischemic brain swelling is closely related to the degree of CBF reduction (CBF threshold), while postischemic brain edema is due to the metabolic disturbances induced by ischemia. It may be that the CBF threshold for ischemic brain cdcma is also thc threshold for the induction of lasting effects on (Na, K)ATPase and serotonin systems, as reflected by postischemic brain swelling.

Acknowledgement. B.M.Dj. was Fogarty International Fellow, Fogarty International Center, National Institutes of Health, Bethesda, MD 20205.

Summary

Edema in the form of brain swelling is common both during ischemia and in the period of reflow. However, ischemic brain swelling is a function of the degree of CBF reduction, which is to say that it appears if a CBF threshold is reached. On the other hand, postischemic brain edema is due to the metabolic disturbances induced by ischemia. It seems likely that the serotonin and (Na, K)ATPase systems are irreversibly altered by ischemia and are involved in the development of postischemic brain swelling.

References

1. Astrup J (1982) Energy-requiring cell functions in the ischemic brain. J Neurosurg 56:482–497
2. Astrup J, Siesjö BK, Symon L (1981) Thresholds in cerebral ischemia – the ischemic penumbra. Stroke 12:723–725
3. Bothe HW, Kerckhoff W, Paschen W, Wallenfang T, Hossmann KA (1984) Dissociation between blood flow and metabolic disturbances in edema associated with experimental abscess in cats. In: Go KG, Baethmann A (eds) Recent progress in the study and therapy of brain edema. Plenum, New York, pp 355–365
4. Cvejić V, Mićić DV, Mršulja BB (1984) Serotonin turnover in reflow following transient brain ischemia in the gerbil: possible relation to oedema. Jugoslav Physiol Pharmacol Acta 20:23–30
5. Eisenthal R, Cornish-Bowden E (1974) Direct linear plot. Biochem J 139:715–720
6. Elliot KAC, Jasper H (1949) Measurement of experimentally induced brain swelling and shrinkage. Am J Physiol 157:122–129
7. Hamer J, Hoyer S, Alberti E, Stoeckel H (1975) Cerebral blood flow and metabolism at different levels of decreased cerebral perfusion pressure induced by raised intracranial pressure and normovolemic arterial hypotension. In: Langfitt TW, McHenry LC, Reivich M, Wollman H (eds) Cerebral circulation and metabolism. Springer, Berlin Heidelberg New York, pp 184–187
8. Hossmann KA (1976) Development and resolution of ischemic brain swelling. In: Pappius HM, Feindel W (eds) Dynamics of brain edema. Springer, Berlin Heidelberg New York, pp 219–227
9. Kirino T (1982) Delayed neuronal death in the gerbil hippocampus following ischemia. Brain Res 239:57–69
10. Laverty R, Taylor M (1968) The fluorimetric assay of catecholamines and related compounds: improvements and extensions to the hydroxyindole techniques. Anal Biochem 22:269–279
11. Lowry OH, Passonneau JV (1972) A flexible system of enzymatic analysis. Academic, New York
12. Mršulja BB, Djuričić BM, Cvejić V, Mršulja BJ, Abe K, Spatz M, Klatzo I (1980) Biochemistry of experimental ischemic brain edema. Adv Neurol 28:217–230
13. Mršulja BB, Djuričić BM, Cvejić V, Mićić DV (1984) Pharmacological approach to postischemic brain edema in gerbils. In: Go GK, Baethmann A (eds) Recent progress in the study and therapy of brain edema. Plenum, New York, pp 683–689
14. Mršulja BB, Ueki Y, Wheaton A, Passonneau JV, Lust WD (1984) Release of pentobarbital-induced depression of metabolic rate during bilateral ischemia in the gerbil brain. Brain Res 309:152–155

15. Pasztor E, Symon L, Branston NM (1973) The hydrogen clearance method in assessment of blood flow in cortex, white matter and deep nuclei of baboons. Stroke 4:556–560
16. Rutledge CO (1980) Effects of metabolic inhibition and ouabain on amphetamine- and potassium-induced release of biogenic amines from isolated brain tissue. Biochem Pharmacol 27:511–516
17. Symon L, Branston NM, Chikovani O (1979) Ischemic brain edema following middle cerebral artery occlusion in baboons: relationship between regional cerebral water content and blood flow at 1 and 2 hours. Stroke 10:184–191
18. Zivin JA, Venditto JA (1984) Experimental CNS ischemia: serotonin antagonists reduce or prevent damage. Neurology (Cleveland) 34:469–474

Serotonin Receptors in Ischemic Brain Edema

B. Wroblewska[1], Y. Ueki, B. B. Mršulja, B. M. Djuričić, and M. Spatz

Key words: Cerebral edema, 5-hydroxytryptamine, [^{3}H]Ketanserin, S_2 receptors

Introduction

The involvement of serotonin (5-hydroxytryptamine, 5-HT) in the development of cerebral edema of both vasogenic and cytotoxic types has been the subject of many investigations since the late 1950s [1, 2, 9–13, 15; Mršulja et al., this volume]. In particular, the studies of Welch first drew attention to the possible relationship of 5-HT to the formation of edema in ischemia [15]. Similar conclusions were also derived from our studies of cerebral edema in ischemic gerbils [9–12; Mršulja et al., this volume]. However, we not only observed a close correlation between the accumulation of water content and the alteration of 5-HT metabolism but also an association of water increment with changes in the activity of Na^+-K^+-ATPase, $Na^+ : K^+$ ratio, and levels of cAMP in the brain [11, 12; Mršulja et al., this volume]. These findings suggested the possibility of interrelated events occurring in ischemia which might affect the cellular membranes and lead to edema. Since the disturbance of the cerebral 5-HT pathway might be one of the main processes involved in the formation of edema, we investigated the kinetic properties of cellular 5-HT (S_2 postsynaptic) receptors in the gerbil model.

This report demonstrates that the characteristics of S_2 postsynaptic receptor binding sites are changed at the time of the greatest accumulation of water in the brain of gerbils recovering from ischemic insult.

Methods

In our previous studies, the greatest formation of ischemic edema in gerbils was found 1–2 h after the release of 15-min bilateral carotid artery occlusion for 15 min. Therefore, groups of five to seven gerbils were subjected to the same experimental procedures, while sham-operated animals served as controls. The quickly dissected cortex was the only brain structure used for these studies.

[1] Laboratory of Neuropathology and Neuroanatomical Sciences, National Institute of Neurological and Communicative Disorders and Stroke, National Institutes of Health, Bethesda, Maryland 20205, USA

Some of the tissues (from each group of animals) were analyzed for both 5-HT content and the properties of S_2 receptors. The levels of 5-HT in the brain homogenates were determined by high-pressure liquid chromatography (HPLC) with an electrochemical detector [4, 9]. The 5-HT data obtained were compared with those observed in corresponding experiments and the 5-HT turnover rate reported elsewhere [4, 9, 12].

S_2-postsynaptic receptors were detected in the cerebrocortical homogenate by binding studies with [^{3}H]Ketanserin (New England Nuclear Corp.), the potent 5-HT antagonist which selectively labels S_2 receptor sites [7]. Tissue was homogenized in 50 m*M* Tris-HCl buffer containing 4 m*M* $CaCl_2$, 0.1% ascorbate, and 1 μ*M* pargyline at pH 7.7 and preincubated for 10 min at 37° C. A further 50 m*M* Tris-HCl buffer (pH 7.7) was used for incubation of the tissue homogenate with [^{3}H]Ketanserin (2–60 n*M*) and methysergide (1 μ*M*) for 30 min at 37° C. Methysergide is the only compound among the known serotonin antagonists which lacks interaction with α_1-adrenergic and histamine (H_1) receptors. Thus, the addition of methysergide eliminates the slight possibility of [^{3}H]Ketanserin binding to α_1-adrenergic or histamine (H_1)-binding sites [7]. The specific [^{3}H]Ketanserin binding was defined by subtracting nonspecific binding determined in assays containing unlabeled methysergide (gift from Sandoz Research Institute, E. Hanover, NJ) in excess of [^{3}H]Ketanserin concentrations. The results obtained were mathematically analyzed according to Scatchard [14] and a computerized nonlinear regression [6]. Protein concentration was determined by the method of Lowry et al. [8].

Results and Comments

Bilateral cerebral ischemia (15 min) reduced (30%) the brain levels of 5-HT, which normalized at 1 h after recirculation, confirming our previous reports.

In general, the ratio of specific binding of [^{3}H]Ketanserin to nonspecific binding (determined in the presence of methysergide) was the same in experimental as in sham-operated and in control brains. The nonspecific binding did not exceed 20% of total binding. As may be seen from Fig. 1, the level of [^{3}]Ketanserin bound to tissue equilibrated at 10 min and did not change significantly during the 30-min incubation of control brain homogenate. However, at 1 and 2 h after the release of occlusion, [^{3}H]Ketanserin-binding equilibrium was disturbed after a longer incubation than 10 min.

The evaluation of kinetic studies with the aid of Scatchard plots showed that [^{3}H]Ketanserin may have more than one binding site in the brain of gerbils subjected to recirculation after 15 min of bilateral arterial occlusion. Indeed, the computerized nonlinear regression analysis confirmed this assumption. The kinetic characteristics of [^{3}H]Ketanserin-binding sites in ischemic brain were similar to those in brains from sham-operated and control animals (Fig. 2). On the other hand, the tissue obtained from gerbils recovering from the ischemic insult revealed two binding sites for [^{3}H]Ketanserin, one with a lower and another with a higher affinity than that observed in brains from sham-operated and ischemic animals (Fig. 2C, D; 15 min of ischemia with 1 h of recirculation). The estimated values after 2 h of recirculation were: $K_{D_1} = 58.0$ n*M*; $K_{D_2} = 13.0$ n*M*; $B_{max} = 1.4$ n*M*.

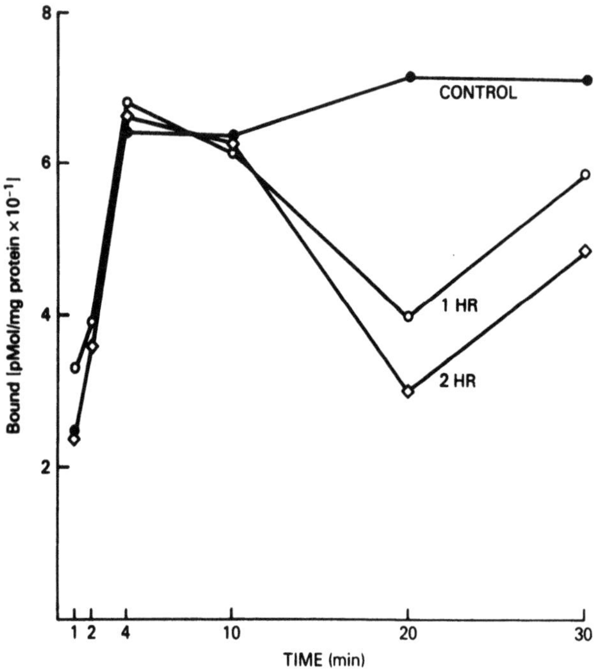

Fig. 1. Association rate of [^{3}H]Ketanserin binding to cerebral cortex homogenate. Specific binding was calculated as the difference between total and nonspecific binding (in the presence of 1 μM methysergide). *Points* represent mean values from two separate experiments each determined in triplicate (SEM ± 10%)

These findings strongly suggest that the properties of S_2 receptor binding sites are altered in cerebral edema induced by ischemia. The demonstrated modulation of [^{3}H]Ketanserin binding sites appears to coincide with the observed attenuated metabolic rate (=increased release) but not with the abnormal levels of 5-HT in the brain. The existing discrepancies in the reported cerebral concentration of 5-HT in ischemia should be stressed at this juncture. Our own and other investigations suggest that the differences observed in the ischemic patterns of 5-HT are most likely related to the type and model of ischemia and/or brain structure studied, as well as

Fig. 2. Characteristics of [^{3}H]Ketanserin binding to cerebral cortex homogenate of sham-operated (**A, B**) and experimental gerbils (**C, D**). Saturation curve (**A**) and linearity of Scatchard analysis (**B**) of the sham control values suggest one binding site. Values estimated from nonlinear regression analysis are: $K_D = 52.0$ and $B_{max} = 1.8$ nmol/mg protein. Similar results were seen after 15 min of ischemia. The biphasic shape of the saturation curve (**C**) and Scatchard analysis (**D**) of the data obtained from experimental animals suggest multiple binding sites. Values estimated from nonlinear regression analysis are: K_{D_1} 18.0 nM, $K_{D_2} = 77.0$ nM and $B_{max} = 1.2$ nmol/mg protein after 15 min bilateral ischemia and 1 h recirculation. The overall values are 10-fold higher than those obtained from tissue homogenate washed three times with 50 mM Tris-HCl buffer. Similar patterns and values were obtained from repeat experiments (5)

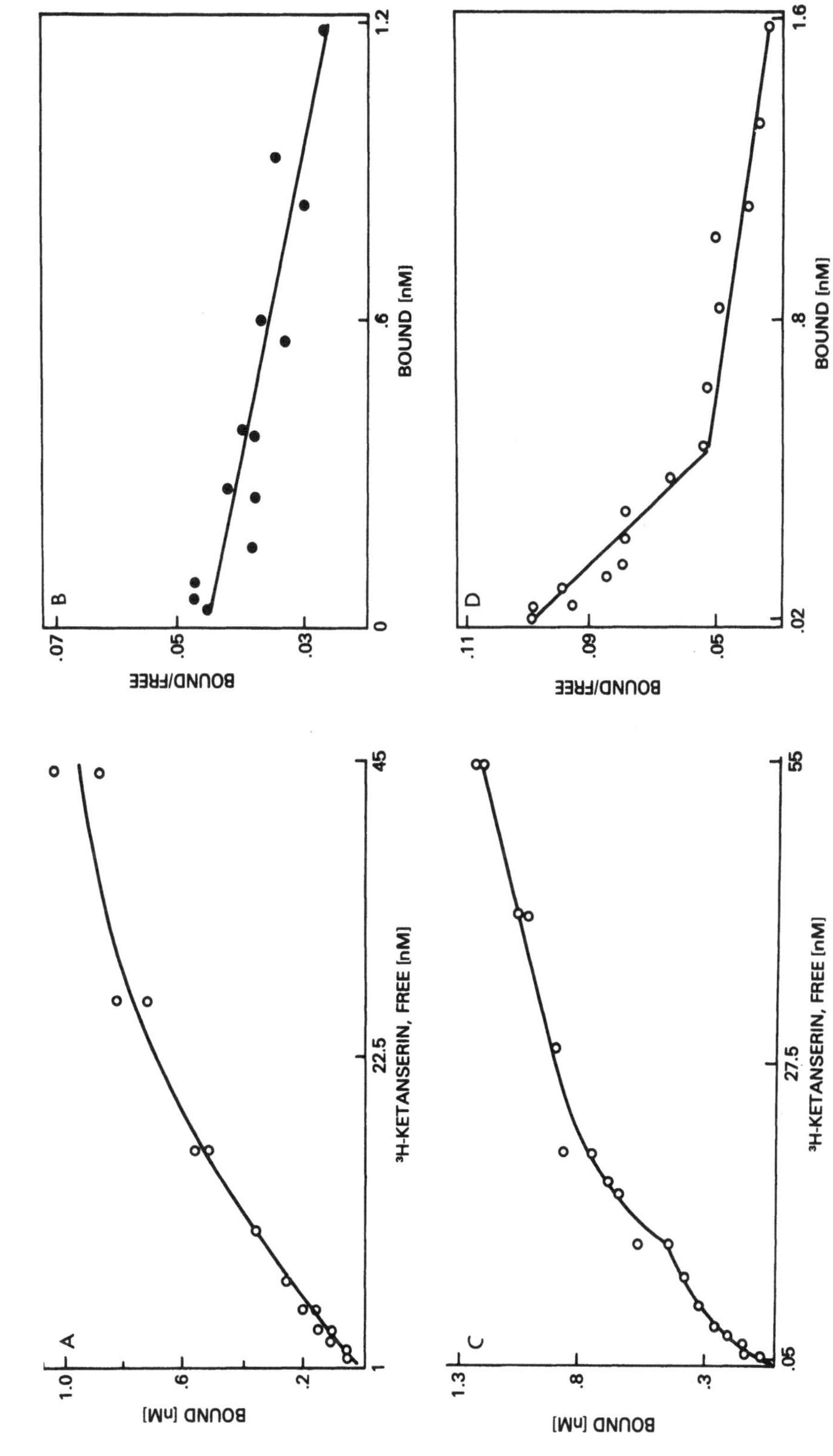
A
BOUND [nM]
1.0
.6
.2
1
22.5
45
³H-KETANSERIN, FREE [nM]
B
BOUND/FREE
.07
.05
.03
0
.6
1.2
BOUND [nM]
C
BOUND [nM]
1.3
.8
.3
.05
27.5
55
³H-KETANSERIN, FREE [nM]
D
BOUND/FREE
.11
.09
.05
.02
.8
1.6
BOUND [nM]

to the method used for detection of 5-HT (for review, see [4]). However, 5-HT metabolism is unquestionably disturbed in the brains of gerbils subjected to 15-min bilateral carotid artery occlusion without recirculation [9–12; Mršulja et al., this volume]. Thus, the absence of obvious changes in the kinetic characteristics of S_2 receptor binding sites might have various reasons, especially if the presynaptic region is considered to be the primary site of the ischemically disturbed 5-HT pathway. The most important of these are: (a) inadequate lapse of time (15 min of ischemia) and/or absence of recirculation, which is needed for development of the postsynaptic changes; and/or (b) presence of altered properties of S_2 receptors in a subcellular compartment that is obscured by examination of the whole cortical homogenate instead of a specific fraction. The modified S_2 receptors may be localized in either neuronal and/or glial and/or vascular postsynaptic membranes.

The detection of S_2 postsynaptic binding sites with lower and higher affinities (indicated by the apparent higher K_D and lower K_D) after 1 h of recirculation than those seen in ischemic and control cortex indicates a desensitization and hypersensitization of the receptor sites, respectively. This may be the result of excessively available 5-HT at the postsynaptic receptor sites due to increased release, decreased uptake and reuptake of 5-HT at the presynaptic regions. On the whole, this phenomenon is consistent with the well-known agonist-specific desensitization of cellular membranes exposed to high levels of hormones and neurohormones, while their depletion results in supersensitization [5]. Besides this, the detected S_2 binding sites with a higher affinity (lower K_D) in the recovery period (recirculation of 1 and 2 h) than those seen in ischemic and control brains may signify either an unmasked preexisting or an additional binding site. In any event, it most probably represents another manifestation of an overall structurally disturbed membrane. Based on the detected changes in the properties of S_2 receptor binding sites, it can be assumed that the existing disturbances of the 5-HT pathway and its adverse effects are not confined to the presynaptic, but also involve the postsynaptic subcellular compartments. Furthermore, it is possible that the 5-HT presynaptically released into the synaptic cleft may also effect the membrane directly. In this way, the overflow of unmetabolized 5-HT may contribute to the increased membrane permeability, allowing a more pronounced passive transfer of ions and accumulation of water in the cells. This supposition is supported by the observed additional increase in Na^+, reduction in K^+ concentration, and decreased activity of Na^+-K^+-ATPase at the time of most marked cellular swelling [3, 11; Mršulja et al., this volume]. The concomitant occurrence of changes in the kinetic properties of S_2 receptors and Na^+-K^+-ATPase activity is of interest especially, since an increase in the levels of $PGF_{2\alpha}$ was also found after the same duration of ischemia and recirculation [12]. The production of $PGF_{2\alpha}$ can be stimulated by 5-HT, since this amine increases the formation of $PGF_{1\alpha}$ in cultured cerebrovascular elements [16; unpublished observations]. On the other hand, substances which inhibit either synthesis or release of 5-HT reduce the formation of edema and reserve the changes in Na^+-K^+-ATPase, $Na^+:K^+$ ratio, and $PGF_{2\alpha}$ [12]. However, it remains to be elucidated whether 5-HT affects (directly or indirectly) the activity of Na^+-K^+-ATPase. Nevertheless, the detected modification of S_2 receptors at the time of most conspicuously increased cellular water in the brain of gerbils subjected to ischemia and recirculation strongly supports the contention of 5-HT involvement in the formation and/or progression of edema.

Summary

Disturbances of 5-hydroxytryptamine (5-HT) metabolism have been associated with the formation and progression of ischemic cerebral edema. To shed more light on the pathogenic mechanisms of edema formation, we investigated the kinetic properties of cellular 5-HT (S_2-postsynaptic receptors) in the cerebral cortex of gerbils subjected to bilateral carotid artery occlusion for 15 min without or with subsequent (1 and 2 h) release. S_2-Receptors were detected in cerebrocortical homogenate by binding studies with [^{3}H]Ketanserin, the potent 5-HT antagonist which selectively labels S_2-receptor sites.

The cerebral cortex obtained from gerbils recovering from the ischemic insult showed two binding sites for [^{3}H]Ketanserin, one with a lower and another with a higher affinity than that observed in control and ischemic brains. The demonstrated modulation of [^{3}H]Ketanserin-binding sites coincided with the observed greatest accumulation of water and the attenuated metabolic rate (=increased release), but not with the abnormal levels of 5-HT in the brain. These findings substantiate the assumed involvement of serotonin in the pathogenesis of ischemic brain edema.

References

1. Bull PH (1957) Effects of reserpine and chlorpromazine in prevention of cerebral edema and reversible cell damage. Proc Soc Exp Biol Med 94:553–556
2. Costa JL, Ito U, Spatz M, Klatzo I, Demirjian C (1974) 5-Hydroxytryptamine accumulation in cerebral injury. Nature 244:135–136
3. Djuricic BM, Micic DV, Mrsulja BB (1984) Phasic recognition of edema caused by ischemia. In: Go KG, Baethmann A (eds) Recent progress in the study and therapy of brain edema. Plenum, New York, pp 491–498
4. Djuricic BM, Ueki Y, Spatz M (1985) Composite technique for regional neurochemical studies. Measurement of energy and neurotransmitter metabolites in single tissue sample. J Neurochem (in press)
5. Iyengar R, Birnbaumen L (1981) Agonist-specific desensitization: molecular locus and possible mechanisms. In: Dumont JB, Greengaid P, Robinson GA (eds) Advances in cycle nucleotide research, vol 14. Raven, New York, pp 93–99
6. Knott GD (1979) MLab – a mathematical modeling tool. Comput Programs Biomed 10:271–280
7. Leysen JE, Niemegeers CJE, Van Neuten JM, Laduron PM (1981) [^{3}H] Ketanserin (R41 468), a selective ^{3}H-ligand for serotonin receptor binding sites. Binding properties, brain distribution and functional role. Mol Pharmacol 21:301–314
8. Lowry OH, Rosenbrough NJ, Farr AL, Randall JR (1951) Protein measurement with folin phenol reagent. J Biol Chem 193:265–275
9. Maruki C, Merkel N, Rausch WD, Spatz M (1984) Brain monoamines in cerebral ischemic edema; the effect of gamma-hydroxybutyrate. In: Go KG, Baethmann A (eds) Recent progress in the study and therapy of brain edema. Plenum, New York, pp 673–681
10. Mrsulja BB, Mrsulja BJ, Spatz M, Klatzo I (1976) Monoamines in cerebral ischemia in relation to brain edema. In: Pappius H, Feindel W (eds) Dynamics of brain edema. Springer, Berlin Heidelberg New York, pp 187–192
11. Mrsulja BB, Djuricic BM, Cvejic V, Mrsulja BJ, Abe K, Spatz M, Klatzo I (1980) Biochemistry of experimental ischemic brain edema. Adv Neurol 28:217–230
12. Mrsulja BB, Djuricic BM, Cvejic V, Micic DV (1984) Pharmacological approach to postischemic brain edema in gerbils. In: Go KG, Baethmann A (eds) Recent progress in the study and therapy of brain edema. Plenum, New York, pp 683–689

13. Osterholm LJ, Bell J, Meyer R, Pyenson (1969) Experimental effects of free serotonin on brain and its relation to brain injury, parts I–III. J Neurosurg 31:408–429
14. Scatchard G (1949) The attraction of proteins for small molecules and ions. Ann NY Acad Sci 51:660–672
15. Welch KMA, Chabi E, Dodson RF, Wang TPF, Nell J, Bergin B (1976) The role of biogenic amines in the progression of cerebral ischemia and edema. In: Pappius H, Feindel W (eds) Dynamics of brain edema. Springer, Berlin Heidelberg New York, pp 193–202
16. Wolfe LS, Ng Ying Kin NMK, Spatz M (1983) Metabolites of arachidonic acid after calcium ionophore stimulation of cultured cerebral capillary endothelial cells and brain tissue: identification of lipoxygenase products. J Neurochem 41:S40

Evaluation of Steroid Treatment of High-Energy Metabolism of Ischemic Brain Edema in Vivo by Means of a Topical Magnetic Resonance (TMR-32) Spectrometer

H. KUCHIWAKI[1], S. TAKADA, N. MISU, H. ISHIGURI, A. IKEDA, N. KAGEYAMA, and H. WATARI

Key words: Methylprednisolone, cerebral infarction, in vivo, high-energy phosphates, topical magnetic resonance

Introduction

During the formation of ischemic brain edema the lesion responsible is thought to influence the metabolism in various ways [12]. The dynamics of metabolism have been studied using steroid treatment to reduce the neurologic deficits induced by edema [2, 3]. However, experimental data on metabolites are frequently evaluated only by means of a statistical analysis by groups that have effected ischemic areas at various locations for each developmental stage of experimental brain edema [2, 7, 9, 11].

It seemed it would be possible to study the dynamics of the metabolism of experimentally induced infarction of the brain in vivo by continuous measurements of metabolites in one animal. Studies based on topical magnetic resonance (TMR-32 spectrometer manufactured by the Oxford Research System, England) provide for such an evaluation of phosphate metabolism in the formation of brain edema [13]. Using the TMR spectrometer we can continuously measure high-energy phosphates influenced by the ischemic insult to the brain, which correlate with the activity of uninjured portion of the brain.

However, the significance of high-energy phosphates determined by TMR techniques should be carefully evaluated, because the phosphates detected by this method are not always all the high-energy metabolites in the living cells of the brain [10]. There are several kinds of high-energy phosphates that have short reaction times under metabolic regulation. One is easily detected by TMR, but the others do not easily appear as signals on the TMR spectrometer. Therefore, the analysis of such data is complicated and the implications of such results are also difficult to determine in the biological system. This is because it is not clear which of the metabolites more clearly reflects the metabolic dynamics involved in the formation of ischemic brain edema. Although there are difficulties, on the basis of the use of incremental scanning times we consider that the changes in signals found with the TMR are a satisfactory reflection of the dynamics of metabolism for ischemic brain edema, as was reported in our previous study [8].

[1] Department of Neurosurgery, Nagoya University School of Medicine, 65 Tsurumai-cho, Showa-ka, Nagoya 466, Japan

On the basis of the changes in high-energy phosphates detected by TMR, we will discuss the dynamics of high-energy metabolites in the brain with a focal ischemic area during the formation of brain edema.

Materials and Methods

Thirteen adult mongrel dogs of 4.5–8 kg body weight were used for this experimental work. They were anesthetized with thiamylal Na 6–8 mg/kg body weight IV during spontaneous respiration with intubation. The neck of each animal was incised on the right side. The right common carotid artery was exposed, followed by the external and internal carotid arteries. The common and external carotid arteries were then ligated.

An 18-gauge Teflon needle was introduced deeply (as near the skull base as possible) into the internal carotid artery with the aid of a guide. A small injector was connected to the needle for embolization. A small amount of bioresin (0.6–0.7 ml) was used in each animal embolization. The other two catheters were placed in the thoracic aorta and the inferior vena cava for measurement of systemic blood pressure (SAP) and IV administration of the anesthetic agent, respectively. The formation of a focal infarction in a brain was identified by infusing carbon black. In this way focal ischemia was induced in the closed skull [8].

At hourly intervals throughout the experiment each animal was placed in the bore of the TMR spectrometer in the position shown in Fig. 1. The animals were placed and fixed in a supine position on a home-made wooden frame to exclude artifacts caused by moving or shifting of the head position due to the anesthesia-induced muscle relaxation and respiration.

Special care was taken during this procedure to prevent the TMR spectrometer from becoming wet owing to exudates or bleeding from the operative wound.

All monitoring apparatuses were disconnected from the body during TMR measurement to avoid interference with the TMR signals. The part of the body protruding from the bore was wrapped in a sheet of aluminium foil connected to the electrical earth. To obtain clearly readable data the resonance condition was estimated by tuning to the radio frequencies corresponding to proton and phosphate. The topical magnetic field was produced by a two-turn home-made surface coil to receive signals from the brain. Its attachment to the skull is shown in Fig. 1. Control signals were obtained before induction of the lesion. Then each animal was temporarily taken out of the bore of the spectrometer for induction of the lesion. The animal was subsequently returned to the frame in the bore in the same position as before, and remained there for the rest of the experimental period. For detection of signals from the infarcted area the coil was adjusted to cover the lesion. The dynamics of the metabolism of the noninfarcted area was recorded by attaching the surface coil to the noninfarcted hemisphere. Every 30 min for 4 h the signals from the brain were scanned 600 times. Following these procedures TMR signals from high-energy phosphates, including creatine phosphate (CrP) as well as inorganic phosphate (Pi), were satisfactorily clear and continuously reproducible. For evaluation of special resolution of the topical magnetic field we used a double-lumen sample tube, which contained phosphates in different buffer solutions and a rat's and a dog's head.

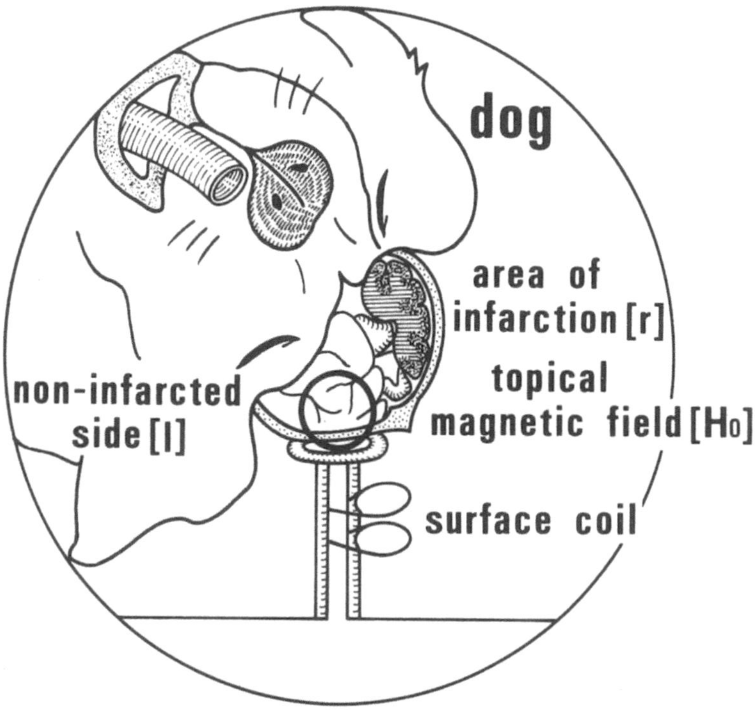

Fig. 1. Schematic illustrating the relation between head and surface coil attachment in the bore of the TMR spectrometer

Two different groups were examined. One group received no steroid treatment (NS group, $n=5$). Animals in the other group received single bolus injections of methylprednisolone 30–40 mg/kg just after induction of the lesion (ST group, $n=5$). The effects of steroid treatment were evaluated by comparing the results in the two groups.

Each high-energy-phosphate signal is displayed on a graph as a proportion of the mean value (=1.0) of all the data throughout the appropriate experimental hour (Figs. 2–5). Equations are shown for calculation of the adenylate energy charge (EC) and the proportion of creatine phosphates (CrP). We considered the signal from adenosine monophosphate (AMP) included that from inorganic phosphate (Pi) [5].

Method of Calculation

Energy charge (EC) = (ATP) + 0.5(ADP)/(ATP) + (ADP) + (AMP)
= 0.5((beta phosphate of ATP)
+ (gamma phosphate of ATP))/((Pi) + (gamma phosphate of ATP)) (Eq. 1)

where (ADP) = (gamma phosphate of ATP) − (beta phosphate of ATP) and (AMP) = (Pi)

Proportion of creatine phosphate (CrP) = (CrP)/(Pi) + (CrP) (Eq. 2)

Results

The infarcted area occupied half to two-thirds of one hemisphere in each experimental model. In the heads of animals we established that a pulse width of 15–21 μs with an interval of 2 s was the best condition for this experiment. The findings for phosphate metabolism in the infarcted area are shown in Fig. 2. After induction of the lesion, signals from beta phosphate of ATP rapidly decreased, while Pi, in contrast, rapidly increased to its maximum value within 2 h. The CrP value fell substantially. In summary, in the course of these experiments the metabolism of the infarcted area rapidly deteriorated and then remained unchanged for the rest of the experimental period.

The levels of beta phosphates of ATP (Fig. 3) varied with increasing amplitude, and the mean slowly decreased with time in the NS group. However, the ST group exhibited smaller variations than the NS group. The levels in the ST group remained at mean values for the 4 h of the experiment. Thus, the level of high-energy phosphates were maintained and relatively stabilized by steroid treatment.

Analysis of the changes in CrP shows that the difference in the amplitude of fluctuation between the two groups was not very pronounced. However, the decline was slightly more marked in the NS group than in the ST group. On evaluating the value for EC we found that it also varied more widely in the NS group than the ST

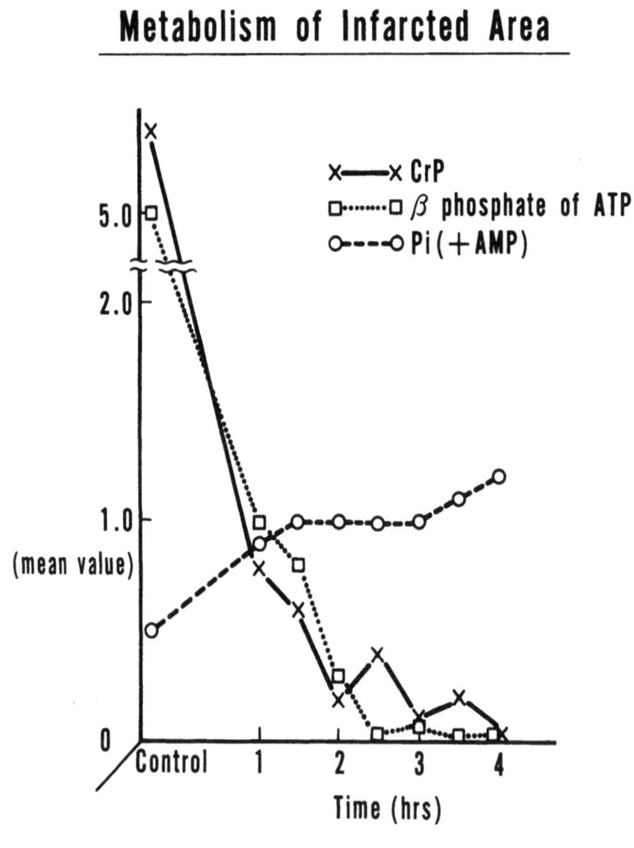

Fig. 2. Graph showing rapid deterioration of high-energy phosphate and proportional increase in inorganic phosphates including AMP in infarcted area of a canine brain

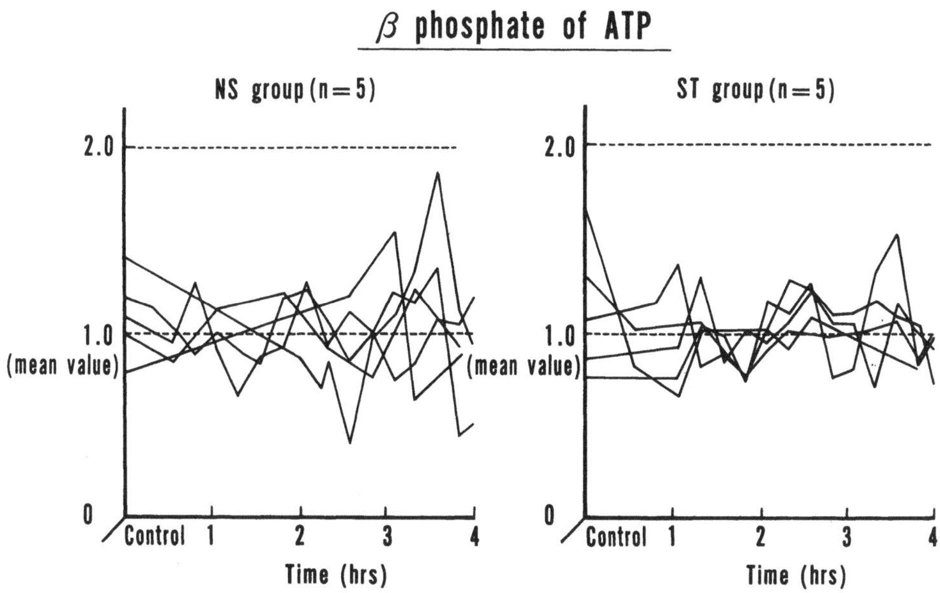

Fig. 3. Graph showing the changes in beta phosphate of ATP. Results from the NS group on the left and from the ST group are demonstrated. Note the greater amplitude of variation in the level of ATP in the NS than in the ST group

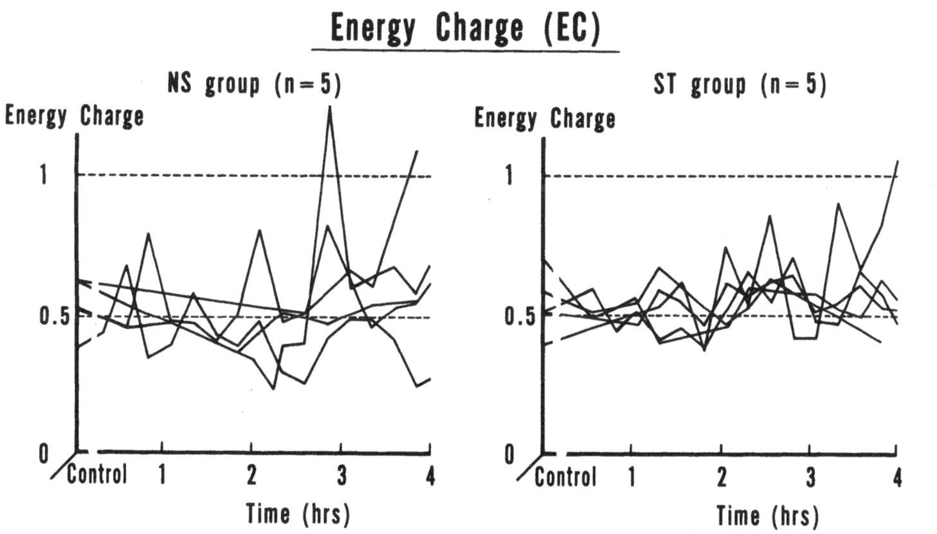

Fig. 4. Graph showing the variation in energy charge. Slightly higher level and reduced variation of the energy charge in the group are easily noticeable

group (Fig. 4). In the last 2 h of the experimental period the EC value was above 0.5 except for a transient decline in the ST group. The EC value became higher in the ST group than in the NS group. From the viewpoint of EC value, steroid treatment also brought about a tendency for a higher stabilized level at the noninfarcted area during the formation of ischemic brain edema. The relationship between EC and pro-

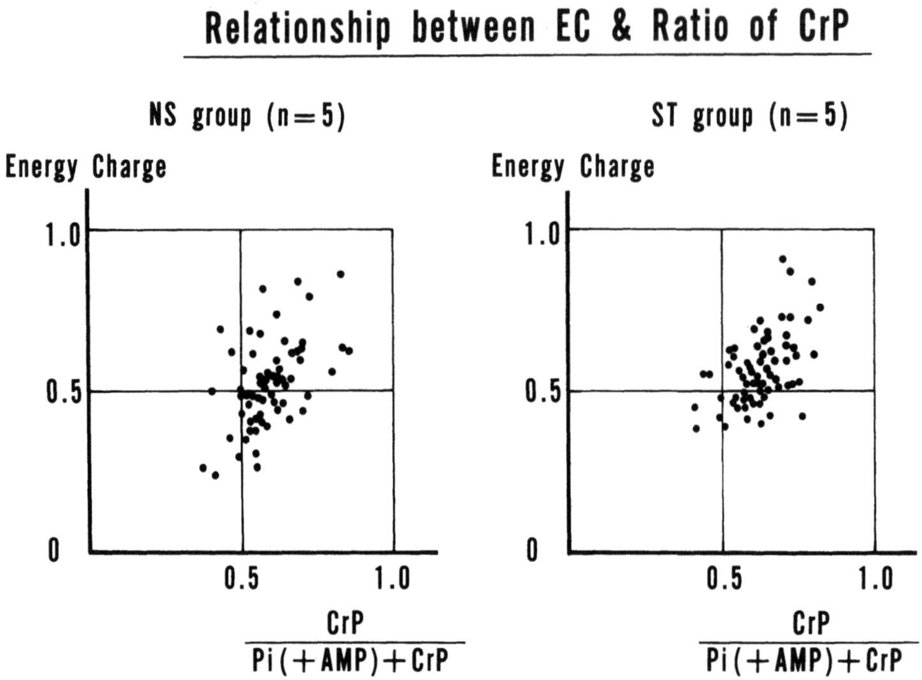

Fig. 5. Graph showing the relation between the energy charge and the proportion of creatine phosphate. Note that in the ST group both are slightly higher than in the NS group, and above 0.5. Correlations are not statistically significant

portion of CrP is shown in Fig. 5. Data displayed in the graph for the NS group vary more widely in their distribution. However, in the ST group variations in distribution were so small that most of the data points were clustered above 0.5. These results seem to indicate that the transformation from the level of CrP to high-energy phosphate metabolites becomes smoother in the ST group than in the NS group. The low values at the control stage were thought to be caused by anesthesia. Control values were recorded both before induction of the lesion and before IV introduction of the steroid. The position of each animal was not the same during the experimental period as during the control period, because the animals were replaced in the bore of the TMR spectrometer after induction of the lesion outside the apparatus. For this reason the control data are not exactly comparable with the data collected after induction of the lesion.

Discussion

Nuclear magnetic resonance (NMR) in vivo, providing continuous measurement of metabolites, might be a good way of evaluating the dynamic aspects of high-energy metabolism [10, 13].

On the other hand, there are many kinds of phosphates, which differ in relaxation times as measured with NMR. Some ATPs, with various relaxation times, are also involved in the metabolism, binding with active materials in the structure of living cells [10]. Evaluation of the changes in phosphate metabolism by the method of NMR might be based upon this limited sample. A rapid disappearance of ATP, associated with a more pronounced increase in Pi including AMP, is typical for the course, in which all kinds of cell activities were lost from the infarcted areas in our subjects [9, 11].

In our previous report an increase of bound water in the gray matter, suggesting edema fluid, was detected in the noninfarcted hemisphere as little as 4 h after the start of the experiment [8]. The movement of such bound water is thought to be so slow that it cannot migrate from the lesion in the infarcted area. These findings suggest that during the formation of edema fluid, bound water may have originated in the adjacent noninfarcted area.

The fluctuation of high-energy phosphates at the noninfarcted site is thought to reflect the metabolic dynamics resulting from diaschisis involving the neural apparatus in the ischemic insult to the brain [6].

Following treatment with the steroid hormone the state of ATP was perceptibly stabilized. In normal metabolism, the same concentration of ATP is simultaneously utilized and produced, resulting in a steady state concentration with a turnover time of 1 s or less [1]. In the cell with an active metabolic process the energy level of the compartment is constant and is supported by the fast-acting ATP-sensing regulatory mechanism [1].

All this shows that fluctuation of ATP is extremely rare. The function of steroid hormone appears to be stabilization of the ATP level during the abnormal metabolism induced by ischemic damage.

Our evaluation of the adenylate energy charge illustrates another problem in the formation of brain edema. Energy charges of the cell in a normal state are constant at 0.8–0.9, except for a rapid fall to 0.55 for several seconds [1, 9, 11, 12]. Bartho et al. [2] evaluated the EC in the formation of brain edema using occlusion of the middle cerebral artery (MCA) in cats as a model. The EC fell at the lesion 30 min after MCA occlusion, while in the perifocal area it did not fall until 240 min after that event. They reported that the decrease in EC could be reduced by steroid treatment only at the lesion. However, the severity of the decrease in EC was less pronounced than in our study. This difference may be caused by the difference in size of the infarcted areas.

In keeping with the theory of Atkinson [1], we speculate that the stabilization of adenylate EC potential by treatment with steroid hormones explains the favorable effects of suppression of the spread of ischemic brain edema by the mechanism presented by Demopoulos et al. [4]. Steroid treatment induces a stable state of high-energy phosphates during the acute stage of cerebral infarction, protecting the normal brain but also inhibiting various invading factors from the adjacent injured tissue.

There are many reports about the ineffectiveness of steroid for the reduction of intracranial pressure [3]. We indeed do not think that the steroid treatment is at all effective in reducing or eliminating all the factors or mechanisms involved in the formation of brain edema.

It is clear that the correlation, or interdependent state, between EC and CrP becomes very marked in normal cells. In Fig. 5 the relation of the two is presented. In the NS group the distribution of EC varies more widely than that of CrP, but in the ST group EC and CrP are both clustered above 0.5. These findings also support the concept of a tendency to return to a normal condition when the EC is smoothly supplied by CrP.

As Kempensky [6] suggested, diaschisis is induced by a neural mechanism, and we also speculate that the mechanism involved in edema formation is part of such a characteristic phenomenon. The normal and abnormal tissue in the infarcted brain has a mosaic configuration, and the areas might affect each other by way of a neural connection or some other unknown mechanism which affects the whole brain in a short time. Possible etiologic mechanisms include the spread of edema fluid by way of hydrostatic pressure [8] and invasion of factors from the lesion, directly or via the systemic circulation.

In conclusion, we speculate that the stabilization mechanism of the energy charge is greatly impaired in both the nonischemic area and the infarcted area. These metabolic changes on the noninfarcted side demonstrate the characteristic findings in the formation of the brain edema. Steroid treatment protected the ischemic brain by the stabilization of energy regulation and maintenance of a higher level of adenylate energy charge.

Summary

The effect of single IV injections of 30–40 mg/kg methylprednisolone were studied in an experimental model of focal ischemia in the canine brain. Animals were divided into two groups, one group receiving treatment and the other not. High-energy phosphate metabolism was analyzed with topical magnetic resonance (TMR) for 4 h after infliction of the lesion. In the infarcted area high-energy phosphate metabolism deteriorated within 2 h, with no subsequent recovery. In the noninfarcted hemisphere high-energy phosphates were slightly reduced, and they fluctuated with greater amplitude in the nontreated group. The adenylate energy charge value also varied in the nontreated group. Both the energy charge and the creatine fraction decreased. In the steroid-treated group there was a tendency for these to stabilize. The energy charge to creatine ratio was maintained at a slightly higher level, above 0.5, in the treated than in the nontreated group.

Steroid treatment seems to be effective for the stabilization of high-energy phosphates and maintenance of a higher adenylate energy charge in the formation of edema in the cerebral infarction. Thus, the potential for the recovery seemed to be conserved by steroid treatment.

References

1. Atkinson DE (1977) Cellular energy metabolism and its regulation. Academic, New York
2. Bartko D, Reulen HJ, Koch H, Schürmann K (1972) Effect of dexamethasone on the early edema following occlusion of the middle cerebral artery in cats. In: Reulen HJ, Schürmann K (eds) Steroid and brain edema. Springer, Berlin Heidelberg New York, p 127
3. Braakman R, Schouten HJA, Dishoeck MB, Minderhoud JM (1983) Megadose steroids in severe head injury. J Neurosurg 58:326–330

4. Dempopoulos HB, Milvy P, Karari S, Ransohoff J (1972) Molecular aspects of membrane structure in cerebral edema. In: Reulen HJ, Schürmann K (eds) Steroid and brain edema. Springer, Berlin Heidelberg New York, p 29
5. Gadian DG (1982) Nuclear magnetic resonance and its applications to living systems. Oxford University Press, Oxford
6. Kempinsky WH (1958) Experimental study of distant effects of acute focal brain injury. Arch Neurol Psychiatr 79:376–389
7. Kogure K, Busto R, Scheinberg P (1974) Energy metabolism and water content in rat brain during the early stage of development of cerebral infarction. Brain 97:103–114
8. Kuchiwaki H, Furuse M, Gonda T, Hirai N, Inao S, Ikeyama A, Kageyama N (1984) Studies on changes in tissue water constitution and focal brain tissue pressure in experimental cerebral infarction. In: Go KG, Baethmann A (eds) Recent progress in the study and therapy of brain edema. Plenum, New York, p 459
9. Nordström C-H, Siesjö BK (1978) Influence of phenobarbital on changes in the metabolites of energy reserve of cerebral cortex following complete ischemia. Acta Physiol Scand 104:271–280
10. Nunnally RL, Hollis DP (1979) Adenosine triphosphate compartmentation in living heart: A phosphorus nuclear magnetic resonance saturation transfer study. Biochemistry 18:3642–3646
11. Siesjö BK (1978) Brain energy metabolism, Wiley, Chichester
12. Sugi T, Schuier FT, Hossmann KA, Zülch KJ (1980) The effect of mild microembolic injury on the metabolism of the cat brain. J Neurol 223:285–292
13. Thulbon K, du Boulay GH, Radda G (1981) Noninvasive measurement of energy metabolism and pH by ^{31}P NMR in experimental stroke: Correlation with cerebral edema. J Cereb Blood Flow Metab [Suppl 1] 1:S80–81

Regional Metabolism and Circulation at Peritumoral Edema Caused by Meningioma and Malignant Glioma

T. TSUBOKAWA [1], T. TSUKIYAMA, H. OHTA, and H. KUMAKAWA

Key words: Brain edema, brain tumor, metabolism, cerebral circulation, PET, matched low perfusion

Introduction

Brain edema fluid develops as a consequence of alterations to the blood-brain barrier in the presence of brain tumor, and edema fluid leaks predominantly into the white matter by way of bulk flow [2, 4, 8].

There are conflicting reports on metabolic dysfunction and alteration of cerebral circulation in peritumoral brain edema. Some workers [1, 6] have reported metabolic dysfunction with either decreased or increased regional cerebral blood flow, while others report that the peritumoral edema area does not interfere with blood flow or flow regulation as long as intracranial pressure is normal [2, 4, 5, 8].

The discrepancy between these findings cannot be explained simply by the absence of intracranial hypertension or of toxic effects of substances released from the tumor.

To examine the changes in both metabolism and cerebral circulation in peritumoral edematous tissue, rCBF, $rCMRO_2$, rOER, rCBV, and rCMRGl were studied by positron emission CT in 30 patients suffering from meningioma or glioma.

Methods and Materials

In 30 patients with primary brain tumor (9 cases of meningioma, 8 cases of astrocytoma grades 1–2, and 13 cases of malignant glioma) and intracranial pressure in the range of 15–30 mmHg, positron emission CT was used to measure rCBF, $rCMRO_2$, rOER, rCBV, and rCMRGl both in the tumor and in the areas of peritumoral édema seen as peritumoral low-density areas on X-ray CT. The positron emission radionuclides used were $^{11}CO_2$ or $^{15}CO_2$ for rCBF, $^{11}CO_2$ for rCBV, and $^{15}O_2$ for r-$CMRO_2$, all given by a continuous inhalation method. In addition, rOER was calculated from $rCMRO_2$ and rCBR. However, to measure rCMRGl, ^{11}C-glucose (oral administration) was used in this study rather than ^{11}C-deoxyglucose or ^{18}F-fluorodeoxyglucose, because the deoxyglucose method indicates only the first-

[1] Department of Neurological Surgery, School of Medicine, Nihon University, Tokyo, Japan

Table 1. Normal ranges recorded with our method using Headtome II

		Normal range
rCBF	(Cortex)	50 ~70 ml/min/100 g
rCBF	(White)	18 ~24 ml/min/100 g
$rCMRO_2$	(Cortex)	4 ~ 6 ml/min/100 g
$rCMRO_2$	(White)	1.5~ 2.0 ml/min/100 g
rOER	(Cortex)	0.5~ 0.6
rOER	(White)	0.4~ 0.5
rCBV		4 ~ 5 ml/100 g
rCMRGl	(Cortex)	100 mg/100 g
rCMRGl	(White matter)	50 mg/100 g

step uptake depending on the activity of hexakinase and cannot detect any specific glycolytic process in the brain tumor that involves a higher rate of synthesis of ribose-5-phosphate and amino acid from the substances produced by anaerobic glycolysis, which is frequently observed in the presence of a brain tumor [9]. The PET scanner used in this study was the Headtome II (Simazu Co.).

Following examinations in ten normal adults, the normal ranges for rCBF, $rCMRO_2$, rOER, rCBV, and products of regional glucose metabolism were recorded and these are shown in Table 1. With PET, not only does the image reveal the most prominent low-density area seen on X-ray CT; in addition each parameter can be calculated at the region of interest (ROI) and compared with the normal value shown in Table 1 or the results recorded in the anatomically equivalent area on the opposite side of the brain.

In six cases of malignant glioma, high-energy phosphates and lactate were fluorometrically measured in surgical specimens taken from the area corresponding to the peritumoral edematous area.

Results

Meningioma Group

In nine cases of meningioma, rCBV increased by about 10%–25% in all parts of the tumor compared with the values in anatomically equivalent areas of the contralateral side of the brain; the products of regional glucose metabolism also increased by 10%–13%, coupled with an increase in rCBF; but $rCMRO_2$ decreased by more than 25% and rOER also decreased. These alterations were observed in regions corresponding to areas shown by enhanced CT to be tumor sites.

At the low-density area of the tumor, both the products of regional glucose metabolism and $rCMRO_2$ decreased without any decrease in rCBF (Fig. 1).

In the area of peritumoral brain edema, rCBF decreased to 25–30 ml/min/100 g and $rCMRO_2$ decreased to 15–22 mg/min/100 g. But rOER was 0.48 (normal level),

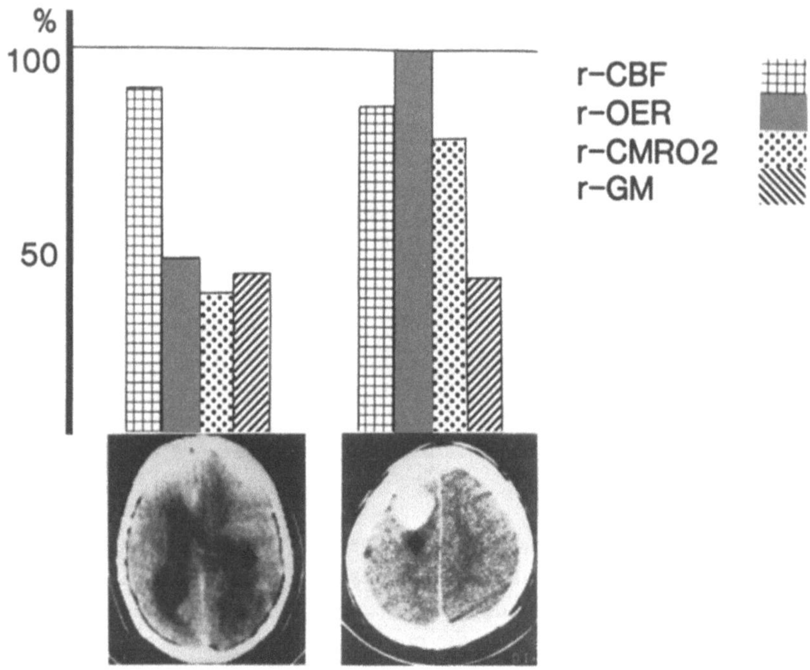

Fig. 1. X-Ray CTs showing alterations in metabolism and cerebral circulation in peritumoral edematous areas (*black diamonds*), reflected in decreased rate compared with the corresponding area on the other side of the brain. *Right,* astrocytoma grade II; *left,* meningioma

and rCBV did not change at all. These findings in the peritumoral edema area on PET indicate the presence of the matched low-perfusion phenomenon, but no anoxic or ischemic alterations were observed. The rate of decrease of rCBF is slower than that of either $rCMRO_2$ or the products of regional glucose metabolism.

After total removal of the tumor this matched low-perfusion phenomenon disappears.

Benign Glioma Group (Astrocytoma Grade 1 or 2)

In eight cases diagnosed histologically as astrocytoma grade 1 or 2, rCBF decreased to 40%–60%, $rCMRO_2$ decreased to 60%–70% with low rOER, and products of regional glucose metabolism also decreased; but the ratio of rCBF to products of regional glucose metabolism was lower than the ratio of rCBF to $rCMRO_2$ in the tumor.

In the area of peritumoral edema the area indicated as a peritumoral low-density area on X-ray CT, rCBF, products of regional glucose metabolism, and $rCMRO_2$ decreased in precisely the same manner as in the presence of a meningioma, but rOER was less than 0.2 (Fig. 1).

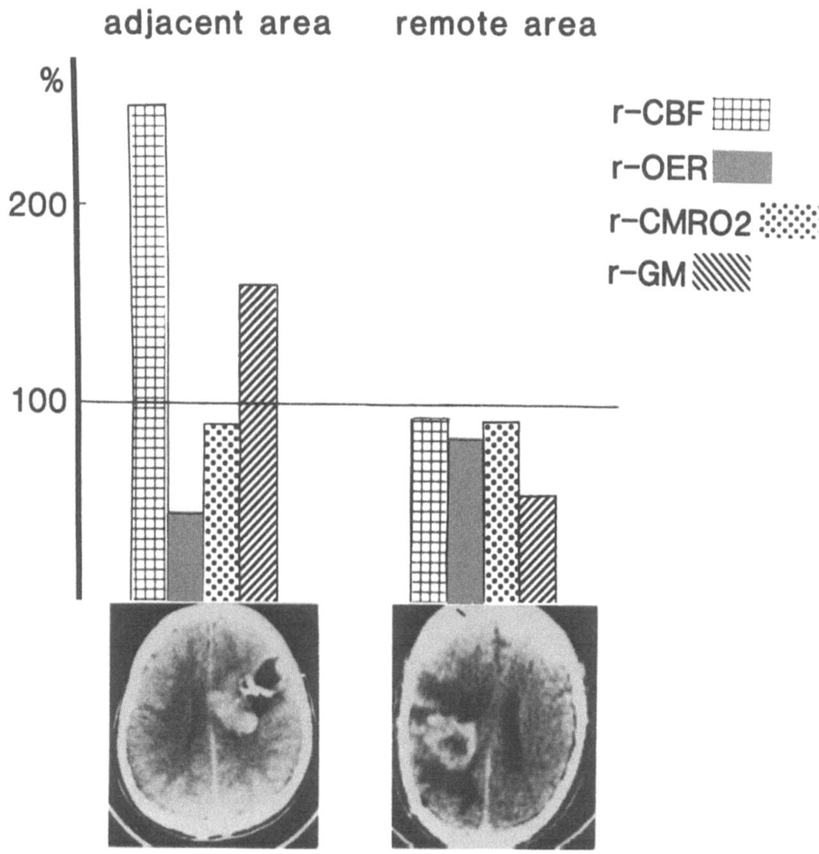

Fig. 2. Two kinds of alterations in metabolism and cerebral circulation in the peritumoral edematous area of glioblastoma. *Right,* metabolic and circulatory changes near the tumor border on enhanced CT; tumor infiltration was found in biopsy specimen. *Left,* metabolic and circulatory changes at outer border of the low-density area on X-ray CT (*black diamond*): no tumor infiltration was found on biopsy, but both total adenirates and energy charge potential were decreased to about 40% of normal

Malignant Glioma Group (Astrocytoma Grade III or IV)

In the 13 cases of malignant glioma, rCBF increased by more than 50% in some areas of the tumors, and by 10%–20% in others, even in the same tumor. Increases and decreases in rCBF in the tumors were heterogeneous, and they did not correlate at all with density changes seen on X-ray CT. $rCMRO_2$ decreased in all tumor areas with low rOER, but the products of regional glucose metabolism increased by more than 10% in all tumor areas, and in some by more than 50%. rCBV increased in some areas of tumors. The rate of these alterations varied from case to case, but their pattern in the PET image was similar. These findings indicate that anaerobic glycolysis without any anoxic or ischemic change must lead to the production of pyrimidine or amino acid in the tumor.

In the area of peritumoral brain edema two kinds of alterations of rCBF and metabolism were revealed by PET (Fig. 2). One type of alteration was observed very close to tumor borders on enhanced CT: rCBF was slightly increased, $rCMRO_2$ decreased and glucose metabolites increased; an increase of rCBV was found in two cases of all those examined. These findings indicate luxury perfusion with vasoparalysis. The other type of alteration was observed at the edge of the outer border of the low-density area on X-ray CT; both rCBF and $rCMRO_2$ decreased at almost the same rate, and regional glucose metabolites also decreased slightly. These findings indicate the matched low-perfusion phenomenon observed in areas of peritumoral edema around meningiomas or benign gliomas.

By using enhanced CT following rapid mannitol infusion for temporary opening of the blood-brain barrier, it was possible to distinguish two areas: the area near the tumor was markedly enhanced, and tumor tissue was observed in biopsy specimens corresponding to the area revealed on PET to contain luxury perfusion and high levels of glucose metabolites, while in the other area neither contrast enhancement nor any tumor infiltration corresponding to the area in which the matched low perfusion phenomenon was observed on PET.

In the peritumoral area of edema, in which the matched low-perfusion phenomenon was seen, total adenylates and the energy charge potential decreased to 40%–50% of the normal values, with no significant increase in lactate.

Discussion and Conclusions

The results presented show no evidence of the anoxic or ischemic brain damage in the area of peritumoral brain edema described by Hossmann et al. [4] and Bothe et al. [2], but decreased rCBF, decreased $rCMRO_2$ with lower rOER, and decreased regional glucose metabolites were observed in the presence of even small meningiomas, while intracranial pressure is not increased above 15 mmHg. Furthermore, this matched low-perfusion phenomenon can be observed in the area of peritumoral brain edema caused by either a benign or a malignant primary brain tumor.

One of the deleterious effects of vasogenic edema fluid on the brain tissue in the edematous area is reversible disturbance of the nerve membrane and capillary epithelium by the plasma transudate content of arachidonic acid [3] or other substances.

The matched low-perfusion phenomenon is often observed in the brain tissue in gradually induced cell death or cell loss caused by a chronic stage of cerebral infarct. But the matched low perfusion in the area of peritumoral brain edema is different from chronic ischemic change insofar as it is reversible; the decrease in total adenylates and energy charge potential with increased lactate is also reversible to normal after removal of the tumor. It is significant that the edema itself is not accompanied by any neurologic signs [7], in spite of the matched low-perfusion phenomenon.

These results might lead to the conclusion that the matched low perfusion observed in the peritumoral edematous area is not only suppressed by increased localized tissue pressure, but that edema fluid also contains substances released from brain tumors and that their noxious effect is reversible after removal of the tumor.

Summary

To demonstrate the alteration of both metabolism and cerebral circulation at peritumoral edematous tissue, rCBF, $rCMRO_2$, rCBV, and rCMRGl were studied by positron emission CT in 30 patients suffering from meningioma or glioma and having intracranial pressure of 15–30 mmHg without disturbance of consciousness.

In all kinds of primary meningioma or glioma, the peritumoral edematous brain tissue corresponded to a peritumoral low-density area on X-ray CT, had decreased rCBF with no increase of rCBV, decreased $rCMRO_2$ with normal to low rOER, and decreased levels of regional glucose metabolites when there was no infiltration of the tumor or any extremely high intracranial pressure of more than 30 mmHg. This is the matched low perfusion phenomenon without anoxia or ischemia, and it is completely reversed with recovery of the normal state after total removal of the tumor.

According to these results, reversible matched low perfusion at the peritumoral edematous brain tissue is not caused solely by increased tissue pressure; in addition, edema fluid contained some substances released from the brain tumor, which had adverse effects on cerebral blood flow and metabolism.

References

1. Bartknowski HM (1984) Peritumoral edema. Prog Exp Tumor Res 27:179
2. Bothe HW, Kerckhoff W, Paschen W, Wallenfang T, Hossmann KA (1984) Dissociation between blood flow and metabolic disturbances in edema associated with experimental abscess in cat. In: Go KG, Baethmann A (eds) Recent progress in the study and therapy of brain edema. Plenum, New York
3. Chan PH, Fishman RA (1984) Phospholipid degeneration and early release of polyunsaturated fatty acids in the evolution of brain edema. In: Go KG, Baethmann A (eds) Recent progress in the study and therapy of brain edema. Plenum, New York
4. Hossmann KA, Bloink M, Wilmes F, Wechsler W (1980) Experimental peritumoral edema of the cat brain. Adv Neurol 28:323
5. Klatzo I, Wisniewski H, Steinwall O, Streicher E (1967) Dynamics of cold injury edema. Brain edema. Springer, New York, p 554
6. Levin UA, Freeman-Dove M, Landahl HD (1975) Permeability characteristics of brain adjacent to tumor in rat. Arch Neurol 32:785–791
7. Penn RD (1980) Cerebral edema and neurological function: CT, evoked responses and clinical examination. Adv Neurol 28:383
8. Reulen HJ, Medzjhradsky F, Enzenbach R, Marguth E, Brendel W (1969) Electrolytes, fluids and energy metabolism in human cerebral edema. Arch Neurol 21:517–525
9. Weber G (1977) Enzymology of cancer cells. New Engl J Med 296:493–496, 541–551

Membrane Events Leading to Glial Swelling and Brain Edema *

B. K. SIESJÖ [1]

Key words: Cytotoxic edema, astrocytes, intracellular pH

Introduction

Although cytotoxic edema is a dreaded complication of cerebral ischemia and trauma, aggravating the impact of the primary insults, its molecular causes are still unknown. No doubt, since this type of edema is caused by loss of control of cell volume, further advances in edema research will require elucidation of the membranous events responsible for regulation of cell volume, and recognition of factors triggering cell swelling. Recent results provide useful information on these issues. First, several studies have shown that regulatory increases in cell volume following osmotic shrinkage involve uptake of Na^+ and Cl^-, with osmotically committed water, via electrosilent Na^+/H^+ and Cl^-/HCO_3^- exchangers [4, 5, 7]. Second, these antiport systems are the ones involved in the regulation of intracellular pH (pH_i); for example, it is recognized that a decrease in pH_i will stimulate Na^+/H^+ exchange, leading to cellular uptake of Na^+, and H^+ extrusion [28]. Third, it is now established that the aggravating effect of hyperglycemia on ischemic brain damage involves gross cellular edema [11, 21].

These findings suggest that tissue acidosis is what precipitates loss of cell volume control in ischemia [31, 32]. The purpose of this article is to discuss the evidence in more detail, and to elaborate on the hypothesis of acidosis-triggered cell swelling. It should be emphasized that the discussion does not cover vasogenic edema (see Rapoport, this volume), nor does it take into account water flux which is secondary to formation or release of osmotically active compounds in the ischemic cell (see Hossmann, this volume). The edema considered, therefore, is that developing in the recovery period following transient ischemia, or that formed in the periphery of an ischemic core during the evolution of stroke. I will begin by describing the origin and the characteristics of this edema, continue by discussing mechanisms of cell volume control, and end by outlining the salient features of the hypothesis of acidosis-triggered cell swelling.

* The study described in this paper was supported by grants from the Swedish Medical Research Council (no. 14X-263), and U.S. Public Health Service (NIH grant no. 2 RO1 NS 07838)
[1] Laboratory for Experimental Brain Research, E-blocket, Lund Hospital, S-22185 Lund, Sweden

Hyperglycemia and Aggravation of Ischemic Brain Damage

Although it had previously been speculated that acidosis might aggravate damage to brain cells, it remained for Myers to provide more definitive proof of a causal relationship. This author made the important observation that fed animals showed more extensive brain damage following ischemia of known density and duration than did fasted ones, and since he was able to reproduce the adverse effects of feeding by preischemic glucose infusion it seemed that enhanced anaerobic glycolysis was responsible [21, 22]. These results were soon confirmed [29].

At the same time, results were published which paradoxically demonstrated that complete ischemia could be followed by a better metabolic recovery than a corresponding period of severe, incomplete ischemia [23, 26]. Since contradictory information was obtained in a subsequent study [34] the field remained controversial for a while. However, the controversy was resolved when new results showed that the outcome of severe incomplete ischemia depended on the nutritional state, notably on blood glucose concentrations [27]. These results and those previously published [18] showed that in both complete and incomplete ischemia, the amount of lactate accumulated in the tissue correlated with blood glucose concentrations. However, the results also made it evident that the outcome depends on both the degree of lactic acidosis and the residual blood flow. As a working hypothesis, then, we can assume that a persisting oxygen supply has a survival value provided that excessive acidosis does not develop; furthermore, such acidosis wrecks the machinery by allowing gross edema to develop (Fig. 1).

So far, I have tacitly assumed, as did Myers [21], that the adverse effect of hyperglycemia is due to enhanced tissue acidosis. The evidence is circumstantial, since it is based on the inverse correlation between tissue lactate content during ischemia and metabolic/functional recovery [6, 25, 27, 36]. However, the assumption of a relationship between acidosis and edema/infarction is strengthened by results obtained in hypoglycemia. Thus, although severe hypoglycemia, a condition which disrupts the cerebral energy state and ion homeostasis in the absence of tissue acidosis, can cause extensive neuronal necrosis, it causes neither gross edema nor infarction [1, 2].

Granting that acidosis is the cause of the enhanced tissue damage, what are the characteristics of the associated edema? In complete cerebral ischemia, impedance measurements demonstrate that extracellular fluid (ECF) volume decreases to about 50% of control while histopathological analyses reveal expansion of astrocytic compartments (for literature, see [10, 30]). Such results suggest that part of the ECF is imbibed by glial cells. However, since circulation has ceased there is neither an increase in tissue water content nor any changes in electrolytes. A similar situation (astrocytic swelling but little sign of tissue edema) is encountered in hypoglycemic coma and in epileptic seizures (literature: [30]). Typically, most of the swelling affects astrocytes surrounding either vessels or neurons which show structural signs of injury.

In contrast, the edema developing in the postischemic period following long periods of complete or near-complete ischemia, or that arising in the periphery ("penumbra") of a densely ischemic core, is associated with net accumulation of water, Na^+, and Cl^-, and usually with loss of potassium (e.g., [10, 12]). At least initially,

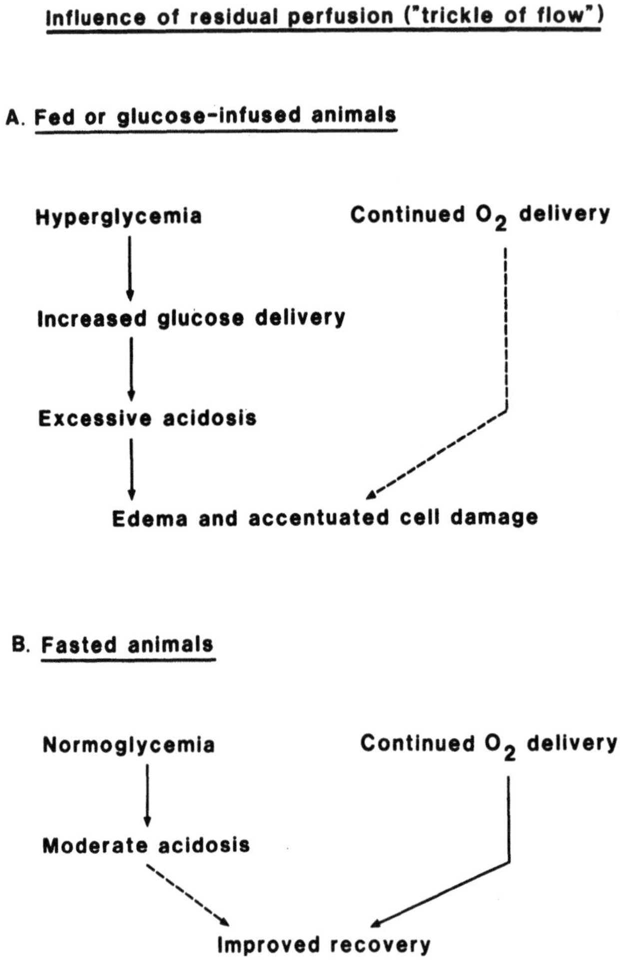

Fig. 1. Tentative schematic explaining why a residual blood flow has a different influence on the outcome of transient ischemia depending on whether animals are fed, glucose-infused, or fasted prior to induction of ischemia

the edema is of the cytotoxic type [16]. Following ischemia in fed rats, the edema manifests itself as a rapid and progressive swelling of glial cells, with eventual rupture of plasma membranes [11, 24]. Obviously, when seeking the relationship between acidosis and brain damage we must focus interest on volume control in glial cells and on its relationship to acid–base changes.

Regulation of Cell Volume

The double Donnan pump-leak hypothesis for control of cell volume has been widely accepted [17, 35]. An elementary description of the hypothesis is given in Fig. 2. Donnan forces due to the presence of impermeant intracellular anions favor influx

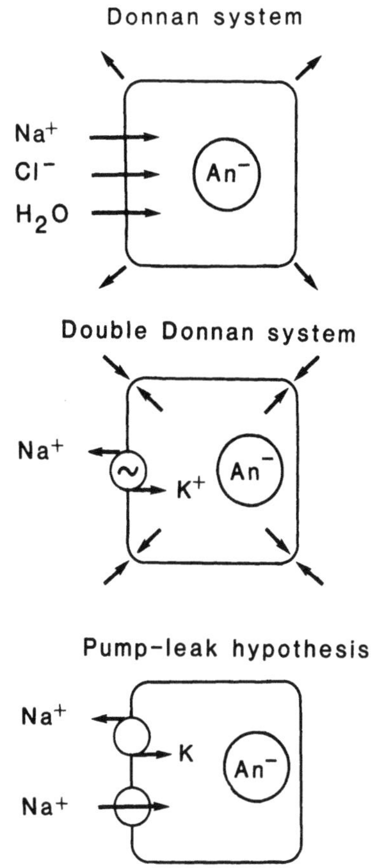

Fig. 2. Elementary schematic describing the double Donnan pump-leak hypothesis for control of cell volume. A Donnan system is one in which cells with permeant anions attract permeant ions and water. In a double Donnan system, cell volume is maintained by active extrusion of Na^+. At steady state, cell volume is a function of the Na^+ leak and the Na^+ pump

of permeant ions and of water. This is counteracted by a membrane pump which, by maintaining Na^+ in a predominantly extracellular position, balances the influence of the intracellular anions. In this situation, cell volume is a function of the balance between the Na^+ pump and the Na^+ leak.

For a long time, the Na^+ leak remained poorly defined. It is now known from experiments on nucleated erythrocytes and other cells which can be studied in vitro, that ion fluxes associated with increases in cell volume are electroneural, and occur as co-transport of Na^+-K^+ and Cl^- into the cell (symport, see [9, 17]) or as countertransport (antiport) of Na^+/H^+ and Cl^-/HCO_3^- [4, 5, 7]. Figure 3 schematically illustrates such coupled ion exchanges in which Na^+ and Cl^- are translocated inward, with osmotically committed water. As demonstrated by Cala [4, 5], the fluxes of H^+ and HCO_3^- are cyclic and therefore osmotically indifferent.

The schematic in Fig. 3 suggests that the Na^+ leak of the classic pump-leak hypothesis is the Na^+/H^+ antiporter. How can its activity be increased? One clue to this problem came when Bourke and Kimelberg and their associates showed that glial swelling could be induced either by high K^+ concentrations or, at constant $[K^+]$, by agonists such as noradrenaline, adenosine, and histamine (see [14, 15]). It seems, therefore, that the antiporters are subject to regulation by exogenous messen-

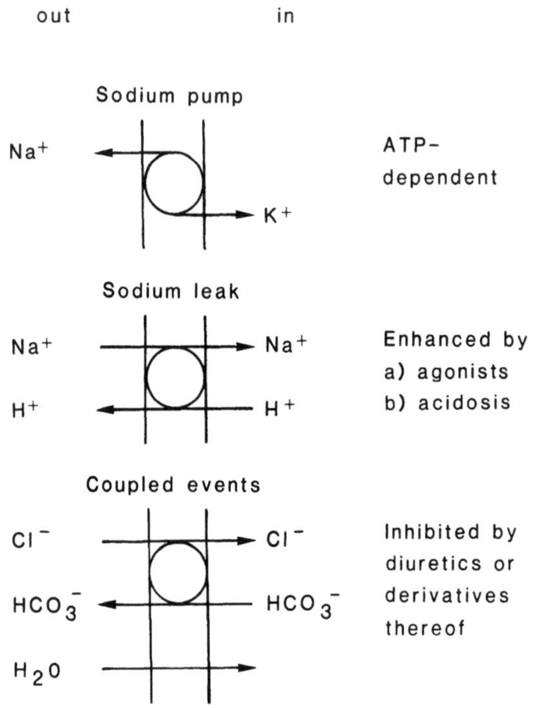

Fig. 3. Schematic illustrating how influx of Na^+ and Cl^-, with osmotically committed water, can occur by coupled Na^+/H and Cl^-/HCO_3^- exchanges. The Na^+/H^+ exchange, which triggers swelling, is shown to be enhanced by certain agonists, and by intracellular acidosis. Coupled Cl^-/HCO_3^- exchange, which is necessary for acidosis to occur, is inhibited by certain diuretics

gers. This is not the only demonstration of such regulation. For example, Moore [20] has suggested that Na^+/H^+ exchange in muscle tissue is enhanced by insulin, and Berridge [3] has cited evidence that agonists which activate phospholipase C and the C-kinase system have a similar end-effect in several cell types. Such enhancement is all that is required, since the normal Na^+ gradient (10:1) provides the necessary driving force for the exchange to occur.

Accepting, at least as a working hypothesis, that the Na^+ leak in the form of Na^+/H^+ exchange can be "induced," how does the Na^+/H^+ antiporter, coupled to Cl^-/HCO_3^- exchange, translocate Cl^- inwards? We recall that, for swelling to occur, both Na^+ and Cl^- must enter the cell. A first requirement to be fullfilled is that the membrane contains an anion exchanger of this type. For glial cells, this seems to be the case [13–15]. A second requirement is that the antiporter operates in the direction indicated, i.e., translocating Cl^- in and HCO_3^- out. To provide a tentative clue to this problem, and indeed to the whole problem of massive enhancement of cell swelling, we must consider the mechanisms of pH_i regulation.

Regulation of Intracellular pH

Although it has been known for almost 15 years that pH_i in brain cells is subject to regulation by mechanisms which must involve both production/consumption of metabolic acids and membrane transport of H^+ or HCO_3^- [33], the actual mechanisms of regulation by membrane transport have been only partly characterized (for

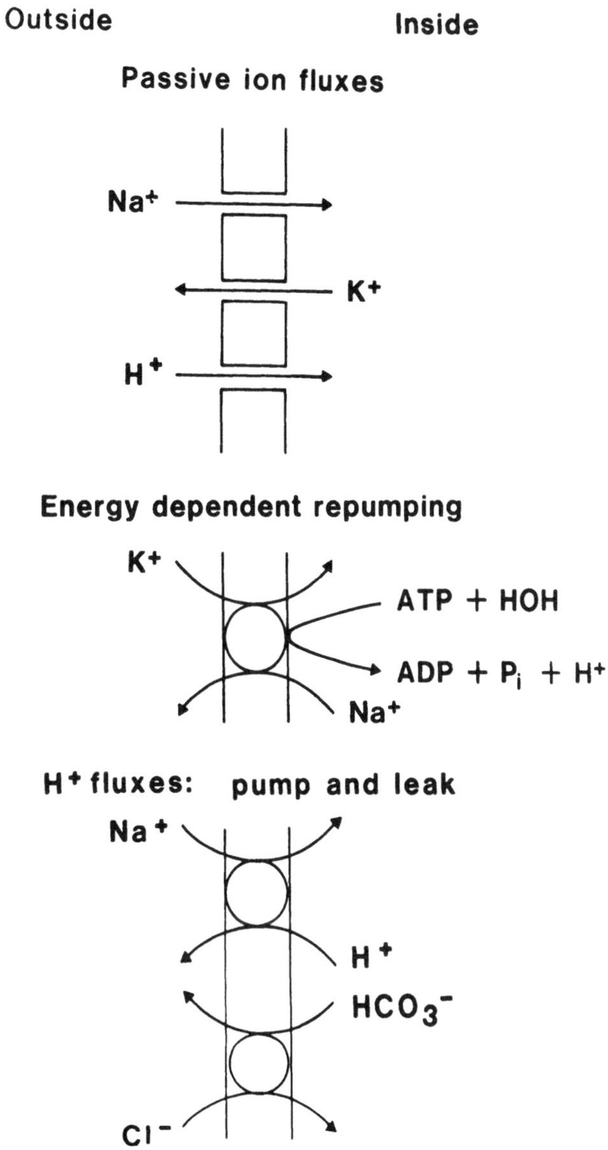

Fig. 4. Tentative schematic showing regulation of pH_i by active extrusion via a Na^+/H^+ antiport, the energy source of which is the Na^+ gradient created by the Na^+, K^+-ATPase. Backflux of H^+ is shown to occur not as conductive H^+ influx, but as HCO_3^- outflux via a Cl^-/HCO_3 antiporter [32]

literature, see [28, 32]). Experiments on a variety of isolated cells, in which pH_i has been measured with H^+-sensitive microelectrodes, suggest that one universal mechanism of pH_i regulation is Na^+/H^+ exchange, the energy source for which is the Na^+ gradient created by Na^+-K^+ ATPase (Fig. 4). I will discuss some of the principal features of this pH_i-regulating ion exchange.

In brain extracellular fluids, pH (pH_e) is around 7.3, and the HCO_3^- concentration, about 22 μmol ml^{-1}. With a negative membrane potential of 60 mV, or more, passive distribution of H^+ would require a pH_i of 6.3 or lower. Likewise, $[HCO_3^-]_i$ would have to be 2 μmol ml^{-1} or lower. Since pH_i is about 7, and $[HCO_3^-]_i$ about 12 μmol ml^{-1}, one must assume that H^+ is constantly and actively extruded from cells, or that HCO_3^- is actively absorbed. By the same token, passive leakage of H^+ must be inward, and that of HCO_3^-, outward. It may be profitable to begin our discussion of ion translocation by assuming that fluxes of H^+ predominate. Then, pH_i is determined by the balance between the rate of extrusion of H^+ (the H^+ pump) and the rate of its back-leakage (the H^+ leak).

Consider a situation in which all, or most, of the transmembrane H^+ flux occurs as coupled Na^+/H^+ exchange. Then, the driving force for the exchange is given by the equation [5]

$$\Delta\mu_{Na^+-H^+} = RT\ln\frac{[Na^+]_i}{[Na^+]_o} - RT\ln\frac{[H^+]_i}{[H^+]_o}. \quad (1)$$

Since the ratio $[Na^+]_e/[Na^+]_i$ is normally 10:1, we have to conclude that H^+ flux is normally outward, not inward, as would be predicted from the Nernst equation if H^+ moved in isolation, i.e., via a conductive pathway. How, then, can we envisage back-leakage of H^+ to occur? One possible explanation is the existence of parallel conductance channels for H^+. Another explanation, though, is that passive H^+ influx occurs as HCO_3^- outflux via the Cl^-/HCO_3^- antiporter. The thermodynamic requirement for this is given by the equation

$$\Delta\mu_{Cl=HCO_3^-} = RT\ln\frac{[Cl^-]_i}{[Cl^-]_o} - RT\ln\frac{[HCO_3^-]_i}{[HCO_3^-]_o}. \quad (2)$$

Since the ratio $[Cl^-]_o:[Cl^-]_i$ is about 10, the coupled exchange will favor influx of Cl^- and outflux of HCO_3^-, i.e., it will presumably function as an H^+ leak. It has been claimed, on the basis of experiments on isolated neurons, that flux via a Cl^-/HCO_3^- antiporter can be the opposite and contribute to pH_i regulation by uphill transport of HCO_3^- (reviewed by [28, 32]). We will assume, though, that at least in glial cells the anion exchanger serves as an H^+ leak.

It has been firmly established that acidification of cells promotes increased Na^+/H^+ exchange (see [8, 28]). In at least one cell type, the isolated thymocyte, lowering of pH_i to 6.2–6.3 has been found to increase Na^+ influx to values of 10 μmol g^{-1} [8]. This is a massive flux of Na^+ (and H^+), capable of rapid regulation of pH_i in situations of acidosis such as ischemia and epileptic seizures [32].

Acidosis and Cell Swelling

Clearly, acidification of the cell interior would lead to at least one of the events which is required for swelling to occur, viz. influx of Na^+ (see Fig. 4). The efficacy of the pH_i regulation will depend on two things: the rate of H^+ extrusion by Na^+/H^+ exchange and the rate of HCO_3^- efflux via the Cl^-/HCO_3^- antiporter. If back-leakage of H^+ via the Cl^-/HCO_3^- antiporter is fast a futile H^+ cycle is created, whose major effect will be accumulation of Na^+ and Cl^-, with osmotically committed water, i.e., cell edema.

It can be concluded, therefore, that sustained acidosis, especially if pronounced, is apt to cause cell swelling. Conceivably, the severity of this edema depends on the behavior of the Cl^-/HCO_3^- antiporter, i.e., on the rate of back-leakage of H^+. If this is high and/or the acid production is sustained, the Na^+/H^+ antiporter will continue to extrude H^+, but at the expense of volume homeostasis. One requirement for continued inward translocation of Cl^- is that a favorable electrochemical gradient is maintained, i.e., that the *ratio* $[Cl^-]_o:[Cl^-]_i$ exceeds the ratio $[HCO_3^-]_o:[HCO_3^-]_i$ (see Eq. 2). The Na^+/H^+ antiporter should by itself maintain this ratio. Thus, by extruding H^+ it will tend to raise $[HCO_3^-]_i$ and lower $[HCO_3^-]_o$. The possibility that Cl^-/HCO_3^- exchange is enhanced by the actions of hormones or other membrane-active compounds cannot be excluded, however.

Admittedly, the hypothesis of acidosis-induced astrocytic edema is based on circumstantial evidence. However, the mere facts that glial cells contain Na^+/H^+ and Cl^-/HCO_3^- antiporters, that these coupled antiporters are involved in both regulatory volume increase, following osmotic shrinkage, and in pH_i regulation, and that intracellular acidosis can trigger massively enhanced Na^+/H^+ exchange, provide strong support for the hypothesis. Nonetheless, these arguments should not be interpreted as suggesting that the mechanisms proposed are the only ones causing "cytotoxic" edema. Rather, they suggest that acidosis is one factor that may precipitate uncontrolled swelling of glial cells in ischemic situations.

Summary

It is now established that hyperglycemia caused by diet or glucose infusion aggravates brain damage incurred as a result of ischemia. Conspicuous features of this damage are edema and infarction. It has been widely concluded that hyperglycemia aggravates ischemic brain damage by enhancing tissue acidosis. Thus, a relationship between acidosis and edema/infarction is suggested. This article discusses the molecular mechanisms that may be involved.

Regulation of cell volume can be explained by the double Donnan pump-leak hypothesis. According to this, cell volume represents the balance between an Na^+ pump and a Na^+ leak. The former has been equated with the Na^+/K^+-ATPase, and recent experiments suggest that the Na^+ leak can be an electrosilent Na^+/H^+ exchanger. In many cells, swelling is induced by the operation of coupled Na^+/H^+ and Cl^-/HCO_3^--exchangers which achieve inward translocation of Na^+ and Cl^-, with osmotically committed water. However, these exchangers are also involved in intracellular pH regulation, and in such a way that acidosis triggers increased Na^+/H^+ exchange, with intracellular accumulation of Na^+. It is proposed that such enhanced exchange, with coupled influx of Cl^- via a Cl^-/HCO_3^- antiporter, is what underlies glial cell swelling in acidotic states.

References

1. Auer RN, Olsson Y, Siesjö BK (1984) Hypoglycemic brain injury in the rat. Correlation of density of brain damage with the EEG isoelectric time: a quantitative study. Diabetes 33:1090–1098

2. Auer RN, Wieloch T, Olsson Y, Siesjö BK (1984) The distribution of hypoglycemic brain damage. Acta Neuropathol (Berl) 64:177–191
3. Berridge MJ (1984) Inositol triphosphate and dialglycerol as second messengers. Biochem J 221:345–360
4. Cala PM (1980) Volume regulation by amphiuma red blood cells. The membrane potential and its implications regarding the nature of the ion-flux pathways. J Gen Physiol 76:683–708
5. Cala PM (1983) Volume regulation by red blood cells. Mechanisms of ion transport. Molec Physiol 4:33–52
6. Gardiner A, Smith M-L, Kågström E, Shohami E, Siesjö BK (1982) Influence of blood glucose concentration on brain lactate accumulation during severe hypoxia and subsequent recovery of brain energy metabolism. J Cereb Blood Flow Metabol 2:429–438
7. Grinstein S, Clarke CA, Rothstein A (1983) Activation of Na^+/H^+ exchange in lymphocytes by osmotically induced volume changes and by cytoplasmic acidification. J Gen Physiol 82:619–638
8. Grinstein S, Cohen S, Rothstein A (1984) Cytoplasmic pH regulation in thymic lymphocytes by an amiloride-sensitive Na^+/H^+ antiport. J Gen Physiol 83:341–369
9. Haas M, Schmidt III WF, McManus TJ (1982) Catecholamine-stimulated ion transport in duck red cells. J Gen Physiol 80:125–147
10. Hossmann K-A (1982) Treatment of experimental cerebral ischemia. J Cereb Blood Flow Metabol 2:275–297
11. Kalimo H, Rehncrona S, Söderfeldt B, Olsson Y, Siesjö BK (1981) Brain lactic acidosis and ischemic cell damage: 2. Histopathology. J Cereb Blood Flow Metabol 1:313–327
12. Katzman R, Clasen R, Klatzo I, Meyer JS, Pappius HM, Waltz AG (1977) Report of Joint Committee for Stroke Resources. IV: Brain edema in stroke. Stroke 8:512–540
13. Kimelberg HK (1983) Primary astrocyte cultures – a key to astrocyte function. Cell Molec Neurobiol 3(1):1–16
14. Kimelberg HK, Bourke RS (1982) Anion transport in the nervous system. In: Lajtha A (ed) Handbook of neurochemistry. Chemical and cellular architecture. 2nd edn, vol 1. Plenum, New York, pp 31–67
15. Kimelberg HK, Bourke RS (1984) Mechanisms of astrocytic swelling. In: Bes A, Braquet P, Paoletti R, Siesjö BK (eds) Cerebral ischemia. Elsevier, Amsterdam, pp 131–146
16. Klatzo I (1967) Neuropathological aspects of brain edema. J Neuropathol Exp Neurol 26:1–14
17. Kregenow FM (1981) Osmoregulatory salt transporting mechanisms: control of cell volume in anisotonic media. Annu Rev Physiol 43:493–505
18. Ljunggren B, Norberg K, Siesjö BK (1974) Influence of tissue acidosis upon restitution of brain energy metabolism following total ischemia. Brain Res 77:173–186
19. MacKnight AD, Leaf A (1977) Regulation of cellular volume. Physiol Rev 57(3):510–573
20. Moore RD (1983) Effects of insulin upon ion transport. Biochim Biophys Acta 737:1–49
21. Myers RE (1979) Lactic acid accumulation as cause of brain edema and cerebral necrosis resulting from oxygen deprivation. In: Korobkin R, Guilleminault G (eds) Advances in perinatal neurology. Spectrum, New York, pp 85–114
22. Myers RE, Yamaguchi S (1977) Nervous system effects of cardiac arrest in monkeys. Arch Neurol 34:65–74
23. Nordström C-H, Rehncrona S, Siesjö BK (1978) Effects of phenobarbital in cerebral ischemia: II. Restitution of cerebral energy state, as well as of glycolytic metabolites, citric acid cycle intermediates and associated amino acids after pronounced incomplete ischemia. Stroke 9:335–343
24. Petito CK, Pulsinelli WA, Jacobson G, Plum F (1982) Edema and vascular permeability in cerebral ischemia: comparison between ischemia neuronal damage and infarction. J Neuropathol Exp Neurol 41:423–436
25. Pulsinelli WA, Waldman S, Rawlinson D, Plum F (1982) Moderate hyperglycemia augments ischemic brain damage: a neuropathologic study in the rat. Neurology 32:1239–1246
26. Rehncrona S, Mela L, Siesjö BK (1979) Recovery of brain mitochondrial function in the rat after complete and incomplete cerebral ischemia. Stroke 10:437–446

27. Rehncrona S, Rosén I, Siesjö BK (1981) Brain lactic acidosis and ischemic cell damage: 1. Biochemistry and neurophysiology. J Cereb Blood Flow Metabol 1:297–311
28. Roos A, Boron WF (1981) Intracellular pH. Physiol Rev 61:296–434
29. Siemkowicz E, Hansen A (1978) Clinical restitution following cerebral ischemia in hypo-, normo-, and hyperglycemic rats. Acta Neurol Scand 58:1–8
30. Siesjö BK (1981) Cell damage in the brain: a speculative synthesis. J Cereb Blood Flow Metabol 1:155–185
31. Siesjö BK (1984) Cerebral circulation and metabolism. J Neurosurg 60:883–908
32. Siesjö BK (1985) Acid-base homeostasis in the brain: physiology, chemistry, and neurochemical pathology. Progr Brain Res (in press)
33. Siesjö BK, Messeter K (1971) Factors determining intracellular pH. In: Siesjö BK, Sørensen SC (eds) Ion homeostasis of the brain. Munksgaard, Copenhagen, pp 244–262
34. Steen PA, Michenfelder JD, Milde JH (1979) Incomplete versus complete cerebral ischemia: improved outcome with a minimal blood flow. Ann Neurol 6:389–398
35. Tosteson DC, Hoffman JF (1960) Regulation of cell volume by active cation transport in high and low potassium sheep red cells. J Gen Physiol 44:169–194
36. Welsh FA, Ginsberg MD, Rieder W, Budd WW (1980) Deleterious effect of glucose pretreatment on recovery from diffuse cerebral ischemia in the cat. II. Regional metabolite levels. Stroke 11:355–363

Early Changes in Blood-Brain Barrier Permeability After MCA Occlusion in Rats

J. Cervós-Navarro [1], Y. Nakagawa, and S. Sampaolo

Key words: Blood-brain barrier, MCA occlusion, focal ischemia, lanthanum, brain edema

Materials and Methods

Surgery

Twenty male Wistar rats weighing approximately 300 g were used. Under ketamine anesthesia (150 mg/kg body weight) the animals were allowed to breathe spontaneously and underwent cannulation of the right femoral artery and vein, which allowed us to monitor physiological parameters and to administer drugs. Body temperature was monitored and kept at 37.5 °C. Once the physiological parameters were within normal ranges the left MCA was exposed according to the procedure of Albanese et al. [1] and occluded by bipolar coagulation. The animals were sacrificed 10, 30, 60, and 180 min after occlusion of the MCA.

Tracers Administered

HRP Groups

Horseradish peroxidase (HRP Sigma II, 100 mg/1 ml PBS) was injected IV to four animals 5 min before occlusion of the MCA. In another group of animals it was injected 5 min after the MCA occlusion. After the given periods of ischemia the animals were perfused via the left cardiac ventricle with 50 ml saline solution followed by a 4% glutaraldehyde-paraformaldehyde solution in 0.1 *M* cacodylate buffer.

$LaCl_3$ Group

Immediately after sacrifice 12 animals were perfused via the left cardiac ventricle with 50 ml saline solution followed by 2% glutaraldehyde-paraformaldehyde fixative solution in a 0.1 *M* sodium cacodylate buffer with a pH of 7.4 at a controlled

[1] Institute of Neuropathology, Free University of Berlin, Hindenburgdamm 30, D-1000 Berlin 45

pressure of 120 mmHg for 5 min. $LaCl_3$ 15 mM was dissolved in the same fixative solution with which it was perfused. The animals were further perfused for 30 min with this new solution. During the last 5 min of perfusion a more concentrated (4%) fixative solution was injected.

Delimitation of the Ischemic Area

In all animal groups 0.1% methylene green was injected at the end of the perfusion to reveal the area of impaired blood supply.

Histology

Light Microscopy

After paraffin embedding 15-μm slices of the brain were stained with H & E and the Nissl technique.

Electron Microscopy

HRP Group. Brain slices 1.5 mm thick were sectioned with a vibratome at a thickness of 50 μm. The slices were then incubated for peroxidase activity by means of a two-step method [2]. After post-fixation five brain areas were selected (Fig. 1) and embedded in araldite. Ultrathin sections were contrasted with uranyl acetate and lead citrate.

$LaCl_3$ Group. Brain slices 1.5 mm thick (Fig. 1) were rinsed and post-fixed in a buffered solution of 1% OsO_4 for 120 min, dehydrated in acetone, and embedded in araldite. Ultrathin sections were observed with a Zeiss EM 10 electron microscope with or without heavy metal staining.

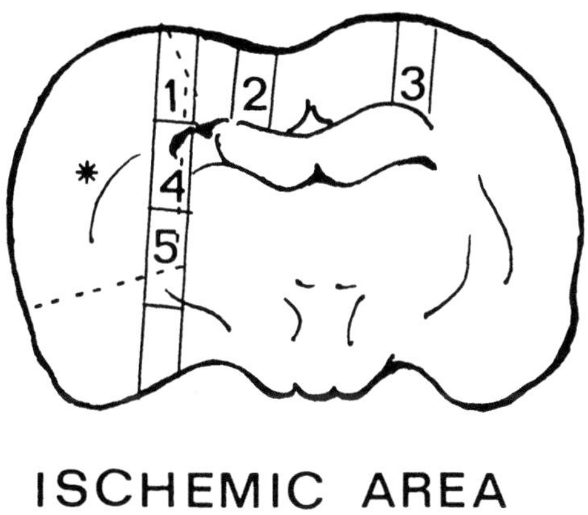

Fig. 1. Areas (*1–5*) selected for embedding in araldite and electron-microscopic examination following post-fixation

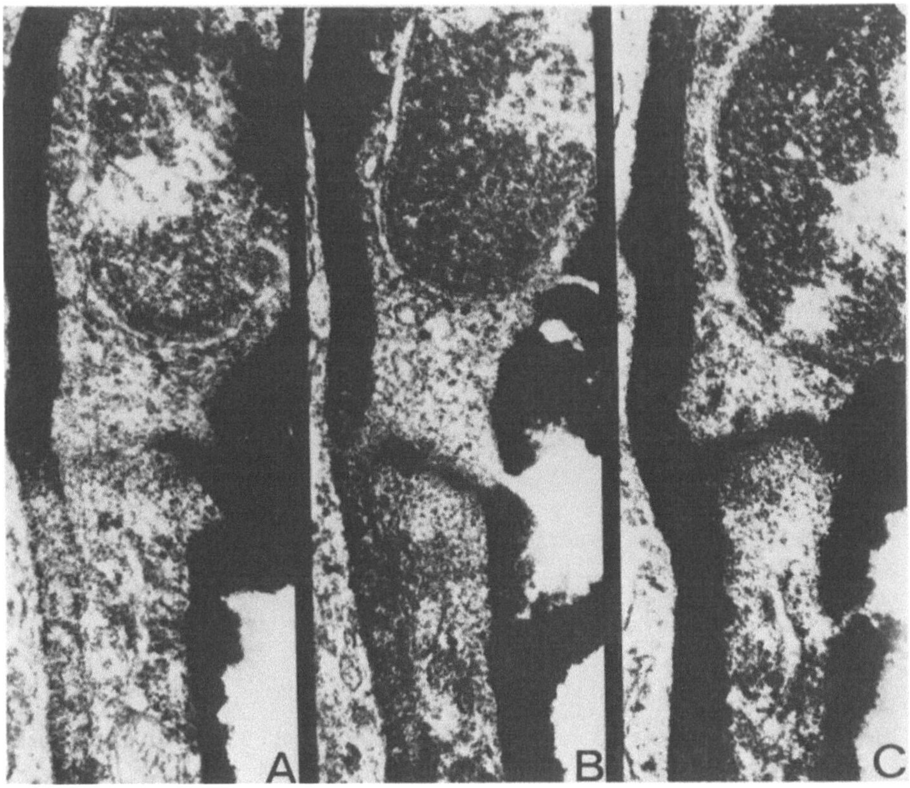

Fig. 2A–C. Serial ultrathin sections prepared after 30 min ischemia. **A** Lanthanum seems to have been stopped by the tight junctions. **B** Lanthanum penetrating into the interendothelial space. **C** Lanthanum has reached the basement membrane

Results

In all the animals an area of ischemia involving the cortex and part of the basal ganglia in the occluded hemisphere was observed. Light microscopy did not reveal ischemic neuronal damage in any of the animals.

With electron microscopy, 10 min after MCA occlusion, lanthanum was only seen in the lumen of the vessels. However, after 30 min ischemia lanthanum penetrated the tight junctions (TJ) and the BM. In specimens 1 and 4 (Fig. 2) lanthanum was sometimes also seen in the ES. After 60 min and 3 h ischemia lanthanum was demonstrated in the TJ, BM, and ES in specimens 1, 4, and 5. In contrast, reactive products of HRP were confined to the lumen of the vessels in every case.

Discussion

Ischemic brain edema is due to a combination of metabolic and vasogenic edema, which occurs early after an ischemic episode. The concept that ischemic edema is cytotoxic in origin has evolved from data demonstrating an increased brain water content concomitant with the inability of large molecules to pass the blood-brain barrier (BBB) [3]. Few reports [4–6] deal with barrier permeability to small molecules in the early stages of ischemia.

Experimental focal cerebral ischemia in the rat is one of the most convenient models for the study of the pathophysiology of this disease [7, 8].

HRP is widely used as an electrodense tracer in ischemia and in other experimental models of BBB disruption [9], because it has a large hydrodynamic diameter (about 5.5 nm) and a high molecular weight (40 000). One of the smallest markers visible with electron microscopy is ionic lanthanum (mol. wt. 138.9, diameter 1.5 nm), In contrast to colloidal lanthanum, which causes blood clotting in vivo, ionic lanthanum can be infused IV to living rodents. However, it is lost from tissue during procedures such as fixation, sectioning, or washing. The safest procedure when $LaCl_3$ is used seems to be to perfuse it together with the fixative solution. Several investigations show that lanthanum does not penetrate the BBB in normal conditions [10–12]. Therefore, we believe that the presence of $LaCl_3$ in the BM and ES after 30 min ischemia is related to an increased permeability of the TJ to water ions.

Shigeno et al. [6], using the same rat model of ischemia as ourselves, observed a decrease in the specific gravity of brain tissue after 30 min of permanent MCA occlusion, but they were not able to find any statistical significance in these changes. However, the water content of the brain tissue was definitely increased after 4 h ischemia.

The same authors [6] report no increase in the BBB permeability to ^{14}C-aminosobutyric acid, a small neutral amino acid (^{14}C-AIB) (mol. wt. 103), up to 4 h after permanent occlusion.

Our data indicate that an increase in the BBB permeability to ionic compounds begins between 10 and 30 min after the ischemic insult. Therefore the lack of significance in the water content calculated by Shigeno et al. [6] may be due to the fact that it was in a very early stage. The different responses of the BBB to ^{14}C-AIB and $LaCl_3$, which are very similar in molecular weight, can be explained when we consider the different transport pathways used by the two tracers [13]. These pathways may have a different sensitivity to the ischemic insult, and therefore the opening of a paracellular pathway for water and ions may play a relevant role in the onset of ischemic edema.

Summary

Blood-brain barrier permeability to ionic lanthanum (La^{3+}) and horseradish peroxidase (HRP) was studied in acute focal ischemia in rats. HRP was injected IV to eight animals before or after the occlusion of the right middle cerebral artery (MCA). Twelve rats were perfused after MCA occlusion with a fixative solution containing 10–20 m*M* $LaCl_3$. The animals were sacrificed at 10, 30, 60, and 180 min of ischemia.

With electron microscopy, 10 min after MCA occlusion $LaCl_3$ was only seen in the lumen of brain vessels. However, after 30 min of ischemia $LaCl_3$ was demonstrated in the interendothelial cleft (IC), in the basal membrane (BM), and in the extracellular space (ES) around the vessels of brain cortex specimens. At 60 and

180 min after MCA occlusion similar results to those at 30 min were observed in specimens from both cortex and basal ganglia. HRP, in contrast was seen only in the lumen of vessels after all periods of ischemia up to 180 min. These findings may indicate that the early phase of ischemia causes increased permeability of the tight junctions of the cerebral microvasculature to water and ions, but not to tracers with higher molecular weight.

References

1. Albanese V, Tommasino C, Spadaro A, Tomasello F (1980) A transbasisphenoidal approach for selective occlusion of the middle cerebral artery in rats. Experientia 36:1302–1304
2. Westergaard E, Deurs B, Brondsted HE (1977) Increased vesicular transfer of horseradish peroxidase across cerebral endothelium, evoked by acute hypertension. Acta Neuropathol 37:141–152
3. Klatzo I (1967) Neuropathological aspects of brain oedema. J Neuropathol Exp Neurol 26:1–14
4. Tyson GW, Teasdale GM, Graham DI, McCulloch J (1982) Cerebrovascular permeability following MCA occlusion in the rat. The effect of halothane-induced hypotension. J Neurosurg 57:186–196
5. Sage JI, Van Uitert RL, Duffy TE (1984) Early changes in blood brain barrier permeability to small molecules after transient cerebral ischemia. Stroke 15:46–50
6. Shigeno T, Teasdale GM, McCulloch J, Mandelow D, Graham DI (1984) Brain edema following focal cerebral ischemia in the rat. In: Go KG, Baethmann A (eds) Recent progress in the study and therapy of brain edema. Plenum, New York, pp 449–459
7. Tamura A, Graham DI, McCulloch J, et al. (1981 a) Focal cerebral ischemia in the rat. 1: Description of technique and early neuropathological consequences following middle cerebral artery occlusion. J Cereb Blood Flow Metab 1:53–60
8. Tamura A, Graham DI, McCulloch J, et al. (1981 b) Focal cerebral ischaemia in the rat: 2. Regional cerebral blood flow determined by (^{14}C) iodoantipyrine autoradiography following middle cerebral artery occlusion. J Cereb Blood Metab 1:61–69
9. Van Deurs B (1980) Structural aspects of brain barriers, with special reference to the permeability of the cerebral endothelium and choroidal epithelium. Cytology 65:117–191
10. Brightman MW, Rees TS (1969) Junctions between intimately apposed cell membranes in the vertebrate brain. J Cell Biol 40:648–677
11. Milhorat TH, Davis DA, Hammock MK (1975) Experimental intracerebral movement of electron microscopic tracers of various molecular size. J Neurosurg 42:315–329
12. Nag S, Robertson DM, Dioensdale HB (1982) Intracerebral arteriolar permeability of lanthanum. Am J Pathol 107:336–341
13. Oldendorf WH (1977) Brain uptake of radiolabeled amino acids, amines and hexoses after arterial injection. Am J Physiol 221:1629–1639

Disturbances of Cerebral Arterial Permeability and Blood-Brain Barrier Following Experimental Subarachnoid Hemorrhage

T. SASAKI[1], N. F. KASSELL, M. YAMASHITA, S. FUJIWARA, and M. ZUCCARELLO

Key words: Blood-brain barrier, subarachnoid hemorrhage, vasospasm, intracranial pressure, computerized tomography

Introduction

Breakdown of the blood-brain barrier (BBB) following experimental subarachnoid hemorrhage (SAH) is currently controversial. Trojanowsky [1] has reported an early profound increase in capillary permeability in cats suffering from SAH. Shigeno et al. [2] have observed extravasation of Evans blue dye only in cats with both SAH and arterial hypertension, while Peterson and Cardoso [3] have recently reported that no demonstrable BBB lesions were observed when cats were rendered hypertensive after SAH.

On the other hand, the effect of SAH on the blood-arterial wall barrier of the major cerebral arteries in the basal cisterns has not been precisely evaluated, though recent clinical studies with contrast-enhanced CT (computered tomography) [4–9] have revealed abnormal post-contrast enhancement in the region of the basal subarachnoid cisterns following SAH. It has been suggested that these abnormalities correlate with the occurrence of angiographic spasm and neurologic deficits, and that contrast-enhanced CT is useful for predicting the occurrence of chronic cerebral vasospasm following SAH. However, the pathophysiology of the abnormal post-contrast enhancement has not yet been clarified.

The present study was undertaken to elucidate the mechanisms responsible for the changes in permeability of both the brain capillaries and the major cerebral arteries in the basal subarachnoid cisterns following SAH.

Materials and Methods

Twelve normotensive dogs of either sex, weighing 4.0–6.8 kg, were anesthetized with sodium pentobarbital, intubated, and ventilated with 60% nitrous oxide and 40% oxygen. Arterial blood gases were frequently checked, and arterial pH, PaO_2, and $PaCO_2$ were maintained within the physiological ranges. Arterial blood pressure and ICP were monitored using pressure transducers.

---

[1] Department of Neurological Surgery, University of Virginia, Charlottesville, Virginia 22908, USA

Table 1. Summary of experimental groups and results

Animal group	Maximum changes in MAP and ICP induced by SAH or saline injection			Barrier breakdown		
	No. of animals	Mean value of ΔMAP (mmHg)	Mean value of ΔICP (mmHg)	ICA	BA	Capillary
I: Control	4	(–)	(–)	(+)	(–)	(–)
II: Saline injection (nonisovolemic)	2	10	142	(++)	(–)	$1/2$
III: SAH (nonisovolemic)	3	77	148	(+++)	(+++)	$1/3$
IV: SAH (isovolemic)	3	12	16	(+++)	(+++)	$2/3$

SAH, subarachnoid hemorrhage; MAP, mean arterial pressure; ICP, intracranial pressure; ICA, internal carotic artery; BA, basilar artery

The animals were divided into four groups, as shown in Table 1. SAH was produced by two injections of 7 ml fresh autologous blood into the cisterna magna, given 72 h apart. In the isovolemic group, 7 ml cerebrospinal fluid was withdrawn immediately before injection of the blood. Animals were sacrificed at 3 days after the second SAH or saline injection.

Evans blued dye (2% solution, 2.5 ml/kg body weight) and horseradish peroxidase (HRP: 200 mg/kg body weight, Sigma type II. RZ: 1.52) were injected IV 20 and 10 min, respectively, before sacrifice of the animals, to assess the integrity of the barrier at 3 days after the second SAH or the saline injection.

The animals were treated with diphenhydramine hydrochloride (5 mg/kg body weight) prior to HRP injection, to prevent HRP-induced hypotension. The animals were perfused and fixed with a mixture containing 2% paraformaldehyde, 2.5% glutaraldehyde in 0.1 *M* phosphate buffer (pH 7.4) at a pressure of 150 cm H_2O. The brain was removed and immersed in a cacodylate-buffered fixative (pH 7.4) for 5 h at 4 °C, and then kept overnight at 4 °C in 0.1 *M* sodium cacodylate buffer (pH 7.3). The clot around the major cerebral arteries was carefully removed under magnification. The brain slices were macroscopically observed to detect whether there was leakage of Evans blue dye. HRP was localized by Graham and Karnovsky's procedure [10]. After osmification and embedding in epoxy resin, ultrathin sections were examined unstained or stained with uranyl acetate and lead citrate in an Hitachi H-600 electron microscope.

Results

Changes of ICP and Arterial Blood Pressure

The results are summarized in Table 1.

Cisternal nonisovolemic injection of 7 ml saline solution transiently elevated the ICP by 142 mmHg, while it elevated the mean arterial pressure (MAP) by only

10 mmHg. Nonisovolemic SAH induced a sudden rise in both ICP and MAP, which lasted for several minutes. On the other hand, isovolemic SAH did not produce any striking changes in either ICP or MAP. At the time of perfusion-fixation, both ICP and MAP of all experimental animals were within the normal ranges.

Morphological Changes

Major Cerebral Arteries

The areas with HRP-reactive products in the major cerebral arteries were easily identified by inspecting the brown-stained area under magnification. The exact location of these HRP-reactive products was identified using electron microscopy.

In control animals, proximal segments extending 1–3 mm from the origin of the intradural segments of both internal carotid and vertebral arteries were stained with HRP-reactive products (Fig. 1). Occasionally, the branching points of the major cerebral arteries were weakly stained.

Cisternal injection of saline solution in a nonisovolemic fashion increased the permeability to HRP in the arteries of the circle of Willis, mainly at the branching points (Fig. 2).

Extensive and marked disturbance of arterial permeability to HRP was consistently observed in the major cerebral arteries in dogs with both isovolemic and nonisovolemic SAH (Fig. 2).

As shown in Fig. 3, electron microscopic studies demonstrated marked corrugation of the elastic lamina. In places, endothelial cells appeared to have degener-

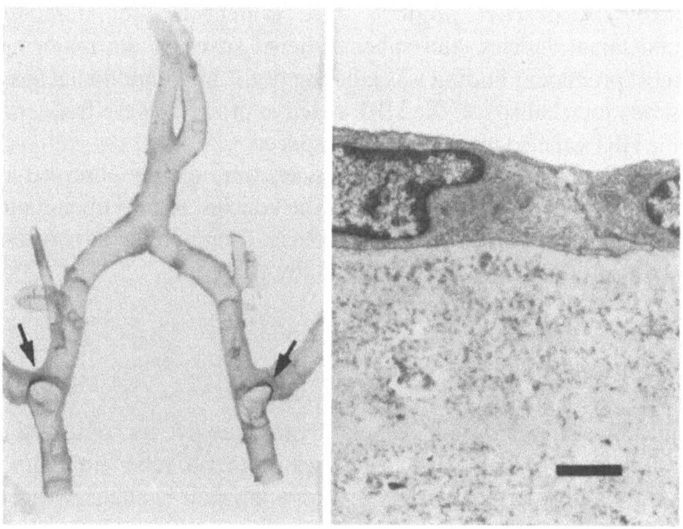

Fig. 1. *Left,* Photomacrograph of the major cerebral arteries in a control dog. *Arrows* indicate the HRP leakage at the proximal parts of the intradural internal carotid arteries. *Right,* electron micrograph of the basilar artery in a control dog. No HRP leakage was observed in the basilar artery. *Bar* = 1 μm

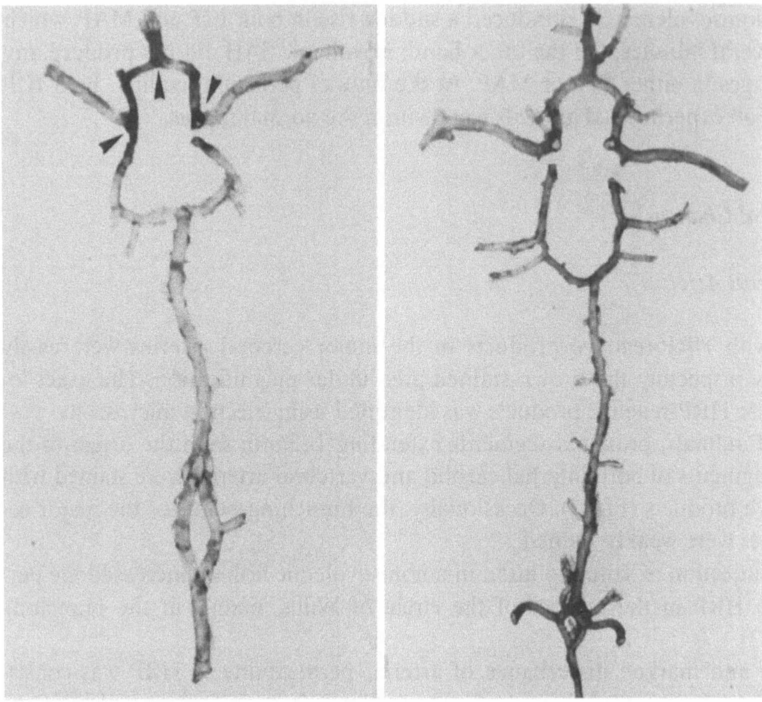

Fig. 2. Photomacrographs of the major cerebral arteries, illustrating the brown-stained area containing HRP-reactive products in dogs after saline injection (*left*) and isovolemic SAH (*right*)

ated. HRP-reactive products were evident in the interendothelial space, plasmalemmal vesicles, and subendothelial space of the major cerebral arteries. The most prominent finding was labeling of the interendothelial spaces with HRP. In the subendothelial space, the HRP-reactive products were frequently localized beneath the HRP-labeled interendothelial space.

HRP-labeled plasmalemmal vesicles were mainly observed at the abluminal face of the endothelial cells (Fig. 3C). The vesicles, or pits, opening to the vascular lumen were devoid of HRP-reactive products. Channel-like structures filled with HRP-reactive products were only occasionally observed.

Brain Capillaries

In control animals, no leakage of Evans blue dye was observed except in areas naturally devoid of BBB, such as the area postrema, tuber cinereum, and choroid plexus. Abnormal leakage of Evans blue dye in brain capillaries was found in one of two dogs in group II and in one of three dogs in group III. No abnormal leakage of the dye was observed in group IV dogs (Table 1).

The areas of cortex in which leakage of Evans blue dye occurred also showed HRP-reactive products within the capillary basement membrane and adjacent ex-

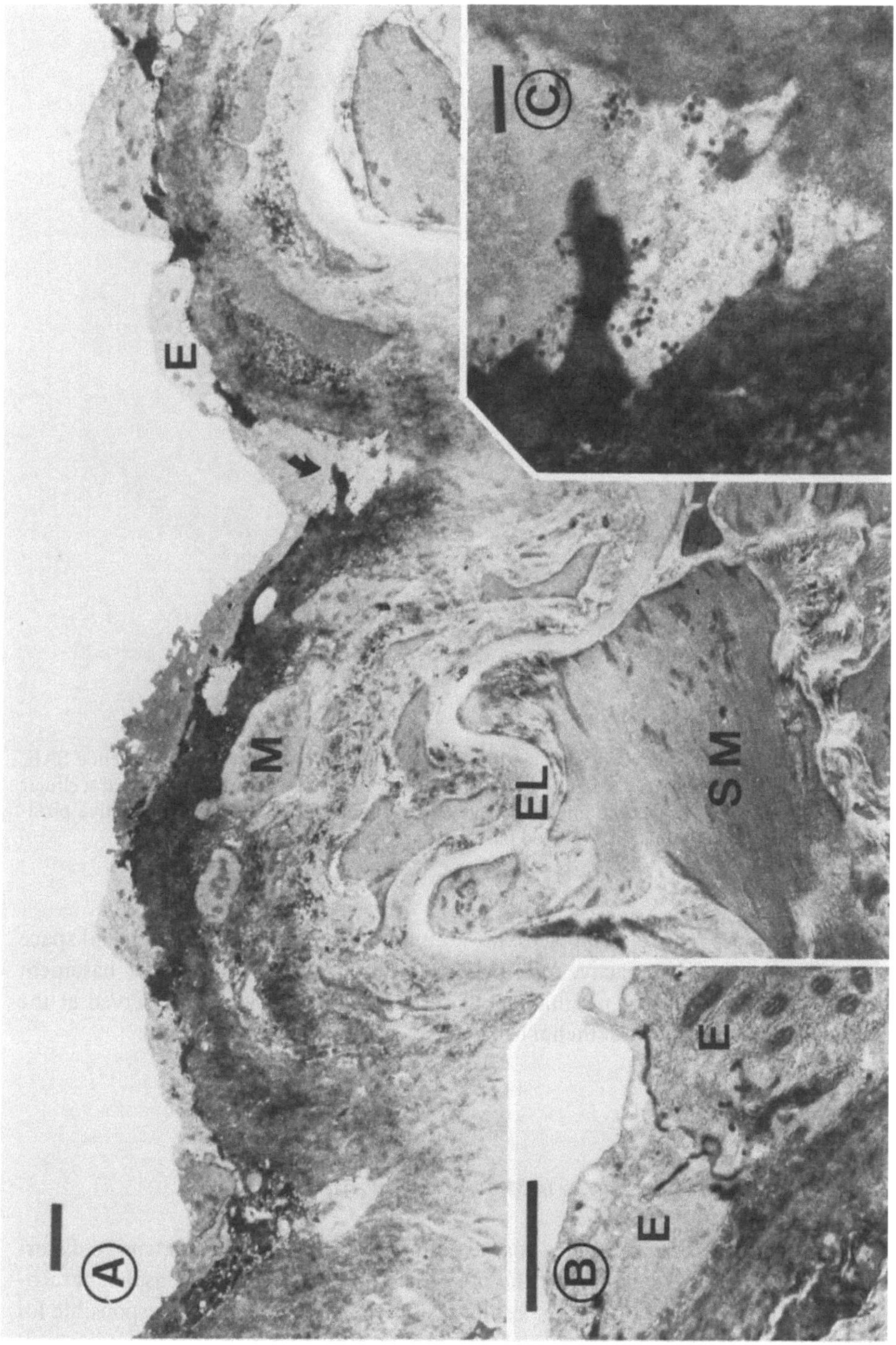

Fig. 3 A–C. Electron micrographs following isovolemic SAH in dogs. **A** A large field at a low magnification, illustrating the HRP-reactive products in the subendothelial space. *Bar* = 2 μm; **B** high magnification of the interendothelial space filled with HRP-reactive products. *Bar* = 0.5 μm; **C** high magnification of HRP-labeled plasmalemmal vesicles at the abluminal front of the endothelium (*arrow*). *Bar* = 0.5 μm. *E*, endothelium; *M*, mesenchymal cell; *EL*, elastic lamina; *SM*, smooth muscle cell

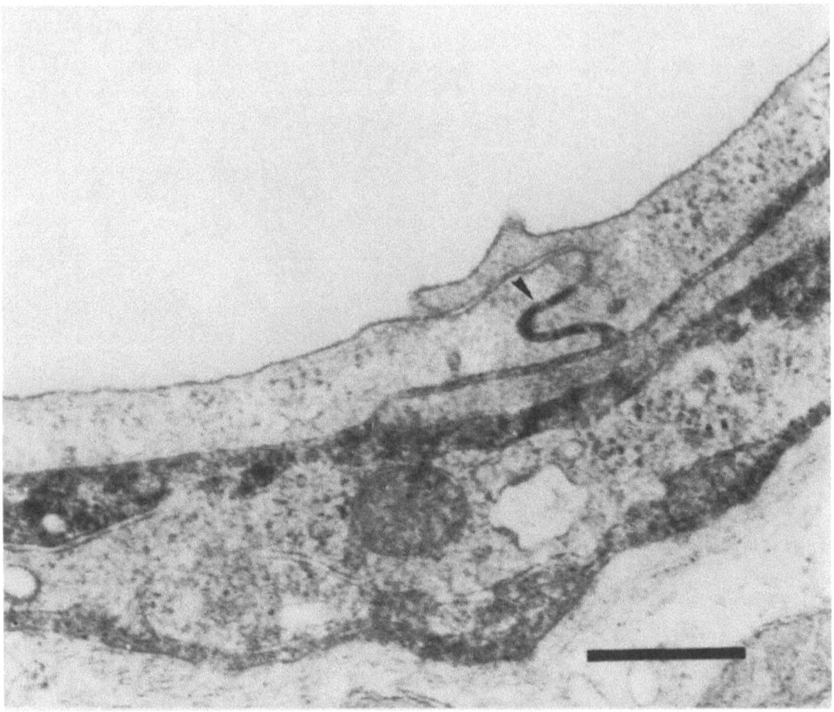

Fig. 4. Electron microscopic view of the brain capillary from a dog after nonisovolemic SAH, showing the HRP-reactive products in the basement membrane and adjacent extracellular space. *Arrowhead* indicates the interendothelial space partly labeled with HRP-reactive products in continuity with the HRP-labeled basement membrane. *Bar* = 0.5 μm

tracellular spaces (Fig. 4). In places, the abluminal part of the interendothelial space was filled with HRP-reactive products in continuity with the labeled basement membrane. HRP-labeled plasmalemmal vesicles were occasionally observed at the abluminal front of the endothelial cells.

Discussion

The Blood-Arterial Wall Barrier in Major Cerebral Arteries

The present experiment revealed that experimental SAH produced extensive disturbance of arterial permeability of the major cerebral arteries in the basal subarachnoid cisterns. On the basis of the present result two important factors responsible for the disturbance of the blood-arterial wall barrier can be proposed: the first is a sudden rise in ICP, since both the cisternal saline injection and nonisovolemic SAH produced a sudden rise in ICP and were followed by increased permeability in the major cerebral arteries; the second important factor is the direct effect of the subarachnoid clot around the arteries. The extensive disturbance of the arterial permeability was even observed in the dogs with isovolemic SAH, in which both the

ICP and the MAP were less markedly elevated. It seems reasonable to assume that the subarachnoid clot was responsible for inducing the breakdown of the blood-arterial wall barrier.

The present electron microscopic studies demonstrate that the opened interendothelial junction is one of the main routes of HRP leakage into the vessel wall. Whether endothelial cell pinocytosis is active in the barrier breakdown is still obscure. HRP-labeled vesicles observed at the abluminal front of the endothelium may represent reverse transport of the HRP from the abluminal front to the lumen. It seems unlikely that transendothelial channels were actively involved in the permeability change, since channel-like structures filled with HRP were only occasionally observed.

Breakdown of the blood-arterial wall barrier in the major cerebral arteries following SAH is of interest with regard to the pathogenesis of cerebral vasospasm. The present results suggest that SAH produces the breakdown of the blood-arterial wall barrier in the major cerebral arteries, which would allow access of vasoactive substances in plasma to the layers of the vessel wall. Some of the plasma factors, such as lipoprotein [11] or a platelet-derived factor [12], are known to stimulate the proliferation of undifferentiated mesenchymal cells, resulting in subendothelial thickening. Furthermore, intravascular vasoconstrictor substances may penetrate into the smooth muscle layer and stimulate vasoconstriction of the cerebral arteries.

The present results may also account for the abnormal post-contrast enhancement in the region of the basal subarachnoid cisterns on contrast-enhanced CT, which has been documented in patients with SAH [4–9]. Although two possible mechanisms for the abnormal enhancement, (a) leakage of contrast medium into the cisterns from the vessels and aneurysmal wall [4], and (b) meningeal hyperemia [5, 6], have been postulated, no evidence has been reported. The present findings support the possibility that contrast medium leaks into cisterns after SAH through the vessel wall of the major cerebral arteries.

The Blood-Brain Barrier

Early breakdown of the BBB has previously been observed in cats suffering from SAH induced by puncture of the internal carotid artery, which led to a marked elevation of ICP [1, 2]. It has also been reported that BBB breakdown was not observed when a marked elevation of ICP was avoided by a slow cisternal injection of blood [3]. In the present experiment, cisternal injection of either saline solution or blood in a nonisovolemic manner produced breakdown of the BBB, while isovolemic SAH did not. Together, these observations suggest that a sudden rise in ICP following SAH is responsible for the early BBB damage, rather than the subarachnoid clot itself.

With respect to the routes of HRP leakage, too few data were obtained in this experiment to allow determination of the role of endothelial pinocytosis, transendothelial channels, or opening of interendothelial junctions. The rupture of brain capillaries might be one possible cause of HRP leakage following SAH. The HRP-reactive products observed within the capillary basement membrane and adjacent extracellular space might have infiltrated from the necrotic area of the brain. The

HRP-reactive products in the interendothelial space or in the plasmalemmal vesicles at the abluminal face of the endothelium may reflect the leakage of HRP from the basement membrane side. Further studies will be necessary to determine the route of HRP leakage following SAH.

Summary

The effects of experimental subarachnoid hemorrhage (SAH) on the blood-arterial wall barrier in the major cerebral arteries and the blood-brain barrier (BBB) were studied in 12 normotensive dogs. Evans blue dye and horseradish peroxidase (HRP) were given IV to assess the integrity of both barriers. Cisternal saline injection produced a transient elevation in the intracranial pressure (ICP) and increased the permeability to HRP in the arteries of the circle of Willis, mainly at the branching points. In both isovolemic and nonisovolemic SAH dogs, extensive disturbance of the blood-arterial wall barrier was consistently observed in the major cerebral arteries. Subarachnoid clot and a sudden rise in the ICP seem to be two important factors responsible for the breakdown of the blood-arterial wall barrier in the major cerebral arteries following SAH. One of the main routes for HRP leakage was shown by electron microscopy to be the opened interendothelial junctions.

Early breakdown of the BBB was occasionally observed in both nonisovolemic SAH dogs and saline-treated dogs, while it was not induced in isovolemic SAH dogs. The early breakdown of BBB seems to be due to a sudden rise in the ICP following SAH rather than to the presence of subarachnoid clot.

Disturbance of arterial permeability in the major cerebral arteries following SAH may account for the abnormal post-contrast enhancement on computerized tomograms seen in some SAH patients, and is probably involved in the pathogenesis of vasospasm.

Acknowledgements. We would like to thank Dr. A. R. Colohan for editorial assistance, and Mrs. Lucille Staiger for typing the manuscript.

References

1. Trojanowski T (1982) Blood-brain barrier changes after experimental subarachnoid haemorrhage. Acta Neurochir (Wien) 60:45–54
2. Shigeno T, Fritschka E, Brock M, et al. (1982) Cerebral edema following experimental subarachnoid hemorrhage. Stroke 13:368–379
3. Peterson EW, Cardoso ER (1983) The blood-brain barrier following experimental subarachnoid hemorrhage. 1: response to insult caused by arterial hypertension. J Neurosurg 58:338–344
4. Fox JL, Ko JP (1978) Cerebral vasospasm: a clinical observation. Surg Neurol 10:269–275
5. Moran CJ, Naidich TP, Gado MH, et al. (1978) Leptomeningeal findings in CT of subarachnoid hemorrhage. J Comput Assist Tomogr 2:520–521
6. Yock DH, Larson DA (1980) Computed tomography of hemorrhage from anterior communicating artery aneurysms, with angiographic correlation. Radiology 134:399–407
7. Hirata Y, Matsukado Y, Fukumura A (1982) Subarachnoid enhancement secondary to subarachnoid hemorrhage with special reference to the clinical significance and pathogenesis. Neurosurgery 11:367–371

8. Tazawa T, Mizukami M, Kawase T, et al. (1983) Relationship between contrast enhancement on computed tomography and cerebral vasospasm in patients with subarachnoid hemorrhage. Neurosurgery 12:643–648
9. Dóczi T, Ambrose J, O'Laoire S (1984) Significance of contrast enhancement in cranial computerized tomography after subarachnoid hemorrhage. J Neurosurg 60:335–342
10. Graham RC, Karnovsky MJ (1966) The early stages of absorption of injected horseradish peroxidase in the proximal tubules of mouse kidney. Ultracytochemistry by a new technique. J Histochem Cytochem 14:291–302
11. Ross R, Glomset JA (1973) Atherosclerosis and the arterial smooth muscle cell. Science 180:1332–1339
12. Ross R, Glomset J, Karya B, et al. (1974) A platelet-dependent serum factor that stimulates the proliferation of arterial smooth muscle cells in vitro. Proc Natl Acad Sci USA 71:1207–1210

Changes in Blood-Brain Barrier Function Associated with Conditioned Fear in Rats

R. L. HAYES[1], C. M. PECHURA, J. T. POVLISHOCK, and D. P. BECKER

Key words: Blood-brain barrier, conditioned fear , horseradish peroxidase

Introduction

Cerebrovascular endothelial cells are joined by tight junctions and lack both fenestrae and significant vesicular activity. Thus, these cells constitute the structural basis for the blood-brain barrier (BBB), which prevents the passage of high-molecular-weight, lipid-insoluble, or charged molecules, including proteins, certain amino acids, and water, into and out of the brain. Interest in BBB research has largely focused on methods to circumvent the barrier for delivery of drugs otherwise prevented from entering the brain and on the mechanisms and consequences (e.g., brain edema) of insults which cause BBB breakdown. These insults include severe hypertension, seizure, and mechanical brain injury [1, 2]. Recently, increased BBB permeability to water has been reported to occur following systemic administration of amitriptyline, an antidepressant drug which has adrenergic effects in the central nervous system [3]. This finding provided additional support for the hypothesis that the permeability of cerebrovascular endothelial cells may be regulated, at least in part, by adrenergic neurons within the central nervous system [4, 5]. Although not uncontested [6–8], the possibility that BBB permeability may be dynamically modulated by neurogenic mechanisms suggests that changes in BBB permeability may occur even in the absence of some extrinsic manipulation or severe insult. Since drugs such as amitriptyline have a powerful influence on affective states, changes in emotionality could be associated with alterations in BBB permeability.

The present report demonstrates that BBB permeability to the protein horseradish peroxidase (HRP) is increased during the emotional state of conditioned fear. The observations further suggest that the BBB is not immutable, but that changes in barrier permeability may rather be normally occurring physiological responses to environmental events.

On each of 3 consecutive days, 14 adult male rats were given scrambled foot shock via an electrified grid (0.5 mA, 10 s) in an operant conditioning chamber. Prior to this conditioning procedure, all animals were habituated to handling and injection procedures by an experimenter who did not participate in the shock sessions. Variations of this procedure are widely used to elicit a conditioned emotional re-

[1] Division of Neurosurgery and Department of Anatomy, Medical College of Virginia, Richmond, VA 23298, USA

sponse through repeated pairing of a fear-producing unconditioned stimulus, foot shock, with initially neutral stimuli (e.g., the operant chamber, shock grid, experimenter and, in this study, the distinctive noise produced by mechanical circuits of the shock scrambler). These initially neutral stimuli subsequently become capable of eliciting a conditioned emotional response in the absence of shock [9].

On the 3rd day, cannulae were implanted, during methoxyflurane anesthesia, in an external jugular vein and exteriorized onto the animals' backs. On the 4th day, 5 min after injection of HRP (Sigma type VI, 50–75 mg/kg, IV), experimental animals ($n=8$) were placed in the operant chamber, in the presence of all conditioned stimuli, but were not shocked. Control animals ($n=6$) also received injections of HRP on the 4th day, but were not re-exposed to any of the conditioned stimuli associated with the foot shock. To assess the effects of foot shock alone, two additional animals received injections of HRP 5 min before a single exposure to the training shock. At 40 min after the HRP injection, all animals were deeply anesthetized with sodium pentobarbitol (30 mg/kg, IV) and perfused transcardially with heparinized saline followed by a mixture of 2% paraformaldehyde and 2.5% glutaraldehyde in 0.1 *M* phosphate buffer. Transverse, vibratome sections (50 μm) from the frontal pole to the lower medulla of each brain were developed with either tetramethylbenzidine histochemistry for visualization of HRP at the light microscopic level [10] or cobalt-glucose oxidase histochemistry for ultrastructural examination [11]. The numbers of HRP extravasation sites in every fifth section were recorded by an observer working blind to the experimental conditions, who performed a light microscopic examination using light and dark field illumination.

The average number of HRP extravasation sites in the brains of animals that experienced conditioned fear was 33.0 ± 1.5, as against 15.7 ± 1.8 sites in control animals ($t=2.95$, two-tailed t-test, $P<0.02$, Table 1). Areas, such as the area postrema,

Table 1. Summary of HRP extravasation

	Experimental ($n=8$)	Control ($n=6$)
Mean extravasation sites (whole brain)	33.0 ± 1.5 [a]	15.7 ± 1.8
Percentage of rats showing extravasation (by region)		
Somatosensory cortex	100% (8)	67% (4)
Caudate putamen	100% (8)	67% (4)
Cingulate cortex	75% (6) [b]	17% (1)
Olfactory cortex	75% (6)	50% (3)
Hippocampal formation	75% (6)	33% (2)
Lateral septum	75% (6)	50% (3)
Trigeminal complex	75% (6)	50% (3)
Motor cortex	63% (5) [c]	0% (0)
Striate cortex	63% (5) [c]	0% (0)
Amygdala	63% (5)	50% (3)

[a] $P<0.02$ (Student's t-test)
[b] $P<0.051$ (Fisher's exact test)
[c] $P<0.028$ (Fisher's exact test)

in which HRP extravasation was seen in all animals due to regional absence of a BBB were not included in these figures. Ultrastructural analysis revealed trans-endothelial transport of HRP via increased vesicular activity and an absence of mechanical disruption of the tight junctions between endothelial cells. A few minute, randomly localized sites of HRP extravasation from small vessels, with diameters of 7–10 μm (the size of precapillary arterioles and venules), were found in the two animals that experienced a single exposure to the training shock. Such sites have been noted in unshocked, normotensive control animals in experiments by others [12].

Table 1 also lists brain regions in which more than 50% (> 4) of the experimental rats showed extravasation. These data are compared with those recorded in the same brain regions of control rats. Differences between experimental and control animals were most prominent in the motor, striate, and cingulate cortices. In contrast, the somatosensory cortex, caudate putamen, olfactory cortex, lateral septum, trigeminal complex, and amygdala exhibited HRP extravasation with notable frequency in both experimental and control animals.

These data indicate that conditioned fear is associated with increased BBB permeability. Thus, changes in BBB permeability may not be associated only with invasive experimental procedures. Rather BBB permeability may change in response to a variety of events that organisms may be expected to encounter normally. Many of those events may be associated with emotional responses. Moreover, during periods of increased BBB permeability, substances which do not normally pass the BBB may exert significant effects within restricted brain regions.

The observation that rats exposed to a single shock failed to show significant HRP extravasation suggests that responses to acutely stressful stimuli may not be related to increased BBB permeability. However, more sensitive, quantitative autoradiographic techniques for assessment of BBB alterations might reveal changes not detected by HRP extravasation [13].

This study did not address the physiological mechanisms mediating BBB changes during conditioned fear. Additional studies could examine the relationship of changes putatively mediated by central adrenergic neurons [4, 5]. Experimentally induced hypertension also produces increased BBB permeability. Since hypertension may accompany conditioned fear, such hypertensive events may be related to increased BBB permeability produced by these paradigms. Although the rather focal patterns of HRP extravasation seen in the present study seem to differ from the more widely distributed extravasation sites seen following experimental hypertension [14], future studies will directly address the contribution of systemic hypertension to increased BBB permeability in conditioned fear paradigms.

Summary

The blood-brain barrier (BBB) can be disrupted by the induction of pathophysiologic events. In contrast, the present study sought to assess the response of the BBB to the environmentally relevant state of classically conditioned fear.

For each of 3 days prior to testing, 20 male Sprague-Dawley rats (350–450 g) were placed in a standard Plexiglas operant chamber with a grid floor through which 0.5 mA of scrambled shock was delivered for 10 s. On the 4th day, experimental animals ($n = 12$) were placed in the chamber in the presence of all other stimulus cues but were not shocked. One day prior to testing, cannulae were placed in the external jugular vein and externalized on the back of each animal under methoxyflurane anesthesia. On the 4th day, experimental animals received 75–100 mg/kg horseradish peroxidase (HRP; Sigma VI) by IV injection 5 min before being placed in the operant chamber. Control animals ($n = 8$) also received HRP but were not placed in the chamber. At 40 min after HRP injection animals were deeply anesthetized with sodium pentobarbital (IV) and perfused with aldehydes. The brains were sectioned at 50 μm and processed for visualization with HRP.

Extravasation of HRP was more prominent in brain sections from experimental animals than in control sections ($P < 0.02$). This extravasation was most often seen, compared with control rats, in motor, striate and cingulate cortices ($P < 0.05$). These data suggest that the physiological components of a normally occurring emotional state such as fear may include altered function of the blood-brain barrier.

References

1. Rapoport SI (1976) Blood-brain barrier in physiology and medicine. Raven, New York
2. Povlishock JT, Becker DP, Sullivan HG, Miller JD (1978) Vascular permeability alterations to horseradish peroxidase in experimental brain injury. Brain Res 153:223–239
3. Preskorn SH, Irwin GH, Simpson S, Friesen D, Rinne J, Jerkovich G (1981) Medical therapies for mood disorders alter the blood-brain barrier. Science 213:469–471
4. Hartman BK, Swanson LW, Raichle ME, Preskorn SH, Clark HB (1980) Central adrenergic regulation of cerebral microvascular permeability and blood flow; anatomic and physiologic evidence. Adv Exp Med Biol 131:113–126
5. Preskorn SH, Hartman BK, Raichle ME, Swanson LW, Clark HB (1980) Central adrenergic regulation of cerebral microvascular permeability and blood flow; pharmacologic evidence. Adv Exp Med Biol 131:127–138
6. Rennels ML, Nelson E (1975) Capillary innervation in the mammalian central nervous system: an electron microscopic demonstration. Am J Anat 144:233–241
7. Swanson LW, Connelly MA, Hartman BK (1978) Further studies on the fine structure of the adrenergic innervation of the hypothalamus. Brain Res 151:165–174
8. Suddith RL, Savage KE, Eisenberg HM (1979) Advances in experimental medicine and biology: the cerebral microvasculature. Plenum, New York
9. Estes WK, Skinner BF (1941) Some quantitative properties of anxiety. J Exp Psychol 29:390–396
10. Mesulam MM (1978) Tetramethylbenzidine for horseradish peroxidase neurohistochemistry: a non-carcinogenic blue reaction product with superior sensitivity for visualizing neural afferents and efferents. J Histochem Cytochem 26:106–117
11. Itoh K, Konishi A, Nomura S, Mizuno N, Nakamura Y, Sugimoto T (1979) Application of coupled oxidation reaction to electron microscopic demonstration of horseradish peroxidase: cobalt-glucose oxidase method. Brain Res 175:341–346
12. Nag S, Robertson DM, Dinsdale HB (1981) Cerebrovascular permeability in mechanically induced hypertension. Can J Neurol Sci 8:215–220
13. Ellison MD, Povlishock JT, Hayes RL (1984) Examining blood-brain barrier permeability to horseradish peroxidase and to α-aminoisobutyric acid following acute hypertension: a comparative, quantitative and morphological study. Neurosci Abstr (in press)
14. Nagy Z, Mathieson G, Huttner I (1979) Blood brain barrier opening to horseradish peroxidase in acute arterial hypertension. Acta Neuropathol (Berl) 48:45–53

Brain Edema in Intracranial Venous Hypertension

K. FUJITA [1], N. KOJIMA, N. TAMAKI, and S. MATSUMOTO

Key words: Brain edema, blood-brain barrier, ICP, sinus occlusion

Introduction

Few reports on experimental brain edema caused by occlusion of the intracranial sagittal sinus have appeared, because there has been no good experimental model of brain edema of venous origin. In the present studies a new experimental model of brain has been attempted by occlusion of the intracranial sinus and investigation of its pathophysiology by means of an embolization technique.

Methods and Materials

Fifteen mongrel dogs were used to make a model of brain edema of venous origin. A small burr hole was made in the anterior one-third of the superior sagittal sinus (SSS), and after introduction of a catheter α-cyanoacrylate monomer was injected into the sinus. This was carried out in 12 dogs as an embolization technique.

These dogs were divided into three groups according to the volume of the embolus injected into the sinus and the extent of the sinus occlusion, as shown in Fig. 1. In group A, the SSS was partially occluded by injecting 0.3–0.5 ml of the embolus; in group B the SSS and the transverse sinus (TS) were occluded by injecting 0.5–0.7 ml of the embolus; and in group C, the SSS, the TS, and the cortical veins were occluded by injecting 0.8–1.0 ml of the embolus. In a control group of 3 dogs, no embolus was injected (sham operation). Intracranial pressure (ICP) at the cisterna magna and SSS pressure (SSSP) were measured with a Statham transducer before and after sinus occlusion. To examine the degree of destruction of the blood-brain barrier (BBB) Evans blue was injected (about 400–500 mg per animal in each group) before autopsy. Histological changes were also studied macroscopically and microscopically after autopsy.

Results

ICP and SSSP Before and After Sinus Occlusion

In the control group, ICP and SSSP were 9 ± 2.2 mmHg and 4 ± 2.5 mmHg, i.e., ICP was higher than SSSP. After the sinus was occluded, ICP and SSSP were

[1] Dept. of Neurosurgery, Kobe University, School of Medicine, 7-chome, Tomogaoka, Suma-ku, Kobe 654, Japan

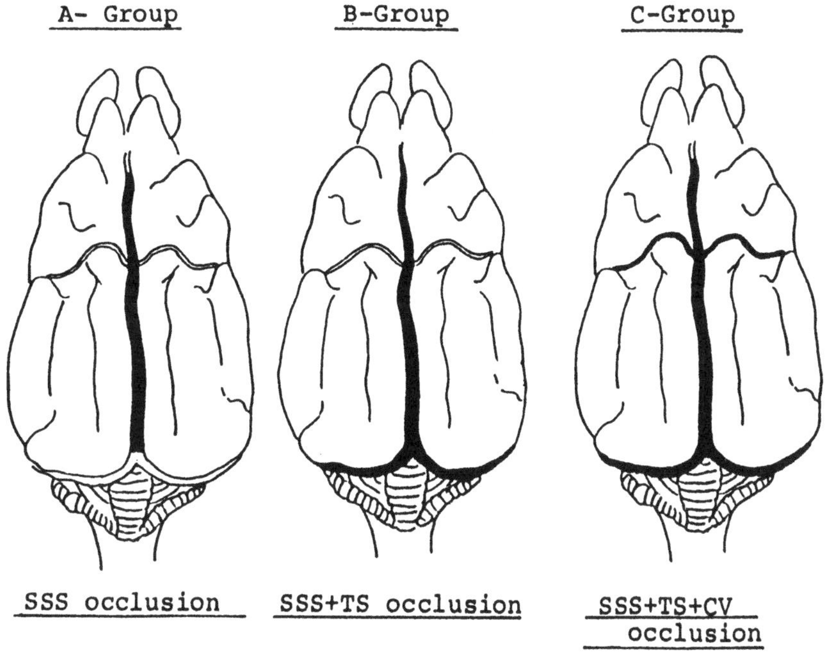

Fig. 1. Classification of the sinus occlusion model according to the extent of sinus occlusion. Only SSS is occluded in group A; SSS and TS in group B; and SSS, TS, and CV in group C. *SSS*, superior sagittal sinus; *TS*, transverse sinus; *CV*, cortical vein

Table 1. ICP and SSSP in each group

Group	ICP (mmHg)	SSSP (mmHg)
A	20±5.5	23±4.5
B	30±5.4	35±5.1
C	65±7.9	72±6.1

20±5.5 mmHg and 23±4.5 mmHg in group A, 30±5.4 mmHg and 35±5.1 mmHg in group B, and 65±7.9 mmHg and 72±6.1 mmHg in group C, respectively. In contrast to the control group, SSSP was higher than ICP in the experimental groups, as shown in Table 1 and Fig. 2.

Change in BBB Permeability After Sinus Occlusion

The change in BBB permeability to Evans blue was examined in each group. In the controls and group A there was no extravasation of the dye from the pial veins. Group B had localized extravasation of the dye from the pial veins along the occluded sinus, but group C showed massive extravasation of the dye from the pial veins and subarachnoid hemorrhage in the cerebral hemisphere, predominantly along the occluded cortical veins and the sinus, as shown in Fig. 3.

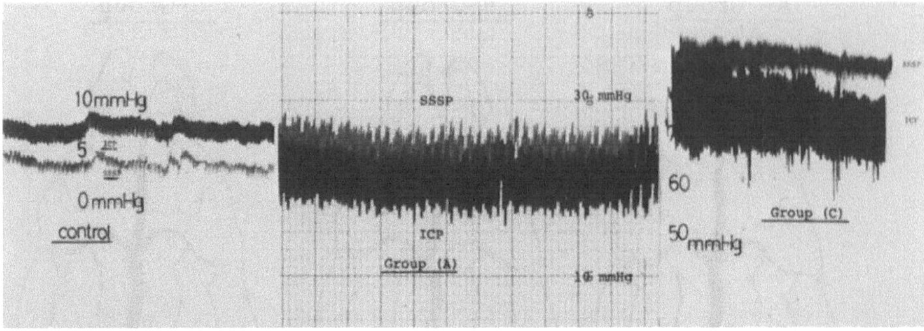

Fig. 2. Changes in ICP and SSSP after sinus occlusion. Before sinus occlusion ICP is higher than SSSP, but after sinus occlusion SSSP exceeds ICP

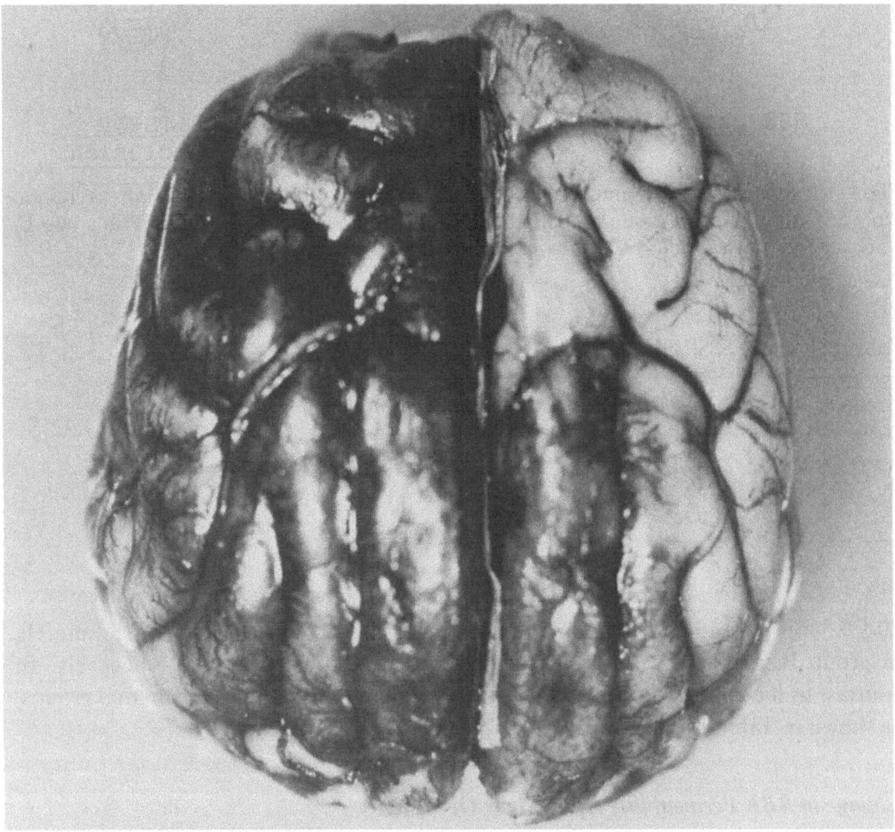

Fig. 3. Massive extravasation of dye from the pial veins along the occluded cortical veins and subarachnoid hemorrhage

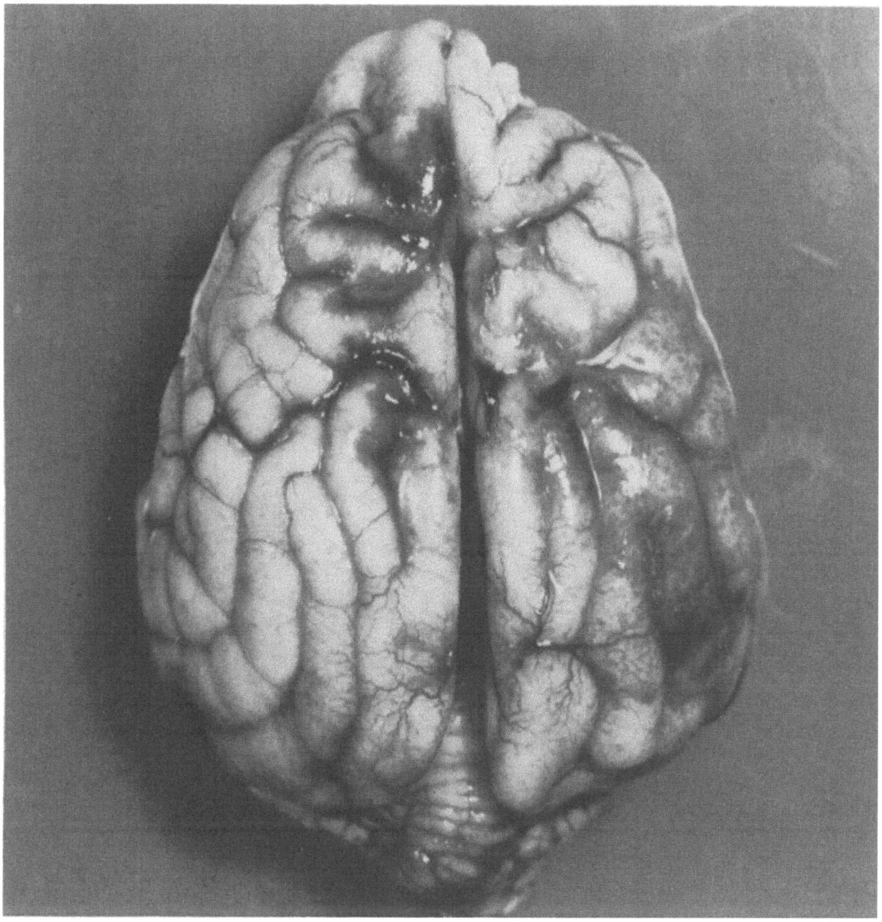

Fig. 4. Autopsy revealed SAH in frontal and parietal area of dogs that died within a few hours after complete sinus occlusion

Autopsy Findings

Gross Anatomy

No pathologic changes were found in group A and only localized petechial hemorrhage in the parietal area along the occluded SSS in group B; but in group C massive brain swelling, subarachnoid hemorrhage, and hemorrhagic infarction in the parietal area along the occluded SSS and cortical veins were found, as shown in Figs. 4 and 5.

Histological Findings

No histological changes were found in group A, and localized subarachnoid hemorrhage with minimal pial vein congestion were the only ones in group B; but group C

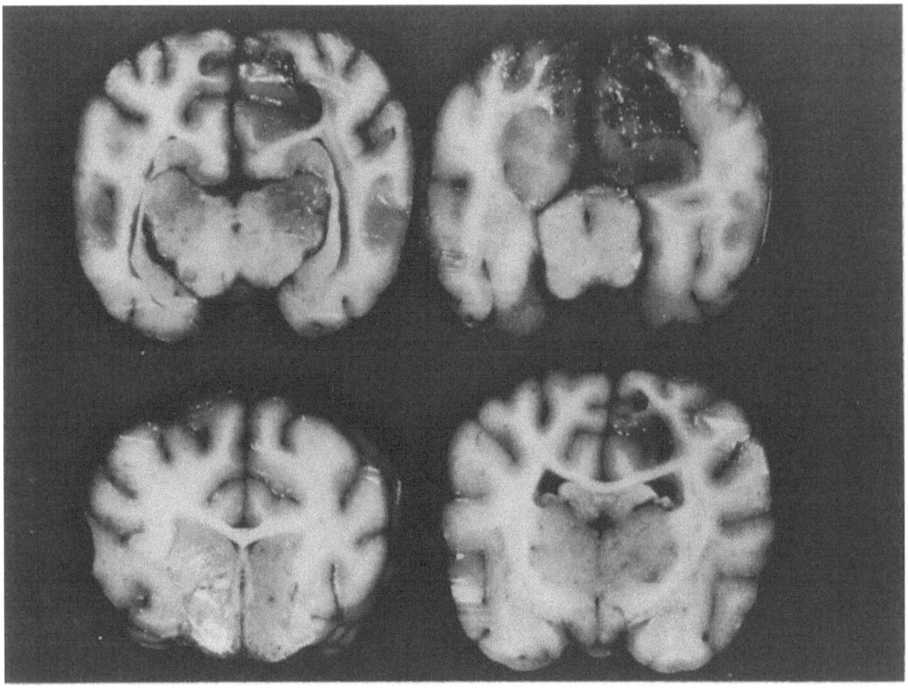

Fig. 5. Hemorrhagic infarction in parietal area near the sinus, also revealed at autopsy

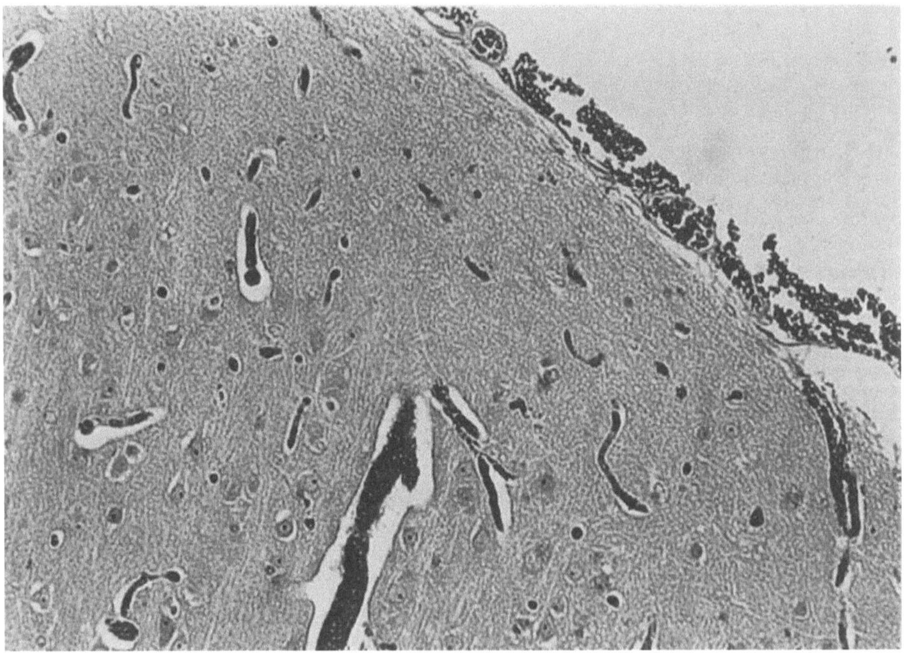

Fig. 6. Micrograph revealing SAH and marked venous dilatation, disruption of the subcortical veins, and degenerative change of the neuron

animals had marked venous congestion in the cortical and subcortical veins with subarachnoid hemorrhage, as shown in Fig. 6.

Discussion

Rives [4] first reported observations in a case of SSS and TS thrombosis in 1825. According to Chiari and Chatterjee [1], the severity of the clinical symptoms due to the dural sinus occlusion are dependent on how much the dural sinus is occluded, and if both the basal dural sinus and the deep cerebral vein are occluded, serious neurologic conditions usually follow. Kalbag et al. [2] also reported that no pathologic findings were present in his autopsy cases in which only the dural sinus was occluded but that in autopsy cases in which dural sinus thrombosis involved the cortical veins or the great vein of Galen, hemorrhagic infarction occurred. Seki et al. [6] confirmed the importance of involvement of the cortical veins from a series of clinical cases with dural sinus thrombosis causing hemorrhagic infarction. Sato et al. [5] investigated the change in the epicerebral microcirculation by fluorescein microangiography before and after sinus occlusion in dogs, and reported that diapedesis of the dye from the pial veins was observed 30 min after the sinus occlusion prior to petechial hemorrhage, and that sinus occlusion led to an increase in the permeability of the pial veins, resulting in subarachnoid hemorrhage. Ray et al. [3] reported that the veins of Trollard and Labbe, orbital and pterygoid plexuses, veins which drain into the cavernosus sinus and the inferior sagittal sinus, superior cerebral veins, and diploic and scalp veins have a role as anastomotic veins following superior sagittal sinus occlusion. From the results of our experiment it may be concluded that cortical veins have an extremely important role as a collateral pathway in sinus occlusion, and BBB destruction first begins in the pial veins, followed by disruption of other cortical and subcortical veins due to the venous hypertension which leads to subarachnoid hemorrhage and hemorrhagic infarction.

Summary

A new experimental model of dural sinus occlusion was devised to study its pathophysiology by an embolization technique. Changes in ICP and SSSP and histological changes were examined after sinus occlusion. In contrast to the control group, SSSP was higher than ICP in all groups of experimental animals. SSSP and ICP exceeded 40 mmHg in group C with cortical vein occlusion. No histological changes were found in group A, and only localized subarachnoid hemorrhage with minimal pial vein congestion in group B, but the animals in group C showed marked venous congestion, subarachnoid hemorrhage, and hemorrhagic infarction.

References

1. Chiari H, Chatterjee RN (1958) Beitrag zur Diagnostik und Therapie der puerperalen Thrombose des Sinus sagittalis superior. Acta Neurochir 6:7–14

2. Kalbag RM, Woolf AL (1972) Thrombosis and thrombophlebitis of cerebral veins and sinuses. Cerebral venous thrombosis. Oxford University Press, London, pp 66–236
3. Ray BS, Dumber HS, Dotter CT (1959) Symposium: Intracranial vascular abnormalities. Dural sinus venography as aid to diagnosis in intracranial diseases. J Neurosurg 8:25–37
4. Ribes F (1825) Des recherches faites sur la phlébite. Rev Med 3:5
5. Sato S, Miyahara Y, Dohmoto Y, Tawase T, Toya S (1983) Cerebral microcirculation in experimental sagittal sinus occlusion in dogs. The cerebral veins. Springer, Wien New York, pp 111–117
6. Seki H, Sonobe M, Higuchi H (1979) A case of sinus thrombosis causing hemorrhagic infarction. Neurologia 19:537–541

The Effect of Sagittal Sinus Occlusion on Blood-Brain Barrier Permeability and Cerebral Blood Flow in the Dog

S. SATO [1], S. TOYA, M. OHTANI, and T. KAWASE

Key words: Blood-brain barrier, brain edema, cerebral blood flow, sinus occlusion, microcirculation

Introduction

In experimental superior sagittal sinus occlusion in dogs, blood-brain barrier (BBB) disruption was monitored by fluorescein angiography and Evans blue extravasation. In addition, CBF in gray and white matter was measured by the hydrogen clearance method. The relation of BBB disruption and CBF will be described here.

Methods

Twenty-one adult mongrel dogs weighing 9.6–14.6 kg were used in the study. They were anesthetized with 25–30 mg/kg pentobarbital sodium. An intratracheal tube was inserted after tracheotomy and connected to an artificial respirator. The experiments were conducted under controlled respiration with room air. Preparatory to fluorescein angiography, a polyethylene tube (inner diameter 0.5 mm) was inserted from the external carotid artery before the bifurcation of the common carotid artery into the internal and external carotid arteries. The tube was fixed in this position for use as an injection channel to deliver the fluorescein sodium. A 1.5×1.5 cm craniectomy was performed in the frontoparietal area at the side on which the polyethylene tube was inserted, and after incision of the dura mater a skull window was made. Before sinus occlusion an initial series of cerebral fluorescein angiograms was obtained. Since the details of the method for fluorescein angiography have been reported previously [4] only an outline is presented here. A Nikon motor-driven camera equipped with a surgical microscope and rechargeable repeating flash was used to take pictures at three frames per second. An Asahi Bunko Kogakusha filter (420–485 mm) was set in front of the flash as an exciting filter and a Kodak-Wrattern no. 12 filter was set in front of the camera as a barrier filter. After the photographic equipment had been assembled, 10 ml fluorescein sodium solution (0.5%) was injected manually at a rapid rate via the polyethylene tube inserted in the common carotid artery. Consecutive shooting was commenced as the injection began,

[1] Department of Neurosurgery, School of Medicine, Keio University, 35 Shinanomachi, Shinjuku-ku, Tokyo 160, Japan

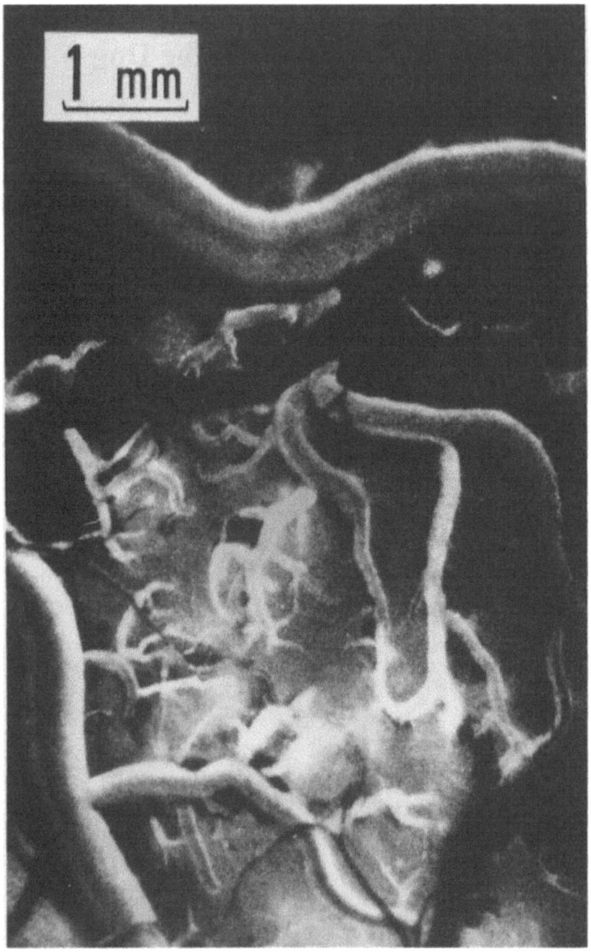

Fig. 1. Fluorescein angiography taken 30 min after sinus occlusion showed diapedesis of fluorescein dye from the pial vein

and a total of 36 photographs were taken. To measure CBF a small burr hole was made in the skull and a needle electrode was inserted into the front parietal brain tissue with the aid of a stereotaxic neurosurgical apparatus. Once the electrode was fixed CBF was measured by the hydrogen clearance method. After completion of the initial fluorescein angiography, a 5-mm-diameter burr hole was made at the vertex, and the superior sagittal sinus was occluded with a neurosurgical clip. Following sinus occlusion it was confirmed that systemic pressure and pulse rate did not change. A series of fluorescein angiographs was subsequently undertaken every 30 min for 3 h. The film was developed at double sensitivity and the photographs were enlarged when detailed analysis was required. After completion of each experiment an autopsy was performed. The brain was fixed in 10% formalin solution. Then tissue samples were prepared and stained with hematoxylin-eosin and Luxol fast blue.

Results

Diapedesis of fluorescein dye was observed in all experiments 5 min after sinus occlusion (Fig. 1). In some of the experiments there was no filling of fluorescein dye in the pial vein, while in others petechial hemorrhage or intravascular sludging was seen after sinus occlusion. Examination of the pathological specimens revealed diapedesis of Evans blue in the cerebral cortex and basal ganglia but not in the white matter (Fig. 2). CBF in the gray matter decreased soon after sinus occlusion and remained low until the end of the experiment (Fig. 3). In contrast, CBF in white matter showed a transient decrease directly after sinus occlusion, but had recovered 2 h after sinus occlusion and some experiments showed hyperemia (Fig. 4). Significant BBB breakdown was observed in the cerebral cortex, and CBF in this area was decreased. In contrast, the BBB of the white matter was well preserved and the CBF in this area showed hyperemia or no change after a transient decrease.

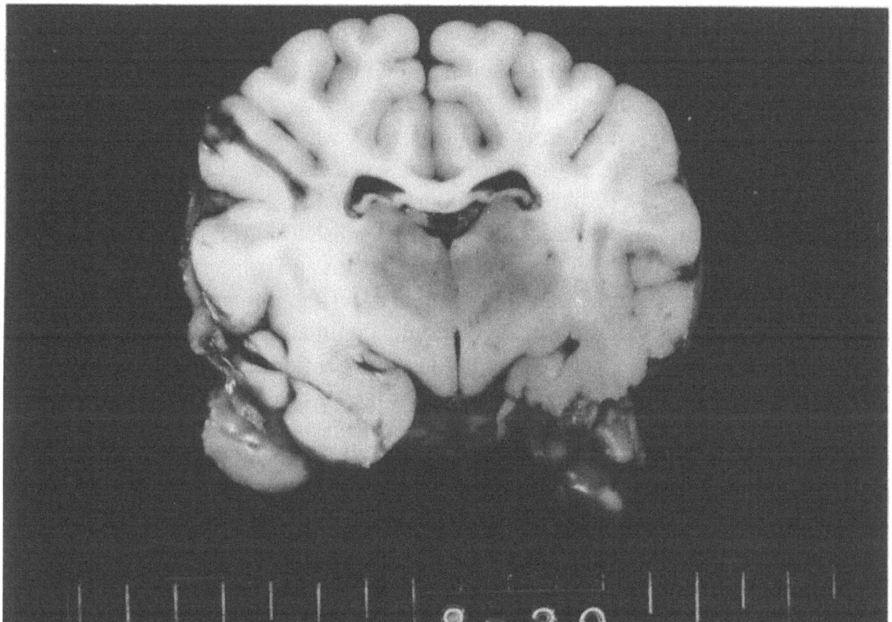

Fig. 2. Pathological specimen: extravasation of Evans blue was observed at the cerebral cortex

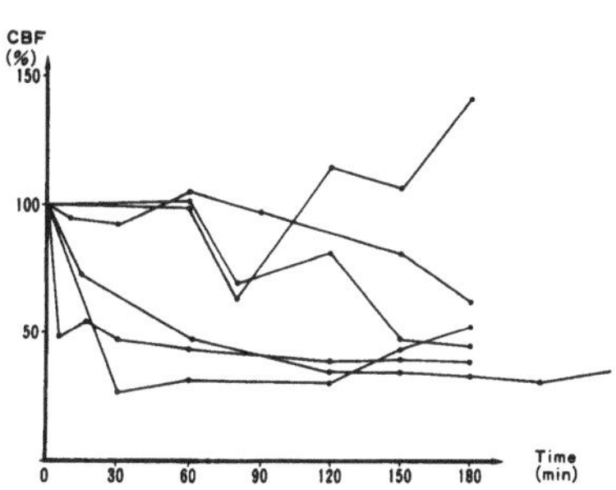

Fig. 3. CBF in gray matter

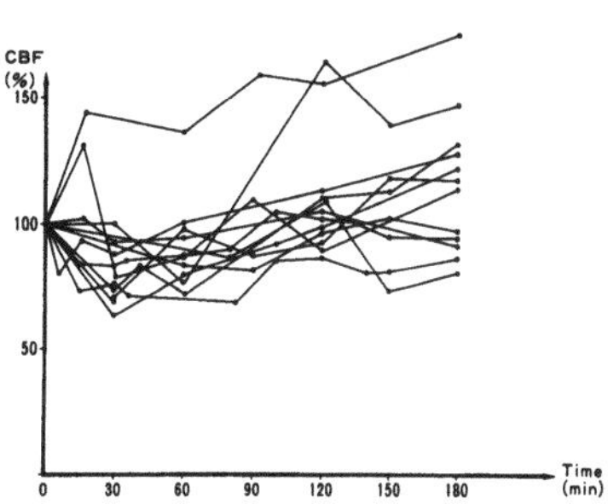

Fig. 4. CBF in white matter

Discussion

Diapedesis of fluorescein sodium was observed prior to petechial hemorrhages, and extravasation of Evans blue was observed before hemorrhagic infarction. Because the molecules of fluorescein sodium and Evans blue are smaller than red blood cells they can pass the dilated endothelial tight junctions created by venous congestion. Petechial hemorrhage was also observed in pial veins in the trauma. This coincidence of instability of pial venous BBB in sinus occlusion and trauma is due to the instability of the pial vein for rheological force, because the pial vein is floating in the subarachnoid space [8]. It is reported that CBF is decreased during sustained high cerebral venous pressure [3]. Clinically, it is also reported that CBF of the cerebral hemisphere is decreased owing to cerebral edema [7]. But as Moyer reported, as long as autoregulation of CBF is maintained, CBF is not changed even when venous pressure is increased [6]. This means that BBB disruption which accompanies brain edema is particularly marked in this area. In this experiment, CBF was decreased in the gray matter and BBB disruption was observed in this area, but in the white matter CBF was well maintained and the BBB was not disrupted. This means that autoregulation was maintained in the white matter but that it disappeared in the gray matter. It is concluded that BBB disruption or brain edema blocks the autoregulation of CBF. After sinus occlusion CBF was relatively well maintained, though it is reported that CBF in white matter is decreased in the intracranial hypertensive state [2]. The difference is autoregulation stability. In other words, autoregulation of the white matter is feeble in response to intracranial hypertension. Physiological changes in the degree of sinus occlusion and intracranial hypertension are quite different, confirming that intracranial hypertension has little to do with the acute stage of the sinus occlusion. Krayenbuhl [5] and Hakmatpanah [1] reported that a disturbance of the cerebrospinal fluid absorption caused intracranial hypertension, and this accelerated the sludging of the cortical cerebral vein after sinus occlusion. But acceleration of cerebral venous thrombosis is a circulatory disturbance rather than intracranial hypertension due to the absorptional disturbance of cerebrospinal fluid.

Conclusion

After sinus occlusion, BBB disruption was first observed in the pial vein. In brain tissue, BBB disruption occurred in the gray matter, where CBF decreased markedly after sinus occlusion. In contrast, the BBB was preserved in the white matter, where CBF decreased only transiently after sinus occlusion. It is concluded that BBB disruption causes brain edema, which then reduces CBF.

Summary

The effect of experimental sagittal sinus occlusion on blood-brain barrier (BBB) permeability and cerebral blood flow (CBF) was studied in the frontal cortex of the dog. The BBB permeability was evaluated with the aid of fluorescein microangiography and Evans blue extravasation. In the gray matter and white matter of the frontal lobe CBF was measured with the hydrogen clearance technique. Diapedesis of fluorescein dye from the pial vein was observed immediately after sinus occlusion, whereas CBF in white matter increased after a transient fall. At the end of the experiment, extravasation of Evans blue-albumin was observed in the cerebral cortex and basal ganglia, but not in the white matter. Thus, disruption of the BBB by occlusion of the sagittal sinus is associated with decreased CBF in the dog.

Acknowledgements. We wish to thank Dr. Quentin R. Smith, Laboratory of Neuroscience, NIA, NIH, for his suggestions and review of the manuscript.

References

1. Hakmatpanah J (1970) Cerebral circulation and perfusion in experimental increased intracranial pressure. J Neurosurg 32:21–29
2. Hayashi N, Tamura M, Inoue H (1973) The cerebral venous mechanism in intracranial hypertension. No Shinkei Geka (Tokyo) 1:143–151 (in Japanese)
3. Jacobson I, Harper AM, McDowall DG (1963) Relationship between venous pressure and cortical blood flow. Nature 200a:173
4. Kawase T, Iisaka Y, Toya S, et al. (1974) Experimental study in cerebral microcirculation. I: Its method and result. Keio Igaku (Tokyo) 51:351–360 (in Japanese)
5. Krayenbühl HA (1967) Cerebral venous and sinus thrombosis (1967) Clin Neurosurg 14:1–23
6. Moyer JH, Miller SI, Shyder H (1954) Effect of increased jugular pressure on cerebral hemodynamics. J Appl Physiol 7:245–247
7. Shinohara Y, Takagi S, Kobatake K, Gotoh F (1982) Influence of cerebral venous obstruction on cerebral circulation in humans. Arch Neurol 39:479–481
8. Smith DM, Ducker TB, Kemp LG (1969) Experimental in vivo microcirculation dynamics of brain trauma. J Neurosurg 30:464–672

Acute Brain Swelling Caused by Stimulation of the Reticular Formation of the Medulla Oblongata

A. NISHIMOTO[1], T. NISHIURA, F. MOMMA, T. MUROTA, M. SUGA, Y. HOMMA, H. KUYAMA, and S. NAGAO

Key words: Acute brain swelling, cerebral blood volume, cerebrovascular tone, intracranial pressure, reticular formation of medulla oblongata

Purpose

It has been proposed that acute brain swelling is caused by vasomotor paralysis secondary to disruption of metabolic and/or neurogenic control of cerebrovascular tone. We experimentally destroyed the dorsomedial nucleus of the hypothalamus (DM) and the reticular formation of the midbrain (MBRF) in 166 cats. Acute brain swelling was produced in 6 of them. In 2 of the 6 animals, acute brain swelling was induced by stimulation of the reticular formation of the medulla oblongata (MORF) with DM and MBRF lesions, suggesting that MORF stimulation decreases cerebrovascular tone. The purpose of the present study is to clarify the effect of stimulation of the MORF on cerebrovascular tone.

Materials and Methods

Thirty-one adult cats were anesthetized with ketamine hydrochloride (10 mg/kg), immobilized, and artificially ventilated with room air. Blood pressure (BP), intracranial pressure (ICP), and cerebral blood volume (CBV) were monitored continuously. ICP was recorded with an epidural pressure sensor, and CBV was measured by a photoelectric method [4]. Electrodes were introduced stereotaxically into the DM ($A_{12.5}$, $L_{\pm 2.0}$, $H_{-4.0}$), MRBF ($A_{4.0}$, $L_{\pm 4.0}$, H_0) and MORF (P_{10}, $L_{\pm 2.0}$, H_{-9}), the atlas of Snider and Niemer [5] being used for guidance. In all animals, the DM and MBRF were first coagulated with 3 mA for 1 min. Then, the animals were divided into four groups. In group 1, ICP was maintained at the normal level. In group 2, ICP was increased to 30 mmHg by an injection of blood into the cisterna magna. Group 3 consisted of animals whose bilateral superior cervical ganglia were resected. In the last group, the spinal cord was transected at the level of C2. In all animals, the MORF was stimulated (5 or 10 V, 10–50 Hz, 1–20 min) unilaterally or bilaterally. At 30 min after the stimulation, the BP was raised by injection of an-

[1] Department of Neurological Surgery, Okayama University Medical School, 2-5-1 Shikatacho, Okayama 700, Japan

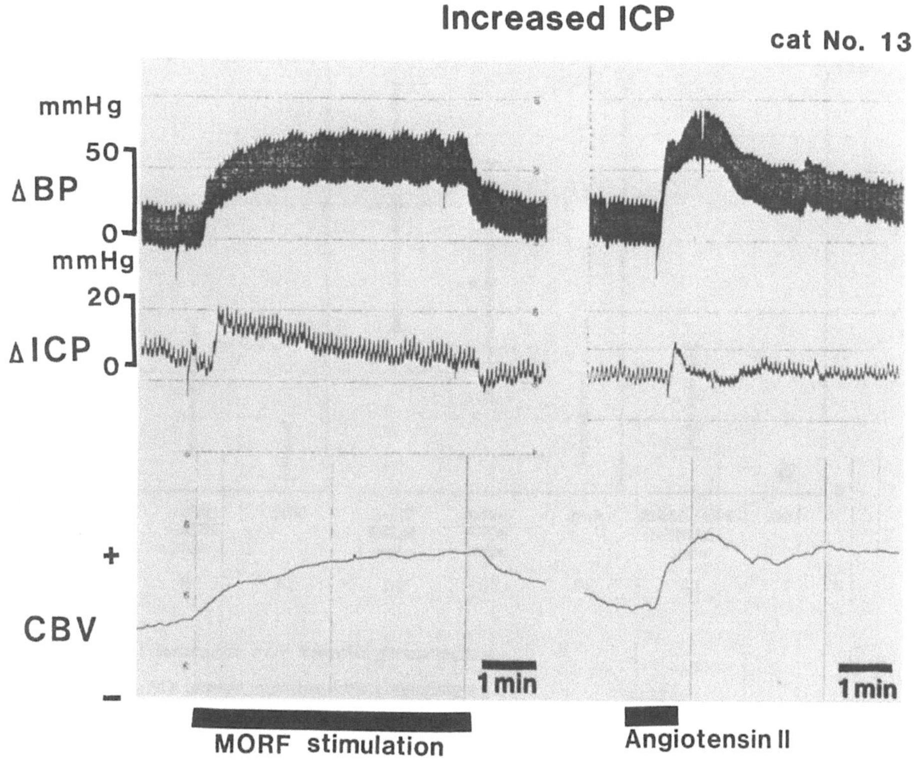

Fig. 1. Effect of stimulation of MORF and injection of angiotensin II on BP, ICP, and CBV in an increased ICP model. Immediately after MORF stimulation, BP, ICP, and CBV increased simultaneously

giotensin II until it reached the same level as with MORF stimulation. The vasomotor index (VI) is defined as $\Delta ICP/\Delta BP$, and thus a high VI means a loss of cerebrovascular tone. The VIs after MORF stimulation and after angiotensin II injection were compared.

Results

The changes in BP, ICP, and CBV following MORF stimulation were essentially the same in all groups except group 4. BP, ICP, and CBV increased simultaneously immediately after MORF stimulation, though the changes in BP and ICP were different in nature. The BP rose slowly and remained elevated during MORF stimulation. On the other hand, ICP increased abruptly and after 10 s or more decreased gradually. After cessation of MORF stimulation, BP, ICP, and CBV returned to the control values. ICP increased slightly and temporarily after injection of angiotensin II. A typical case of increased ICP following experimental subarachnoid hemorrhage is illustrated in Fig. 1. Figure 2 shows the VI values under MORF stimulation and after injection of angiotensin II in three groups. In these groups, the VIs upon MORF stimulation were significantly higher than the VIs upon injection with an-

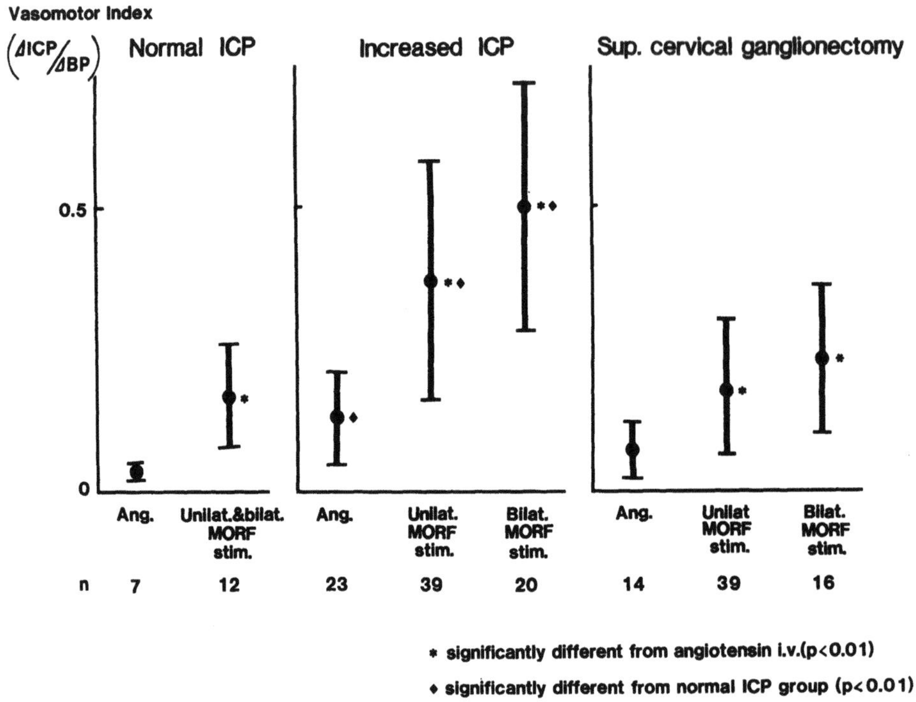

Fig. 2. Comparison of the vasomotor index among the groups with normal and increased ICP and those subjected to bilateral superior cervical ganglionectomy

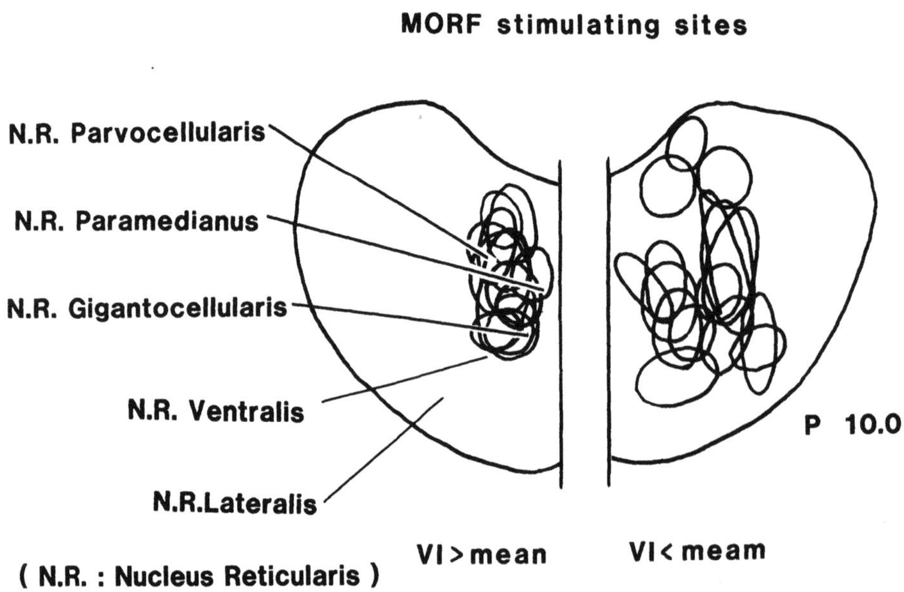

Fig. 3. Map of MORF-stimulating sites. Sites where VI upon MORF stimulation was higher than the mean value are shown on the *left*, and those where VI was lower than the mean, on the *right*

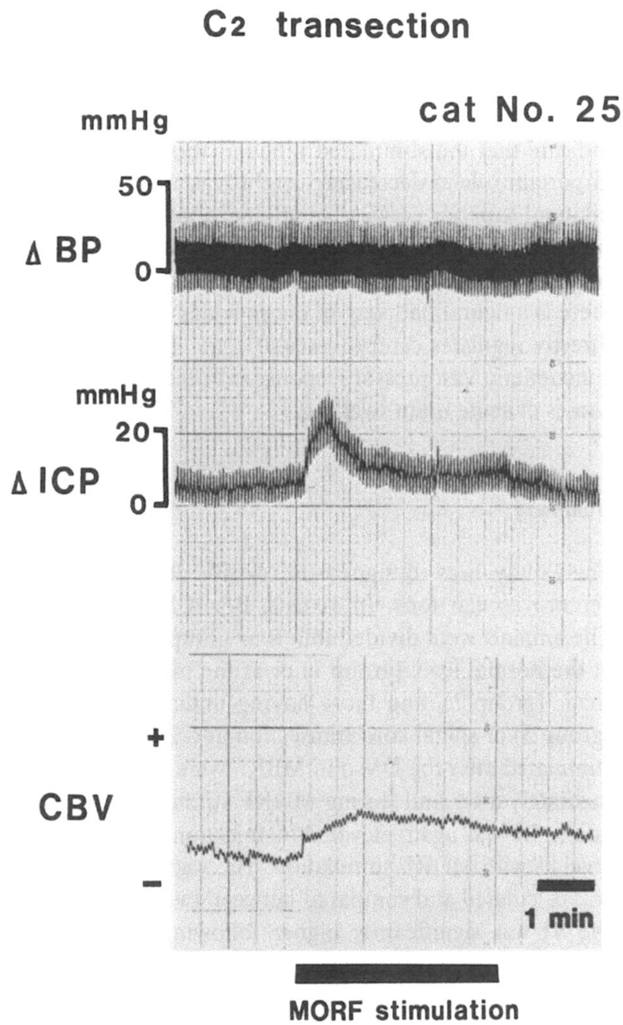

Fig. 4. The effect of stimulation of the MORF on BP, ICP, and CBV after transection of spinal cord at C2

giotensin II ($P < 0.01$). There were no significant differences in the effect of MORF stimulation on the VI between ganglionectomized and control groups. In macroscopically observed brain sections the sites of high VI values upon stimulation of the MORF were located in the paramedian area (Fig. 3). After transection of the upper spinal cord (C2) ICP increased with the stimulation of the MORF in the same manner as in groups 1, 2 and 3, although no change was found in BP (Fig. 4).

Discussion

Many clinical and experimental studies have suggested that dysfunction of the vasomotor center in the brain stem is one of the major factors causing acute brain swelling [1–3]. In this study, BP, ICP, and CBV increased simultaneously immediately after MORF stimulation. The increase in ICP was not secondary to the increase in BP, because the VI value under MORF stimulation was significantly higher than the VI value upon administration of angiotensin II. Furthermore, in animals with the spinal cord transected at C2, ICP increased without changes in BP. These findings indicate that the stimulated reticular formation of the medulla oblongata plays an important role in decreasing cerebrovascular tone. This effect was not influenced by bilateral superior cervical ganglionectomy, indicating that there is an intrinsic neural pathway which regulates cerebrovascular tone directly. The elevation of BP associated with MORF stimulation results in a further increase in ICP. In conclusion, there is a neural pathway in the reticular formation of the medulla oblongata which directly regulates cerebrovascular tone. The reduction of cerebrovascular tone and concomitant vasopressor response induced by MORF stimulation may be one of the causes of acute brain swelling.

Summary

This study was designed to clarify the effect of stimulation of MORF on cerebrovascular tone. In 31 cats, BP, ICP, and CBV were measured continuously. The animals were divided into four groups: those in which the ICP was maintained at the normal level (group 1) or at the higher level following subarachnoid hemorrhage (group 2), and those having undergone a superior cervical ganglionectomy (group 3) or spinal cord transection at C2 (group 4). In all animals, the MORF was stimulated after the DM and MBRF were destroyed. Both BP and ICP increased immediately after and during MORF stimulation. At 30 min after cessation of stimulation, BP was again elevated by injection of angiotensin II until it reached the same level as with MORF stimulation. The vasomotor index (VI), defined by $\Delta ICP/\Delta BP$, was calculated and compared between two different situations. In groups 1, 2, and 3, the VI was significantly higher following MORF stimulation than following angiotensin II. The increase in ICP with MORF stimulation in group 4 was similar to that observed in groups 1, 2, and 3. In conclusion, the stimulated MORF plays an important role in lowering the cerebrovascular tone via intrinsic pathways.

References

1. Bruce DA, Alavi A, Bilaniuk L, Donlinskas C, Obrist W, Uzzell B (1981) Diffuse cerebral swelling following head injuries in children: the syndrome of "malignant brain edema". J Neurosurg 54:170–178
2. George B, Thurel C, Pierron D, Ragueneau JL (1981) Frequency of primary brain stem lesions after head injuries. A CT scan analysis from 186 cases of severe head trauma. Acta Neurochirurgica 59:35–43
3. Ishii S (1966) Brain-swelling. Study of structural, physiologic and biochemical alterations. In: Caverness WF, Walker AE (ed) Head injury. Conference proceedings, chap 24. Lippincott, Philadelphia, pp 276–299
4. Kuyama H, Fujimoto S, Nishimoto K, Ninomiya K, Akioka T, Matsumoto A, Nishimoto A (1978) Measurement of regional cerebral blood volume by photoelectric method. Neurol Med Chir (Tokyo) 18(II):655–664
5. Snider RS, Niemer WT (1961) A stereotaxic atlas of the cat brain. University of Chicago, Chicago

Restriction of Cellular Swelling and Spontaneous Increase in the Osmolality of the Intracellular Fluid in a Simplistic Cell Model

M. TOMITA [1], F. GOTOH, M. KOBARI, T. SHINOHARA, Y. TERAYAMA, B. MIHARA, and P. TURCANI

Key words: Cytotoxic edema, cellular swelling, iso-osmotic osmosis, hyperosmotic osmosis, osmolality

Introduction

As a possible mechanism of the cellular swelling in cytotoxic edema, fluid shift from the extracellular compartment to the intracellular compartment due to isothermal, isobaric, and iso-osmotic osmosis was demonstrated experimentally by Tomita [3] in a simplistic cell model. This process would proceed iso-osmotically if the cell membrane were sufficiently flaccid not to impede the cellular swelling. However, cellular swelling in situ is restricted by the tension developed by the surrounding tissue of the glial layers, the constraint of the pia and dura, and finally the rigidity of the closed calvarium.

The purpose of this investigation was to examine the changes in osmolality of the intracellular fluid of a simplistic cell model employing an unstretchable membrane to prevent "free" cellular swelling.

Methods

The a priori assumptions for cellular swelling are that (a) the intracellular and extracellular fluids are iso-osmotic [2]; (b) the net activity of small ions in the extracellular fluid (mostly Na^+ and Cl^-) is higher than that inside the cell (mostly K^+ and negative small ions in lesser quantities); and (c) in pathologic conditions in which cytotoxic edema would develop the cell membrane is selectively permeable to small ions, but not to proteins. Based on these assumptions, the following cell model was constructed to reproduce such cytotoxic edema.

Two solutions consisting of ion-free aqueous polyethylene glycol (PEG, hydrophilic long-chain molecules of mol. wt. 6000) at a concentration of 170 g/liter and physiologic saline, representing the intra- and extracellular fluids, respectively, were prepared. The Na^+ and Cl^- in the saline solution represented the surplus ionic activity in the extracellular fluid in an exaggerated manner. Both solutions were iso-osmotic at 0.54 °C in freezing point depression. A piece of seamless, unstretchable

[1] Department of Neurology, School of Medicine, Keio University, 35 Shinanomachi, Shinjaku-ku, Tokyo 160, Japan

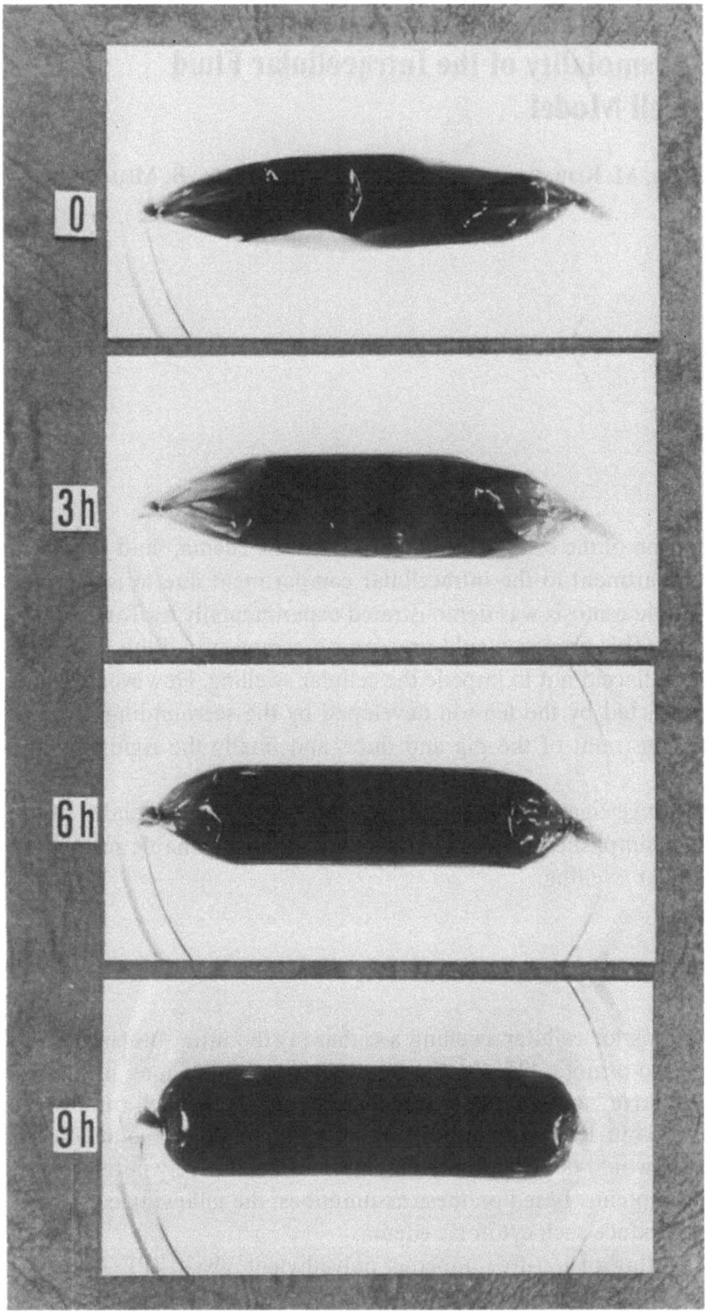

Fig. 1. Simulated cell model with an intracellular fluid composed of 170 g/l polyethylene glycol 6000 (PEG) solution in a Visking tube. The "cell" is immersed in extracellular fluid composed of saline under isothermal, isobaric, and iso-osmotic conditions. The Visking tube represents an unstretchable, uncharged membrane permeable to water and sodium chloride, but not to PEG molecules. After immersion, the cell gradually became swollen with time, as shown by the photographs taken at 3 h and at 6 h. The swelling at 9 h appeared to be restricted. It was found that the osmolality of the intracellular fluid (estimated from the freezing point depression) was increased at 9 h

cellulose tubing 15 mm in diameter and 80 mm in length, with pores 24 Å in size (Visking Company) was used as the ischemic cell membrane which was permeable to small ions but impermeable to colloid molecules. The PEG solution was tinted with black ink for visualization, and 8 ml was introduced into the Visking tubing, both ends of which were tightly ligated so that the membrane was flaccid (see the cell model at 0 h in Fig. 1). This ischemic cell model was bathed in 30 ml saline in a test glass vessel at room temperature. Thus, the two iso-osmotic solutions were in contact with each other via the membrane under isothermal and isobaric conditions. In the control situation and at 9 h after commencement of the experiment, the osmolality of the "extra-" and "intracellular" fluids was determined from the freezing point depression by means of a Fiske osmometer, and their ion concentrations of Na^+ and Cl^-, with a Beckmann flame photometer and a chloride meter, respectively.

Results

The Visking tube became swollen with time, as shown in Fig. 1. However, at 9 h the swelling appeared to be restricted because of the tension in the unstretchable membrane. The volume of fluid that had moved into the "cell" across the membrane was calculated as 3.8 ml at 9 h after commencement of the experiment. The changes in ionic concentrations and osmolality concomitant with the cell swelling at 9 h are summarized in Table 1. The intracellular fluid was concentrated, whereas the extracellular fluid became more dilute with time. This must have been due to small ion influx. The quantity of small ions gained by the intracellular fluid or lost by the extracellular fluid was calculated as 1.26 m*M* salt (Na^+ and Cl^-). Since 1.26 m*M* salt and 3.8 ml fluid were transported across the membrane during the same period of time, the average concentration of the fluid, like the volume flow, was simply calculated at twice that of the saline (approx. 150 m*M*/liter), with 1.26 m*M*/3.8 ml or 330 m*M*/liter. In other words, the fluid shifting across the membrane was apparently hyperosmotic compared with the extracellular fluid, resulting in an increase in osmolality of the intracellular fluid.

Table 1. Changes in ionic concentrations and osmolality after 9 h

	Volume (ml)	Osmolality (mosmol/liter)	Na^+ (mEq/liter)	Cl^- (mEq/liter)
	Extracellular fluid, $n=7$			
Control	30.0	290.0±1.6	156.7±1.3	150.6±1.3
9 h	24.8±0.25	251.5±3.1*	131.7±1.9**	131.5±1.3**
	Intracellular fluid, $n=7$			
Control	8.0	290.3±2.1	0	0
9 h	11.8	358.3±7.3*	96.1±1.5**	102.7±1.1**

Values are presented as means±standard errors. * $P<0.05$, ** $P<0.01$, against corresponding control values (Student's *t*-test)

Discussion

The rapid increase in osmolality in ischemic cerebral tissue has been attributed to autolysis of cellular constituents, or catabolic products in the damaged cells [1]. The present simplistic experiment suggests that at least part of the increase in osmolality could be due to the influx of hyperosmotic fluid across the cell membrane, whose extensibility was somehow restricted. Such paradoxical phenomena as the spontaneous increase in osmolality may be explained as follows. The diffusional process of iso-osmotic fluid demonstrated in the previous experiment must be impeded by the tension of the membrane (T), which is equal to $P \times R$ according to Laplace's law, where P is the pressure developed in the cell and R the radius of the cell. At the time of no volume flow across the selective membrane, P is equivalent to the difference in osmotic pressure between the extra- and intracellular fluids. Thus, the osmolality must be higher in the intracellular fluid than in the extracellular fluid for thermodynamic equilibrium. These fundamental observations are supported by the experimental data of Zimmermann and Hossmann [5], which showed that after reperfusion of the ischemic brain, the intracranial pressure of animals increased to more than 75 mmHg, with an accompanying influx of sodium and chloride, and passive water shift from the extracellular into the intracellular compartment.

How high, then, could the intracranial pressure become in cytotoxic edema? Assuming that a tissue block freshly excised from the mammalian brain could be regarded as a conglomerate of numerous ischemic cells, or as a large single cell with a hypothetical damaged cell membrane at the surface, Tomita et al. [4] reported that a pressure of 578 mmHg was required to counteract the swelling of a cat brain tissue block in Ringer's solution. This pressure may be equivalent to the intracellular colloid osmotic pressure, therefore reflecting the maximum potential inherent in the brain tissue.

Summary

A cell model consisting of seamless, unstretchable cellulose tubing (Visking) and an intracellular fluid of polyethylene glycol 6000 (PEG) solution was immersed in saline as the extracellular fluid. The cell gradually became swollen, indicating a fluid shift from the extra- to the intracellular compartment in isothermal, isobaric, and iso-osmotic conditions, as demonstrated in a previous communication. However, the swelling became restricted with time through the tension in the cell membrane. This restriction resulted in an increase in the osmolality of the intracellular fluid together with the development of a high intracellular pressure. Such a spontaneous event would be potentiated in the system by the energy of uneven distribution of small ions and high molecular colloids separated by a membrane that was permeable to small ions but not to the colloids. Such a self-perpetuating process may be pertinent to the development of cytotoxic edema.

References

1. Katzman R, Pappius HM (1973) Brain electrolytes and fluid metabolism. Williams and Wilkins, Baltimore, pp 6–8
2. Leaf A (1956) On the mechanism of fluid exchange of tissues in vitro. Biochem J 62:241–248
3. Tomita M (1985) Mechanism of cytotoxic edema. In: Mchedlishvili GI, et al. (eds) Pathophysiological mechanisms of brain edema development. Akadémiai Kiadó, Budapest (in press)
4. Tomita M, Gotoh F, Sato T, Yamamoto M, Amano T, Tanahashi N (1979) Determination of the osmotic potential for swelling of cat brain in vitro. Exp Neurol 65:66–77
5. Zimmermann Z, Hossmann K-A (1975) Resuscitation of the monkey brain after one hour's complete ischemia. II: Brain water and electrolytes. Brain Res 85:1–11

Experimental Model of Cytotoxic Brain Edema: Systemic Administration of Kainic Acid

F. SEITELBERGER [1], H. LASSMANN, K. KITZ, U. PETSCHE, H. BARAN, and O. HORNYKIEWICZ

Key words: Kainic acid, brain edema, epilepsy

Introduction

Kainic acid (KA), a rigid analogue of glutamic acid, is a cytotoxic agent causing strong excitation of neurons of the mammalian central nervous system [2, 5]. Systemic administration of KA leads to a clinical picture of secondarily generalized limbic seizures, accompanied by nerve cell loss and reactive gliosis mainly in the hippocampus (the CA1 and CA3 sector) and in the entorhinal and pyriform cortex [1, 4, 6]. Although it is generally believed that KA-induced brain damage is due to mechanisms directly related to the action of the drug [1, 4], we recently found evidence that brain edema with subsequent disturbance of brain microcirculation may play an essential role in its pathogenesis [3, 6].

Materials and Methods

Experimental epilepsy was induced in rats by SC injection of KA (10 mg/kg). The clinical severity of seizure activity was scored [3, 6] and the animals were sampled for neuropathological and neurochemical studies at various time intervals between 1 h and 20 days after injection of the drug. Morphological studies included light and electron microscopy and blood-brain barrier studies with sodium fluorescein, Evans blue, horseradish peroxidase, and endogenous albumin [3]. In addition, neurotransmitters (noradrenaline, dopamine, serotonin), transmitter metabolites (homovanillic acid, 5-hydroxyindoleacetic acid), and neuronal transmitter enzymes (glutamate decarboxylase, choline acetyltransferase) were determined neurochemically [6]. Treatment of KA-induced brain edema was performed with dexamethasone or mannitol at various doses and schedules [3].

Results and Conclusions

Systemic injection of KA resulted in long-lasting secondarily generalized limbic seizures. The first seizures appeared 1–1.5 h after SC injection of the drug, reaching

[1] Neurological Institute of the University of Vienna, Schwarzspanierstraße 17, A-1090 Wien

their maximal intensity 2 and 3 h after the injection. During the next few hours epileptic seizures gradually diminished in frequency, and after 1 day only rare seizures were noted, which either occurred spontaneously or were induced by noise or handling of animals [6].

Neurochemical testing during the stage of generalized status epilepticus revealed a massive turnover of neurotransmitters, expressed in a decrease in noradrenaline and dopamine and an increase in transmitter metabolites such as 5-hydroxyindoleacetic acid and homovanillic acid [6]. On neuropathological testing at this stage some dark condensed neurons were found, together with massive swelling of astrocytes in the limbic system, resulting in compression of local blood vessels in edematous areas [3]. Three days after KA injection and later, neurotransmitter levels and transmitter metabolites returned to normal values, indicating normalization of transmitter turnover [6]. However, neuronal transmitter enzymes such as glutamate decarboxylase were permanently decreased in the limbic system, which suggests degeneration of nerve cells in this region. In neuropathology nerve cell loss and incomplete parenchymal necrosis were present, especially in the hippocampus, the amygdala, and the entorhinal/pyriform cortex. In addition, multiple perivenous hemorrhages were found in the necrotic areas, suggesting herniation damage due to brain edema during status epilepticus [3, 6]. Treatment of brain edema with dexamethasone did not change the clinical appearance of KA-induced seizures and had no effect on the incidence and severity of KA-induced permanent brain lesions. However, mannitol treatment had a clear-cut therapeutic effect. In fact, irreversible brain lesions due to KA, according to both neuropathological and neurochemical examinations, were completely prevented in more than 50% of the animals treated with mannitol [3]. Our results suggest the following conclusions: Kainic acid induces strong excitation of neurons in the limbic system (secondarily generalized limbic seizures), accompanied by a massive turnover of neurotransmitters. Neuronal excitation leads to focal cytotoxic brain edema (swelling of astrocytes), which by compressing local blood vessels may result in disturbance of local microcirculation and herniation damage. Irreversible brain damage following KA is brought about by an imbalance of increased metabolic demand of overactive neurons and focal ischemia, due to edema-induced decreased microcirculation. Mannitol treatment of brain edema results in partial or complete prevention of irreversible brain damage after KA toxification.

Summary

Kainic acid (KA)-induced epilepsy is accompanied by widespread irreversible lesions in the limbic system. Our present observations suggest that cytotoxic brain edema plays an essential role in the pathogenesis of brain damage following status epilepticus.

References

1. Ben Ari Y, Tremblay E, Riche D, Ghillini G, Naquet R (1981) Electrographic, clinical, and pathological alterations following systemic administration of kainic acid, bicuculline or

pentetrazole: metabolic mapping using deoxyglucose method with special reference to the pathology of epilepsy. Neuroscience 6:1361–1391
2. Johnston GAR, Curtis DR, Davies J, McCulloch RM (1974) Spinal interneurone excitation by conformationally restricted analogues of L-glutamic acid. Nature 248:804–805
3. Lassmann H, Petsche U, Kitz K, Baran H, Sperk G, Seitelberger F, Hornykiewicz O (1984) The role of brain edema in epileptic brain damage induced by systemic kainic acid injection. Neuroscience 13:691–704
4. Schwob JE, Fuller T, Price JL, Olney JW (1980) Widespread patterns of neuronal damage following systemic or intracerebral injection of kainic acid: a histological study. Neuroscience 5:991–1014
5. Shinozaki H, Konishi S (1970) Action of several antihelminthics and insecticides on rat cortical neurones. Brain Res 24:368–371
6. Sperk G, Lassmann H, Baran H, Kish SH, Seitelberger F, Hornykiewicz O (1983) Kainic acid induced seizures: neurochemical and histopathological changes. Neuroscience 10:1301–1315

Vasogenic Brain Edema and Cortical Neural Function

S. Nagao[1], F. Momma, T. Nishiura, T. Murota, M. Suga, Y. Homma, T. Tanimoto, H. Kuyama, and A. Nishomoto

Key words: Vasogenic brain edema, air exposure, direct cortical response, water content, cortical blood flow

Abbreviations

lCBF	local cortical blood flow
DCR	direct cortical response
MP	methylprednisolone
BBB	blood brain barrier

Purpose

In head-injury patients, vasogenic edema results from damage to cerebral cortical vessels, which permits the extravasation of plasma ultrafiltrate into the surrounding extracellular space. Although the electrophysiological effects of white matter edema have been studied [3, 6, 8], it remains unclear whether the exudation of plasma into the cerebral cortex results in any direct impairment of cortical function. The present experiment was carried out to study the effects of cortical edema and ischemia on cortical neural activity. The air-exposure edema used does not induce direct cortical injury comparable to that caused by cold injury or brain compression. Effects of a high dose of steroid on cortical neural function were also investigated.

Materials and Method

In 40 cats, vasogenic brain edema was produced by exposure of the brain surface to room air (approximately 26 °C, humidity 60%) for 12 h. The water content and local cortical blood flow (lCBF) were measured by gravimetry and hydrogen clearance, respectively, 3, 6, 9, and 12 h after air exposure. The direct cortical response (DCR) [1, 2], which represents the synaptic potential of apical dendrites of pyramidal cells, was used to evaluate cortical neurophysiological activity. Sequential changes in the amplitude of the 7–15 ms surface-negative wave were measured after direct stimu-

[1] Department of Neurological Surgery, Okayama University Medical School, 2-5-1 Shikata-cho, Okayama 700, Japan

lation of the suprasylvian gyrus. An IV injection of 2% Evans blue (2 ml) was given to allow evaluation of BBB (blood-brain barrier) disruption. To determine the steroid effect on cortical edema, a high dose of methylprednisolone (MP 30 mg/kg) was given at the beginning of the exposure.

Results

At 6 h after air exposure, extravasated Evans blue was observed macroscopically in the gray and white matter, and by the end of the experiments herniation of the cortex had occurred through the craniotomy in some animals. Figure 1 depicts the changes in the water content and lCBF in the air-exposure and air-exposure plus MP groups as a function of time after exposure of the brain surface. In animals subjected to exposure for 12 h, there were stepwise increases in the water content to 81.0% ± 0.6% g water/g tissue ($n = 14$) (control value = 79.1% ± 0.3%, $n = 25$) and decreases in lCBF to 71.5% ± 14.5% ($n = 17$) of the control. In contrast, animals receiving a high dose of MP had a slight increase in water content to 79.7% ± 0.6% g wa-

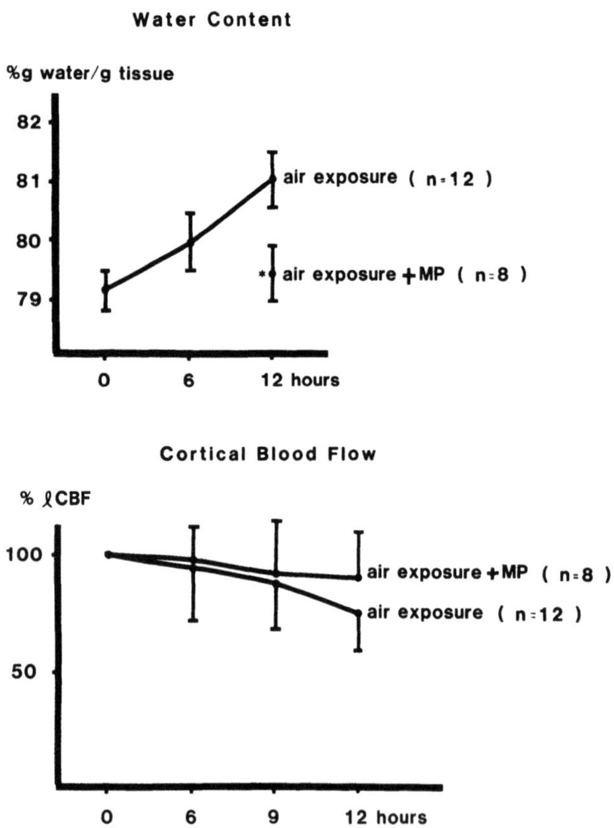

Fig. 1. Mean water content (g water/g tissue) as a percentage (*above*) and cortical blood flow as a percentage of control value (*below*) against time after exposure of the brain to air

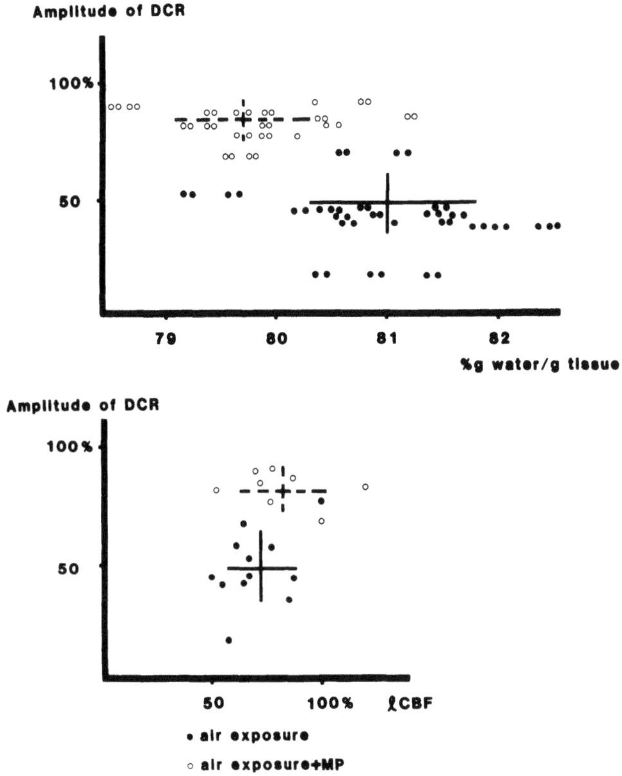

Fig. 2. Relationship between water content, lCBF and DCR amplitude 12 h after exposure to air, with (*open circles* and *dashed line*) and without methylprednisolone (MP) treatment

ter/g tissue ($n = 8$), which was significantly less than in the nontreated group, and a mild decrease in lCBF to 82.6% ± 19.1% ($n = 8$) of the control value. Correlations between changes in the water content and lCBF and the DCR amplitude after 12 h of exposure are shown in Fig. 2. An increase in water content and decrease in lCBF of the cortex were associated with suppression of the DCR amplitude. In the MP-treated group there appeared to be a significant decrease in the water content and an increase in lCBF compared with the nontreated group. The DCR amplitude was maintained at more than 80% of the control. As shown in Fig. 3, exposure of the brain surface to air produced a stepwise suppression of the DCR amplitude, which was 49.0% ± 14.5% ($n = 12$) of control 12 h after exposure. MP produced a significant improvement in the DCR amplitude 6 h after exposure, and at 12 h it was still 83.0% ± 6.8% ($n = 8$) of control.

Discussion

In experimental exposure of the brain surface to air, Prados et al. [7] found disturbances of cortical microcirculation, such as venous congestion, collapsed capillaries, and loss of tonicity of the vessel wall, and confirmed the presence of cortical isch-

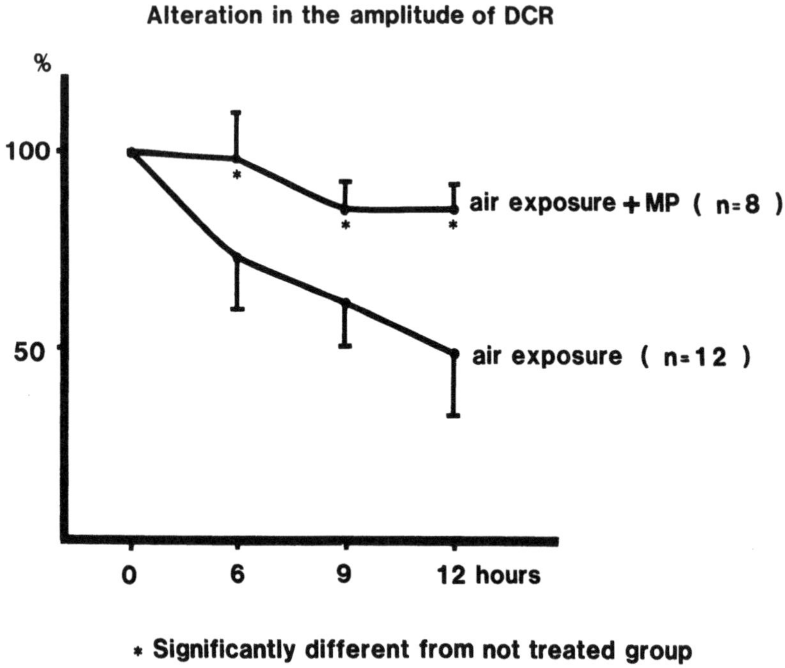

Fig. 3. Mean changes in the DCR amplitude during 12 h of exposure to air, with and without methylprednisolone (MP) treatment

emia by the use of benzidine stain. Vällfors et al. [9] also observed extravasation of Evans blue in the leptomeninges during exposure to air for as little as 15 min. Thus, exposure of the brain surface to air has been thought to produce serious cortical damage secondary to ischemia of the gray matter and BBB disruption. However, we were unable to find a previous report concerning the changes in the water content and lCBF of the cortex in long-term air exposure. Our data indicated that the water content increased by 1.9% from the control, and lCBF decreased to 71% of the control after 12 h of exposure, presumably due to BBB disruption and cortical microcirculatory impairment. Marmarou et al. [5] concluded that white matter edema did not result in regional white matter ischemia in the infusion edema model, and white matter edema itself is thought to have no or little influence on electrophysiological alterations [3, 6, 8]. However, it has been proposed that neurophysiological function in the cerebral cortex, assessed by the DCR, is mediated through changes in lCBF in acute intracranial hypertension [4] and global ischemia [10]. Our results clearly showed that both increased cortical water content and decreased lCBF were responsible for the suppression of cortical neural function. A high dose of MP seemed to provide protection against cortical edema and ischemia and resulted in a marked improvement in cortical electrophysiological function. In conclusion, this study demonstrates the importance of immediate administration of high doses of steroids for the treatment of vasogenic cortical edema.

Summary

To study the effect of vasogenic brain edema on cortical neural function, the surface of the cat brain was exposed to air for 12 h while serial measurements of cortical water content (gravimetric method) and blood flow (lCBF, hydrogen clearance method) were made. The amplitude of the direct cortical response (DCR) was measured to assess the local cortical neurophysiological activity. The water content of the cortex significantly increased by 1.9% (mean value, $n = 14$) during the 12 h of exposure, and lCBF decreased to 71.5% ($n = 17$) of control. The DCR amplitude was suppressed significantly after 6 h exposure, and was 49.0% ($n = 12$) of control after 12 h. Methylprednisolone (30 mg/kg) given at the beginning of exposure resulted in significantly less severe cortical edema after 12 h of exposure. The DCR amplitude remained at 83% ($n = 8$) of control. It was concluded that in vasogenic brain edema both cortical edema and ischemia are responsible for the suppression of cortical neural function, and high doses of steroids are effective in improving cortical neural activity.

References

1. Chang HT (1951) Dendritic potential of cortical neurons produced by direct electrical stimulation of the cerebral cortex. J Neurophysiol 14:1–21
2. Eccles JC (1951) Interpretation of action potentials evoked in the cerebral cortex. Electroencephalogr Clin Neurophysiol 3:449–464
3. Gastaut JL, Michel B, Hassan SS, Cerda M, Bianchi L, Gastaut H (1979) Electroencephalography in brain edema (127 cases of brain tumor investigated by cranial computerized tomography). Electroencephalogr Clin Neurophysiol 46:239–255
4. Grossman RG, Turner JW, Miller JD, Rowan JD (1973) The relationship between cortical electrical activity, cerebral perfusion pressure and cerebral blood flow during increased intracranial pressure. Stroke 4:346–347
5. Marmarou A, Takagi H, Shulman K (1980) Biomechanics of brain edema and effects on local cerebral blood flow. Adv Neurol 28:345–358
6. Penn RD (1980) Cerebral edema and neurological function: CT, evoked responses, and clinical examination. Adv Neurol 28:383–394
7. Prados M, Strowger B, Feindel WH (1945) Studies on cerebral edema. I: Reaction of the brain to air exposure; pathologic changes. Arch Neurol Psychiatr 54:163–174
8. Sutton LN, Bruce DA, Welsh F (1980) The effect of cold-induced brain edema and white-matter ischemia on the somatosensory evoked response. J Neurosurg 53:180–184
9. Wällfors B, Hansson HA, Srensson J (1980) Experimental exposure of the cat brain surface to neurosurgical irrigation fluids and air: study of blood-brain barrier damage. Neurosurg 7:53–56
10. Yamagata S, Carter LP, Erspamer R (1982) Cortical ischemia: Effect upon direct cortical response. Stroke 13:680–686

Simultaneous Topographic Analysis of Brain Edema, Parenchymal Energy Metabolisms (NAD/NADH Redox State, Reduced Cytochrome aa_3, ATP), and Intracellular Calcium During Cerebral Ischemia

N. Hayashi[1], T. Tsubokawa, S. Kimura, Y. Makiyama, and M. Toeda

Key words: Cerebral ischemia, brain edema, intracellular Ca, mitochondrial energy metabolism, laser photospectrometric analysis

Introduction

In cases of brain edema caused by cerebral ischemic insult it has been documented that cytotoxic edema occurs before vasogenic edema [3, 8] and that both types promote the development of secondary brain edema with concomitant metabolic changes and microcirculatory disturbances [5]. As a consequence, studies of brain edema have focused on the correlations between metabolic changes, intracellular ion changes, and vasogenic edema following cerebral ischemia. These parameters were simultaneously subjected to topographic analysis with reference to the same sliced brain by a laser photographic, computer-assisted method developed in our laboratory in collaboration with NIIC Laser Co. (4-16-13 Nishi Azabu Minato-ku, Tokyo, Japan). The block diagram is shown in Fig. 1.

Materials and Method

An experimental model of cerebral ischemia (incomplete) was induced in spontaneously hypertensive rats (SHRs) by bilateral carotid ligations. The persistent and qualitative topographic changes in oxyhemoglobin, NAD/NADH redox state, ATP, reduced cytochrome aa_3, and intracellular calcium related to the blood-brain barrier (BBB) were studied simultaneously, following the induction of cerebral ischemia in the SHR. The experimental sliced brain specimens were prepared according to the head cup frozen technique described previously [10]. The cut surface of the brain tissue block immersed in liquid nitrogen was exposed to N_2 laser-ultraviolet light (337 nm) for excitation and/or absorption of metabolic factors and luminescent probes in the brain tissue. Previous light emission and/or reflection values in the NAD/NADH redox state (λ 450 nm), reduced cytochrome aa_3 (λ 605–590 nm), oxyhemoglobin [1/3 (λ 578–0.5 λ 457 nm)], Na fluorescein (λ 500 nm) and Evans blue (λ 610 nm) were computed and analyzed for evaluation

[1] Department of Neurosurgery, Nihon University, 30-1 Oyaguchi Kamimachi, Itabashi-ku, Tokyo 173, Japan

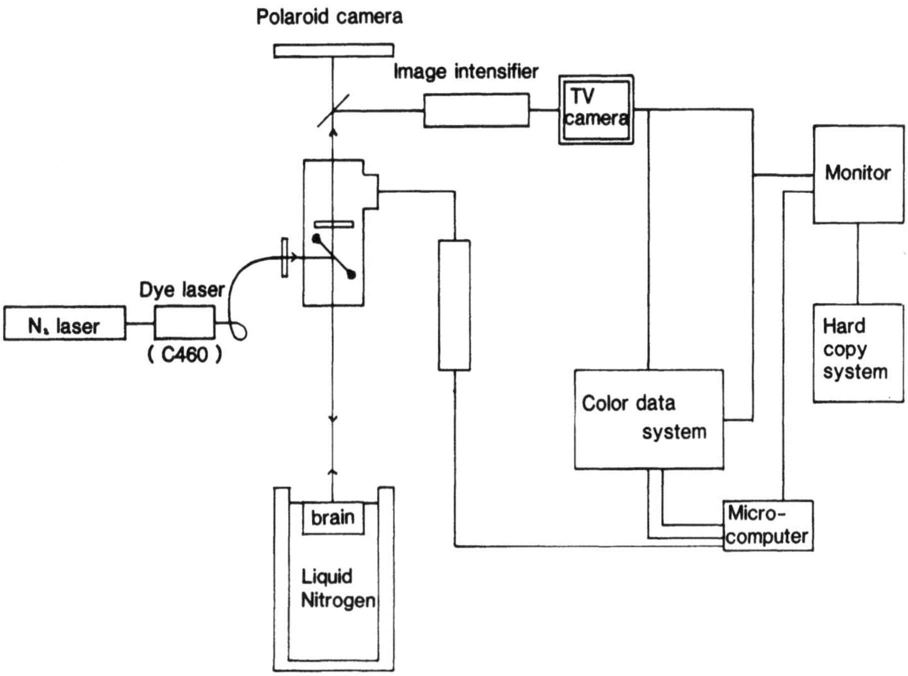

Fig. 1. Block diagram of the laser photospectrometric computer-assisted system for simultaneous analysis of cerebral ischemia, energy metabolism, intracellular ions, and blood-brain barrier

of regional changes in cerebral metabolism, ischemia, and vasogenic edema, respectively. The topographic changes in intracellular calcium were analyzed by using specific intracellular calcium luminescent probes as described previously [9]. In these studies the intensity of NADH fluorescence was used for calibration (λ 450–500 nm) to avoid the overestimation possible with intracellular calcium fluorescence. The regional cerebral ATP changes have been studied by means of an enzyme photoluminescent technique described previously [4].

Results and Discussion

The parenchymal cerebral ischemia following bilateral carotid ligation in the SHR occurred in different areas in different animals. As a consequence, simultaneous topographic studies of cerebral metabolism, intracellular calcium and vasogenic edema revealed the correlations between these parameters very clearly.

Changes in Cerebral Energy Metabolism and Intracellular Calcium

The initial changes in the hydrogen electron transport system, as reflected in activated NADH fluorescence, were observed at 10–30 min after cerebral ischemia, after which the of cytochrome aa_3 level fell. After 1 h of cerebral ischemia, areas of loca-

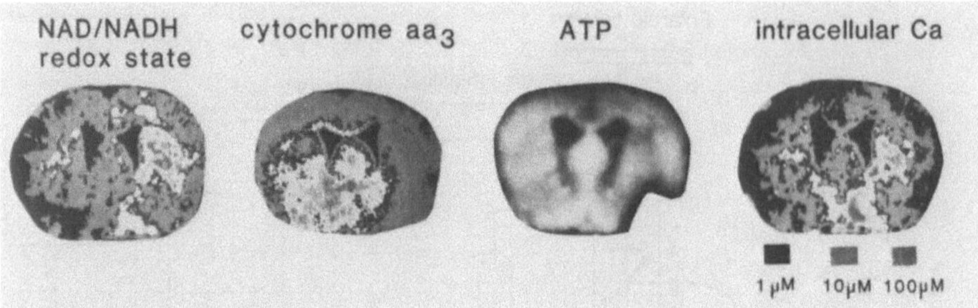

Fig. 2. Alterations of cerebral energy metabolism and intracellular Ca in the brain of the SHR following 1 h of ischemia

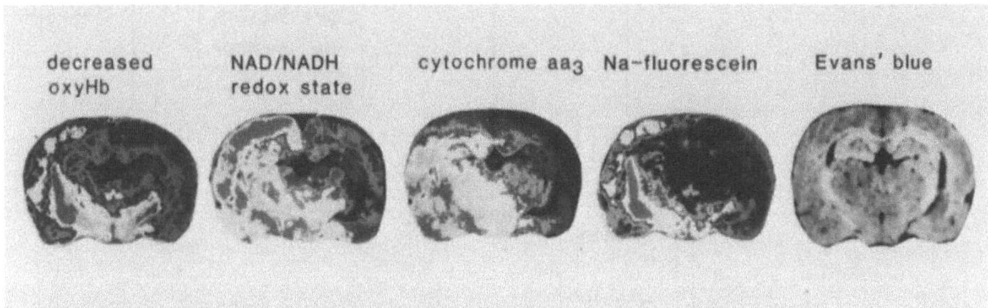

Fig. 3. Simultaneous topographic analysis of cerebral ischemia, metabolism, and vasogenic edema in the brain of the SHR following 4 h of ischemia

lized ATP loss were observed, with reduced cytochrome aa_3 and accumulation of free calcium in the cells, as shown in Fig. 2. Severe ATP loss and a pronounced reduction in cytochrome aa_3 were observed at 3–4 h after the onset of cerebral ischemia. At this stage, intracellular calcium increased to over 100 μM. This suggests that the mitochondrial intracellular calcium buffer capacity might be severely decreased [1]. One consequence of this is cytotoxic edema, because ATP loss and blocking of the Na-K pump by increased intracellular calcium [2, 6, 7] change the cellular membrane's permeability.

Changes in Vasogenic Edema and Cerebral Energy Metabolism

No vasogenic edema developed until 4 h after cerebral ischemia, even though the hydrogen electron transport system was already damaged as previously described. Vasogenic edema, evaluated with reference to the extravasation sodium of fluorescein developed in the white matter more than in the gray matter, with or after ATP loss, reduction of cytochrome aa_3, and increased intracellular calcium, which cause intracellular water extraction to decrease. Double-tracer study of vasogenic edema with sodium fluorescein and Evans blue showed this difference between the gray and white matter. High intensities of sodium fluorescein (mol. wt. 332) have been observed in the white matter; a high intensity of Evans blue (mol. wt. 960) was observed more in the gray matter, as shown in Fig. 3.

In this study, the mechanisms of formation of these different vasogenic edemas in the gray and white matters were not estimated; they might involve different forms of pinocytosis in the vascular wall and different bulk flows of interstitial proteins and water.

Conclusion

Simultaneous topographic analysis of cerebral ischemia, intracellular Ca^{2+}, energy metabolism, and the blood-brain barrier in the same sliced brain by means of a laser photographic computer-assisted technique provided clear documentation of the process of cellular damage and of specific localizations of tissue damage correlated with changes to the blood-brain barrier during cerebral ischemia.

Summary

Simultaneous topographic analysis of cerebral energy metabolism, intracellular calcium, and vasogenic edema following cerebral ischemia in the spontaneously hypertensive rat was performed by means of a laser photographic computer-assisted method developed in our laboratory.

The results show that the hydrogen electron transport system was initially disturbed, with increased NADH and reduced cytochrome aa_3. Persistent cerebral ischemic insult (longer than 3 h) produced ATP loss and an increase in intracellular calcium as a consequence of reduced mitochondrial intracellular calcium buffer capacity. These metabolic and ionic changes could be considered one reason for cytotoxic edema formation.

Vasogenic edema, evaluated by measurements of sodium fluorescein, developed 4–5 h after ATP crisis and high intracellular calcium had been recorded. This means that vasogenic edema was always accompanied by cytotoxic edema in the presence of cerebral ischemia. Double-tracer study of vasogenic edema with sodium fluorescein and Evans blue showed the difference between the edema in gray and that in white matter. Higher intensities of sodium fluorescein (mol. wt. 332) were observed in the white matter than in the gray matter, while Evans blue (mol. wt. 960) was observed more in the gray matter.

References

1. Blaustein MP, Ratzlaff RW, Schweitzer ES (1980) Control of intracellular calcium in presynaptic nerve terminals. Fed Proc 39:2790–2795
2. Crompton M, Moser R, Lüdi H, Carafoli E (1978) The interrelations between the transport of sodium and calcium in mitochondria of various mammalian tissues. Eur J Biochem 82:25–31
3. Katzman R, Clasen R, Klatzo I, Meyer JS, Pappius HM, Waltz AG (1977) Report of joint committee for stroke resources. 4: Brain edema in stroke. Stroke 8:512–540
4. Kogure K, Alonso OF (1978) A pictorial representation of endogenous brain ATP by a bioluminescent method. Brain Res 154:273–284

5. Little JR, Kerr FWL, Sundt TM Jr (1976) Microcirculatory obstruction in focal cerebral ischemia: an electron microscopic investigation in monkeys. Stroke 7:25–30
6. Nathanson JA (1977) Cyclic nucleotides and nervous system function. Physiol Rev 57:157–256
7. Nicholls DG, Crompton M (1980) Mitochondrial calcium transport. FEBS Lett 111:261–268
8. Schuier FJ, Hossmann KA (1980) Experimental brain infarcts in cats. II: Ischemic brain edema. Stroke 11:591–601
9. Tsien RY, Rozzant T, Rink TJ (1982) Calcium homeostasis in intact lymphocytes: cytoplasmic free calcium monitored with a new intracellularly trapped fluorescent indicator. J Cell Biol 94:325–334
10. Welsh FA (1980) In situ freezing of cat brain. In: Passonneau JV et al. (eds) Cerebral metabolism and neuronal function. Williams and Wilkins, Baltimore

Local Cerebral Blood Flow and Oxygen Metabolism in Hydrocephalus After Subarachnoid Hemorrhage

M. ISHIKAWA [1], H. HANDA, Y. YONEKAWA, W. TAKI, A. KOBAYASHI, K. TORIZUKA, Y. YONEKURA, S. TANADA, M. SENDA, H. FUKUYAMA, N. FUJIMOTO, K. HARADA, and Y. SHIMIZU

Key words: Cerebral oxygen metabolism, cerebral blood flow, misery perfusion, hydrocephalus, subarachnoid hemorrhage

Introduction

Hydrocephalus that develops after subarachnoid hemorrhage is of particular interest in relation to some forms of dementia. Various studies, including examination of cerebrospinal fluid (CSF) circulation, X-ray CT, and monitoring of cerebral blood flow and intracranial pressure, have been performed. However, little is known about the changes of oxygen metabolism, which is closely related to brain function. Cerebral oxygen metabolism and blood flow were studied by means of positron emission CT (PET) to elucidate the involvement of cerebral oxygen metabolism in the pathophysiology of normal- and high-pressure hydrocephalus after subarachnoid hemorrhage.

Methods and Materials

A new PET scanner (Positologica III) at Kyoto University Hospital [4] makes it possible to obtain seven slices simultaneously with a spatial resolution of 7.6 mm FWHM (full width at half maximum). This scanner was used with continuous inhalation of ^{15}O-labeled O_2 gas and CO_2 gas, and multiple images recording cerebral blood flow (CBF), cerebral oxygen consumption ($CMRO_2$), and oxygen extraction fraction (OEF) were obtained. Six cases were studied, three of normal-pressure hydrocephalus (NPH) and three of high-pressure hydrocephalus (HPH). Four cases were studied after removal of 20 ml CSF and three were also studied after surgery: The shunt operation was performed in five cases, and it was effective in all but one. Spontaneous improvement was noted in one case.

Result

Multiple images of CGF, $CMRO_2$, and OEF were reviewed in each case. There was a general tendency for CBF and $CMRO_2$ to decrease, especially in the frontal lobe.

---

[1] Departments of Neurosurgery, Kyoto University Hospital, 54 Shogoin Kawahara-cho, Sakyo-ku, Kyoto 606, Japan

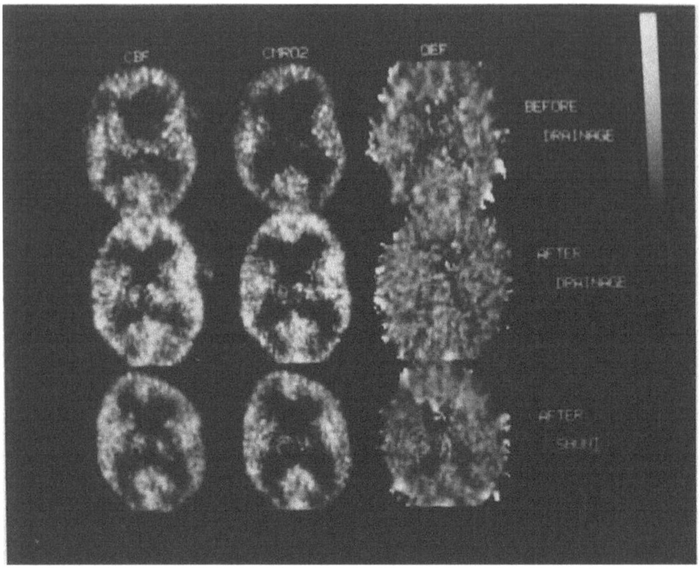

Fig. 1. Changes in CBF, $CMRO_2$, and OEF after CSF removal and after shunt operation in high-pressure hydrocephalus (shunt effective)

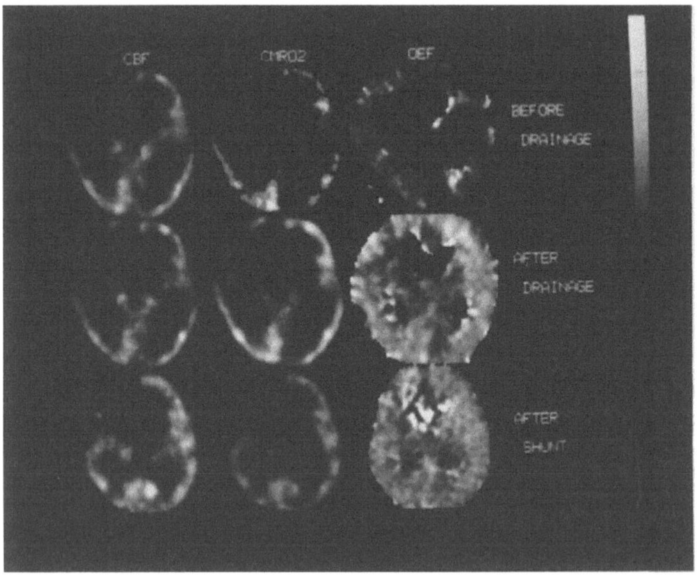

Fig. 2. Changes in CBF, $CMRO_2$, and OEF after CSF removal in high-pressure hydrocephalus (shunt not effective)

OEF increased diffusely in the cerebral hemisphere. Quantitative changes were evaluated in the frontal cortex. In normal volunteers, CBF were 40–60 ml/100 ml/min; $CMRO_2$ 3.1–4.4 ml O_2/100 ml/min; and OEF 0.31–0.48. In hydrocephalus after subarachnoid hemorrhage, the mean CBF in the both frontal cortices was 27.8 ± 8.5; $CMRO_2$ 2.16 ± 0.45; OEF 0.61 ± 0.06 in NPH and 29.4 ± 10.4,

1.80 ± 0.63, 0.46 ± 0.11 in NPH. Thus, OEF was higher in NPH than in HPH, although CBF was almost the same in both conditions. $CMRO_2$ was higher overall in NPH, which is due to a very low value in one patient with HPH whose shunt was not effective.

The response to CSF removal was examined in one case of NPH and three cases of HPH. CBF and $CMRO_2$ were increased (Fig. 1), but by different degrees in the two cases. The increase in CBF and $CMRO_2$ was more prominent in two cases of NPH. In the one case with a noneffective shunt, $CMRO_2$ and OEF increased markedly, but $CMRO_2$ was still low in the brain as a whole (Fig. 2). The postoperative status was also examined in three cases. All had higher CBF and $CMRO_2$ than in the preoperative state.

Discussion

In subarachnoid hemorrhage, Grubb [3] reported decreased CBF and $CMRO_2$. Grubb et al. [2] also reported that these were decreased in primary normal-pressure hydrocephalus or that secondary to subarachnoid hemorrhage. Their results are highly consistent with those obtained in the present study. Furthermore, the present study reveals the regional differences in these parameters; there is a more pronounced decrease in the frontal cortex. It is interesting to note that OEF is higher than normal throughout the brain in most of cases. OEF is a ratio of oxygen consumption to blood flow, and the term "misery perfusion" has been coined by Baron et al. [1] for a rise in this ratio. A high OEF means that blood flow is inadequate to meet oxygen demands, and the tissue can still be viable even in the cerebral ischemic lesion. The present findings are closely correlated with the effectiveness of the shunting operation in hydrocephalic patients after subarachnoid hemorrhage. Response to CSF removal appeared to be more pronounced in HPH, although it is too early to draw any conclusions. A further study is planned to elucidate the role of oxygen metabolism in the pathophysiology of hydrocephalus after subarachnoid hemorrhage.

Summary

Cerebral oxygen metabolism and cerebral blood flow were studied with positron emission CT in six cases of hydrocephalus after subarachnoid hemorrhage. There was a general tendency for CBF and $CMRO_2$ to decrease and for OEF to rise. The decrease in CBF and $CMRO_2$ was more prominent in the frontal cortex. The increase of OEF was diffuse throughout the cerebral hemisphere, which reflects the misery perfusion that occurs in the presence of a cerebral ischemic lesion. This finding can be correlated with the effectiveness of shunting operation. In one patient, in whom the shunt operation was not effective, $CMRO_2$ was low throughout the brain; it responded with an increase to CSF removal, but it was still low. A further study is planned to elucidate the functional role of cerebral oxygen metabolism in the hydrocephalus after subarachnoid hemorrhage.

References

1. Baron JC, Bousser MG, Comar D, et al. (1981) Noninvasive tomographic study of cerebral blood flow and oxygen metabolism in vivo. Eur Neurol 20:273–284
2. Grubb RL, Raichle ME, Gado MH, et al. (1977) Cerebral blood flow oxygen utilization, and blood volume in dementia. Neurology 27:905–910
3. Grubb RL (1982) Cerebral hemodynamics and metabolism in subarachnoid hemorrhage. In: Hopkins LN, Long DM (eds) Clinical management of intracranial aneurysms. Raven, New York, pp 163–176
4. Senda M, Torizuka K, Yonekura Y, et al. (1985) Performance characteristics of Positologica III, a newly designed wholebody multi-slice positron computed tomograph. J Comput Assist Tomogr (submitted)

Local Blood Flow and Oxygen Metabolism in Glioma and Its Surrounding Brain

W. TAKI[1], H. HANDA, M. ISHIKAWA, A. KOBAYASHI, J. YAMASHITA, Y. YONEKAWA, S. TANADA, M. SENDA, Y. YONEKURA, K. TORIZUKA, T. FUJITA, H. FUKUYAMA, K. HARADA, N. FUJIMOTO, and M. KAMEYAMA

Key words: Brain tumor, cerebral circulation, metabolism, brain edema

Purpose

The purpose of this study was to examine the circulation and metabolism in various brain tumors and the brain tissues surrounding them by means of a PET scan.

Materials and Methods

Eight subjects with brain tumors and eight normal volunteers were included in the present study. The histological diagnoses were obtained either by stereotaxic biopsy or by craniotomy. There were two low-grade gliomas (astrocytoma grades I and II), three high-grade gliomas, and two meningiomas. One subject had a mixture of glioblastoma and radiation necrosis.

The continuous inhalation technique with $^{15}O\text{-}O^2$and $^{15}O\text{-}CO_2$ gases were used to obtain local cerebral blood flow (lCBF), local oxygen extraction fraction (lOEF), and local oxygen consumption ($lCMRO_2$). The $^{15}O\text{-}CO$ single breathing technique was used to obtain local cerebral blood volume (lCBV). To provide visual as well as quantitative records of lCBF and $lCMRO_2$, the transverse section measurements of tissue concentration were utilized together with the measurements of arterial concentration in the equations of Subramanyam et al. [4] to compute CBF, OEF, and $CMRO_2$ on a pixel-to-pixel basis. A correction was also made for the presence of intravascular oxygen-15 in the steady state technique, according to the equation of Lammertsma et al. [3]. The physiological parameters were measured with the normal values.

Results

For evaluation of the cerebral blood flow and oxygen metabolism in brain tumor, local physiological parameters were compared with the normal values. The analysis focused upon brain tumor, perifocal gray and perifocal white matter, and remaining

[1] Dept. of Neurosurgery, Kyoto University Medical School, 54 Kawaharacho Shogoin, Sakyo-ku, Kyoto 606, Japan

Table 1. Parameters in tumors vs normal control tissue

	CBF	OEF	$CMRO_2$	CBV
Normal gray matter	47.2+10.3	0.398+0.078	3.49+0.74	3.98+1.16
Low-grade glioma				
1	52.4+11.3	0.198+0.05	1.58+0.53	2.10+0.60
2	17.0+ 0.3	0.260+0.04	0.67+0.17	1.40+0.07
M	34.7 (74%)	0.229 (58%)	1.13 (32%)	1.75 (44%)
High-grade glioma				
1	28.8+ 4.3	0.224+0.050	1.10+0.35	3.6 +0.8
2	57.6+12.0	0.185+0.048	1.71+0.59	2.7 +0.59
3	18.9+ 1.7	0.255+0.066	0.76+0.20	5.8 +0.99
M	35.1 (74%)	0.221 (56%)	1.09 (31%)	4.03 (101%)
Meningioma				
1	35.2+ 2.5	0.205+0.089	1.14+0.48	15.1 +3.1
2	28.1+ 8.7	0.298+0.068	1.43+0.73	5.6 +1.5
M	31.7 (67%)	0.252 (63%)	1.29 (37%)	10.35 (260%)
Necrosis				
1	2.1+ 1.4 (4%)	0.016+0.072 (4%)	0.04+0.08 (1%)	0.60+0.70 (15%)

Numbers in parentheses give the values as percentages of the normal mean values in gray matter

gray and remaining white matter. Perifocal gray and white matter were defined as the gray and white matter in the vicinity of the tumor. Remaining gray and white matter were defined as matter contralateral to the tumor site or remote from the medially situated tumor, and with a normal appearance on X-ray CT. Table 1 shows the physiological parameters in the brain tumors. The mean values in each group were divided by the normal values for gray matter. Although the mean value for lCBF was about 70% of the normal value, in two tumors blood flow was increased. Also, the distribution of blood flow was heterogeneous in each tumor. Each tumor group showed a similar degree of suppression of oxygen utilization in brain tumor tissue, and each value was about 33% of that in normal gray matter. This suppression of oxidative metabolism was more pronounced than the reduction in blood flow, and the OEF declined by about 40% in each group. A clear difference among the groups was noted in lCBV, the meningioma group showing the highest value, followed in declining order by the high-grade glioma group and the low-grade glioma group.

The perifocal white matter was characterized by the suppressed oxygen consumption associated with decreased blood flow (Tables 2 and 3). Although oxygen utilization in the perifocal gray matter was suppressed, the blood flow decreased more markedly in the meningioma group. The lCBV in the high-grade glioma group

Table 2. Parameters in perifocal gray matter vs normal gray matter

	CBF	OEF	$CMRO_2$	CBV
Normal gray matter	47.2 + 10.3	0.398 + 0.078	3.49 + 0.74	3.98 + 1.16
Low-grade glioma				
1	51.9 + 11.1	0.324 + 0.045	2.60 + 0.47	4.30 + 1.89
2	28.8 + 6.4	0.403 + 0.048	1.91 + 0.52	2.60 + 1.17
M	40.4 (85%)	0.364 (91%)	1.81 (52%)	3.45 (87%)
High-grade glioma				
1	23.7 + 4.2	0.503 + 0.059	2.07 + 0.39	1.9 + 0.68
2	36.2 + 5.1	0.410 + 0.103	2.39 + 0.59	1.7 + 0.56
3	14.8 + 2.1	0.499 + 0.074	1.20 + 0.28	2.0 + 0.5
M	24.9 (53%)	0.471 (118%)	1.89 (54%)	1.87 (47%)
Meningioma				
1	44.5 + 4.8	0.608 + 0.072	4.55 + 0.43	4.7 + 1.25
2	22.8 + 4.4	0.423 + 0.054	1.60 + 0.45	4.1 + 1.44
M	33.7 (71%)	0.516 (130%)	3.08 (88%)	4.4 (111%)

Table 3. Parameters in perifocal matter vs normal white matter

	CBF	OEF	$CMRO_2$	CBV
Normal white matter	23.1 + 6.1	0.394 + 0.096	1.88 + 0.37	1.78 + 0.33
Low-grade glioma				
1	23.4 + 3.8	0.396 + 0.045	1.43 + 0.25	1.6 + 0.78
2	–	–	–	–
M	(101%)	(100%)	(76%)	(89%)
High-grade glioma				
1	–	–	–	–
2	16.1 + 2.1	0.438 + 0.060	1.09 + 0.12	0.7 + 0.14
3	15.9 + 3.2	0.459 + 0.095	1.18 + 0.31	2.1 + 1.09
M	16.0 (69%)	0.449 (114%)	1.14 (60%)	1.4 (79%)
Meningioma				
1	16.7 + 2.8	0.552 + 0.069	1.47 + 0.29	2.5 + 1.27
2	11.6 + 2.2	0.301 + 0.075	0.51 + 0.18	1.2 + 0.65
M	14.2 (61%)	0.427 (108%)	0.99 (53%)	1.9 (104%)

Table 4. Parameters in remaining gray matter vs normal gray matter

	CBF	OEF	$CMRO_2$	CBV
Normal gray matter	47.2+10.3	0.398+0.078	3.49+0.74	3.98+1.16
Low-grade glioma				
1	48.5+ 6.4	0.421+0.030	3.25+0.45	3.3 +0.7
2	34.2+ 5.2	0.450+0.050	2.64+0.40	4.2 +1.0
M	41.4 (88%)	0.436 (109%)	2.95 (84%)	3.8 (94%)
High-grade glioma				
1	28.6+ 3.1	0.518+0.051	2.61+0.36	3.4 +0.9
2	38.0+ 3.6	0.500+0.043	3.16+0.47	1.1 +0.4
3	30.6+ 3.6	0.512+0.046	2.66+0.40	2.76+0.63
M	32.4 (69%)	0.510 (128%)	2.81 (81%)	2.42 (61%)
Meningioma				
1	32.2+ 3.9	0.652+0.053	3.51+0.45	4.7 +2.0
2	36.8+ 5.2	0.48 +0.04	3.0 +0.6	3.4 +0.8
M	34.5 (73%)	0.566 (142%)	3.26 (93%)	4.1 (102%)

Table 5. Parameters in remaining white matter vs normal white matter

	CBF	OEF	$CMRO_2$	CBV
Normal white matter	23.1+6.1	0.394+0.096	1.88+0.37	1.78+0.33
Low-grade glioma				
1	28.8+2.1	0.409+0.035	1.82+0.33	1.80+0.60
2	20.0+3.4	0.45 +0.05	1.50+0.28	1.7 +1.0
M	24.4 (106%)	0.430 (109%)	1.66 (88%)	1.75 (98%)
High-grade glioma				
1	17.7+2.9	0.469+0.087	1.42+0.35	1.8 +0.38
2	22.4+3.0	0.491+0.051	1.78+0.31	0.43+0.21
3	18.3+2.7	0.436+0.074	1.34+0.36	1.63+0.46
M	19.5 (84%)	0.465 (118%)	1.51 (80%)	1.29 (72%)
Meningioma				
1	18.1+1.3	0.657+0.057	1.91+0.30	2.2 +0.65
2	21.9+3.4	0.39 +0.04	1.4 +0.3	1.8 +0.4
M	20.0 (87%)	0.523 (133%)	1.66 (88%)	2.0 (112%)

was the smallest in all three groups. In the remaining brain tissue contralateral to the brain tumor or remote from a medially situated brain tumor, oxygen utilization was slightly decreased in both the gray and the white matter (Tables 4 and 5). In each tumor group the remote brain tissue had decreased blood flow. The extent of this decrease differed among groups, and in the high-grade glioma and meningioma groups the blood flow decreased by a greater amount than the oxygen utilization.

Discussion

Oxygen utilization of the brain tumors was low in all tumor groups and the extent of the suppression was equivalent in all three groups. The suppression of oxygen consumption did not correlate with the decrease in blood flow. This might correlate with anaerobic breakdown of glucose in brain tumors [1, 2]. In our limited series there was no correlation between oxidative metabolism and the histological grade of gliomas. The clear difference between low-grade and high-grade glioma was an increase in lCBV in the high-grade glioma group, which was considered to correlate either with higher vascularity observed in the angiogram or with positive contrast enhancement in X-ray CT. The CBV increase was not associated with a blood flow increase in all cases. The perifocal brain tissue showed a decrease of about 50% in oxygen utilization associated with decreased blood flow. The gray and the white matter remote from the tumor showed the decrease in oxygen metabolism of the perifocal brain tissue. This suppression in the remote brain may be consistent with the suppressed glucose metabolism in remote brain in the experiment of Hossmann et al. [1]. This suppression of glucose metabolism was slight, but the decrease in the blood flow was greater in the meningioma and the high-grade glioma groups. Although the decrease was partly related to functional suppression of a remote effect, the elevated OEF in the meningioma and the high-grade glioma groups may suggest that this suppression is partly due to the increased intracranial pressure. Since the size of our series was limited, our conclusions are tentative and further studies are required.

Summary

Eight subjects with brain tumors and eight normal volunteers were included in the present study. There were two low-grade gliomas, three high-grade gliomas and two meningiomas. One subject had a mixture of glioblastoma and radiation necrosis. ^{15}O-labeled gases were used to obtain lCBF, lOEF, $lCMRO_2$, and lCBV. The oxygen utilization of the brain tumors was low in all tumor groups, and the extent of the suppression was equivalent among three groups. There was no correlation between oxidative metabolism and histological grade of gliomas. The clear difference between low-grade and high-grade glioma was that there was an increase of lCBV in the latter group. This increase in lCBV was not associated with increased blood flow in all cases. The perifocal brain tissue showed about a decrease of 50% in oxygen utilization, associated with decreased blood flow. The gray and the white matter remote from the tumor showed a decrease in oxygen metabolism. Although this suppression was small, the decrease in blood flow was greater in the meningioma group and in the high-grade glioma group. Although the decrease was related to functional suppression of remote effects in some cases, elevated OEF in the meningioma and high-grade glioma groups may suggest this suppression is due partly to increased intracranial pressure.

References

1. Hossmann KA, Niebuhr I, Tamura M (1982) Local cerebral blood flow and glucose consumption of rats with experimental gliomas. J Cereb Blood Flow Metab 2:25–32
2. Warburg O (1930) Metabolism of tumors. Constable, London
3. Lammertsma AA, Jones T (1984) Correction for the presence of intravascular oxygen-15 in the steady-state technique for measuring regional oxygen extraction ratio in the brain: I. Description of the method. J Cereb Blood Flow Metab 3:416–424
4. Subramanyan R, Albert NM, Hoop B Jr, Brownell GL, Tareras JM (1978) A model for regional cerebral oxygen distribution during continuous inhalation of $^{15}O_2$, $C^{15}O$ and $C^{15}O_2$. J Nucl Med 19:48–53

Changes in Local Cerebral Blood Flow and Oxygen Metabolism with Glycerol Infusion in Various Pathologic States

A. KOBAYASHI[1], H. HANDA, M. ISHIKAWA, W. TAKI, Y. YONEKAWA, S. TANADA, Y. YONEKURA, M. SENDA, T. FUJITA, K. TORIZUKA, H. FUKUYAMA, N. FUJIMOTO, K. HARADA, and M. KAMEYAMA

Key words: CBF, $CMRO_2$, glycerol loading

Introduction

Local cerebral blood flow (CBF) and oxygen metabolism were studied before and after drip infusion of glycerol in seven patients and two normal volunteers.

Materials and Method

The patients were 35–63 years old (two men and five women): two had meningiomas, three gliomas, one cerebellar infarction, and one putaminal hemorrhage. Normal volunteers were men aged 33 and 35 years. The physiological parameters monitored were $PaCO_2$, PaO_2, and blood pressure. Patients showing large differences in each parameter between before and after glycerol loading were excluded.

CBF, oxygen extraction fraction (OEF), cerebral metabolic rate for oxygen ($CMRO_2$), and cerebral blood volume (CBV) were measured with continuous inhalation of ^{15}O-labeled O_2 gas and CO_2 gas using positron emission CT (Positrosica III). $CMRO_2$ and OEF were corrected for CBV, according to the method of Lammertsma. After the first control by measurements of CBF, OEF, $CMRO_2$, and CBV, 300 ml 10 w/v% glycerol was given by IV infusion over 20 min. At 30 min after the infusion a second series of measurements was taken. The patients were resting with their eyes closed.

Each absolute value for CBF, OEF, and $CMRO_2$ was calculated with the region of interest (ROI) set in the lesion, perifocal area, the remaining gray matter, and the remaining white matter. The number of pixels in each ROI was about 50–100.

Results

In the remaining gray matter, CBF increased in most of the patients. Moreover, $CMRO_2$ increased in five patients with meningioma, glioma, cerebellar infarction, or

[1] Department of Neurosurgery, Kyoto University Medical School, 54 Kawaharucho Shogoin, Sakyo-ku, Kyoto 606, Japan

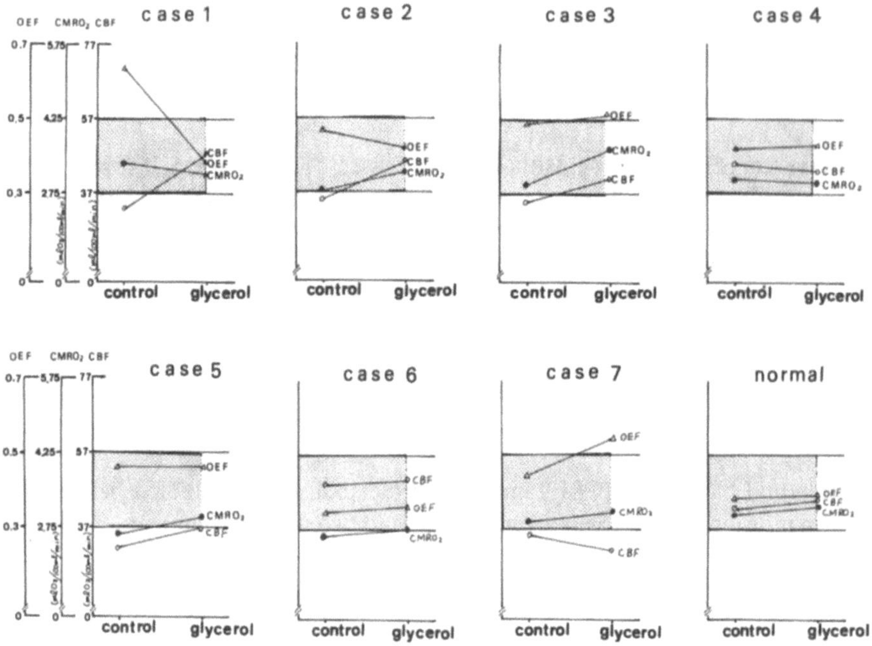

Fig. 1. Changes in each parameter in the remaining gray matter. Of the patients with brain tumors (cases 1–5), CBF increased in cases 1, 2, 3, and 5. In cases 2, 3, and 5 $CMRO_2$ also increased. In the patients with cerebellar infarction and putaminal hemorrhage, $CMRO_2$ tended to increase (cases 6 and 7). In normal volunteers, CBF increase paralleled that in $CMRO_2$. *Spotted areas* show normal range (mean ± SD)

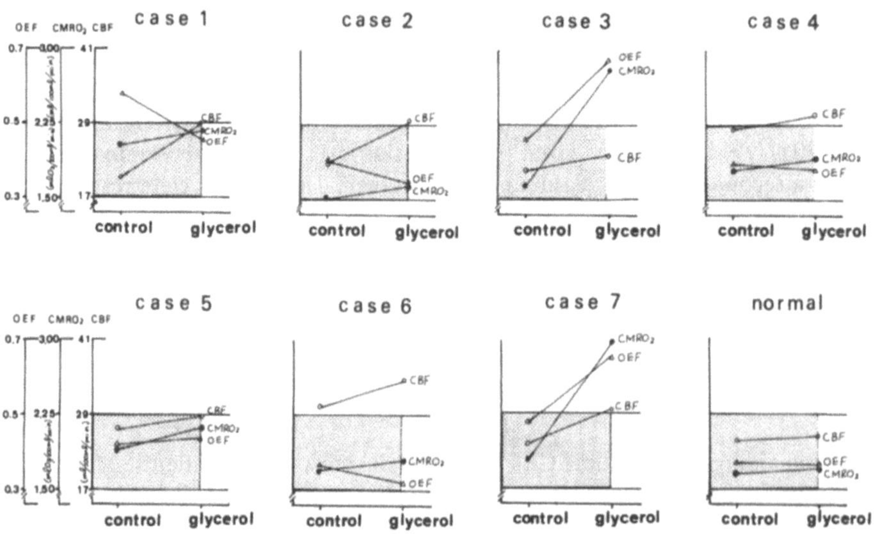

Fig. 2. Changes in each parameter in the remaining white matter. In all cases, CBF and $CMRO_2$ increased markedly. In cases 3, 5 (glioma cases), and 7 (putaminal hemorrhage), the changes in $CMRO_2$ were greater than those in CBF. In normal volunteers, CBF increase paralleled that of $CMRO_2$. *Spotted areas* show normal range (mean ± SD)

putaminal hemorrhage. In normal volunteers the CBF increase parallelled that in $CMRO_2$ (Fig. 1).

In the remaining white matter, CBF and $CMRO_2$ increased more markedly than in the remaining gray matter in all cases. In some cases (two of glioma and one of putaminal hemorrhage), the changes in $CMRO_2$ were greater than those in CBF. In normal volunteers the CBF increase paralleled that in $CMRO_2$ (Fig. 2).

In the lesions, the changes in CBF and $CMRO_2$ were varied. No definite tendency was recognized in the changes.

In the perifocal region, however, CBF and $CMRO_2$ increased after the infusion of glycerol.

Discussion

Various findings have been reported as effects of glycerol [2–4]. It was found that the intracerebral water content was decreased and microcirculation was improved after infusion of glycerol. In animal experiments, some glycerol was reported to be taken up in the brain and metabolized [1, 6].

In this study, the influence of glycerol on the lesions had no fixed tendency. In the remaining region, CBF and $CMRO_2$ tended to increase. The effect of glycerol was considered to be greater in the remaining white matter than in the remaining gray matter. It is interesting to note that the response to glycerol was marked in the white matter in which no brain edema was seen on X-ray CT.

In some of our cases, the improvement in $CMRO_2$ was greater than that in CBF. Such data may indicate that glycerol was taken up in the brain and metabolized.

Thus the efficacy of glycerol was considered to result from increases not only in CBF but also in $CMRO_2$ in the remaining region, especially in the remaining white matter.

Summary

Local cerebral blood flow (CBF), oxygen extraction fraction (OEF), and cerebral metabolic rate for oxygen ($CMRO_2$) were studied before and after drip infusion of glycerol in five patients with brain tumors, one with cerebellar infarction, one with putaminal hemorrhage, and two normal volunteers.

In each lesion, the changes in CBF and $CMRO_2$ varied. No general tendency was recognized in the changes.

In the perifocal region, CBF and $CMRO_2$ increased after drip infusion of glycerol.

In the remaining gray matter CBF increased in most of the patients, but in one with glioma and one with putamine hemorrhage, CBF decreased slightly. $CMRO_2$ increased in five patients with meningioma, gliomas [2], cerebellar infarction, or putaminal hemorrhage. In normal volunteers, the CBF increase paralleled that in $CMRO_2$.

In the remaining white matter, CBF and $CMRO_2$ increased markedly in all cases. In some cases, the changes in $CMRO_2$ were greater than those in CBF. In normal volunteers the CBF increase paralleled that of $CMRO_2$.

Thus, the efficacy of glycerol was considered to result from increases not only in CBF but also in $CMRO_2$ in the remaining site, especially in the remaining white matter.

References

1. Ackermann RH, Bassler K, Wagner K (1974) The relation between the blood-level of a substrate and enzyme kinetics studied with glycerol in rat. Hoppe-Seyler's Z Physiol Chem 355:576
2. Freund G (1968) The metabolic effects of glycerol administered to diabetic patients. Arch Intern Med 121:123–129
3. Meyer JS, Fukuuchi Y, Shimazu K, Ohuchi T, Ericssen AD (1972) The effect of intravenous infusion of glycerol on hemispheric blood flow and metabolism in patients with acute cerebral infarction. Stroke 13:168–180
4. Sacks W (1976) Human brain metabolism in vivo. In: Himwich HE (ed) Brain metabolism and cerebral disorders. Spectrum, New York, pp 89–127
5. Senda M, Torizuka K, Yonekura Y, et al. (1985) Performance characteristic of Positrosica III, a newly designed whole body multi-slice positron computed tomograph. J Comput Assist Tomogr (in press)
6. Sloviter HA, Suhara K (1967) A brain infusion method for demonstrating utilization of glycerol by rabbit brain in vivo. J Appl Physiol 23:792–797
7. Tanada S, Yonekura Y, Senda M, et al. (1984) The measurement of sequential changes in cerebral blood flow and oxygen metabolism by positron computed tomography with continuous inhalation of oxygen-15 labelled gases. J Nucl Med 25(5):P50

Protective Effects of Glycerol and Perfluorochemical in Experimental Cerebral Ischemia Demonstrated by In Vivo ^{31}P-NMR *

S. NARUSE [1], Y. HORIKAWA, C. TANAKA, K. HIRAKAWA, H. NISHIKAWA, and H. WATARI

Key words: In vivo ^{31}P-NMR, cerebral ischemia, EEG, glycerol, perfluorochemical

Introduction

The treatment of cerebral ischemia has been a matter of concern for some years [12]. Although many drugs have been suggested, there are none that have proved to be definitely superior. Recently, perfluorochemicals (PFCs) with or without the addition of glycerol have been used experimentally as one of the most effective groups of drugs for this condition [2, 10]. However, their mechanism of action is not yet clearly understood. Further studies based on new techniques are necessary to solve this problem.

We reported previously that the energy metabolism in the living rat brain could be observed during the course of cerebral ischemia by means of in vivo ^{31}P-NMR spectrum measurement [7, 8]. Our results clearly demonstrated that the levels of high-energy phosphorus compounds phosphocreatine (PCr) and ATP declined immediately after the induction of ischemia, with rapid flattening of EEG activities, and returned to normal 30 min after the restoration of circulation to the ischemic brain despite delayed recovery of the EEG. We also recognized that in vivo ^{31}P-NMR spectrum measurement was useful for the evaluation of therapeutic effects on various diseases. Therefore, we applied this method for the examination of the efficacy of PFC and glycerol on cerebral ischemia.

Materials and Methods

Forty-six Wistar rats weighing about 200 g each were used for the experiment. Cerebral ischemia was induced in the rats by a four-vessel occlusion method [11] during anesthesia attained by IP injection of sodium pentobarbital at a dose of 35 mg/kg. After various periods of ischemia ranging from 30 to 240 min, circulation was restored to the ischemic brain by untying the ligated common carotid arteries bilater-

---

* The work described in this paper was supported in part by Grants-in-Aid for Scientific Research (58440059, 58570597, and 59570623) from the Ministry of Education, Science and Culture, Japan.

[1] Department of Neurosurgery, Kyoto Prefectural University of Medicine, Kawaramachi-Hirokoji, Kamigyo-Ku, Kyoto 602, Japan.

ally. Rats were divided into two main groups, untreated and treated ones, numbering 28 and 36, respectively. The treated group was subdivided into three groups according to the drugs administered: glycerol alone, PFC alone, and a combination of PFC and glycerol. Eleven rats received IV injections of 10% glycerol at a dose of 1 g/kg 30 min before recirculation. Sixteen rats received IV injections of 20% Fluosol DA (PFC) at a dose of 20 ml/kg before the induction of ischemia. Six rats treated with PFC had injections of 10% glycerol in the same manner as mentioned above in addition. Half the rats in each group were maintained by spontaneous respiration with room air and the other half with a gas mixture of 95% oxygen and 5% carbon dioxide in a specially devised plastic chamber. In all rats, in vivo ^{31}P-NMR spectra were measured sequentially during the course of preischemic, ischemic, and recirculated periods by using a TMR-32 spectrometer (Oxford Research Systems, UK; 1.8 Tesla). Scalp EEGs were monitored simultaneously during the ^{31}P-NMR measurements. These methods have been reported in detail in previous papers [7, 8]. Recovery rates of the ^{31}P-NMR spectrum after the recirculation were compared among each subgroup.

Results

All the rats showed the same sequential changes in the ^{31}P-NMR spectrum, irrespective of respiration method and experimental group. There were several peaks in the spectrum of the normal and preischemic brain: β-ATP, α-ATP and α-ADP with NAD^+/NADH, γ-ATP and β-ADP, phosphocreatine (PCr), phosphodiesters, inorganic phosphate (Pi), and phosphomonoesters (PME) (Fig. 1). Within a few minutes after the induction of ischemia, PCr and ATP peaks decreased and a Pi peak increased remarkably. These changes reached their maximum within 15 min and remained constant thereafter during the ischemic periods. Tissue pH calculated from the chemical shift of the Pi peak decreased to 6.25 from the normal value of 7.27 during the ischemic period. In the untreated 30-min ischemia group all 16 rats showed rapid recovery of PCr and ATP and decrease of Pi after the circulation was restored. The ^{31}P-NMR spectrum pattern became identical with that seen in the preischemic state 30 min after recirculation, while recovery of the EEG pattern was delayed until 12 h after recirculation. In the untreated 60-min ischemia group, 3 of 6 rats showed recovery of the ^{31}P-NMR spectrum about 1 h after recirculation. In the untreated 120-min ischemia group none of the rats showed recovery of the ^{31}P-NMR spectrum after the recirculation (Fig. 2), and they died within 24 h.

In the treated group with glycerol alone, all 4 rats in the 30-min ischemia and 5 of 7 rats in the 60-min ischemia showed rapid recovery of the ^{31}P-NMR spectrum after the recirculation. However, none of the 4 rats exposed to 120-min ischemia showed recovery of the spectrum.

In the group treated with PFC alone, all 4 rats in 60-min ischemia showed rapid recovery of the ^{31}P-NMR spectrum and delayed recovery of the EEG. Even in the 120-min ischemia group treated with PFC, all 8 rats showed recovery of the ^{31}P-NMR spectrum about 1 h after recirculation (Fig. 3). In this last group, however, the EEG did not recover at all, and the rats became inactive and finally died 2 or 3

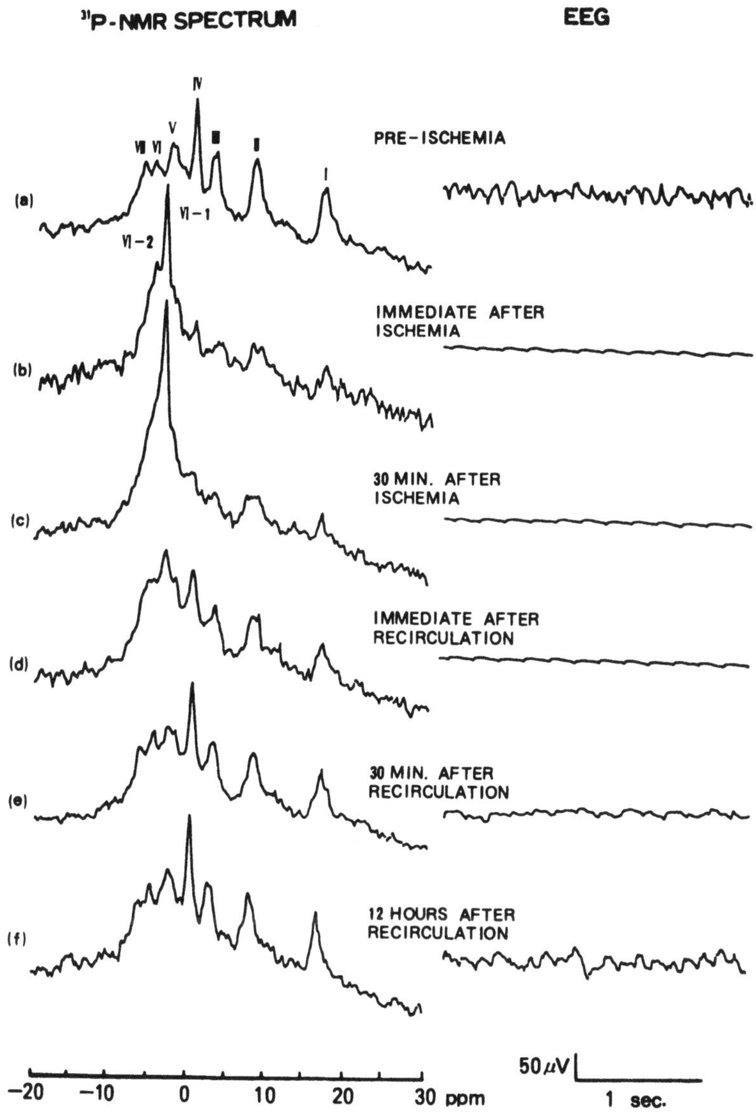

Fig. 1a–f. Sequential changes in ^{31}P-NMR spectra and EEGs during experimental cerebral ischemia of untreated rat brain [9]. **a** ^{31}P-NMR spectrum and EEG in the preischemic stage. The assignments of the ^{31}P-NMR spectrum are: *I*, β-ATP; *II*, α-ATP and α-ADP with NAD^+/NADH; *III*, γ-ATP and β-ADP; *IV*, phosphocreatine (PCr); , *V* phosphodiesters; *VI*, inorganic phosphate (Pi); *VII*, phosphomonoesters (PME). **b** Immediately after the induction of ischemia: ATP and PCr levels have declined and the Pi level increased markedly in the NMR spectrum, and the EEG is flattened. **c** Status 30 min after ischemia. **d** Immediately after recirculation: ATP and PCr have begun to recover and Pi has decreased rapidly in the NMR spectrum, but the EEG has a flat pattern. **e** By 30 min after recirculation the NMR spectrum has recovered but the EEG has not. **f** By 12 h after recirculation both the NMR spectrum and the EEG have recovered. (Reproduced from Naruse, S., et al., *Neurological Research,* 1984, 6, 169–175, by permission of the publishers, Butterworth & Co. Ltd.)

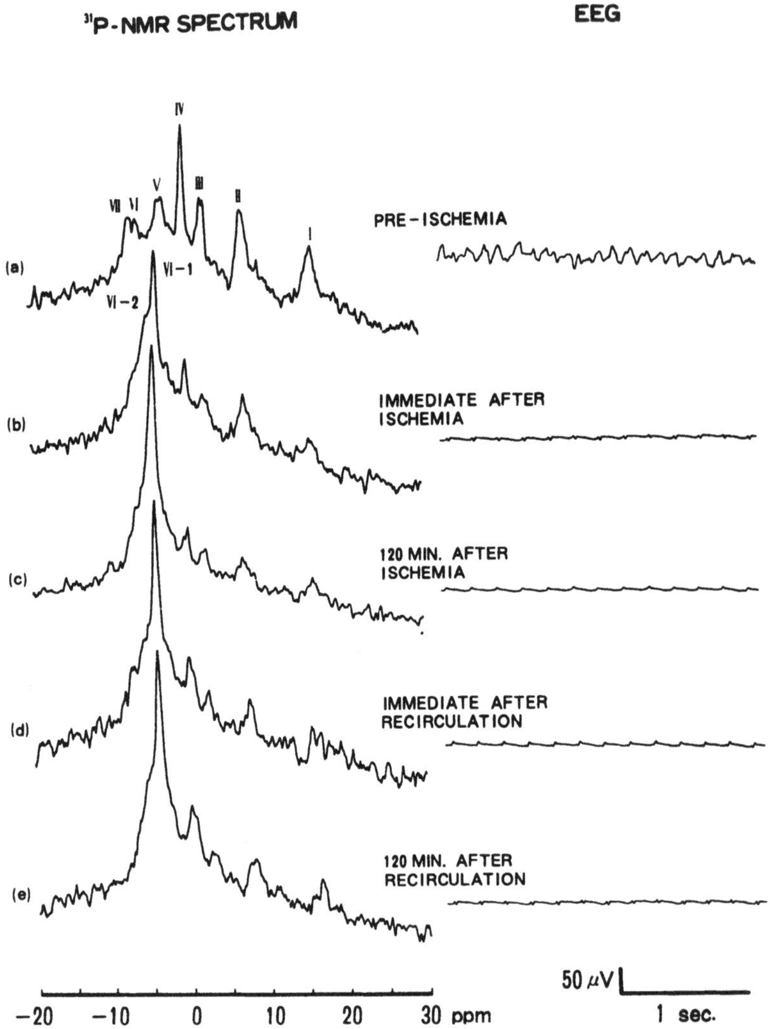

Fig. 2a–e. Sequential changes of ^{31}P-NMR spectra and EEGs in the untreated rat brain for a 120-min duration of ischemia [9]. **a** Preischemic stage; **b** immediately after the induction of ischemia; **c** 2 h after ischemia; **d** immediately after recirculation; **e** 2 h after recirculation; neither the NMR spectrum nor the EEG has recovered. (Reproduced from Naruse, S., et al., *Neurological Research,* 1984, 6, 169–175; by permission of the publishers, Butterworth & Co. Ltd.)

days later. When the ischemic period was prolonged to 240 min recovery of the spectrum was not observed in any of the 4 rats treated with PFC alone.

In the group treated with the combination of PFC and glycerol, in 4 of the 6 rats there was a temporary recovery of the ^{31}P-NMR spectrum for several hours even after 240-min ischemia (Fig. 4). The EEG, however, did not recover at all, and all rats died around 24 h after recirculation. The number of cases in which recovery was observed in the NMR spectrum after recirculation is summarized in Table 1.

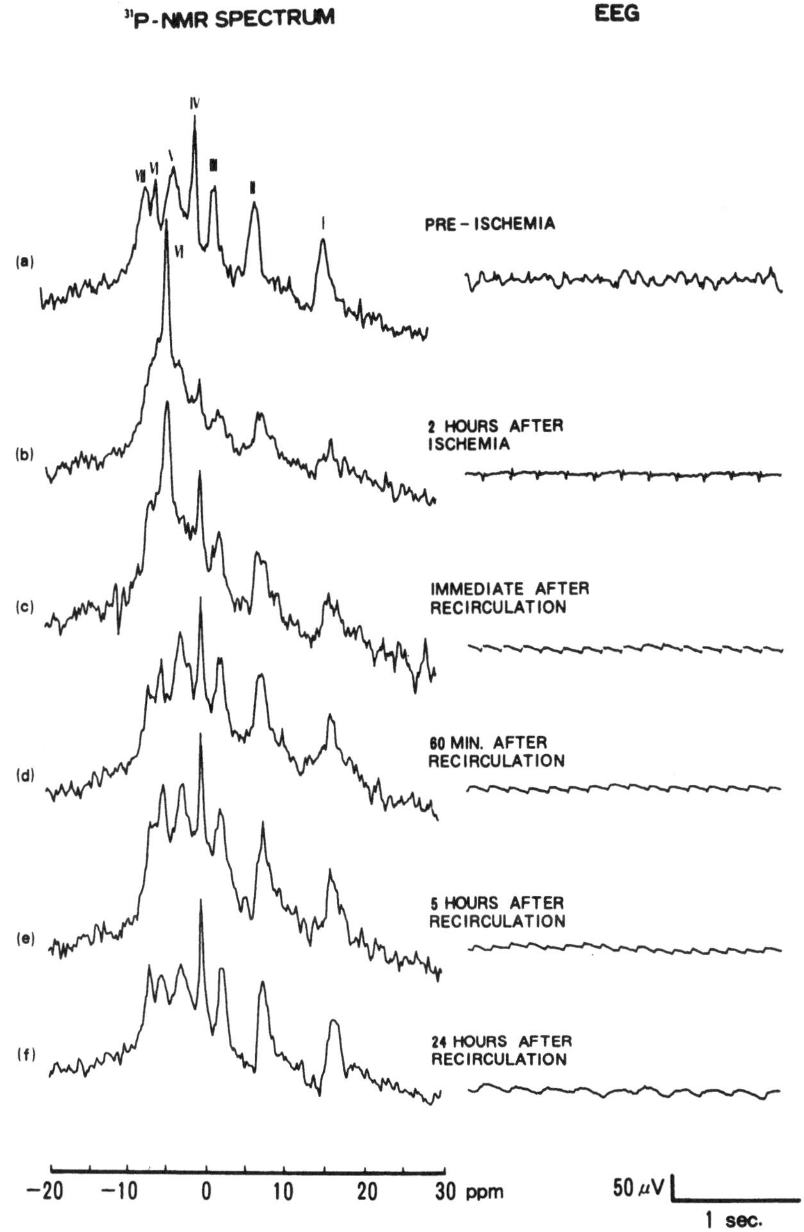

Fig. 3a–f. Sequential changes of ^{31}P-NMR spectra and EEGs in experimental cerebral ischemia of rat brain treated with 20% Fluosol DA [9]. **a** Preischemic stage. **b** At 2 h after the induction of ischemia, levels of ATP and PCr have declined and that of Pi increased markedly. **c** Immediately after recirculation: ATP and PCr have begun to recover and Pi has declined in the NMR spectrum, but the EEG does not yet show any signs of recovery. **d** At 60 min after recirculation the NMR spectrum pattern has recovered but the EEG still shows no signs of recovery. **e** By 5 h after recirculation the NMR spectrum has completely recovered but the EEG still has a flat pattern. **f** At 24 h after recirculation the NMR spectrum has a normal pattern, but the EEG has not recovered and shows very low activity. (Reproduced from Naruse, S., et al., *Neurological Research,* 1984, 6, 169–175, by permission of the publisher, Butterworth & Co. Ltd.)

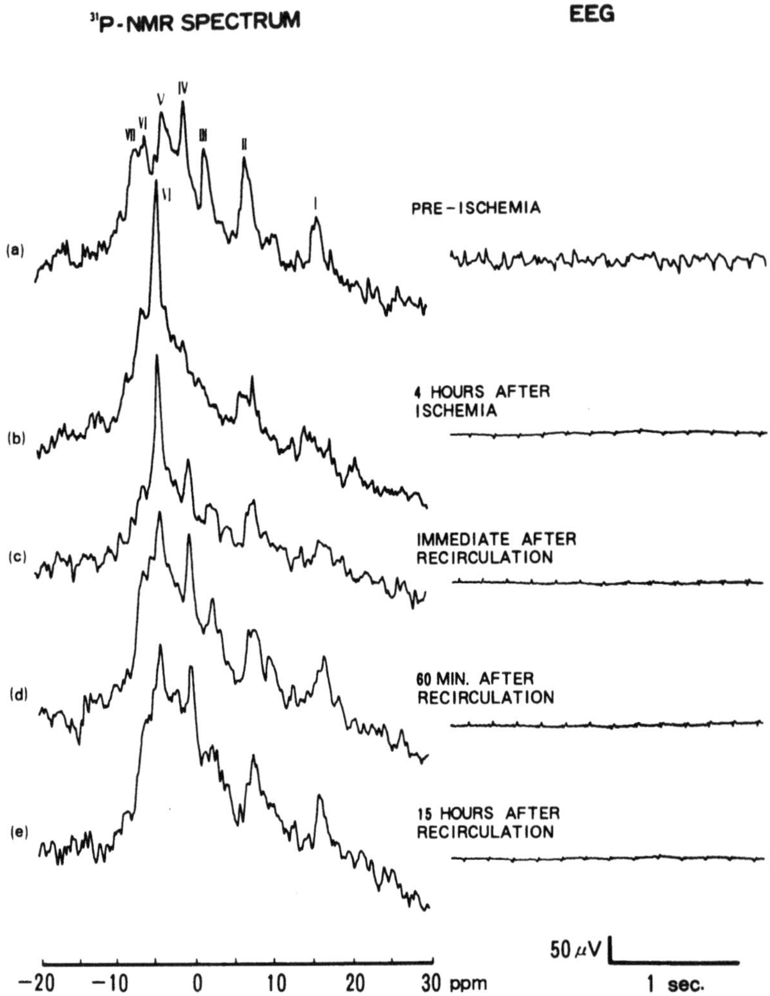

Fig. 4a–e. Sequential changes in the ^{31}P-NMR spectra and EEGs in the experimental cerebral ischemia of rat brain treated with 20% Fluosol DA and glycerol [9]. **a** Preischemic stage. **b** At 4 h after the induction of ischemia the NMR spectrum has a Pi-dominant pattern and the EEG, a flat pattern. **c** Immediately after recirculation ATP and PCr have begun to recover in the NMR spectrum despite the long duration of ischemia. The EEG does not show any signs of recovery. **d** At 60 min after recirculation ATP and PCr are recovering gradually but there is still a large Pi peak in the NMR spectrum. The EEG has not recovered. **e** At 15 h after recirculation the degree of recovery of the NMR spectrum has not changed since 60 min after recirculation. The EEG has a flat pattern. (Reproduced from Naruse, S., et al., *Neurological Research,* 1984, 6, 169–175, by permission of the publisher, Butterworth & Co. Ltd.)

Discussion

Our previous report indicated that changes of energy metabolism in the experimental cerebral ischemia could be examined sequentially by in vivo ^{31}P-NMR spectrum measurement [7, 8]. It was also demonstrated that energy metabolism in the ischemic brain could be reversed when circulation was restored within a certain period.

Table 1. Cases with recovery of ^{31}P-NMR spectrum after recirculation

Duration of ischemia	Untreated	Treated with glycerol	Treated with PFC	Treated with PFC and glycerol
30 min	15 (15)	4 (4)	–	–
60 min	3 (6)	5 (7)	4 (4)	–
120 min	0 (6)	0 (4)	8 (8)	–
240 min	–	–	0 (4)	4 (6)

PFC, fluosol DA 20 ml/kg IV, 30 min before the induction of ischemia; glycerol: 1 g/kg IV, 30 min before recirculation; ( ) no. of cases examined

The critical period for reversibility of the energy metabolism was consistent, about 30–60 min, in the experimental model.

In this experiment, we evaluated the effects of PCF and glycerol on the cerebral ischemia, observing the prolongation of the critical period for reversibility of the energy metabolism. A dramatic effect was seen in the group treated with PFC. Even if the ischemic period was prolonged to 120 min recovery of the ^{31}P-NMR spectrum was seen after recirculation in all rats treated with PFC alone. This was good evidence for a strong protective effect of PFC on ischemic brains. This effect of PFC might be attributable to its high oxygen-carrying capacity, which is the most characteristic property of this drug. Our data, however, suggested that the protective effects of this drug were not so simple. A high oxygen tension is usually necessary for PFC to work as an effective oxygen carrier [4]. In this experiment with PFC administration, the critical period for reversibility of the energy metabolism could be prolonged to the same degree regardless of whether room air or high-oxygen gas was used for respiration. An additional experiment with the same conditions as those in which the in vivo ^{31}P-NMR measurements were carried out demonstrated that blood oxygen tension actually rose to about 300 mmHg in the rats respirated with a gas mixture of 95% O_2 and 5% CO_2. It was threefold that of the group respirated with room air. Therefore, the protective effect of this drug on the cerebral ischemia cannot be completely explained by the high oxygen-carrying capacity; other causes must be suspected. Possible explanations are [3, 10]: (a) Decreased blood viscosity; (b) prevention of narrowing of the arterior and capillary lumen; (c) increase in cerebral blood flow; (d) small-particle oxygen and carbon dioxide carriers which can reach low-perfusion areas. With this combination of factors, a capacity for recovery can be retained for an ischemic region even during long periods of ischemia.

In comparison with the dramatic effect of PCF, glycerol had a less pronounced effect on the energy metabolism in the cerebral ischemia. That is, there were no statistically significant effects on the recovery of energy metabolism in either the 60-min or the 120-min ischemia group treated with glycerol alone. However, the treatment was effective in more cases in the 60-min ischemia group. It might be difficult to detect the real effectiveness by ^{31}P-NMR spectrum measurement alone, because the effect of glycerol was referred to the prevention of ischemic brain edema [1]. As our previous reports concerning brain edema indicated [5, 6], measurement of

^{1}H-NMR relaxation time would be a suitable way of determining the real effectiveness.

Furthermore, it is surprising that energy metabolism recovered even after 240-min ischemia in four of six cases treated with both PFC and glycerol. Recovery of energy metabolism after such a long duration of ischemia was not observed in the groups treated with either PFC or glycerol alone. Therefore, PFC and glycerol appear to have a synergistic effect. This finding has previously been suggested by results obtained with other methods [2, 10].

It was clearly proved that PFC had remarkable protective effects on the ischemic brain. Moreover, a curative effect of this drug on the ischemic brain was also suggested by our additional experiment in which the same results were obtained; that is, recovery of the ^{31}P-NMR spectrum was observed even after 120-min ischemia when PFC was administered within 60 min after the induction of ischemia.

Despite the drastic recovery of the energy metabolism after a long ischemic period with PFC and glycerol, the EEG did not return to normal. Energy metabolism indicates direct cell activity, while the EEG represents a higher function, that is, integration of the electrical activities of cells. Thus, it seems that dissociation may take place in the recovery process between the direct activities of cells and the higher function. This is also supported by the delayed recovery of the EEG in the untreated rats with 30-min duration of ischemia [7].

In vivo ^{31}P-NMR measurement provides new knowledge not only about the analysis of various diseases but also about the effects of drugs. The NMR devices available now have some limitations. One is that the target area is still too large to detect small topographical changes. Another is that quantitative analysis for each phosphorus compound has so far been impossible owing to poor resolution of the spectrum and/or to the vagueness of the areas detected. These problems will hopefully be solved in the future with further development of new technology. Even with these faults, this method is still very valuable both experimentally and clinically.

Summary

Effects of glycerol and perfluorochemical (PFC) on energy metabolism in cerebral ischemia were examined by sequential measurements of the in vivo ^{31}P-NMR spectrum with a TMR-32 spectrometer (Oxford Research Systems, UK). Experimental cerebral ischemia was induced in 64 Wistar rats by a four-vessel occlusion method. Several peaks were identified in the ^{31}P-NMR spectrum of the preischemic brain; β-ATP, α-ATP, γ-ATP, phosphocreatine (PCr), phosphodiesters, inorganic phosphate (Pi), and phosphomonoesters. The PCr and ATP peaks declined and the Pi peak rose immediately after the induction of ischemia. The chemical shift of the Pi peak decreased, showing acidosis of the brain tissue. When circulation was restored following 30-min ischemia, recovery of the ^{31}P-NMR spectrum occurred within 30 min in all 16 untreated rats. In half the 6 rats in the untreated group the spectrum recovered after 60-min ischemia. The spectrum did not recover after 120-min ischemia in any of the 6 rats in the untreated group. When 10% glycerol was administered at a dose of 1 g/kg 30 min before recirculation, in 5 of 7 rats the spectrum recovered after 60-min ischemia. When 20% Fluosol DA was administered at a dose of

20 ml/kg before the induction of ischemia, there was recovery of the spectrum after 120-min ischemia in all 8 rats. Moreover, 4 of 6 rats treated with both PFC and glycerol had a temporary recovery even after 240-min ischemia. The protective effects of glycerol and PFC on cerebral ischemia were proved by the in vivo ^{31}P-NMR spectrum measurements.

References

1. Meyer JS, Fukuuchi Y, Shimazu K, Ohuchi T, Ericsson AD (1972) Effect of intravenous infusion of glycerol on hemispheric blood flow and metabolism in patients with acute cerebral infarction. Stroke 3:168–180
2. Mizoi K, Yoshitomo T, Suzuki J (1981) Experimental study of new cerebral protective substances – Functional recovery of severe, incomplete ischemic brain lesions pretreated with mannitol and fluorocarbon emulsion. Acta Neurochir 56:157–166
3. Nagasawa S, Handa H, Yonekawa Y, Oda Y, Tsuda Y, Yokoyama K (1983) Effects of a transfusion with a blood substitute (Fluosol-DA, 20%). II: Human cerebral blood flow. Neurol Res 5:19–30
4. Naito R, Yokoyama K (1978) Physical and chemical properties of Fluosol-DA after mixing with annex solution. In: Naito R, Yokoyama K (eds) Perfluorochemical blood substitutes. Green Cross Corporation, Osaka, pp 73–79
5. Naruse S, Horikawa Y, Tanaka C, Hirakawa K, Nishikawa H, Yoshizaki K (1982) Proton nuclear magnetic resonance studies on brain edema. J Neurosurg 56:747–752
6. Naruse S, Horikawa Y, Tanaka C, Hirakawa K, Nishikawa H (1982) Nuclear magnetic resonance studies of effects of glycerol on brain edema. Brain Nerve (Tokyo) 34:805–809
7. Naruse S, Horikawa Y, Tanaka C, Hirakawa K, Nishikawa H, Watari H (1984) In vivo measurement of energy metabolism and the concomitant monitoring of electroencephalogram in experimental cerebral ischemia. Brain Res 296:370–372
8. Naruse S, Takada S, Koizuka I, Watari H (1983) In vivo ^{31}P-NMR studies on experimental cerebral infarction. Jpn J Physiol 33:19–28
9. Naruse S, Horikawa Y, Tanaka C, Hirakawa K, Nishikawa H, Watari H (1984) Measurements of in vivo energy metabolism in experimental cerebral ischemia using ^{31}P-NMR for the evaluation of protective effects of perfluorochemicals and glycerol. Neurol Res 6:169–175
10. Peerless SJ, Ishikawa R, Hunter IG, Peerless MJ (1981) Protective effect of Fluosol-DA in acute cerebral ischemia. Stroke 12:558–563
11. Pulsinelli WA, Brierly JB (1978) A new model of bilateral hemispheric ischemia in the unanesthetized rat. Stroke 10:267–272
12. Selman WR, Spetzler RF (1980) Therapeutics for focal cerebral ischemia. Neurosurgery 6:446–452

The Continuing Search for Mechanisms Underlying Functional Disturbances in Traumatized Brain *

H. M. PAPPIUS [1]

Key words: Brain injury, functional deficits, LCGU, serotonin, Ca modulator drugs

Introduction

At the 5th International Symposium on Brain Edema held in Groningen in 1982, I presented a working hypothesis developed on the basis of our earlier work [5–9], according to which prostaglandins and/or serotonin and/or catecholamines released in the injured brain, probably in an interrelated fashion, induced changes in the distribution of calcium, which in turn caused widespread functional depression [10]. The studies reported in this paper represent three aspects of a continuing search by myself and my colleagues for mechanisms which underlie functional disturbances in traumatized brain.

Behavioral Studies in Rats with Freezing Lesions

In our studies the functional state of the rat brain was assessed by metabolic mapping using the ^{14}C-deoxyglucose technique [15], and we have interpreted the hemispheric depression in cortical local cerebral glucose utilization (lCGU) in focally lesioned brain as a manifestation of widespread cerebral dysfunction [5]. The close relationship between physiological function and energy metabolism in the normal central nervous system is now widely accepted [14]. Whether this holds in pathologic conditions is not as clear. The assumption that the depression in lCGU resulting from trauma reflects functional disturbances is crucial to our concept of using metabolic mapping to assess the functional state of the brain in studies on the neurochemical sequelae of brain damage and their role in the associated cerebral dysfunction. Accordingly, in an attempt to validate this assumption, in collaboration with L. Holmes and L. Colle (The Center for Research in Behavioral Neurobiology, Department of Psychology, Concordia University, Montreal), behavioral studies were carried out on rats with the standard freezing lesion [3].

---

* The work described in this paper was supported in part by grant MT-3021 from the Medical Research Council of Canada, and by the Canadian Donner Foundation.
[1] The Goad Unit of The Donner Laboratory of Experimental Neurochemistry, Montreal Neurological Institute and Hospital and the Department of Neurology and Neurosurgery, McGill University, Montreal, Quebec, Canada

Methods

Freezing lesions standardized to produce superficial focal cortical injury in the rat were made as described previously [5]. For behavioral testing, both sham-operated and lesioned rats were studied at least once, but usually twice, prior to craniotomy and on each of the 3 days after. The rats were tested in four behavioral paradigms described in detail elsewhere [3]. Those who tested the animals were unaware which rats were lesioned and which were sham-operated. On completion of the testing on the 3rd day after infliction of the lesion or sham operation, ^{14}C-deoxyglucose studies were carried out in awake rats as described previously [5].

Results and Discussion

The best correlation between cortical glucose utilization and behavioral deficits in lesioned animals was found with the bilateral adhesive removal test, which has been shown to detect somatosensory asymmetry independent of motor bias [13]. Thus, this was the only test that demonstrated a progressive deficit over the 3 postlesion days; its progression resembled the time course of lCGU changes as reported previously [5]. Furthermore, linear regression analysis showed a statistically significant correlation ($r = -0.70$, $P < 0.05$) between average cortical lCGU and the latency of tape removal from the contralateral forepaw in individual lesioned animals 72 h after infliction of the lesion.

We believe that the finding in rats with freezing lesions of definite somatosensory deficits significantly correlated with the cortical metabolic depression supports the interpretation that the diminished lCGU reflects functional disturbances in this model of brain injury.

Serotonin Turnover in Injured Brain

The involvement of the serotonergic system in functional depression that develops as a result of injury was indicated by the fact that inhibition of serotonin (5-HT) synthesis with *p*-chlorophenylalanine resulted in a significant amelioration of the decrease in lCGU seen 3 days after infliction of the lesion in traumatized brain [9, 10]. For further elucidation of the role of the perturbations in this neurotransmitter system, 5-HT and 5-HIAA were measured with time after injury in cortical areas of both hemispheres of unilaterally lesioned brain.

Methods

Standardized freezing lesions were made as described previously [5]. Normal and lesioned rats were decapitated into liquid nitrogen at specified times after the lesion was made. Animals were not anesthetized, except those killed at 1 min, since the lesion is made under halothane anesthesia. The heads were kept at $-25\,°C$ for 30 min, after which the brains were removed and areas of the cortex dissected and

Table 1. Serotonin turnover in injured brain (5-HIAA : 5-HT)

Normal (17)	0.40±0.08	
Time after lesion	Lesioned side	Contralateral side
1 min (8)	0.44±0.02	0.41±0.03
4 h (6)	0.78±0.17*	0.46±0.05
24 h (7)	1.40±0.14**	0.74±0.09**
72 h (9)	0.98±0.12**	0.42±0.02

Averages ± SEM, number of animals in brackets
* $P<0.05$; ** $P<0.01$ (Bonferroni method for calculation of conservative critical value for modified *t*-statistics [16])

quickly weighed. Frozen tissue was extracted with 0.2 *M* perchloric acid. 5-HT and 5-HIAA were measured in the extract by high-performance liquid chromatography, with electrochemical detection by a modification of the method of Mefford [4] using an internal standard for quantitation.

Results and Discussion

The content of 5-HT and 5-HIAA in rat cerebral cortex was found to be quite variable with time after lesion, so that it was difficult to demonstrate any consistent changes. In contrast, when the results were expressed as a ratio of the metabolite to the neurotransmitter (5-HIAA/5-HT), which can be considered as a measure of serotonin turnover, clear-cut increases with time became apparent (Table 1). At 1 min after infliction of the lesion the ratio of 5-HIAA : 5-HT was unchanged. By 4 h after, a statistically significant increase in the ratio was apparent on the lesioned side, with a further increase at 24 h and continued elevation at 72 h. On the side contralateral to the lesion the serotonin system was also affected, but to a lesser extent, as shown by a significant but moderate rise in 5-HIAA : 5-HT ratio at 24 h but not at other times.

These results confirm that the serotonin system is perturbed in injured brain and show that the changes in turnover develop with time and persist while ever the functional disturbances, as reflected by metabolic depression, are present. With the data available at this time it appears that the peak increase in serotonin turnover (24 h after lesion) precedes the peak of the depression in lCGU (72 h after lesion). Further studies are required to determine whether normalization of the serotonergic system precedes recovery of the functional state of a traumatized brain or whether the two processes resolve in parallel.

Effects of Calcium Antagonist PY 108-068 in Injured Brain

An alteration in calcium distribution has been postulated to play an integral part in the chain of events leading from brain injury to functional disturbances [10]. To test this part of our hypothesis the effects of PY 108-068 (Sandoz), a potent calcium modulator drug of the dihydropyridine type [2], were studied in rats with cold lesions [1].

Methods

Standard cold lesions were made in rats and 3 days later lCGU or local cerebral blood flow (lCBF) was measured by autoradiographic techniques [12, 15]. The animals were untreated or given PY 108-068. The drug was administered according to two regimens. One group of animals, in which lCGU was measured 3 days later, received a bolus IV injection of 20 μg/kg 30 min before the lesion was made and then 10 μg/kg/h for 2 h (total dose 40 μg/kg over 2.5 h). Other animals were given the drug 3 days after the lesion was made, in a bolus IV injection 30 min before a ^{14}C-deoxyglucose or ^{14}C-iodoantipyrine study with a dose of either 10 or 20 μg/kg. In all cases the dosage schedule provided stable hemodynamic conditions during lCGU or lCBF measurements.

Results and Discussion

Results summarized in Table 2 show that PY 108-068 had no effect on lCGU in traumatized brain, whether given at the time of injury or 3 days later when the metabolic depression was at its peak. We have no data on what effect PY 108-068 might have if given throughout the 3-day postlesion period.

PY 108-068 had an unexpected effect on lCBF in injured brain. In normal animals a highly significant correlation between the rate of glucose utilization and

Table 2. Effect of PY 108-068 on lCGU in injured brain

Hemisphere	Lesioned side		Contralateral side	
Areas and structures	Cortical (5)	Subcortical (12)	Cortical (5)	Subcortical (12)
Conditions	lCGU as percentage of normal			
72 h after lesion				
Untreated (13)	54±3	81±3	84±3	89±2
PY, day of lesion:				
40 μg/kg over 2.5 h (4)	62±3	77±3	75±4	78±2
PY, 3 days after lesion:				
10 μg/kg (3)	44±2	78±6	80±3	88±1
20 μg/kg (3)	45±3	84±4	88±3	93±1

Averages ± SEM; numbers of animals in parentheses
Results in 5 cortical areas and 12 subcortical structures were expressed as percentages of normal and averaged for each animal. The group averages were then calculated. Differences from untreated group not statistically significant

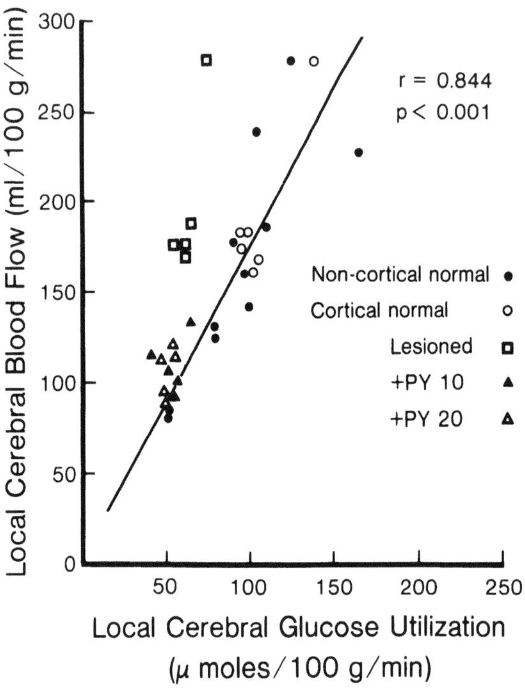

Fig. 1. Relationship between lCGU and lCBF in normal brain and the effect of PY 108-068 on this relationship in lesioned brain. Each *point* represents an individual area or structure. The *regression line* for normal brain was drawn from data for 17 structures. Data for five cortical areas only are given for lesioned brain, untreated brain, and brain treated with PY 108-068

blood flow in different structures of the brain has been demonstrated [8, 11]. The normal relationship between cerebral blood flow and cerebral metabolism was disturbed in injured brain, since lCBF was globally, though not significantly, increased 3 days after a freezing lesion while lCGU was depressed particularly in cortical areas of the traumatized hemisphere. In animals given 10 or 20 μg PY 108-068 3 days after the lesion the relative hyperemia in areas of depressed glucose utilization was abolished, although in normal or ischemic conditions this and other calcium antagonists are known to increase cerebral blood flow [17]. The relationships between lCGU and lCBF under the different experimental conditions are summarized in Fig. 1. In untreated traumatized brain the points representing the five cortical areas in which lCGU and lCBF were measured are clearly displaced to the left of the normal regression line, as lCGU decreased with little or no change in lCBF. Both doses of PY 108-068 used produced a depression of lCBF compared with results in untreated animals with no change in lCGU. Thus, the points for the cortical areas in the treated animals fell back to the regression line, but at a lower level than previously (both lCGU and lCBF depressed). These results suggest that in traumatized brain vasodilatation occurs independently of metabolic depression, masking the usual coupling between metabolism and blood flow. The finding that the relative hyperemia in injured brain was blocked by the administration of a potent calcium antagonist implicates calcium in the mechanism of the postulated vasodilatation.

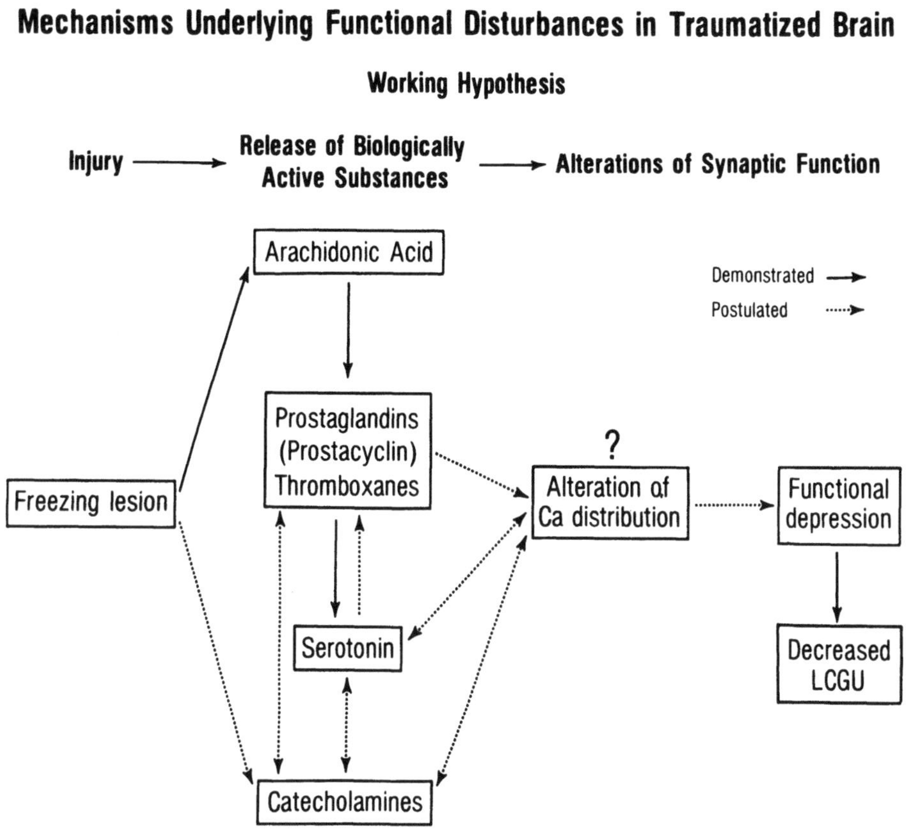

Fig. 2. Update schematic of working hypothesis linking brain injury to alteration in function

Conclusion

An updated version of the working hypothesis for the study of mechanisms underlying functional disturbances in traumatized brain is presented in Fig. 2.

The release of arachidonic acid and synthesis of prostaglandins has been demonstrated previously [7, 8], and the importance of these processes in the development of functional depression is indicated by normalization of lCGU in traumatized brain by nonsteroidal anti-inflammatory drugs [8]. Inhibition of serotonin and catecholamine synthesis was shown to ameliorate the depression of glucose utilization in injured brain [9], indicating involvement of these neurotransmitter systems in the development of functional disturbances resulting from trauma. The increased serotonin turnover demonstrated following a freezing lesion in the results presented here provides additional evidence that the serotonergic system is indeed affected in traumatized brain. The postulated involvement of changes in calcium distribution in the overall process leading from injury to alterations in synaptic function must be reassessed in view of the failure of a calcium antagonist to modify the metabolic response of the lesioned brain. Finally, the assumption that metabolic mapping can be used to assess the functional state of lesioned brain has been strengthened by our studies on the behavioral status of lesioned rats which showed close correlation between somatosensory deficits and lCGU following infliction of a freezing lesion.

Summary

To validate the use of the deoxyglucose technique as a measure of the functional state of injured brain behavioral studies were carried out in lesioned rats. The results showed definite somatosensory deficits in rats with standard freezing lesions, which correlated with the demonstrated metabolic depression. This lends support to the interpretation that diminished cortical glucose utilization reflects a functional disturbance in this model of brain injury.

Serotonin turnover in rat brain increased with time after infliction of a freezing lesion. The changes were most pronounced in the lesioned hemisphere, where the serotonin turnover reached a peak at 24 h and was still elevated at 72 h. The side contralateral to the lesion was also affected but to a much lesser extent and only at 24 h.

The role of calcium, as postulated initially in a working hypothesis for a study of mechanisms underlying functional disturbances in traumatized brain, may have to be reexamined, as calcium modulators of the dihydropyridine type were shown to have no effect on the depressed glucose utilization in the freezing lesion model of brain injury. Surprisingly, blood flow was decreased by these drugs in those parts of injured brain where glucose utilization was diminished, implying that changes in calcium distribution may play a part in the vasodilatation, which apparently occurs with time after trauma in the cold lesion model of injury.

Acknowledgements. I wish to express my appreciation to Dr. L. S. Wolfe for his continued interest in this work, his fruitful collaboration on some aspects of it, and many stimulating discussions.

I am indebted to Hanna Szylinger, Michael McHugh, and Ralph Dadoun for technical assistance and to Linda Michel for clerical assistance.

References

1. Archer DP, Pappius HM (1985) The effect of calcium antagonists on local cerebral glucose utilization and blood flow in injured brain (in preparation)
2. Hof RP, Hof A, Neumann P (1982) Effects of PY 108-068, a new calcium antagonist, on general hemodynamic and regional blood flow in anesthetized cats: a comparison with Nifedipine. J Cardiovasc Pharmacol 4:352–362
3. Holmes L, Colle L, Pappius HM (1985) Correlation between behavioral status and cerebral glucose utilization in rats following freezing lesion. Brain Res (submitted for publication)
4. Mefford IN (1981) Application of high performance liquid chromatography with electrochemical detection to neurochemical analysis: measurement of catecholamines, serotonin and metabolites in rat brain. J Neurosci Methods 3:207–224
5. Pappius HM (1981) Local cerebral glucose utilization in thermally traumatized rat brain. Ann Neurol 9:484–491
6. Pappius HM (1982) Dexamethasone and local cerebral glucose in freeze-traumatized rat brain. Ann Neurol 12:157–162

7. Pappius HM, Wolfe LS (1983) Functional disturbances in brain following injury: search for underlying mechanisms. Neurochem Res 8:61–70
8. Pappius HM, Wolfe LS (1983) Effects of indomethacin and ibuprofen on cerebral metabolism and blood flow in traumatized brain. J Cereb Blood Flow Metab 3:448–459
9. Pappius HM, Wolfe LS (1983) Involvement of serotonin and catecholamines in functional depression of traumatized brain. J Cereb Blood Flow Metab 3 [Suppl 1]:S226–S227
10. Pappius HM, Wolfe LS (1984) Effects of drugs on local cerebral glucose utilization in traumatized brain: Mechanisms of action of steroids revisited. In: Go G, Baethmann A (eds) Recent progress in the study and therapy of brain edema. Plenum, New York, pp 11–26
11. Pickard JD (1981) Role of prostaglandins and arachidonic acid derivatives in the coupling of cerebral blood flow to cerebral metabolism. J Cereb Blood Flow Metab 1:361–384
12. Sakurada O, Kennedy C, Jehle J, Brown JD, Carbin GL, Sokoloff L (1978) Measurement of local cerebral blood flow with iodo (^{14}C)antipyrine. Am J Physiol 234:H59–H66
13. Schallert T, Upchurch M, Lobaugh N, Farrar SB, Spirduso WW, Gilliam P, Vaughn D, Wilcox RE (1982) Tactile extinction: distinguishing between sensorimotor and motor asymmetries in rats with unilateral nigrostriatal damage. Pharmacol Biochem Behav 16:455–462
14. Sokoloff L (1977) Relation between physiological function and energy metabolism in the central nervous system. J Neurochem 29:13–26
15. Sokoloff L, Reivich M, Kennedy C, Des Rosiers MH, Patlak CS, Pettigrew KD, Sakurada O, Shinohara M (1977) The (^{14}C)deoxyglucose method for the measurement of local cerebral glucose utilization: theory, procedure and normal values in the conscious and anesthetized albino rat. J Neurochem 28:897–916
16. Wallenstein S, Lucker CL, Fleiss JL (1980) Some statistical methods useful in circulation research. Circ Res 47:1–9
17. Wiernsperger N, Gygax P, Hofmann A (1984) Calcium antagonist PY 108-068: Demonstration of its efficacy in various types of experimental brain ischemia. Stroke 15:679–685

Inhibition of the Kallikrein-Kinin System in Vasogenic Brain Edema *

A. UNTERBERG [1], C. DAUTERMANN, W. MÜLLER-ESTERL, and A. BAETHMANN

Key words: Kallikrein-kinin system, aprotinin, SBTI, posttraumatic brain swelling, vasogenic brain edema

Introduction

Evidence of a role of the kallikrein-kinin (KK) system as mediator in vasogenic brain edema is impressive, albeit not complete [1]. Experimental findings demonstrate that kinins, the active peptides of the KK system, induce brain edema of gray and white matter [10]. Cerebral administration of kinins opens the blood-brain barrier for small molecules, which may be viewed as a mechanism leading to interstitial fluid accumulation [11, 12]. Moreover, experimental injury to the brain (cold lesion) is associated with the formation of kinins in and around the primary insult [6]. However, no evidence is available so far to indicate whether specific inhibition of the release or function of kinins is therapeutically beneficial in brain edema.

The purpose of the current investigations was to study the effect of inhibition of the KK system by aprotinin and soybean-trypsin inhibitor (SBTI), on the development of cold injury brain edema. The compounds are protease inhibitors, which interfere with the enzyme (kallikrein)-catalyzing formation of kinins [3, 4].

Materials and Methods

The experiments were performed in rabbits weighing 3.3 ± 0.6 kg, anesthetized with ketamine and xylazine. A circular craniectomy was performed over the left hemisphere for induction of cold injury by means of a copper cylinder (dia 10 mm) cooled with a dry-ice and acetone mixture. Treatment with inhibitors given by IV injection was started 15 min after trauma and was continued until termination 24 h later. Control animals ($n = 12$) received physiological saline. The following regimens were used:

1. Soybean-trypsin inhibitor (6 mg kg^{-1} h^{-1}; SBTI; $n = 9$)
2. Aprotinin (6 mg kg^{-1} h^{-1} = 42 000 KIU kg^{-1} h^{-1}; $n = 14$)
3. SBTI + aprotinin (3 mg kg^{-1} h^{-1} each; $n = 10$)

---

* The work described in this paper was supported by grant no. Ba 452/6-5 from the Deutsche Forschungsgemeinschaft

[1] Institute for Surgical Research, Klinikum Großhadern, Division of Surgery, University of Munich, D-8000 Munich 70

Arterial blood pressure was monitored for 2 h after the induction of cold injury, or longer. Partial thromboplastin time (PTT) and aprotinin concentrations were determined in addition in blood samples at various intervals before and after trauma. The animals were anesthetized again for exsanguination 24 h after cold injury. The brain was removed for meticulous separation of the experimental (left) and the control (right) hemispheres in the median plane. Hemispheric swelling (as a percentage) was determined as the difference in weight between the traumatized and contralateral hemispheres. The cerebral water content of both hemispheres was obtained by dry/wet weight measurements. Tissue Na^+ and K^+ contents were determined in desiccated brain specimen. The cerebral uptake of aprotinin into edematous brain tissue was investigated in a limited number of experiments after in situ fixation with liquid N_2. Aprotinin concentrations in plasma and tissue were measured by ELISA according to Müller-Esterl [7].

Results

Cold injury to the brain led to an increase of 13.0% ± 2.6% (mean + SD) in the weight of traumatized hemispheres over the nondamaged hemispheres. Infusion of aprotinin reduced the swelling of injured hemispheres to 10.1% ± 2.5% ($P < 0.01$ vs untreated controls), and aprotinin plus SBTI reduced it to 10.4% ± 2.1% ($P < 0.02$ vs controls). Animals receiving SBTI had only a marginal reduction of hemispheric swelling to 11.7% ± 1.6%, however, which did not attain statistical significance (Table 1). A reduction of hemispheric swelling from 13.0% to 10.1% is equivalent to a 22% decrease in edema. Traumatized cerebral hemispheres had a significant increase in tissue water content, which was most pronounced in control animals and smallest in rabbits that received infusions of aprotinin. The differences, however, did not reach a statistically significant level. An increased amount of water in lesioned hemispheres was associated with an increase in Na^+ and a decrease in K^+ content.

Table 1. Increase in weight of traumatized hemispheres (mean ± SD) over the corresponding contralateral hemispheres of animals with and without treatment

	Weight increases	
	g	%
Controls ($n = 12$)	0.47 ± 0.10	13.6 ± 2.6
Aprotinin ($n = 14$)	0.37 ± 0.09*	10.1 ± 2.5***
Aprotinin + SBTI ($n = 10$)	0.39 ± 0.08	10.4 ± 2.1*
SBTI ($n = 9$)	0.43 ± 0.05	11.7 ± 1.6

* $P < 0.05$; ** $P < 0.02$; *** $P < 0.01$ vs controls

Table 2. Aprotinin concentrations (KIU/ml, or KIU/g f.w.) in plasma and in damaged brain tissue (mean ± SEM)

Plasma	
0.5 h after trauma	144 ± 22
2 h after trauma	160 ± 26
6 h after trauma	178 ± 31
24 h after trauma	428 ± 64
Cerebral tissue	
Focus	494 ± 173
Perifocal edema	172 ± 59

Since the formation of vasogenic edema may be influenced by arterial hypotension [5, 8], the effect of treatment on arterial blood pressure was monitored. Systemic blood pressure, however, was affected neither by cold injury nor by treatment with aprotinin. On the other hand, treatment had a marked influence on coagulation. Infusion with SBTI had increased PTT from 20 to 42 s by 30 min after trauma. PTT continued to rise, reaching 72 s by 24 h after trauma. PTT was also delayed in animals receiving aprotinin, in which PTT rose to 38 s by 24 h after trauma. However, the decrease in coagulatory capacity by aprotinin did obviously not affect its therapeutic effect on edema, although interference with coagulation may promote edema influx [9]. Table 2 gives the aprotinin concentrations in blood and cerebral tissue 24 h after cold lesion. At 45 min after the start of the infusion, 120 kallikrein-inactivator units/ml (KIU) were found in the plasma. At termination, the mean plasma concentration was 450 KIU/ml. A concentration of 500 KIU/g f.w. (fresh weight) was found in focal necrotic tissue, and 170 KIU/g f.w. in perifocal edematous brain. The concentrations are considered sufficient for effective inhibition of the KK system [4].

Discussion

Inhibition of the KK system by aprotinin in association with a reduction of posttraumatic brain swelling can be considered as final proof of a mediator function of kinins in vasogenic brain edema. Yet, the level of specificity of inhibition of the KK system by aprotinin or SBTI in brain edema is an important point in this context, since other proteolytic enzymes, such as trypsin, can also be inhibited [3, 4]. However, evidence has not been provided for an involvement of trypsin, plasmin, or other proteases in the formation and spread of vasogenic brain edema. Inhibition of brain swelling by aprotinin is unlikely to have resulted from decreased arterial blood pressure. In fact, blood pressure was barely affected by the inhibitor. Arterial hypotension secondary to aprotinin might, however, be an important mechanism in other species, such as cats. According to our experience, cats develop hypotension during infusion of aprotinin. This may explain the beneficial effects of aprotinin on cerebral edema in cats studied by Czernicki [2]. In these experiments, less than a third of the dose used in the present investigations was found sufficient to reduce brain edema.

Although it has not been directly assessed, effective inhibition of the KK system in the damaged brain can be inferred from the aprotinin concentrations found in plasma and samples of focal and perifocal cerebral tissue. Aprotinin concentrations of 125 KIU/ml in plasma can be expected to antagonize serum kallikrein completely [4]. Such concentrations were present even as little as 1 h after cold injury. Failure of SBTI to influence brain edema may be explained by side effects of the compound on coagulation, e.g., a marked increase in the partial thromboplastin time. The conclusion is based on findings that interference with coagulation, such as platelet inhibition, enhances cerebral edema [9].

In conclusion, inhibition of the KK system was found to reduce formation of post-traumatic brain swelling secondary to cold injury significantly. The results can be considered as a piece of evidence so far lacking, but necessary for a final identification of kinins as mediators in brain edema. It remains to be shown whether treatment with aprotinin genuinely prevents the formation of kinins in cerebral damage. Nevertheless, the progress made in the field thus far is easily enough to justify the initiation of clinical trials on inhibition of the KK system for treatment of cerebral edema.

Summary

The kallikrein-kinin system is considered to be a mediator of vasogenic brain edema. Evidence has been provided that kinins, the active peptides of the system, induce edema by opening of the blood-brain barrier. Moreover, kinins are formed in brain tissue under pathophysiologic conditions. The present study was designed to investigate whether specific inhibition of formation of kinins in cerebral trauma (cold injury) by blocking of the activating enzyme kallikrein has a therapeutic function in brain swelling. The findings definitely demonstrate a role of kinins as mediators in secondary processes arising from cerebral lesions. Administration of inhibitors commenced 15 min after trauma. Treatment with aprotinin or with aprotinin plus SBTI caused a significant reduction in hemispheric swelling, from 13.0% (controls) to 10.1%, or 10.4% ($P < 0.01$ or $P < 0.02$), respectively. Infusion of SBTI only was not effective in reducing post-traumatic brain swelling. Attenuation of cerebral edema by aprotinin was associated with a reduction of the tissue water content. Nonspecific therapeutic effects of aprotinin by way of a reduction in blood pressure can be ruled out; this was hardly affected during infusion of the inhibitor. A therapeutic failure of SBTI may be attributable to interference with coagulation. Animals with SBTI had a marked increase of the partial thromboplastin time. The current findings provide final experimental evidence for a role of the KK system in post-traumatic brain swelling. Pertinent clinical trials in acute forms of traumatic vasogenic brain edema appear worthwhile.

Acknowledgements. We are indebted to Ulrike Goerke, Angelika Konrad, Barbara Stöpfel, Ruth Demmer, and Friederike Helmes, who provided invaluable technical and secretarial help.

References

1. Baethmann A, Oettinger W, Rothenfußer W, Kempski O, Unterberg A, Geiger R (1980) Brain edema factors: current state with particular reference to plasma constituents and glutamate. Adv Neurol 28:171–195
2. Czernicki Z (1979) Treatment of experimental brain oedema following sudden decompression, surgical wound, and cold lesion with vasoprotective drugs and the proteinase inhibitor "Trasylol". Acta Neurochir 50:311–326
3. Erdös EG (ed) (1979) Bradykinin, kallidin and kallikrein. Handbook of experimental pharmacology, vol 25 [suppl]. Springer, Berlin Heidelberg New York
4. Fritz H, Wunderer G (1983) Biochemistry and applications of aprotinin, the kallikrein-inhibitor from bovine organs. Arzneimittelforsch 33:479–494
5. Klatzo I (1967) Presidential address. Neuropathological aspects of brain edema. J Neuropathol Exp Neurol 26:1–14
6. Maier-Hauff K, Baethmann A, Lange M, Schürer L, Unterberg A (1984) The kallikrein-kinin system as mediator in vasogenic brain edema. 2: Studies on kinin formation in focal and perifocal brain tissue. J Neurosurg 61:97–106
7. Müller-Esterl W, Oettel A, Truscheit E, Fritz H (1984) Monitoring of aprotinin plasma levels by an enzyme-linked immunosorbant assay (ELISA). Fresenius Z Anal Chem 317:718–719
8. Pappius HM (1974) Fundamental aspects of brain edema. In: Vinken PJ, Bruyn GW (eds) Tumors of the brain and skull. Handbook of clinical neurology, vol 16, part 1. North-Holland, Amsterdam, pp 167–185
9. Segawa H, Patterson RH (1981) Role of platelets in vasogenic brain edema: I. Significance of thrombus formation in the damaged vessels. Arch Neurol 38:265–270
10. Unterberg A, Baethmann A (1984) The kallikrein-kinin system as mediator in vasogenic brain edema. 1: Cerebral exposure to bradykinin and plasma. J Neurosurg 61:87–96
11. Unterberg A, Wahl M, Baethmann A (1984) Effects of bradykinin on permeability and diameter of pial vessels in vivo. J Cereb Blood Flow Metab 4:574–585
12. Unterberg A, Hack U, Baethmann A (1985) Blood flow, metabolism and function of the brain during cerebral administration of bradykinin. In: Dietz H, Brock M, Klinger K (eds) Advances in neurosurgery, vol 13. Springer, Berlin Heidelberg New York (in press)

Thromboxane Synthetase Inhibition in Ischemic Brain Injury *

N. A. MOUFARRIJ [1], J. R. LITTLE, V. SKRINSKA, F. V. LUCAS, J. P. LATCHAW, R. M. SLUGG, and P. LESSER

Key words: Cerebral ischemia, thromboxane synthetase inhibitor (TSI), platelet function, lipoxygenase products

Introduction

The purpose of this investigation was to study the effects of a selective thromboxane A_2 (TXA_2) synthetase inhibitor U.K. 38,485 (TSI) upon the evolution of cerebral infarction in the cat.

Method

This model has been used extensively in our laboratory [1]. Briefly, adult cats lightly anesthetized with nitrous oxide were subjected to right middle cerebral artery (MCA) occlusion for 4 h, followed by a 2-h period during which perfusion was reestablished before the end of the experiment. Ten cats were not treated, ten cats received TSI 3 mg/kg IV immediately before MCA occlusion, and ten cats received TSI 3 mg/kg IV immediately after MCA occlusion. The bleeding time was determined at baseline and at the end of each experiment. Electroencephalographic recordings (EEG) were obtained before and after MCA clipping, before and after MCA release, and at hourly intervals thereafter. An EEG percentage index was derived by comparing the average wave amplitude of the ischemic right hemisphere (numerator) with the average wave amplitude of the intact left hemisphere (denominator) [1]. Regional cerebral blood flow (rCBF) was measured by the xenon-133 (^{133}Xe) clearance technique before and after MCA occlusion, before and after MCA release, and before the termination of each experiment. In each cat, 30 min before perfusion 5 cm^3 arterial blood was drawn for measurement of thromboxane B_2 (TXB_2), and Evans blue (1 ml 10% solution) and sodium fluorescein (1 ml 10% solution) were given IV. At 6 h after MCA occlusion and 2 h after MCA release the cats were then perfused with colloidal carbon and buffered formaldehyde. The brain of each cat was removed and evaluated for midline shift, Evans blue and sodium fluorescein extravasation, carbon staining, and infarct size. Ten further cats subjected to MCA occlusion and reperfusion were used for pharmacological studies. Five of them received TSI 3 mg/kg IV immediately after MCA occlusion, and serial TSI

* The work described in this paper was supported by a grant from the Cleveland Foundation.
[1] Departments of Neurosurgery, Cleveland Clinic, Cleveland, Ohio, USA

and thromboxane B_2 (TXB_2) levels (a stable metabolite of TXA_2) were measured. Another five cats were not treated and serial TXB_2 levels were plotted.

Results

The three treatment groups did not differ significantly in bleeding time, arterial blood pressure, rCBF changes, EEG changes, brain swelling, or vital dye extravasation.

Substantial failure of carbon filling was recorded in five control, seven post-treated, and eight pretreated cats. The difference between the control and the pretreated group achieved the lowest *P*-value, with 0.20. The mean infarct sizes in the control, pretreated, and post-treated group were 28%, 43%, and 32%, respectively. The *P* values obtained by comparing the control and the post-treated groups, the control and the pretreated groups, and the post-treated and the pretreated groups were 0.85, 0.25, and 0.30, respectively. Therefore, carbon staining and infarct size differences between the three groups also failed to reach statistical significance, but there was a suggestion that these parameters were adversely affected in the cats pretreated with TSI.

Thromboxane production was inhibited by 95% in the cats receiving TSI either immediately before or immediately after MCA clipping as opposed to untreated animals. In the pharmacological studies, the mean TSI serum levels in five cats after MCA occlusion 15 min after the TSI IV administration was 6 μg/ml. It declined during the first 3.5 h and then stabilized, reaching a mean of 1 μg/ml at 6 h. The concomitant changes in TXB_2 serum levels reveal a precipitous fall, from a mean level of 185 ng/ml before treatment to mean values between 0.6 and 4 ng/ml at 30 min after the administration of TSI, where they remained. The plasma TXB_2 levels in the five untreated cats did not significantly change with time and were below 4 ng/ml.

Discussion

The inhibition of TXA_2 production was thought to have potential beneficial effects upon the evolution of cerebral infarction [3, 7]. In this study, U.K. 38,485, a selective thromboxane synthetase inhibitor, was used in an established model of acute focal cerebral ischemia. This compound is 3-(1*H*-imidazol-1-yl-methyl)-2-methyl-1*H*-indole-1-propanoic acid, the imidazole ring being the active moiety of the molecule [2].

The rCBF changes were not affected by treatment with TSI. This suggests that release of TXA_2 by platelets in untreated cats does not substantially increase the resistance in collateral arterial channels to the ischemic zone. In addition, the findings recorded in the rCBF and carbon perfusion studies do not support the hypothesis that intravascular platelet aggregation induced by TXA_2 release obstructs the microcirculation in the ischemic zone and thereby impairs perfusion.

Pretreatment with TSI tended to produce larger infarcts (43%) than were seen without treatment (28%) or with treatment started after MCA occlusion (32%). When the EEG curves were examined the TSI-pretreated group seemed to recover less well after reperfusion than the untreated and the post-treated groups. Although these two observations did not attain statistical significance they are worth noting, because of their possible pathophysiologic implications. Indeed, preservation of some degree of platelet function in the setting of cerebral infarction may have a protective function. Conversely, the severe abolition of platelet aggregation achieved by TXA_2 synthetase inhibition may be detrimental and hence may be unmasking a hitherto unsuspected beneficial role of platelets in cerebral infarction.

One possible mechanism that could explain the largest infarcts in cats pretreated with TSI is that inhibition of TXA_2 production leads to redirection of its precursors into the leukotriene and other lipoxygenase products, which may promote tissue damage. The two fundamental premises of such a mechanism are: (a) The recent demonstration that platelet derived lipoxygenase byproducts may be taken up by other cells, in particular neutrophils [6]; and (b) the recent implication of neutrophils in the propagation of infarction in several myocardial infarction models, as recently reported [4, 5, 8]. Why results with pretreatment and post-treatment are different is unclear.

Summary

Thromboxane synthetase inhibition failed to have any favorable influence on the evolution of cerebral infarction in cats subjected to middle cerebral artery (MCA) occlusion. When the inhibitor of thromboxane synthetase was given before MCA occlusion cerebral infarction tended to be more extensive.

Acknowledgements. Dr. P. R. Urquilla from the Pfizer Company kindly provided the thromboxane synthetase inhibitor U.K. 38,485.

We thank Sarah B. Forsythe, M.Sc. from the Department of Biostatistics for her help in the analysis of the results.

References

1. Awad I, Little Jr, Lucas F, et al. (1983) Modification of focal cerebral ischemia by prostacyclin and indomethacin. J Neurosurg 58:714–719
2. Cross PE, Dickinson RP, Parry MT, et al. (1981) 3-(1-Imidazolylmethyl) indoles: potent and selective inhibitors of human blood platelet thromboxane synthetase. Agents Actions 11:274–280
3. Hossmann KA, Hossmann V (1977) Coagulopathy following experimental cerebral ischemia. Stroke 8:249–254
4. Jolly SR, Kane WT, Bailie MB, et al. (1983) Reduction of reperfusion injury after canine myocardial ischemia by superoxide dismutase plus catalase. Circulation 68 [Suppl 3]: 185 (abstract)
5. Ksiezycka E, Hastie R, Maroko RP, et al. (1983) Reduction in myocardial damage after experimental coronary artery occlusion by two techniques which deplete neutrophils. Circulation 68 [Suppl 3]: 185 (abstract)
6. Marcus AJ (1983) Recent progress in the role of platelets in occlusive vascular disease. Stroke 14:475–479
7. Randall MT, Parry MT, Hawkeswood E, et al. (1981) UK-37,248, a novel, selective thromboxane synthetase inhibitor with platelet anti-aggregatory and anti-thrombotic activity. Thromb Res 23: 145–162
8. Rao PS, Cohen MV, Mueller HS (1983) Transcardiac production of thromboxane: prostacyclin and free radicals in early experimental myocardial ischemia. Circulation 68 [Suppl 3]: 185 (abstract)

The Role of Adrenergic Activity and Histamine in Ischemic Brain Edema

H. MOROOKA [1] and A. NISHIMOTO

Introduction

It has been noted that irreversible membrane disturbance is caused by the peroxy radical, which is formed by the reaction of active oxygen (O_2, OH, O_2, H_2O_2) with unsaturated fatty acids, during the development of cerebral ischemia [1]. In recent experiments the peroxidation reaction in the cell membrane has been proved biochemically to occur only after exposure to O_2 [2].

This study was designed to elucidate the pathomechanisms of cerebral microcirculatory disturbance caused by a free radical reaction in the dynamics of cerebral ischemia and subsequent cerebral edema by simultaneous examination of the role of active oxygen formed in the blood platelets and the adrenergic system [3–5] in this free radical reaction and the involvement of catecholamines and histamine in the changes of cerebrovascular permeability.

Materials and Methods

The experimental animals used were male Wistar strain rats weighing approx. 300–350 g.

For the experiment the rats were divided into two groups, the first being the control group ($n=50$) and the second group being treated with 0.2 mg 6-hydroxydopamine (6-OHDA) injected by the cisternal puncture method 48 h before the experiment ($n=7$). Under ether anesthesia intratracheal intubation was performed; 70% N_2O and 30% O_2 were used to maintain anesthesia with adjusted respiration. The experimental animals were immoblized by IV injection of 0.1 mg/kg pancronium bromide (Myoblock). Blood gases were measured by means of a polyethylene tube inserted into the femoral artery. PCO_2 was maintained at approx. 35–40 mmHg, PO_2 above 100 mmHg, pH at about 7.35–7.45, and body temperature at 37 °C. For the preparation of an experimental cerebral infarction model, a polyethylene tube was inserted into the right internal carotid artery, and plastic microspheres (35 μm in diameter) and arachidonic acid (5 m*M*, 25 μl) were injected slowly over 10 s. The brain was fixed by freezing with liquid nitrogen before injection of the microspheres and then 15 min, 1 h, 2 h, 3 h, and 4 h after the injection, after which it was subjected to biochemical examinations.

---

[1] Dept. of Neurological Surgery, Okayama University Medical School, 2-5-1, Shikata-cho, Okayama 700, Japan

The excised brain tissue was weighed at 0 °C, homogenized with 0.1 *M* potassium phosphate buffer at pH 7.4, and centrifuged for 30 min at 0 °C and 25 000 *g*. The supernatant was used for measurements of α-tocopherol concentration, glutathione concentration, dopamine β-hydroxylase (DBH) activity, malonyldialdehyde (MDA) concentration, and histamine concentration. (a) Tissue DBH activity was measured by the partially modified method of Nagatsu et al. [6] and expressed as micrograms of octopamine per minute at 37 °C per gram. (b) Tissue α-tocopherol concentration was measured by the method of Abe et al. [7], and expressed as micrograms per gram wet weight. (c) Tissue glutathione concentration was measured by the method of Hissin [8], and expressed as GSSG/GSH%. (d) Tissue MDA concentration was measured by the method of Ohkawa et al. [9], and expressed as nanomoles of MDA per gram of tissue. (e) Tissue histamine concentration was measured by the method of Anton et al., and expressed as nanograms per gram of tissue. For the measurement of water content in the brain the lyophilization method was used, and for pathological examinations 30 min after injection of the microspheres 10% formaldehyde solution was used to fix the brain tissue by perfusion at a pressure of 150 cmH_2O; the specimens were observed both macroscopically and by light microscopy after hematoxylin and eosin staining.

For the examination of disturbance of the blood-brain barrier the method of dye leakage following IV injection of 3 ml Evans blue was used immediately before injection of the microspheres. Cases with microspheres in the left cerebral hemisphere were excluded from the analysis.

Results

DBH activity in the brain tissue of rats treated with 6-OHDA ($n = 7$) was 0.06 ± 0.04 units, markedly lower than that in the controls ($n = 7$), which was 1.15 ± 0.09 units ($P < 0.001$). Macroscopically visible pathologic findings in rats with infarction treated with 6-OHDA were slight ischemic areas in the cerebral hemisphere on the embolic side and good transfer of microspheres into the cortical perforating arteries. The light-microscopic pathologic findings were slight edematous change around the blood vessels occupied by microspheres only. Macroscopic pathologic findings in rats with infarction and no treatment were marked ischemic areas in the cerebral hemisphere on the embolic side, and microspheres tending to occupy the origin of the middle cerebral artery, where marked cerebral vasospasm was noted in all cases.

The light-microscopic pathologic findings included extensive edematous changes, with marked swelling of nerve cells and interstitial tissue around the cortical perforating arteries occupied by microspheres. The water content of the brain tissue on the embolic side in rats with infarction and no treatment increased gradually after the infarction, and 4 h after the infarction reached $81.5\% \pm 1.8\%$, which was higher than that of the controls, with $77\% \pm 1.0\%$ ($P < 0.05$) (Fig. 1). The concentration of α-tocopherol in the brain tissue on the embolic side decreased markedly after the infarction, to become 62% ($P < 0.01$) 15 min after the infarction, and showed a slightly decreasing tendency thereafter. GSSG : GSH increased to 1.3 times the value before infarction 15 min after infarction ($P < 0.01$), showed a peak 2 h after, when it had increased to 1.8 times the value before infarction ($P < 0.001$), and decreased gradu-

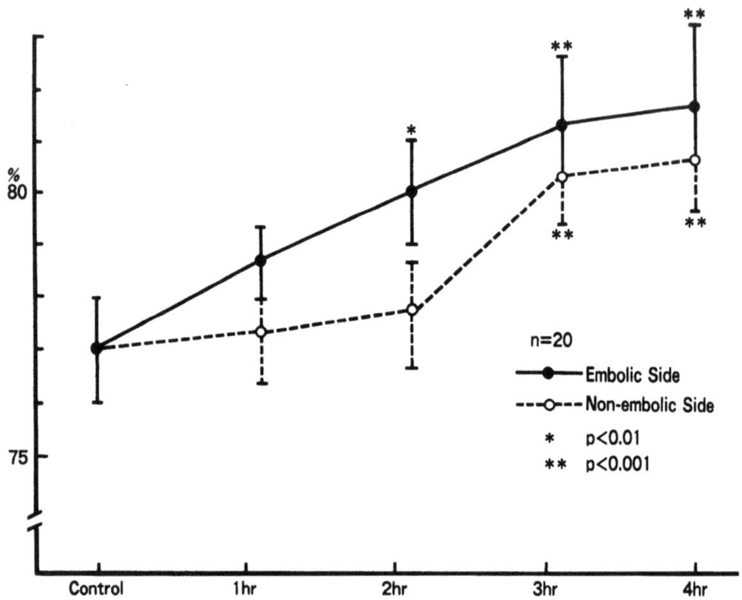

Fig. 1. Changes in water content in the rat cerebral cortex following ischemic stroke

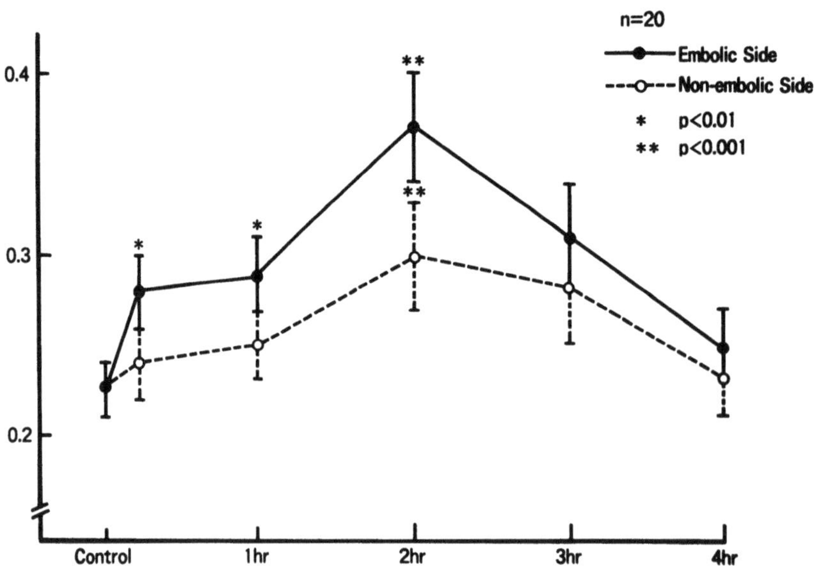

Fig. 2. Changes in GSSG : GSH ratio in the rat cerebral cortex following ischemic stroke

ally thereafter, returning to a value close to that recorded before the infarction by 4 h after (Fig. 2). The concentration of MDA in the brain tissue on the embolic side showed a peak 2 h after the infarction, when it was 1.5 times the value before the infarction ($P<0.001$), decreased markedly thereafter, and by 4 h after the infarction it had declined to 80% of the value before infarction ($P<0.01$) (Fig. 3).

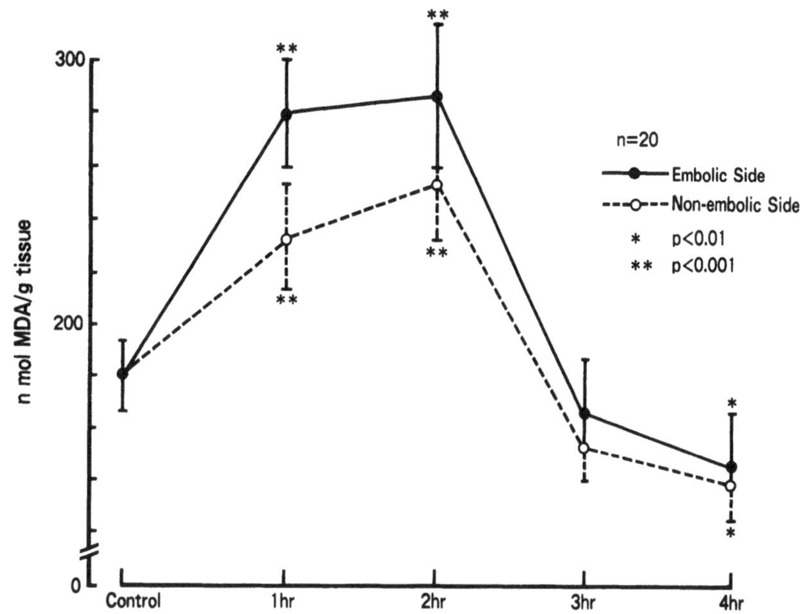

Fig. 3. Changes in malonyldialdehyde concentration in the rat cerebral cortex following ischemic stroke

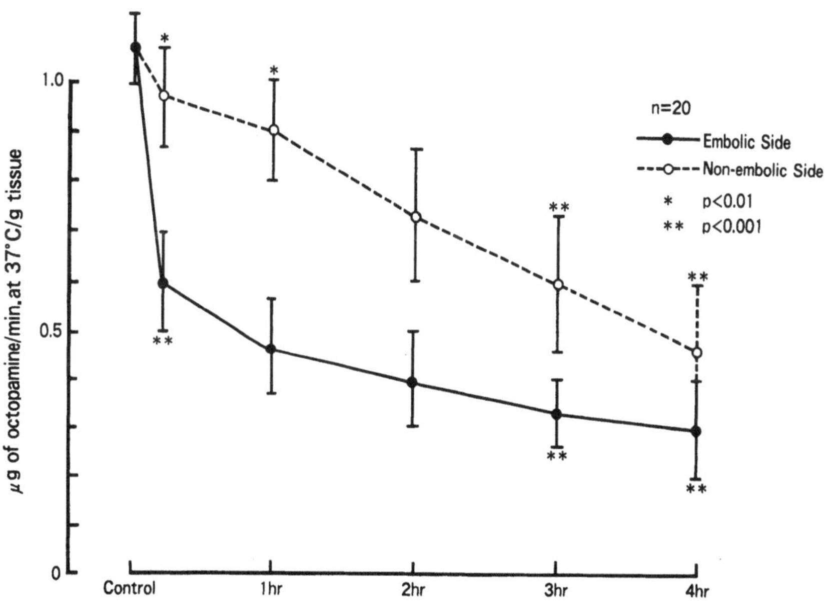

Fig. 4. Changes in dopamine-β-hydroxylase activity in the rat cerebral cortex following ischemic stroke

DBH activity in the brain tissue on the embolic side decreased markedly by 15 min after the infarction, when it was 50% of the value before infarction ($P<0.001$), subsequently decreasing gradually until 4 h after the infarction it was 25% of the value before the infarction ($P<0.001$) (Fig. 4). The concentration of histamine in the brain tissue on the embolic side increased after infarction, and 4 h after the in-

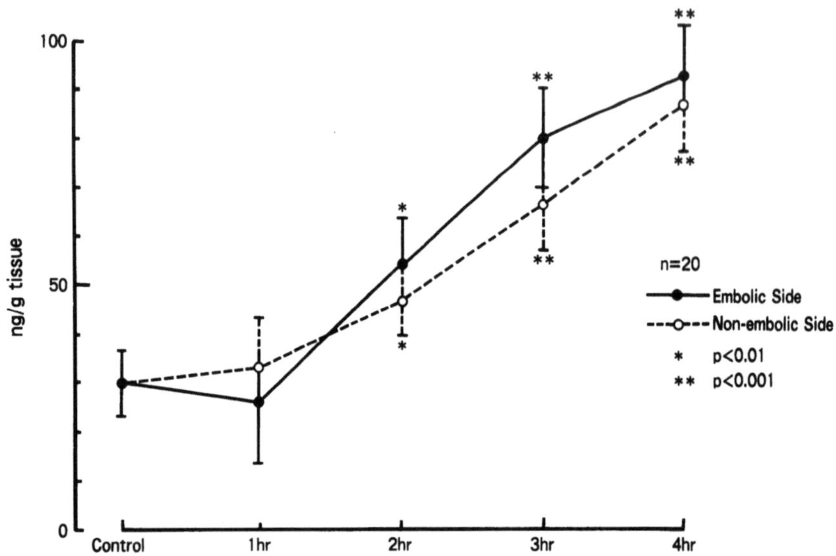

Fig. 5. Changes in histamine concentration in the rat cerebral cortex following ischemic stroke

farction it was three times the value before infarction ($P<0.001$) (Fig. 5). Water content in the brain tissue of the nonembolic side increased from 2 h after the infarction, and 4 h after infarction it was 1.04 times the value before it ($P<0.001$). The changes in α-tocopherol concentration, GSSG : GSH, MDA concentration, DBH activity, and histamine concentration in the brain tissue on the nonembolic side showed changes similar to those on the embolic side, but were quantitatively slight compared with the values on the embolic side. In the examination of disturbance of the blood-brain barrier, the leakage of Evans blue was noted from 3 h after infarction, corresponding to the site of infarction.

Discussion

In experimental cerebral infarction caused by platelet aggregation with arachidonic acid (AA) as substrate in rats subjected to chemical denervation with 6-OHDA, edematous changes in the area of infarction and around the blood vessels were totally absent or slight compared with those in rats with infarction and no treatment, and on the basis of this fact it was suggested that not only the AA cascade but also the sympathetic nervous system are closely concerned with the disturbance of the cerebral microcirculation. Platelet phospholipase A_2 is activated by such chemical stimuli as AA, norepinephrine (NE), epinephrine, ADP, thrombin, and collagen. As a result, AA is released from phospholipid, a constituent of the membrane, being converted to PGG_2 by the action of cyclo-oxygenase, and this PGG_2 forms further PGH_2 and active oxygen by the action of PG hydroperoxide [3]. From this PGH_2, TXA_2 with strong actions of platelet aggregation and vasoconstriction [10] is synthesized by TX synthetase. TXA_2, ADP, and 5HT are released from platelets by the mechanism of Ca^{2+}-dependent actomyosin contraction [11], and platelets are aggregated successively in a chain reaction in cooperation with the activated oxygen formed [12].

The active oxygen formed damages endothelial cells by way of a free radical reaction, inhibits the formation of PGI_2, with its actions of platelet aggregation inhibition and vasodilatation, and forms thrombi. As a result of an increase in the sympathetic nervous activity in the vascular wall, NE and DBH are released from the nerve endings into the blood by the mechanism of exocytosis [13], and these NE and DBH systems also form active oxygen [4, 5]; NE also causes vasospasm [6]. In addition, in our experimental results α-tocopherol and GSH, which were radical scavengers, were consumed after ischemia, while MDA in the brain tissue increased for more than 2 h after ischemia, which suggests that lipid peroxidation by a free radical reaction lasted for more than 2 h after ischemia, causing membranous damage. In the central part of the ischemic region energy depletion causes cytotoxic edema and impairment of the Na-K pump [14]. Around the ischemic part or at other, distant sites, not only may vasospasm occur owing to the increase of sympathetic nervous activity, but also the endothelial cell may be damaged by a free radical reaction caused by the active oxygen formed, causing microcirculatory damage by way of platelet aggregation.

In our experimental results, the concentration of cerebral histamine increased, corresponding to the increase of cerebral water content after ischemia, following the free radical reaction. On the basis of this it was assumed that the formation of histamine was accelerated by free radicals and/or the reduction of sympathetic activity, and as a result increased histamine caused increased macromolecular permeability

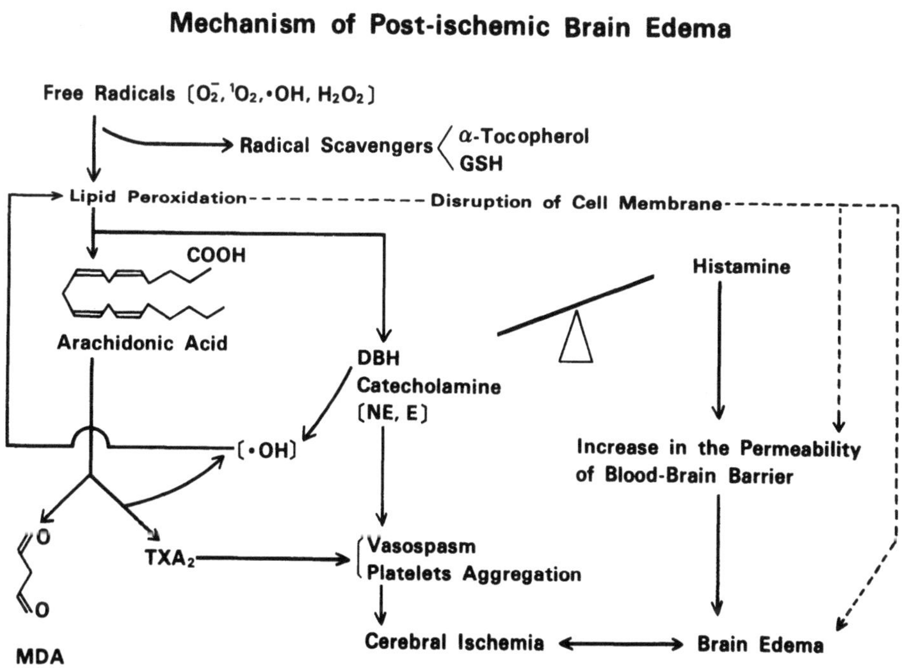

Fig. 6. Schematic showing a suggested mechanism for the genesis of postischemic brain edema

of the blood-brain barrier and vasodilatation [15], which was responsible for the vasogenic edema consequent on an increase in the osmotic pressure of interstitial fluid protein associated with the destruction of the blood-brain barrier induced by the radicals (Fig. 6).

Summary

Cerebral ischemia was produced in rats by a right intracarotid injection of microspheres (35 μ∅) and arachidonic acid (5 m*M*, 25 μl). Microscopic findings demonstrated markedly edematous changes in the nontreated rat brain 30 min after the ischemic stroke, while pathologic changes in the 6-OHDA-treated rats after stroke were absent or minimal. The water content of the embolized brain increased gradually up to 4 h after the ischemic stroke. DBH activity and α-tocopherol concentration in the embolized hemisphere decreased immediately after the stroke and remained low for the entire 4 h. MDA concentration and GSSG : GSH ratio in the embolized hemisphere gradually increased up to 2 h and then returned to normal by 4 h after the stroke. In addition, the histamine concentration in the embolized hemisphere gradually increased to three times that of the control level by 4 h after the stroke. In all instances there was a quantitatively similar but slightly smaller alteration in the substances measured in the nonembolized contralateral hemisphere.

These results suggest that an adrenergic mechanism may play an important part in the occurrence of microcirculatory damage induced by lipid peroxidation following stroke and the accumulation of histamine in the brain tissue may cause increased macromolecular permeability of the BBB leading to the vasogenic edema associated with free radical cell damage.

References

1. Demopoulos H, Flamm E, Seligman M, Power R, Pietronigro D, Ransohoff J (1977) Molecular pathology of lipid in CNS membranes. In: Jöbsis FF (ed) Oxygen and physiological function. Professional Information Library, Dallas, pp 491–508
2. Kogure K, Morooka H, Busto R (1979) Involvement of lipid peroxidation in postischemic brain damage. Neurology (Minneap) 29:546
3. Kuehl FA, Humes JL, Egan RW (1977) Role of prostaglandin endoperoxide PGG_2 in inflammatory processes. Nature 265:170–172
4. Bors W, Saran M, Lengtelder E, Michel C, Fuchs C, Frenzel C (1978) Detection of oxygen radicals in biological reactions. Photochem Pathobiol 28:629–638
5. Liu TZ, Shen JT, Ganong WF (1974) Evidence for the involvement of superoxide anion in dopamine-β-hydroxylase system. Proc Soc Exp Biol Med 146:37–40
6. Morooka H (1978) Cerebral arterial spasm I. Adrenergic mechanism in experimental cerebral vasospasm. Acta Medica Okayama 32:23–37
7. Abe K, Yukuchi Y, Katui G (1975) Quantitative determination of tocopherols by high-speed liquid chromatography. J Nutr Sci Vitaminol (Tokyo) 21:183–188
8. Hissin P, Hilf R (1979) A fluorometric method for determination of oxidized and reduced glutathione in tissues. Anal Biochem 74:214–226
9. Ohkawa H, Ohishi N, Yagi K (1979) Assay for lipid peroxides in animal tissues by tiobarbituric acid reaction. Anal Biochem 95:351–358

10. Hamberg M, Svensson J, Samuelsson B (1975) Thromboxanes: a new group of biologically active compounds derived from prostaglandin endoperoxides. Proc Natl Acad Sci USA 72:2994–2998
11. Lebowitz EA, Cooke R (1978) Contractile properties of actomyosin from human blood platelets. J Biol Chem 253:5443–5447
12. Handin RI, Karabin R, Boxer GJ (1977) Enhancement of platelet function by superoxide anion. J Clin Invest 50:954–965
13. Viveros OH, Arqueros L, Kirshner N (1968) Release of catecholamines and dopamine-β-hydroxylase from the adrenal medulla. Life Sci 7:609–618
14. Klatzo I (1981) Interrelationships between cerebral blood flow and brain edema. In: Minderhoud JM (ed) Cerebral blood flow: basic knowledge and clinical implications. Excerpta Medica, Amsterdam, pp 160–173
15. Gross PM, Harper M, Teasdale GM (1981) 1. Participation of vascular H_1- and H_2-receptors in vasodilatory responses to carotid arterial infusion. J Cereb Blood Flow Metab 1:97–108

Cerebrovascular Injuries and Brain Edema Following Activation of Platelets

T. FUJIMOTO[1], H. SUZUKI, K. TANOUE, Y. FUKUSHIMA, and H. YAMAZAKI

Key words: Cerebrovascular injury, brain edema, platelet aggregation, ADP, thromboxan A_2

Introduction

Recently, physiologically active substances released from activated platelets have attracted attention because of their pronounced effect on circulating platelets and vessel walls. The possibility that these vasoactive substances from platelets might injure the vessels has been suggested by several investigators [1]. Jørgensen [2], Furlow and Bass [3], and Fischi [4] observed intravascular platelet aggregation and disturbances of cerebral circulation after the injection of platelet-aggregating agents such as ADP or arachidonic acid. But vascular changes associated with platelet thrombi were not observed. We have previously reported the appearance of vascular injuries in cerebral arteries induced by intravascular platelet aggregation in vivo [5–7]. In this paper we describe the vascular injury and give our analysis of the mechanisms of these vascular changes and of brain edema.

Vascular Injuries Induced by Intravascular ADP Injection

Twenty-two white male rabbits were used. Under general anesthesia with sodium pentobarbital (50 mg/kg IP) a polyethylene catheter was inserted into the right external carotid artery and its tip was advanced to the carotid bifurcation. At 5 min after an IV injection of 100 units/kg heparin, 40 mg/kg ADP (Sigma, concentration 60 mg/ml) was injected through the catheter into the right internal carotid artery over 1 min. Immediately after and at 5, 15, and 60 min after the ADP injection, animals were sacrificed. At 30 min after the injection of ADP, 1 ml/kg 2% Evans blue was used as a marker to show disturbance of the BBB. Small pieces of the middle cerebral artery in the subarachnoid space were taken and fixed with 1% glutaraldehyde-2% paraformaldehyde in 0.1 *M* phosphate buffer (pH 7.4). They were postfixed with 1% osmium tetroxide in the buffer for 90 min at 4 °C. Ultrathin sections were double-stained with uranyl acetate and lead citrate and observed in an electron microscope (JEM-100S, JEOL, Japan) at 80 kV.

---

[1] Department of Neurosurgery, Showa University Fujigaoka Hospital, 1-30 Fujigaoka, Midori-ku, Yokohama 227, Japan

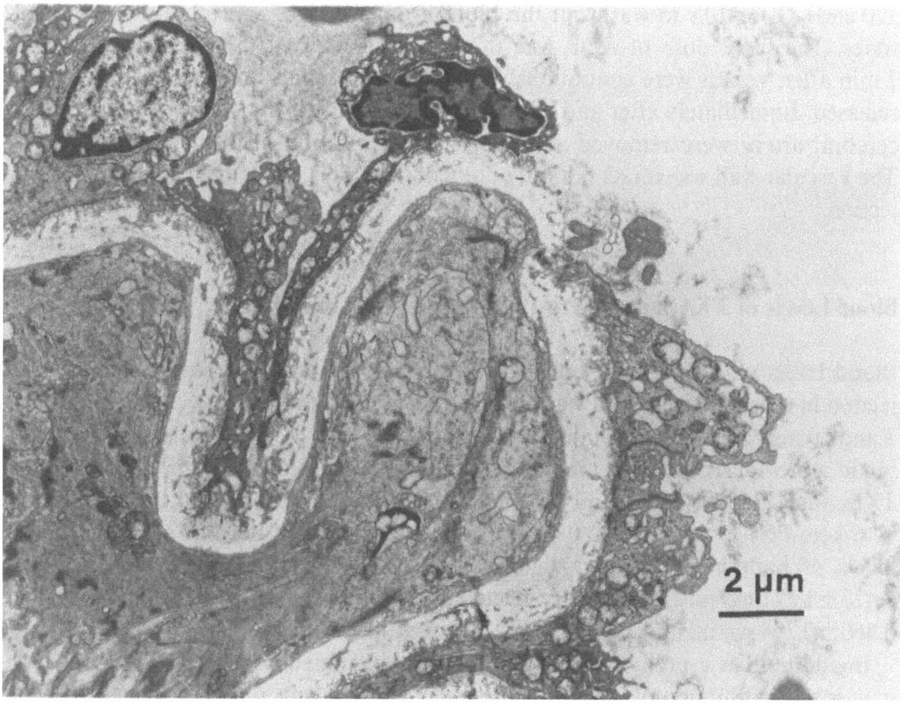

Fig. 1. Middle cerebral artery 60 min after an injection of ADP. Vacuolizations in the endothelial cells and tortuosity of internal elastic lamina are obvious. Vacuole formations and edematous changes in subendothelial and muscular layers are also seen

One hour after the injection of ADP, blue staining with Evans blue was seen only on the injection side of the hemisphere in 80% of the animals. This suggests that the BBB is impaired.

Electron microscopic examination revealed small aggregates of platelets immediately after the injection in the middle cerebral artery, but the vascular wall was intact. Five minutes later, sporadic formation of intracytoplasmic vacuoles (1.0–2.0 µm in diameter) in the endothelial cells was seen. Slight tortuosity of the vessel wall was also observed. By 1 h after the injection pronounced tortuosity of internal elastic lamina and abundant intracytoplasmic vacuole formation were seen (Fig. 1). De-endothelialization was observed in parts and platelets had adhered in such regions. Edematous changes in the subendothelial layer and smooth muscle cells were also observed. Endothelial junctions were still well preserved. These changes were noticed only at the injection side.

Intravascular ADP Injection in Absence of Blood

To clarify the role of platelets in this model, we injected ADP in the absence of blood. The right common carotid artery was clamped, and warmed physiological saline was injected through the catheter into the internal carotid artery at a pressure of

120 cmH_2O for 10 s to wash out the blood from the right carotid and cerebral arteries. The same dose of ADP was then injected. During the injection and until 1 min after, vessels were continuously irrigated with saline, and the clamp was then released. Immediately after and at 5 and 60 min after the injection pieces of middle cerebral artery were removed and prepared for electron-microscopic observation. The vascular wall was intact not only immediately after but also 60 min after the injection.

Blood Levels of TXA_2 and 6-Keto-$PGF_{1\alpha}$ After ADP Injection

Blood levels of TXB_2 and 6-keto-$PGF_{1\alpha}$ were measured before and after ADP injection in nine rabbits. Blood was collected from the right jugular vein before and at 3 and 60 min after the ADP injection. TXB_2 and 6-keto-$PGF_{1\alpha}$ were assayed according to a previously reported method [8]. Before the ADP injection, the blood level of TXB_2 was 0.346 ± 0.143 ng/ml (mean and standard deviation), and the blood level of 6-keto-$PGF_{1\alpha}$ was 0.833 ± 0.403 ng/ml. By 3 min after the injection, the blood levels of both had increased significantly, to 1.266 ± 0.741 ng/ml ($P<0.02$) and 5.427 ± 1.521 ng/ml ($P<0.001$), respectively. By 60 min after, they had returned to 0.460 ± 0.294 ng/ml and 1.342 ± 0.707 ng/ml, respectively.

In addition, as a preliminary experiment we examined whether OKY-046, which is a specific inhibitor of TXA_2 synthetase, provided any protection against these vascular injuries. In only one of five animals pretreated with OKY-046 was there some slight extravasation of Evans blue. In contrast, in four of the five animals not pretreated marked extravasation was observed.

Mechanisms of the Vascular Injury and Brain Edema

With the object of analyzing the mechanisms of this reaction, and especially of observing the appearance of brain edema, we injected horseradish peroxidase (HRP, Type VI, Sigma, USA) as a tracer to 12 rabbits. The procedure for this experiment was the same. Small pieces of middle cerebral artery and brain cortex were removed and fixed with 1% glutaraldehyde-2% paraformaldehyde. Sections (40 μm) of the samples were cut off with a vibratome. These sections were incubated for 60 min in modified Graham-Karnowsky medium (0.05 *M* Tris-HCl buffer, pH 7.6, 10 ml containing 0.002% H_2O_2 and 5 mg 3-3′-diaminobenzidine tetrahydrochloride DBA, grade II, Sigma, USA). They were postfixed with 1% osmium tetroxide. After embedding in Epon 812, ultrathin sections stained with uranyl acetate and lead citrate or unstained sections were examined under electron microscope.

By 5 min after the injection of ADP, numbers of small vesicles (0.05–0.2 μm in diameter) containing black HRP reaction products were seen on the injection side. Vacuoles (1.0–2.0 μm in diameter) were seen sporadically in the cytoplasm of the endothelial cells. These vacuoles did not contain HRP reaction products. Over five times as many vesicles were present on the injection side as on the noninjection side. By 60 min after the injection, many intracytoplasmic vacuoles were observed in the endothelial cells on the injection side only. In these endothelial cells, the cytoplasm

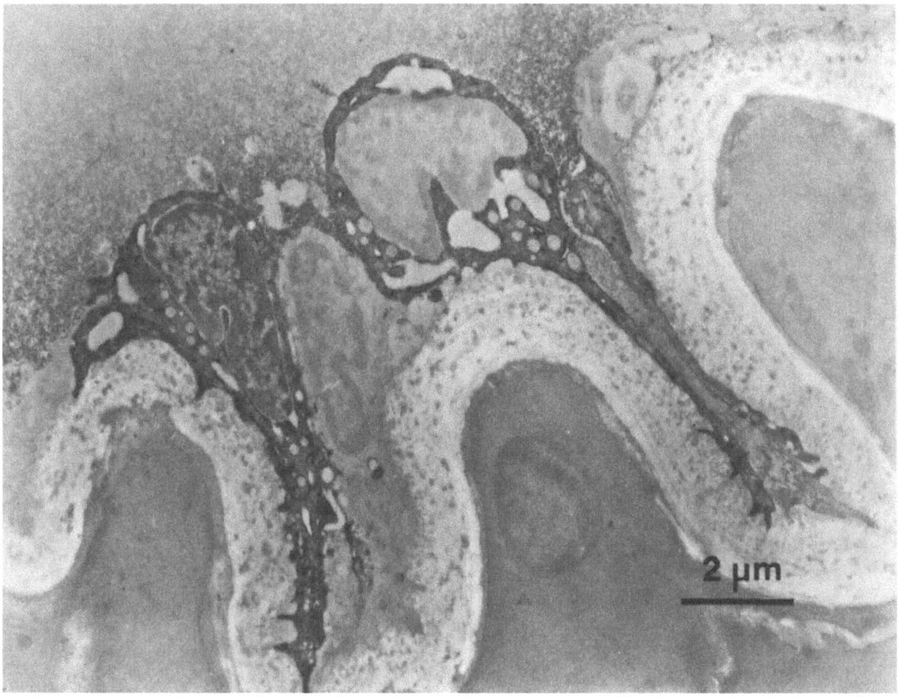

Fig. 2. Middle cerebral artery 60 min after injection, nonstaining condition. Many intracytoplasmic vacuoles can be observed in the endothelial cells and the cytoplasm of these endothelial cells is filled with black HRP reaction products. Even in these arteries, extravasation of HRP reaction products is not clear

was filled with black HRP reaction products. Tortuosity of the internal elastic lamina was prominent. Even in these arteries, extravasation of HRP reaction products into the subendothelial and muscular layers was not clear in nonstaining sections (Fig. 2). On the other hand, in the capillaries in the cortex, endothelial cell damage seemed to be different from that observed in the middle cerebral artery. At 15 min after the injection, the numbers and sizes of HRP-positive vesicles in endothelial cells were increased, but vacuoles were rarely observed. At 60 min after an injection, various sizes and numbers of HRP-positive vesicles were increased in the endothelial cells, while HRP-negative vacuoles were rarely seen. Prominent extravasation of black HRP reaction products into the perivascular area with edematous changes was seen only on the injection side. Extravasated HRP reaction products were diffusely distributed in the interstitial space (Fig. 3). Even in these capillaries, tight junctions were well preserved (Fig. 4). These changes were never seen in the noninjection side.

Discussion

The injuries were not produced when the blood was washed out with physiological saline. In attempting to decide what the main causes of these vascular injuries are it

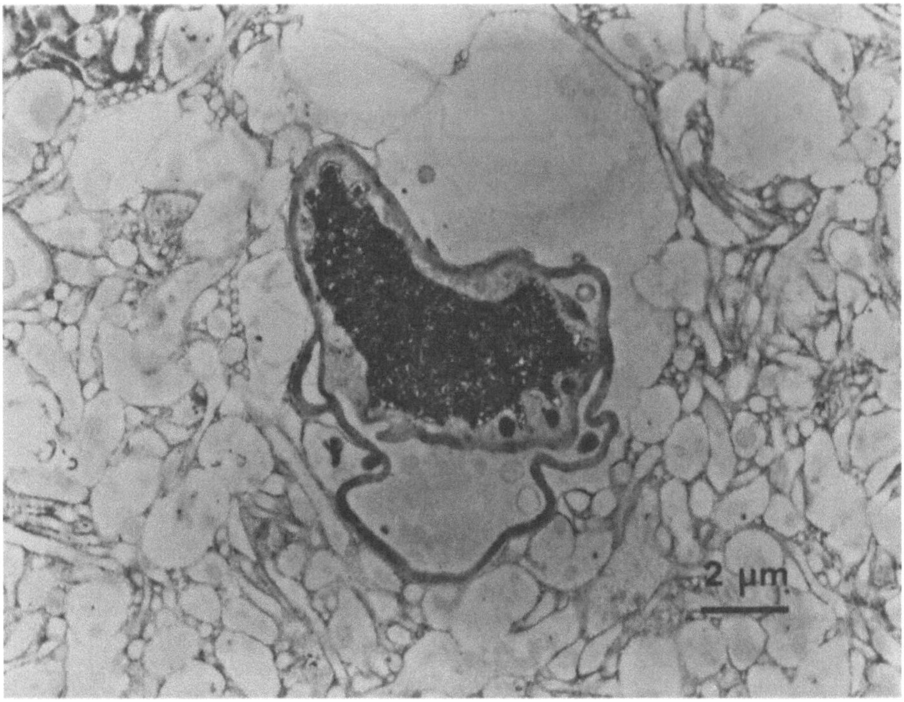

Fig. 3. Capillary in the cortex on the injection side 60 min after an injection. Nonstaining section. Various sizes and numbers of HRP-positive vesicles are increased in endothelial cells, but few HRP-negative vacuoles are present. Prominent perivascular edematous changes are revealed

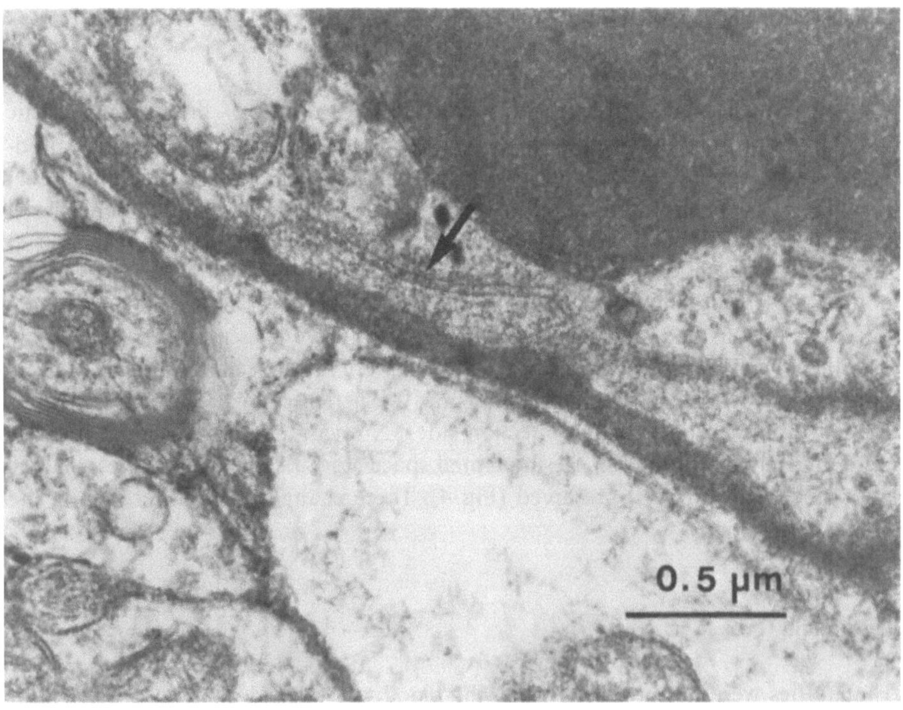

Fig. 4. The same case as in Fig. 3, nonstaining condition. Extravasation of HRP reaction product is obvious, but the tight junction (*arrow*) is well preserved

may be necessary to consider the involvement of ischemia induced by platelet aggregation and thrombus. However, the platelet aggregates were easily disaggregated within a short time, and we could not find any obstruction in blood vessels with platelet aggregate, even at 5 min after the injection. Thus, ischemia seemed not to be the main cause.

Substances released from platelets must be considered as one of the important causes of these vascular injuries, because of their strong vasoactive effects. The blood level of TXB_2, which is the terminal product of TXA_2, increased to four to five times the preinjection level. Simultaneously, 6-keto-$PGF_{1\alpha}$ which is a terminal product of PGI_2, was also found to increase markedly. This phenomanon may provide a protective mechanism against thrombus formation.

Our results suggest that vasoactive substances resulting from activation of platelets in vivo may play an important part in the production of these vascular injuries and brain edema. Platelet aggregation may commonly occur not only in cerebral infarction, but also in various pathologic conditions. Understanding of the pathophysiologic mechanism and treatment of various vascular diseases will require careful attention to this phenomenon.

Summary

Vasoactive substances which are released from activated platelets are considered because of their marked effects. We have observed the details of cerebrovascular injuries and brain edema produced by intravascular platelet aggregation induced by ADP injection into the carotid artery of rabbits. Intracytoplasmic vacuole formation and partial de-endothelialization were characteristic changes in the middle cerebral artery. These vacuoles did not contain horseradish peroxidase, which was used as a marker for changes in vascular permeability. Compared with these phenomena, increased vesicular transport in capillaries and perivascular edema were prominent in the cortex, and vacuole formation was rarely seen. Endothelial cell damage seemed to be more prominent in large arteries, but only the capillaries showed remarkable perivascular edematous changes. Blood levels of TXB_2 and 6-keto-$PGF_{1\alpha}$ were significantly increased 3 min after the ADP injection and returned to preinjection levels at 60 min after. Our results suggest that vasoactive substances released from activated platelets may play an important role in producing these cerebrovascular injuries and brain edema.

References

1. Mustard JF, Packham MA (1975) The role of blood and platelets in atherosclerosis and the complication of atherosclerosis. Thromb Diath Haemorrh 33:444–456
2. Jørgensen L, Rowsell HG, Hovig T, Glynn MS, Mustard JF (1976) Adenosine diphosphate-induced platelet aggregation and myocardial infarction in swine. Lab Invest 17:616–644
3. Furlow TW, Bass NH (1975) Stroke in rats produced by carotid injection of sodium arachidonate. Science 187:658–660
4. Fischi C, Battistini N, Volante F, Zanette E, Weber G, Passere S (1975) Animal model of TIA: an experimental study with intracarotid ADP infusion in rabbits. Stroke 6:617–621

5. Fujimoto T, Inaba Y, Motomiya T, Yamazaki H (1980) Intravascular aggregation of platelets and cerebrovascular insufficiency. In: Spatz M (ed) Circulatory and developmental aspects of brain metabolism. Plenum, New York, pp 169–180
6. Yamazaki H, Motomiya T, Fujimoto T (1980) Vascular injuries induced by intravascular platelet aggregation. Acta Hematol Jpn 43:208–216
7. Fujimoto T, Suzuki H, Tanoue K, Fukushima Y, Yamazaki H (1985) Cerebrovascular injuries induced by activation of platelets in vivo. Stroke 16:245–250
8. Yamazaki H, Isohisa I, Tanoue K (1983) Sudden death induced by intracoronary platelet aggregation. Jpn Circulation J 47:596–607

Oxygen-Free Radicals: Potential Edema Mediators in Brain Injury *

P. H. CHAN [1], S. LONGAR, and A. FISHMAN

Introduction

During the past few decades, a large body of experimental data has accumulated indicating that the biological reduction of molecular oxygen could yield dangerously reactive-free radical intermediates [14]. In mammalian cells, various subcellular membranous structures and cytosolic compartments are sites of production of oxygen radicals [15]. It has been demonstrated that about 2%–5% of the electron flow in isolated mitochondria goes to produce superoxide ($O_2\cdot-$) and hydrogen peroxide (H_2O_2) [3]. Under normal metabolic conditions, these oxygen radicals formed by mitochondria and other sources are constantly scavenged by endogenous enzymes (superoxide dismutase, catalase, glutathione peroxidase, etc.) and antioxidants (vitamin E, glutathione, vitamin C, etc.). However, pathologic insults such as ischemia and injury cause perturbation of this defense mechanism and the overproduction of oxygen radicals and lipid peroxidation [4, 12, 13, 20]. Moreover, the release of free polyunsaturated fatty acids (PUFAs) from phospholipids of damaged membranes also contributes to the formation of oxygen radicals. The conversion of PGG_2 to PGH_2, HPETE to HETE, and HPETE to leukotriene A_4 (LTA_4) will produce the active oxygen radical species [21, 23]. The pathologic role of these oxygen radicals in CNS injury is not clear. Using cortical brain slices as an in vitro bioassay system, we have demonstrated that oxygen radicals produced by an exogenous xanthine oxidase system induce lipid peroxidation and the development of cellular (cytotoxic) edema [6]. Furthermore, membrane phospholipids of synaptosomes were degraded and the levels of free fatty acids, arachidonic acid (20:4) and docosahexaenoic acid (22:6), in particular, were increased significantly following the incubation of oxygen radicals [6, 11]. These data led us to propose the hypothesis that oxygen radical-induced membrane perturbation and activation of membrane phospholipase A_2 may play an important role in the pathogenesis of brain edema following brain ischemia and injury [5]. The purpose of the present study is to investigate the focal effects in vivo of intracerebral enzymatically generated oxygen radicals on membrane phospholipid degradation, free fatty acid accumulation, and the development of vasogenic brain edema. The beneficial effects of dexamethasone, a membrane-stabilizing agent and inhibitor of phospholipase A_2, on both membrane phospholipid degradation and edema development were also investigated.

---

* The work described in this paper was supported by the NIH Brain Edema Research Center (grant no. 2 POI-14 543-07).

[1] Brain Edema Clinical Research Center, Department of Neurology, University of California, School of Medicine, San Francisco, CA 94143, USA

Materials and Methods

Male Sprague-Dawley rats, weight 200±20 g, were anesthetized with pentobarbital (50 mg/kg body weight IP). These spontaneously breathing animals were placed in a stereotaxic head-frame (Trent Wells, Inc., South Gate, Calif). One of the following: saline (0.1 ml, pH adjusted to 7.4 with NaOH); a mixture of xanthine oxidase (0.4 units); hypoxanthine (0.1 m*M*); ADP (0.1 m*M*) and $FeCl_3$ (0.01 m*M*) solution in saline buffer (pH 7.4); or a mixture of hypoxanthine, ADP, and $FeCl_3$ in the absence of xanthine oxidase, was infused into the caudate putamen of the right hemisphere through a 22-gauge spinal needle at a rate of 6.7 µl per min for 15 min, regulated by a Harvard pump. The coordinates measured from the bregma were anterior 1.4 mm, lateral 3 mm and ventral 6 mm. The body temperature was maintained at 37 °C by a heating lamp according to our previous method [10]. The mean arterial blood pressure (MABP), blood gases, and blood pH were monitored. The animals were killed by in situ rapid freezing with liquid nitrogen. The frozen brain was dissected by an Orthopower reciprocating saw and irrigated with liquid nitrogen during the dissecting process. Approximately 200 mg tissue was dissected and quickly immersed in liquid nitrogen for further biochemical analysis [10]. One group of animals ($n=7$) received injections of dexamethasone (10 mg/kg body weight IM) 24 h before the infusion of xanthine oxidase. Another group ($n=5$) was injected with dexamethasone 2 h after infusion of the xanthine oxidase system.

Separation of Phospholipids and Free Fatty Acids

Membrane phospholipids were extracted with chloroform and methanol (2:1, v/v). The various phospholipids, free fatty acids, and neutral lipids were further separated by high-performance liquid chromatography (1082B liquid chromatography, Hewlett Packard, Palo Alto, Calif) using a silica column (Micro-Pak Si-5, 30 cm ×4 mm ID, Varian Assoc., Palo Alto, Calif) according to the method already described elsewhere [8]. The HPLC was equipped with a variable wavelength detector (190–600 nm) and a stop-flow scanning spectrophotometer. The gradient began with an initial mobile phase of 4% H_2O in hexane/2-propanol (3:4, v/v), and was increased to 9% H_2O at 10 min and maintained at 9% H_2O for another 10 min, followed by 4% H_2O at 25 min as described previously [8]. Flow rate was maintained at 1 ml/min. Elution was monitored at 206 nm with recorder response at 0.0512 AU (absorbance units)/cm.

Fatty Acid Analysis

The free fatty acid peaks eluted from the HPLC were pooled and subjected to methylation [8]. The fatty acid methylesters were analyzed by means of a gas chromatograph (Hewlett Packard 5830A) equipped with a silica capillary column (0.25 mm ID×30 m, Supelco). The flow rate was 1 ml/per min. The initial column temperature was 40 °C for 0.5 min and was then increased to 210 °C and held at this level for 9 min. Injector and detector were both set at a temperature of 250 °C. A known concentration of heptadecanoic acid (17:0) was routinely added to the samples as an internal standard [8].

Results

Oxygen-Free Radicals and Brain Edema

Two hours after the infusion of xanthine oxidase (0.4 units/0.1 ml), hypoxanthine, ADP, and Fe^{3+}, the H_2O content of the infused right hemisphere rose to 80.6% from 78.7%, a 1.9% increase ($P < 0.001$; Table 1). The edema progressed to reach a maximum at 24–48 h, and had later significantly declined at 1 and 2 weeks (data not shown). The Na^+ content of the caudate putamen, infused with xanthine oxidase and substrates, was increased significantly, and there was a concomitant slight decrease in K^+ content at 2 h. The sodium content of the contralateral caudate putamen increased to a lesser extent, indicating possible bulk flow of Na^+-containing edema fluid across the corpus callosum from the region of injury. There were no changes in Na^+, K^+, or water content in hemispheres infused with saline or with the substrates without xanthine oxidase.

Oxygen-Free Radicals and Membrane Phospholipid Degradation

Table 2 shows the total phospholipid phosphorous content in both control and oxygen radical-infused caudate putamen. The membrane phospholipid was degraded by 11%, 8%, and 9% at 30 min, 2 h, and 24 h, respectively, following the infusion of oxygen radicals. The effects of oxygen radicals on the total fatty acids at 24 h are shown in Table 3. The cerebral levels of saturated fatty acids, palmitic acid (16:0) and stearic acid (18:0), were slightly decreased. The monounsaturated oleic acid (18:1) was not affected. Among the PUFAs, the level of docosahexaenoic acid (22:6) was significantly decreased, whereas that of arachidonic acid (20:4) was slightly affected. Table 4 shows the levels of free fatty acids in caudate putamen following exposure to the oxygen-free radicals. The levels of free fatty acids were increased four- to sevenfold. Arachidonic acid (20:4) and docosahexaenoic acid (22:6) were the most markedly affected free fatty acids in brain. These data indicate

Table 1. Effects of oxygen-free radicals on cerebral H_2O, Na^+, and K^+ contents

Time	H_2O	Na^+ (mEq/kg dry wt)	K^+ (mEq/kg dry wt)
Control (11)	78.6±0.3	300±11	434± 8
2 h (5)	80.6±0.1*	571±62	385± 6*
24 h (11)	84.5±0.5*	811±53*	260±23*
48 h (5)	83.5±0.2*	627±23*	360±56

Means±SEM. Figures in parentheses give number of animals in each case
* Statistically significant difference from control group ($P < 0.01$)

Table 2. Effects of intracerebral infusion of xanthine oxidase/ Fe^{3+} on levels of total phospholipid phosporus

Time	Total phospholipid phosphorus (nmol mg protein^{-1})	Change (%)
Control (zero)	473± 7 (20)	–
30 min	420±31 (4)*	–11%
2 h	435±25 (4)*	– 8%
24 h	431±30 (8)*	– 9%

Means±SEM. Figures in parentheses give number of animals in each case
* Statistically significant difference from control group ($P<0.01$)

Table 3. Effects of oxygen radicals on total fatty acid contents in caudate putamen

	Fatty acid content (nmol mg protein^{-1})				
	16:0	18:0	18:1	20:4	22:6
Control (22)	210±29	253±20	186±29	95±12	119±0
Xanthine oxidase + Fe^{3+} (4)	129±20	208±36	183±23	72±10	67±7*

Means±SEM. Figures in parentheses give number of animals in each case
* Statistically significant difference from control group ($P<0.01$)

that phospholipases A_2 and A_1 were both affected by oxygen radicals. These data thus confirmed the results obtained in our in vitro studies, which showed that enzymatically generating oxygen-free radicals stimulate the release of free fatty acids from synaptosomal membrane preparations [9, 11].

Effects of Dexamethasone on Oxygen Radical-Induced Brain Edema and Levels of Free Fatty Acids

The effects of glucocorticoids upon free radical-induced injury was studied by pretreatment with dexamethasone (10 mg/kg) given 24 h before the infusion of xanthine oxidase –Fe^{3+}. Twenty-four hours later, a slight reduction of free arachidonic acid and a significant reduction of docosahexaenoic acid was noted with a concomitant significant reduction in cerebral edema (Table 5). Furthermore, the cerebral levels of Na^+ were decreased associated with the increase in K^+. Dexamethasone was not effective in ameliorating brain edema and free PUFAs when the animals were treated 2 h after the infusion of xanthine oxidase –Fe^{3+}.

Table 4. Effects of oxygen radicals on free fatty acid contents in caudate putamen

	Free fatty acid content (nmol mg protein^{-1})				
	16:0	18:0	18:1	20:4	22:6
Control (22)	0.35±0.02	0.37±0.04	0.16±0.02	0.06±0.02	0.05±0.01
Xanthine oxidase/ Fe^{3+} (11)	1.50±0.26*	1.52±0.26*	0.60±0.01*	0.37±0.01*	0.36–0.05*
Increase (fold)	4.3	4.1	3.8	6.2	7.2

Means ± SEM. Figures in parentheses give number of animals in each case
* Statistically significant difference from control group ($P < 0.05$)

Table 5. Effects of dexamethasone on brain water, sodium, potassium and polyunsaturated fatty acids in oxygen radical-injured rat brain

Components	No treatment	Treatment 2 h after infusion	Treatment 24 h before infusion
H_2O (%)	84.45± 0.5 (11)	85.4 ± 0.4 (5)	80.8 ± 0.8 (7)**
Na^+ (mEq/kg dw)	811 ±33 (11)	1072 ±11 (5)	507 ±34 (7)*
K^+ (mEq/kg dw)	260 ±23 (11)	232 ±21 (5)	382 ±32 (7)*
20:4	0.37± 0.01 (22)	0.26± 0.04 (4)	0.29± 0.04 (4)
22:6	0.36± 0.05 (22)	0.20± 0.04 (4)	0.13± 0.02 (4)**

Means ± SEM. Figures in parentheses give number of animals in each case
Free fatty acids content is given in nanomoles per milligram of protein
* $P < 0.05$, ** $P < 0.01$, for difference from no-treatment group

Discussion

The present data demonstrate that enzymatically generated oxygen-derived free radicals, when infused intracerebrally into rats, induce both cellular injury and edema as well as changes in membrane integrity. The time course of cellular injury and edema was similar to that of the edema induced by cold injury [9] or intracerebral infusion of arachidonic acid [7]. Our previous fluorescence microscopy studies have shown that abundant extravasation of Evans blue was found in the injured caudate putamen area 2 h after the infusion of oxygen radicals [10]. These studies suggest that endothelial cells of capillaries may be important targets for the action of free radicals. However, they do not address the question as to whether free radicals directly cause an increase in brain endothelial cell permeability or, less probably, whether the change in the blood-brain barrier is a result of glial or neuronal injury with secondary effects on endothelial permeability.

Our studies have also demonstrated that pretreatment with a high dose of dexamethasone exhibits beneficial effects in ameliorating brain edema and the reduction of the free docosahexaenoic acid content. It has been suggested that dexamethasone and other glucocorticoids may intercalate into membrane phospholipids and stabilize the membrane against free radical attack [16]. On the other hand, glucocorticoids stimulate the production of lipomodulin from the leukocytes and the production of macrocortin from macrophages and lung cells [2, 17]. The two proteins are immunologically similar and act as potent inhibitors of membrane phospholipase A_2. Our early in vitro work has demonstrated that phospholipase A_2, the rate-limiting enzyme in deacylation of arachidonic acid and docosahexaenoic acid from membrane phospholipids, has been shown to be activated by free radicals [11]. Thus, glucocorticoids may exert their antiedema effect through the inhibition of the release of arachidonic acid [19]. This view has been questioned by Pappius and Wolfe, who have shown that glucocorticoids fail to reduce the high level of the arachidonic acid accumulated in cold-injured rat brain [22]. However, the recent work of Bazan et al. [1] has clearly demonstrated that dexamethasone at a dose about five to ten times higher than the dosage used by Pappius and Wolfe reduced both the cerebral edema and the free arachidonic acid content in cold-injured rat brain. The discrepancy in the data obtained from these two groups seems to have resulted from differences in dosage regimen and in the times chosen for the endpoint measurements. Our present studies demonstrate the beneficial effects of glucocorticoids on the reduction of the level of PUFAs, docosahexaenoic acid in particular, in oxygen radical-injured rat brain. These effects are analogous to the effects of steroids on the vasogenic edema induced by intracerebral arachidonic acid or by a freezing lesion. The therapeutic value of glucocorticoids on brain edema may result from a combination of membrane-stabilizing effects and by stimulating the synthesis of phospholipase A_2 inhibitory protein. Further studies are necessary to elucidate these possibilities.

Acknowledgements. We thank Mrs. Sheryl Colwell for editorial assistance.

Summary

Superoxide anion ($O_2{\cdot}-$), hydrogen peroxide (H_2O_2) and hydroxyl radicals ($\cdot OH$) are produced in biological systems by the single-electron reduction of oxygen. These oxygen radicals are highly reactive and cause the peroxidation of membrane phospholipids and the oxidation of cellular protein and DNA. It has been suggested that these oxygen radicals may play a role in brain injury, ischemia, reperfusion, hypoxia and other pathologic insults. The present investigation deals with the direct effects of oxygen radicals on membrane phospholipid degradation and the development of brain edema. Intracerebral injection of oxygen radicals generated from an enzymatic system (xanthine oxidase/hypoxanthine/ADP-Fe^{3+}) caused a time-dependent evolution of brain edema with early changes in vascular permeability. Free fatty acids, arachidonic acid (20:4) and docosahexaenoic acid (22:6) in particular, were increased 11.9-fold and 7.6-fold at 24 h concomitant with decreases in the 20:4 and 22:6 fatty acid constituents of various phospholipids as measured by high-performance liquid chromatography (HPLC) and gas chromatography (GC). Thus, oxygen-free radicals induce rapid release of polyunsaturated fatty acids (PUFAs) from membrane phospholipids. Pretreatment with a high dose of dexamethasone reduced the free-radical-induced brain edema and the release of free PUFAs. We propose that oxygen-free radicals activate membrane phospholipase A_2 and the subsequent development of edema and necrosis.

References

1. Bazan NG, Rodriguez de Turco EB, Politi E (1984) Dexamethasone inhibits the production of free arachidonic acid in cryogenic brain edema. Trans Am Soc Neurochem 15:105
2. Blackwell GJ, Carnuccio R, Di Rosa M, Flower RJ, Parente L, Persico P (1980) Macrocortin: a polypeptide causing the anti-phospholipase effect of glycocorticoids. Nature 287:147–149
3. Boveris A, Chance B (1973) The mitochondrial generation of hydrogen peroxide. Biochem J 134:707–716
4. Chan PH, Fishman RA (1980) Transient formation of superoxide radicals in polyunsaturated fatty acid-induced brain swelling. J Neurochem 35:1004–1007
5. Chan PH, Fishman RA (1985) Free fatty acids, oxygen free radicals and membrane alterations in brain ischemia and injury. In: Plum F, Pulsinelli W (eds) Cerebrovascular disease (14th Princeton-Williamsburg Research Conference on Cerebrovascular Diseases). Raven, New York, pp 161–169
6. Chan PH, Yurko M, Fishman RA (1982) Phospholipid degradation and cellular edema induced by free radicals in brain cortical slices. J Neurochem 38:525–531
7. Chan PH, Fishman RA, Caronna J, Schmidley JW, Prioleau G, Lee J (1983a) Induction of brain edema following intracerebral injection of arachidonic acid. Ann Neurol 13:625–632
8. Chan PH, Fishman RA, Chen S, Chew S (1983b) Effects of temperature on arachidonic acid-induced cellular edema and membrane perturbation in rat brain cortical slices. J Neurochem 41:1550–1557
9. Chan PH, Longar S, Fishman RA (1983c) Phospholipid degradation and edema development in cold-injured rat brain. Brain Res 277:329–337
10. Chan PH, Schmidley JW, Fishman RA, Longar SM (1984) Brain injury, edema and vascular permeability changes induced by oxygen-derived free radicals. Neurology 34:315–320
11. Chan PH, Fishman RA, Schmidley JW, Chen SF (1984) Release of polyunsaturated fatty acids from phospholipids and alteration of brain membrane integrity by oxygen-derived free radicals. J Neurosci Res 12:595–605
12. Demopoulos HB, Flamm E, Seligman M, Pietronigro DD (1982) Oxygen free radicals in central nervous system ischemia and trauma. In: Autor AP (ed) Pathology of oxygen. Academic, New York, pp 127–155
13. Flamm ES, Demopoulos HB, Seligman ML, Poser RG, Ransohoff J (1978) Free radicals in cerebral ischemia. Stroke 9:445–447
14. Fridovich I (1982) Superoxide dismutase in biology and medicine. In: Autor AP (ed) Pathology of oxygen. Academic, London, pp 1–17
15. Freeman BA, Crapo JD (1982) Biology of disease. Free radicals and tissue injury. Lab Invest 47:412–426
16. Hall ED, Braughler JM (1982) Effects of intravenous methylprednisolone on spinal cord lipid peroxidation and ($Na^+ + K^+$)-ATPase activity. J Neurosurg 57:247–253
17. Hirata F, Schiffman E, Venkatasubramanian K, Salomon D, Axelrod J (1980) A phospholipase A_2 inhibitory protein in rabbit neuropils induced by glucocorticoids. Proc Natl Acad Sci USA 77:2533–2536
18. Hirata F, Notsu Y, Iwata M, Parente L, Di Rosa M, Flower RJ (1982) Identification of several species of phospholipase inhibitory protein(s) by radioimmunoassay for lipomodulin. Biochem Biophys Res Commun 109:223–230
19. Hong SC, Levine L (1976) Inhibition of arachidonic acid release from cells as the biochemical action of anti-inflammatory corticosteroids. Proc Natl Acad Sci USA 73:1730–1734
20. Kogure K, Watson BD, Busto R, Abe K (1982) Potentiation of lipid peroxides by ischemia in rat brain. Neurochem Res 7:437–454
21. Kuehl FA, Egan RN (1980) Prostaglandins, arachidonic acid, and inflammation. Science 210:978–984
22. Pappius HM, Wolfe LS (1983) Functional disturbances in brain following injury. Search for underlying mechanisms. Neurochem Res 8:63–72
23. Samuelsson B (1983) Leukotrienes: mediators of immediate hypersensitivity reactions and inflammation. Science 220:568–575

Reduction of Experimental Acute Ischaemic Cerebral Oedema with Zy15051

B. S. ASPEY [1], T. J. STEINER, and F. CLIFFORD ROSE

Key words: Cytotoxic oedema, vasogenic oedema, cerebral microembolism, cerebral ischaemia, catechin

Introduction

Cerebral microembolism of atherothrombotic elements is common and may be an important cause of cerebral infarction [6]. Emboli that are physically stable occlude small arteries or arterioles and, depending on their number, ischaemia may ensue. The relative importance of cytotoxic as opposed to vasogenic oedema in the subsequent series of pathological events is equally determined by the number and the distribution of occlusive lesions [3]. Both may be important to clinical outcome, and active measures against them would be therapeutically beneficial.

Zy15051 (Bencianol: Zyma), a catechin derivative, reduces microvascular permeability and oedema, and increases blood supply, in various noncerebral experimental models (Zyma SA Internal Reports). In this study, its effects on acute development of cerebral oedema, blood-brain barrier (BBB) breakdown, regional cerebral blood flow (rCBF) and ischaemic cellular death were assessed in a conscious animal model of microembolic cerebral ischaemia and infarction.

Methods

Animals

In all, 62 adult CFY albino rats (350–450 g) of either sex were used. The technique for conscious cerebral embolisation in this animal has been reported before [1], and will only be outlined here.

Under halothane anaesthesia, the left external carotid artery was cannulated, the tip of the cannula placed at the carotid bifurcation so that infusions would necessarily enter the common to internal carotid artery blood stream (Fig. 1). The cannula, led through a subcutaneous tunnel to a dorsal skin opening in the neck, passed through a protective wire tube and was infused with normal saline at 2 mg/h (Fig. 2) to maintain patency.

---

[1] The Reta Lila Weston Institute of Neurological Studies, The Middlesex Hospital, London, Great Britain

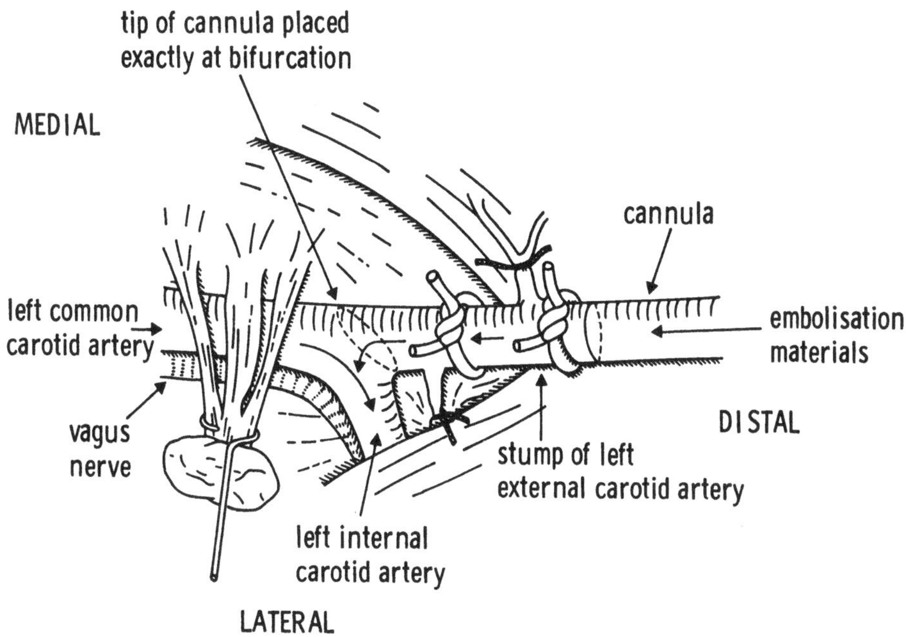

Fig. 1. Cannulation procedure. The view is of the ventral aspect of the neck with the head to the right

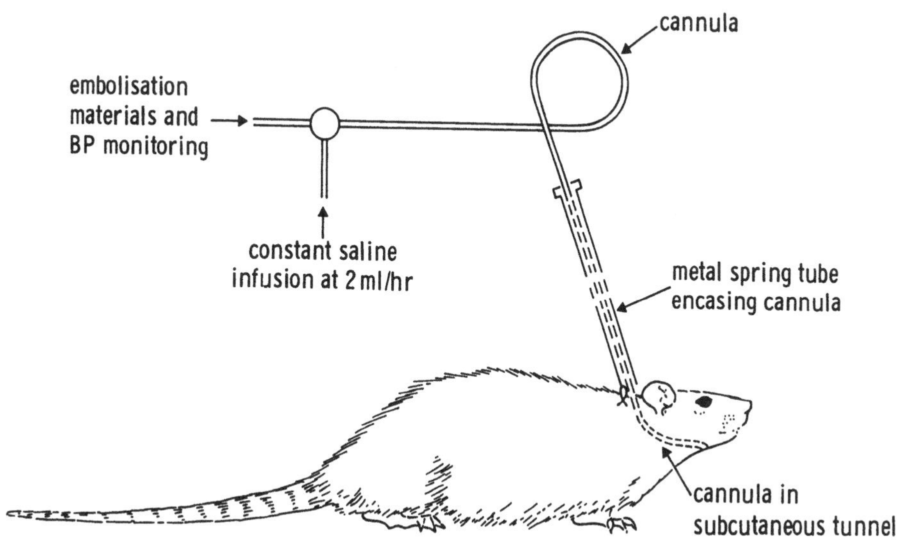

Fig. 2. Arrangement of cannula for free movement of the conscious animal

Approximately 24 h after recovery, animals were ready to be embolised. Blood pressures of all animals immediately beforehand ranged between 100 and 120 mmHg.

Embolic Material

The embolic material was human atheromatous material (HAM) from mature lesions in aortae obtained post mortem, suspended in sterile saline and homogenised to pass freely through a 30-gauge needle.

Administration of Zyl5051

Zyl5051 was administered IP in the recommended single dose of 50 mg/kg body weight, suspended in 10% cremophore (in saline) at a concentration of 25 mg/ml. The drug quickly settled in this suspension, and slight variations in delivery were unavoidable. The drug, or cremophore control, was administered 30 min after embolisation to give peak blood levels at approximately 1 h.

Assessment of Cerebral Oedema

Eighteen rats were embolised with approximately 2.0 mg HAM (dry weight). Nine later received Zyl5051 and nine the cremophore vehicle, and 6 h after embolisation all animals were decapitated and the brains removed rapidly. In a modification of the method of Elliot and Jasper [2], each cerebral hemisphere was weighed, dried at 110 °C for 24 h, and reweighed to determine water content.

Assessment of Blood-Brain Barrier Damage

Another 18 rats were embolised with approximately 1.75 mg HAM, and 9 were treated with Zyl5051, 9 with cremophore. At 4 h after embolisation all animals received a 0.5-ml intracarotid injection of Evans blue dye solution in saline (40 mg/ml) and 2 h later [8] they were decapitated; the brains were removed and photographed, first whole and then coronally sectioned in the middle cerebral artery territory.

Regional Cerebral Blood Flow Study

Eighteen rats embolised with approximately 1.75 mg HAM were treated 30 min later, nine with Zyl5051 and nine with cremophore. Indian ink infusion followed a modification of the method of Yamaguchi et al. [8]. Approximately 1 h after drug administration each animal was reanaesthetised with urethane (3.5 ml of 18% IP), and body temperature maintained. Via a laparotomy, the dorsal aorta was cannulated so that infusions would enter both common carotid and both vertebral arteries. Approximately 30 min later (2 h after embolisation), with blood pressure stable, 5 IU heparin and then 5 ml ink were infused at 100 mmHg and both external jugular veins were sectioned. After 2 min the animal was decapitated and the brain removed into 10% neutral formalin (in saline). The cerebrum was coronally sectioned at three levels through the middle cerebral artery territory and photographed.

Histological Assessment

Eight further rats were embolised with approximately 2.0 mg HAM, and four were treated with Zyl5051 and four with cremophore. After 6 h they were killed with barbiturate. The brains of these animals, together with ten brains embolised with 1.75 mg HAM (4 treated and 6 control) from the BBB study, were fixed in 10% neutral formal saline. A coronal slice in the middle cerebral artery territory of each, at the level of the optic chiasm, was embedded in paraffin, sectioned at 5 μm, and stained with haematoxylin and eosin. Infarcted areas were mapped and measured.

Results

Cerebral Oedema

The water contents of both cerebral hemispheres are given in Table 1. There was evidence of oedema in all cases on both sides, but it was much more pronounced in the embolised left hemisphere. Water contents were lower bilaterally in Zyl5051-treated animals, and significantly lower ($P=0.05$) on the left side. The net difference was about 5%, but assuming a baseline water content of 3.7 g per g dry tissue, this represents a reduction of more than 30% in the increase in water content (presumed to equate to oedema formation).

Table 1. The effect of Zy15051 on cerebral water content after embolisation

No. of rats	Embolic dose (mg HAM)	Treatment	Average water content of cerebrum (g H_2O/g dry tissue)	
			Left hemisphere	Right hemisphere
9	2.0	Zy15051	4.23 SD=0.21	3.72 SD=0.13
9	2.0	Cremophore control	4.46 SD=0.26 $P=0.05$	3.84 SD=0.17 $P<0.1$

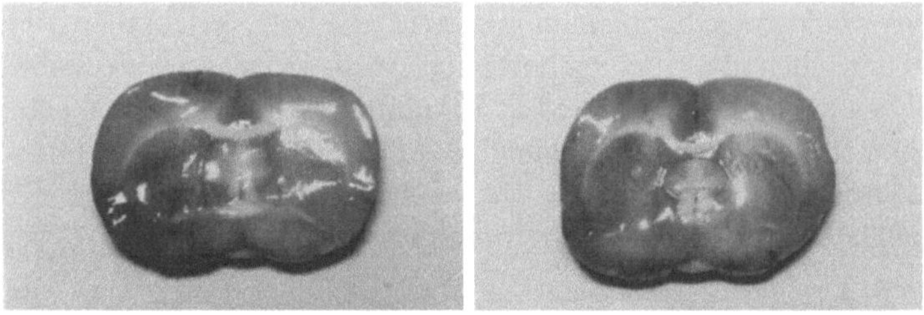

Fig. 3. Coronal sections, viewed from the posterior aspect, of (*left*) control and (*right*) Zyl5051-treated brains. Extravasation of Evans blue dye into the embolised left hemisphere is more severe in the control brain

Blood-Brain Barrier Damage

Intensity of staining varied quite widely in brains, whether Zyl5051-treated or control. Figure 3 shows coronal sections of two brains (treated and control) selected for a moderate degree of staining. Black-and-white photographs do not allow appreciation of the more subtly stained areas evident in colour slides, which revealed the presence of markedly more interstitial dye in the left hemispheres of all brains. In the control brains, most of the left cortex and basal ganglia were stained light blue, and more concentrated staining occurred in the dorsal and ventrolateral cortex. Despite a similar distribution of dye in the drug-treated brains and a variable intensity of staining within both groups, the amount of dye was noticeably less overall in Zyl5051-treated coronal sections, especially in the left ventrolateral cortex, than in control brains.

Regional Cerebral Blood Flow

The extent and location of the pale ischaemic areas also varied widely in brains from both groups. The left cortex was always much paler, especially dorsally and ventrolaterally. Occasional areas of the left caudate putamen nucleus were also affected. Areas in the left thalamus and hippocampus were noticeably involved. The extent and variability of this evidence of ischaemia were very similar in both groups of animals: no consistent differences could be observed.

Histology

Differences in the extent of ischaemic damage between treatment groups were not significant for either hemisphere or for either dose of HAM (Table 2). The location of damage was always similar, but it was more extensive with the higher dose of HAM. The dorsal cortex of the left hemisphere was most severely affected, but damage was recognisable in the other areas of observed ischaemia.

Table 2. The effect of Zy15051 on cerebral infarction

No. of rats	Embolic dose (mg HAM)	Treatment	Average percentage area of ischaemic damage	
			Left hemisphere	Right hemisphere
4	1.75	Zy15051	8.68 SD=4.42	0.31 SD=0.41
6	1.75	Cremophore control	5.72 SD=2.61	0.07 SD=0.17
4	2.0	Zy15051	13.08 SD=7.03	0.55 SD=0.64
4	2.0	Cremophore control	11.89 SD=5.67	0.43 SD=0.36

Discussion

In various non-cerebral experimental models, Zyl5051 has been shown to reduce oedema and microvascular permeability and to improve blood flow. Its effects on cerebral oedema have not previously been studied. Cerebral oedema in the ischaemic brain has been classified as cytotoxic or vasogenic [4], the relative importance of the two types in cerebral microembolism depending on the magnitude (size and number) of the embolic load [3]. Experimentally, massive microembolisation has initially produced cytotoxic oedema, which was later complicated by vasogenic oedema [5], whereas after a less severe insult vasogenic oedema resulting from microvascular damage has been the primary event [7]. Clinically, a variable combination of the two may be expected.

In previous studies in the conscious rat model (unpublished data), HAM emboli lodged in small arteries and arterioles, mainly in the distribution system of the middle cerebral artery. Of the two doses of HAM used here, the lower dose (1.75 mg) produced minor ischaemic damage in control animals but the higher dose (2.0 mg) caused death within 6–12 h. The cause was thought to be progressive cerebral oedema.

In the group of experiments assessing acute oedema, when the high dose of HAM was used Zyl5051 caused a mean reduction of about 30%, which was statistically significant ($P=0.05$). An association with other beneficial effects (on BBB and blood flow) might be expected. In the assessments of BBB damage and rCBF the lower dose of HAM was used, so that primary effects of Zyl5051 on these could be observed without massively complicating oedema. Zyl5051 may have given minor protection to the BBB, perhaps contributing to its anti-oedema properties (vasogenic). In the rCBF study, Indian ink was perfused only 2 h after embolisation to preclude extensive microvascular damage. Ischaemic areas were often larger than corresponding areas with the histological features of infarction, implying that some tissue was surviving after 6 h with a reduced blood supply. However, Zyl5051 had no evident effect on ischaemia or infarction during this time.

These experiments were not designed to observe long-term effects, but early histological assessment of the degree of infarction is an insensitive measure. The salient finding has been that acute cerebral oedema formation in ischaemic brain is inhibited, and a secondary benefit, implying improved prognosis in ischaemic stroke, may be apparent in the ultimate outcome, to be measured later.

Summary

Zyl5051 (Zyma), a catechin derivative, has anti-oedema effects in several experimental models. To assess its potential for use in stroke therapy, its activity was examined in a conscious animal model of embolic cerebral infarction.

Homogenised human atheromatous material was embolised, via an implanted cannula, into the left internal carotid artery of conscious rats 30 min before IP administration of 50 mg/kg Zyl5051[1] or inactive vehicle. In separate experimental groups of 18 animals the following were studied: acute cerebral oedema formation, by measurement of cerebral water content; breakdown of the blood-brain barrier, by extravasion of Evans blue dye; and regional cerebral blood flow, by intra-aortic injection of Indian ink. Histological changes were also observed.

References

1. Aspey BS (1983) Animal models of stroke – recent advances. In: Greenhalgh RM, Clifford Rose F (eds) Progress in stroke research, vol 2. Pitman, London, pp 37–47
2. Elliot KAC, Jasper H (1949) Measurement of experimentally induced brain swelling and shrinkage. Am J Physiol 157: 122–129
3. Hossmann K-A (1982) Review: treatment of experimental cerebral ischaemia. J Cereb Blood Flow Metab 2: 275–297
4. Klatzo I (1967) Presidential address: neuropathological aspects of brain edema. J Neuropathol Exp Neurol 26: 1–14
5. Kogure K, Busto R, Scheinberg P, Reinmuth OM (1974) Energy metabolites and water content during the early stage of development of cerebral infarction. Brain 97: 103–114
6. Rail DLH, Steiner TJ, Clifford Rose F (1981) Differential contributions of major lipid components of atheroma to outcome of cerebral atheroembolism. Stroke 12: 445–453
7. Vise WM, Schuier FJ, Hossmann K-A, Takagi S, Zulch KJ (1977) Cerebral microembolisation. I. Pathophysiological studies. Arch Neurol 34: 660–665
8. Yamaguchi M, Shirakata S, Yamasaki S, Matsumoto S (1976) Ischaemic brain edema and compression brain edema. Stroke 7: 77–82

[1] Zyl5051 produced a significant fall ($P = 0.05$) in cerebral water content, implying a 30% reduction in oedema formation, and a minor reduction in the extravasation of Evans blue dye. It had no beneficial effect on the extent of cerebral infarction apparent histologically at 6 h, or on the distribution of Indian ink at 2 h, both of which are insensitive measures of outcome. Although lacking measurable effects on tissue death or blood flow in this experimental model, Zyl5051 nevertheless had activity that might improve prognosis in some cases of stroke.

Brain Edema, Brain Water, and Aging

F. COHADON[1] and P. DESBORDES

Key words: Aging, brain edema, brain osmotic responses

Introduction

Some clinical features are characteristic of brain lesions in elderly patients: most of the time clinical signs of high intracranial pressure are absent; even large tumors develop without major displacements of brain structures and midline shifts: the edematous reaction surrounding the lesions is rarely significant, and for some lesions there is an age-dependent reduction in edema formation: for example, in a series of hemispheric metastases there is a significant negative correlation between the amount of edema and the age of the patient ($P<0.001$). On the other hand there is a striking susceptibility of the brain to osmotic stress: even limited variations of serum osmolarity can result in severe and long-lasting clinical disorders.

Most of these features commonly encountered in old age can be explained by the well-documented age-related reduction of brain mass with concomitant enlargement of highly compliant CSF spaces [11]. However, a number of clinical observations suggest that abnormal brain water responses might also be involved.

In an attempt to increase our understanding of these problems a simple experiment was designed to compare the response of brain water and Na/K/ATPase activity in two groups of rats (Long Evans) aged 60 ± 5 days (group I) and 630 ± 10 days (group II) subjected to (a) a cryogenic lesion of the right hemisphere, (b) acute hypernatremia, and (c) acute hypo-osmotic loading.

Result

Control Groups

Water Content

In control animals the water content of the brain was lower in group II ($P<0.005$). Brain water content related to age has been assessed in a number of animal species and in humans with inconsistent results. In the rat, the present results are in keeping with those already published [3, 8].

[1] Laboratoire de Neuro-chirurgie Expérimentale et Neurobiologie E.R.A. C.N.R.S. n° 843 – Université de Bordeaux II, B.P. 48 33076, Bordeaux, France

Na/K/ATPase
Ouabain-sensitive Na/K/ATPase of the plasmic membrane plays a major role in cation transport, and hence in the regulation of intracellular water balance. In this laboratory, in adult normal animals a highly significant correlation has been found between brain water content and enzyme activity [2]. In this study, Na/K/ATPase activity was lowered in group II ($P<0.02$). Similar results have already been found in rats [9, 10].

Cryogenic Lesions

Following a classical cryogenic lesion, the total amount of edema at 24 h was smaller in group II ($P<0.05$). Conversely, the reduction of Na/K/ATPase activity is much more pronounced in group II ($P<0.01$) (Table 1).

In group I and group II there is a significant correlation between the total amount of edema and Na/K/ATPase activity (group 1: $P<0.05$; group II: $P<0.001$). The slopes of linear regression in the two groups are different ($P<0.01$), however.

Hypernatremia

Acute hypernatremia (IP injection of 150 ml of 7.5% NaCl, sacrifice 60 min later) produced a severe osmotic shift of water from the brain (Table 2).

The increase in natremia and the decrease in brain water were more pronounced in old age, the two phenomena being roughly proportional. Na/K/ATPase activities remained unaffected. Observation suggested that younger rats remained normal until sacrifice, whereas in all cases old rats appeared severely ill with profound lethargy and ataxia.

Hyponatremia

Acute hyponatremia [IP injection of 1% glucose (10% of body weight) plus arginine vasopressin, sacrifice 120 min later] produced a decrease in serum osmolarity and brain edema. Hypo-osmolarity was more severe in group II, but with a less pronounced increase in the brain water content. In both groups Na/K/ATPase activities remained normal (Table 3).

Brain Water and Natremia

In both groups there was a highly significant correlation ($P<0.001$) between the full range of natremic states (hypo-osmotic stress, control, hyperosmotic stress) and the brain water response. The two regression lines were strictly parallel.

Table 1. Changes in brain water and Na/K/ATPase following infliction of a cold lesion

	2 Months		21 Months	
	Control	Cold lesion	Control	Cold lesion
Brain water	3.72±0.16	4.22±0.24	3.39±0.11	3.94±0.31
	└	┘ $P<0.01$	└	┘ $P<0.001$
	└		┘ $P<0.05$	
		└		┘ $P<0.05$
Na/K/ATPase	138 ±21	156 ±18	131 ±28	134 ±12
	└	┘ $P<0.05$	└	┘ $P<0.01$
	└		┘ $P<0.05$	
		└		┘ $P<0.01$

Table 2. Natremia and brain water following NaCl loading

	2 Months		21 Months	
	Control	Hyper	Control	Hyper
Natremia	147±15	203 ±11	147 ±	211 ±11
	+38%		+44%	
	└	┘ $P<0.01$	└	┘ $P<0.01$
	└		┘ NS	
		└		┘ $P<0.01$
Brain water	3.72±0.16	3.14±0.09	3.39±0.11	2.71±0.14
	−15.6%		−20%	
	└	┘ $P<0.01$		$P<0.01$
	└		┘ $P<0.05$	
		└		┘ $P<0.01$

Table 3. Natremia and brain water following hypo-osmotic loading

	2 Months		21 Months	
	Control	Hypo-osmosis	Control	Hypo-osmosis
Natremia	147±15	137 ±8	147 ±8	125 ±6
	−7%		−15%	
	└	┘ $P<0.01$	└	┘ $P<0.01$
	└	┘ NS		
		└		┘ $P<0.01$
Brain water	3.72±0.15	3.95±0.7	3.39±0.11	3.48±0.13
	+6%		+3.5%	
	└	┘ $P<0.01$		$P<0.01$
	└		┘ $P<0.05$	
		└		┘ $P<0.01$

Discussion

These experimental results are in keeping with clinical findings in humans: the increase in brain water content was reduced in old age following cryogenic injury, and this is somewhat comparable to the reduced amount of edema around brain tumors or traumatic contusions in elderly patients.

In cryogenic edema the impairment of Na/K/ATPase activity has been ascribed to membrane damage probably due to phospholipidic breakdown [2]. Here the deleterious effect of this damage on enzyme function is more pronounced in the older group. A number of publications have speculated on membrane damage in old age [5–7], and Na/K/ATPase has been found to be more susceptible to ethanol inhibition in preparations from murine or human brains from elderly individuals [9]. In old age a larger decrease in Na/K/ATPase activity is correlated with a lesser degree of brain edema: we have no straightforward explanation for these paradoxical findings.

The susceptibility of serum osmolarity to osmotic stress in elderly subjects is well known [1–6], as is the susceptibility of the aging brain to both hypo- and hypernatremia [6]. Following hypernatremia the loss of brain water is severe and can lead to major clinical disorders. Since it is normal for the brain water content to be lowered in rats in old age, the further reduction caused by hypernatremia is likely to reach a level of dehydratation incompatible with ionic transport and normal brain function. The reason for the limited increase of brain water content following hyponatremia is not clear. Nevertheless, the responses of brain water to all degrees of natremia are exactly parallel in adult and old animals. This probably means that, given the initial difference in water content in control animals, the osmotic response of the brain follows the same basic mechanisms in both age groups.

Conclusion

Our experimental data are somewhat comparable to what is known from clinical observations. The water content around a lesion is lower in an aged brain, but at least in rats this can be accounted for by an initial difference between young and old control brains; the percentage edema formation in the two groups is similar.

Following an osmotic stress the shift of water into or out of the brain is more severe in old animals, but this can be explained by a larger difference in the serum osmolarity response.

Finally, we may assume that the intrinsic responses of brain water to these experimental insults are essentially similar in young and old animals, and that the actual differences in brain water content are mainly due to age-related structural changes or systemic disorders.

Summary

Brain water content and Na/K/ATPase activity were compared in two groups of rats aged 60±5 days (group I) and 630±10 days (group II). In control animals brain water content and Na/K/ATPase activity were found significantly reduced in group II.

Following a cryogenic lesion of the brain the increase in water content was more pronounced in group I, whereas impairment of Na/K/ATPase activity was much more pronounced in group II.

Following a hyperosmotic stress the increase in serum natremia was more marked in group II, as was the shift of water from the brain, leading to severe clinical disorders.

Following a hypo-osmolar stress, the decrease in serum natremia was more pronounced in group II but the increase of brain water content remained limited.

These results are in keeping with clinical observations in humans.

References

1. Arieff AI (1984) Central nervous system manifestations of disordered sodium metabolism. Clin Endocrinol Metab 13:269–294
2. Cohadon F, Rigoulet M, Averet N (1983) Alterations of membrane-bound enzymes in vasogenic edema. In: Go KG, Baethmann A (eds) Recent progress in the study and therapy of brain edema. Plenum, New York, pp 223–232
3. Donaldson HH (1916) A preliminary determination of the part played by myelin in reducing the water content of the mammalian nervous system (albino rat). J Comp Neurol 26:443–451
4. Holliday MA, Kalayci MN, Harrah J (1968) Factors that limit brain volume changes in response to acute and sustained hyper- and hyponatremia. J Clin Invest 47:1916–1928
5. Grinna LS (1977) Changes in cell membranes during aging. Gerontology 23:452–464
6. Lye M (1984) Electrolytes disorders in the elderly. Clin Endocrinol Metab 13:377–398
7. Nagy IZ (1978) A membrane hypothesis of aging. J Theor Biol 75:189–195
8. Nagy IZ, Nagy K, Lustyik G (1982) Protein and water contents of aging brain. In: Hoyer S (ed) Experimental brain research: the aging brain, suppl. 5. Springer, Berlin Heidelberg New York, pp 118–122
9. de Soussa BN, Kendrick ZV, Roberts J, Baskin SI (1978) Na^+/K^+/ATPase in rat brain and spinal cord during aging. Adv Exp Med Biol 97:255–258
10. Sun AY, Samorajski T (1975) The effects of age and alcohol on Na^+/K^+/ATPase activity of whole homogenate and synaptosomes prepared from mouse and human brain. J Neurochem 24:161–164
11. Zatz LM, Jernigan TL, Ahumada AJ (1982) Changes on computed cranial tomography with aging: intracranial fluid volume. AJNR 3:1–11

Enhancement of the Na, K-ATPase Activity of the Brain Microvessel by Arachidonic Acid and Its Hydroperoxide, 15-HPAA

T. ASANO[1], T. KOIDE, H. MATSUSHITA, and K. TAKAKURA

Key words: Ischemic brain edema, arachidonate cascade, brain microvessel, hydroperoxides, arachidonic acid, Na, K-ATPase free radicals

Introduction

In the prepared brain microvessel (MV), it has been shown that the endothelial cells of the brain capillary play a vital role in the transport function of the blood-brain barrier (BBB) [3, 6, 20, 22]. It was also shown that there is a unipolar transport mechanism of sodium across the BBB, which is due to the anteluminal localization of the Na, K-ATPase in the endothelium [2, 3]. This mechanism may be important in the regulation of ion homeostasis as well as the volume control of the extracellular fluid (ECF) in the physiological state [2, 4] it may also be relevant to the mechanism of ischemic brain edema, since the sodium influx across the BBB was shown to correlate closely with the edema formation [2, 11]. In this regard, we have shown that production of hydroxy acids in the MV is enhanced following regional ischemia in rats [1], and that some radical scavengers, such as AVS, suppress both the lipoxygenase activity of the MV and edema formation [10, 15]. These results suggest that the production of hydroperoxides by the MV lipoxygenase is related to edema formation following ischemia. In this respect, lipid peroxides are known to reduce the activity of the Na, K-ATPase activity of the synaptosomes [17, 23]. However, since their effects on the Na, K-ATPase of the MV are unknown, the present study was carried out to study the effect of AA and its hydroperoxide, 15-HPAA, on the activity of the Na, K-ATPase of the MV.

Materials and Methods

The preparation of the rat MV or synaptosomes was carried out as previously reported [15]. For the determination of ATPase activity, aliquots of MV (15 μg protein) or synaptosomes (about 20 μg protein) were preincubated at 37 °C for 10 min in the presence or absence of drugs. The incubation medium contained 100 m*M* NaCl, 10 m*M* KCl, 5 m*M* $MgCl_2$, 2 m*M* vanadium-free Na_2-ATP, 30 m*M* Tris-HCl (pH

[1] Department of Neurosurgery, University of Tokyo Hospital, 7-3-1, Hongo, Bunkyo-ku, Tokyo 113, Japan

7.4), or NaCl and KCl were replaced by 1 m*M* ouabain (total volume of 1.0 ml). After 30 min of incubation, the reaction was terminated by the addition of 300 μl of 30% trichloroacetic acid, and the inorganic phosphate was determined by the phosphomolybdate method. The Na, K-ATPase activity was obtained by subtracting the ouabain-insensitive activity (Mg-ATPase) from the total activity in the presence of Na and K, and the absence of ouabain. Throughout this experiment, an incubation mixture containing no protein was used as a blank and was subtracted from the activity. The protein concentration was determined according to the method of Lowry et al. [19]. Chemically purified 15-HPAA was synthesized according to the method previously reported by ourselves [14]. Vanadium-free Na_2-ATP, sodium dodecyl sulfate (SDS), palmitic acid, linoleic acid, arachidonic acid (AA), dexamethasone, quinacrine, indomethacin, caffeic acid, D-α-tocopherol acid succinate, superoxide dismutase (SOD), catalase, mannitol, sodium benzoate, and hydroquinone were purchased from Sigma. Eicosatetraynoic acid (ETYA) was purchased from Hoffmann La Roche (Netley, NJ).

Results

Effects of 15-HPAA on the Na, K-ATPase Activity in the MV and Synaptosomes

As shown in Fig. 1, 15-HPAA stimulated the ATPase activity from the concentration level of 1×10^{-8} *M* to one of 1×10^{-5} *M* in the MV. In the synaptosomes, in contrast, dose-dependent inhibitions of the ATPase activity was observed.

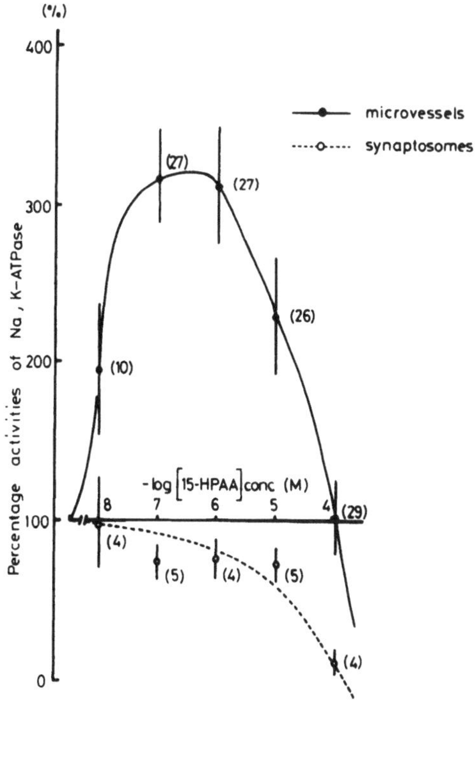

Fig. 1. Effects of 15-HPAA on the Na, K-ATPase activity of the rat brain microvessels and synaptosomes. Each value represents the mean (± SEM) percentage of control ATPase activity. The number of experiments is shown in parentheses in each case. The basal activity of ATPase in microvessels and synaptosomes was 5.53 ± 0.81 and 3.08 ± 0.38 (μmol Pi/mg/protein/h), respectively

Table 1. Effects of fatty acids on the ATPase activity of the rat brain microvessel

ATPase	Fatty acids	Concentration of each fatty acid (M)			
		1×10^{-7}	1×10^{-6}	1×10^{-5}	1×10^{-4}
Na, K-ATPase	Sodium dodecyl sulfate (12:0) ($n=7$)	0.97±0.14	0.44±0.19	0.23±0.08	0.09±0.01
	Palmitic acid (16:0) ($n=4$)	0.86±0.03	0.77±0.29	0.62±0.03	0.59±0.07
	Linoleic acid (18:3) ($n=4$)	0.93±0.15	0.47±0.07	0.24±0.06	0.07±0.03
	Arachidonic acid (20:4) ($n=5$)	2.15±0.51	1.98±0.61	1.79±0.17	0.68±0.12

Each value represents the mean (± SEM) percentage of control values. The asal activity of Na,K-ATPase and Mg-ATPase was 6.47±0.94 and 10.27±0.17 (μmol Pi/mg protein/h), respectively

Table 2. Effects of radical scavengers on the enhanced ATPase activity induced by 15-HPAA

ATPase	Radical scavengers	Concentration of 15-HPAA (M)			
		1×10^{-7}	1×10^{-6}	1×10^{-5}	1×10^{-4}
Exp 1	Control ($n=7$)	3.37±0.41	5.56±1.58	4.50±1.90	1.78±0.92
	+Mannitol (2×10^{-2} M) ($n=6$)	6.58±2.60	4.57±1.45	5.40±2.30	1.57±0.60
	+Na benzoate (2×10^{-2} M) ($n=6$)	4.03±0.81	2.96±1.45	3.04±1.64	1.66±1.22
Na/K-ATPase	+SOD (50 μg ml) ($n=4$)	8.94±3.36	5.80±0.78	6.80±4.35	0.58±0.32
	+Catalase (50 μg ml) ($n=4$)	7.49±3.12	5.56±1.20	3.02±0.58	0.62±0.38
	+SOD plus catalase ($n=4$)	6.85±2.49	3.68±1.01	3.55±0.55	1.25±0.79
	+α-tocopherol (1×10^{-4} M) ($n=9$)	1.80±0.77	2.57±0.70*	2.23±0.35**	1.38±0.53
	+Hydroquinone (1×10^{-4} M) ($n=5$)	1.23±0.46**	0.46±0.23*	0.38±0.08*	0.38±0.17
Exp 2	Control ($n=6$)	3.18±0.30	3.12±0.38	2.29±0.38	1.02±0.24
	+AVS (5×10^{-5} M) ($n=6$)	1.64±0.29*	2.05±0.55*	1.49±0.23	0.77±0.18
	+AVS (5×10^{-4} M) ($n=6$)	1.66±0.26*	1.42±0.22*	1.20±0.23*	1.03±0.40
	+Mannitol (2×10^{-2} M) ($n=6$)	3.05±1.63	4.35±1.76	3.73±2.23	1.57±0.60

Each value represents the mean (± SEM) ratio to the controls' baseline activity. The number of the experiments is shown in parentheses in each case. Baseline basal Na, K-ATPase activities were 5.52±0.59 and 5.53±0.81 (μmol Pi/mg protein/h), respectively

* $P<0.05$, ** $P<0.01$

Effects of Fatty Acids on the Na, K-ATPase Activity in the MV

The effects of various fatty acids on the ATPase activity in the MV are shown in Table 1. Among these fatty acids, only AA stimulated, whereas the others inhibited, ATPase activity.

Effects of Several Types of Arachidonate Cascade Inhibitors on the Na, K-ATPase Enhanced by 15-HPAA

Pretreatment of the MV with quinacrine significantly suppressed the ATPase activity enhanced by 15-HPAA (Fig. 2). Dexamethasone also had a similar suppressive effect. As shown in Fig. 3, ETYA and caffeic acid significantly inhibited the enhancement of ATPase activity by 15-HPAA, whereas indomethacin had no effect. None of the above compounds affected the basal ATPase activity in the MV.

Effects of Radical Scavengers on the Enhancement of ATPase Activity by 15-HPAA

As shown in Table 2, among the various radical scavengers tested, α-tocopherol, hydroquinone, and AVS each caused a significant reduction of the enhancement of ATPase activity by 15-HPAA.

Discussion

In the present study, 15-HPAA enhanced the activity of Na, K-ATPase in the rat MV perceptibly, whereas it diminished that of synaptosomes. It is unlikely that the

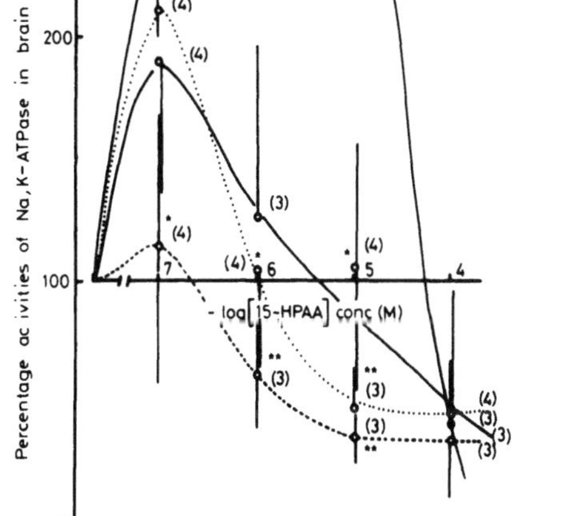

Fig. 2. Effect of phospholipase-A_2 inhibitor, quinacrine, on the enhanced Na, K-ATPase activity induced by 15-HPAA. Each value represents the mean (± SEM) The number of experiments is shown in parentheses. * $P<0.05$; ** $P<0.01$. ——, control; - - - -, 1×10^{-5} *M*; - - · - -, 1×10^{-4} *M*; · · · · · 1×10^{-3} *M*. The basal Na, K-ATPase activity was 5.92±0.12 (μmol Pi/mg/protein/h)

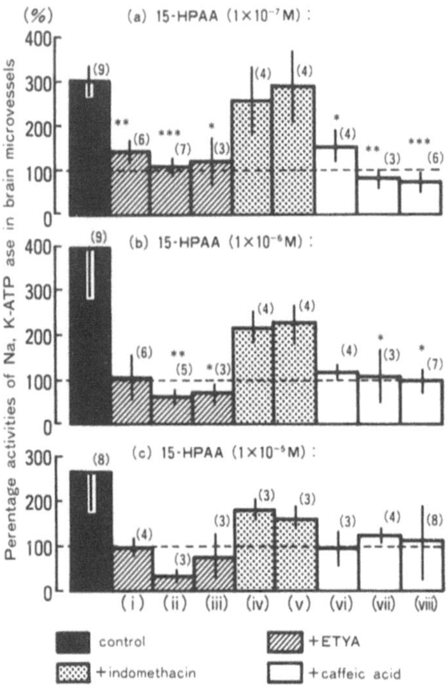

Fig. 3. Effects of ETYA, indomethacin, and caffeic acid on the enhanced Na, K-ATPase activity induced by 15-HPAA. Each value represents the mean (± SEM) percentage of control activity. The number of experiments are shown in parentheses in each case. (*i*), 1×10^{-5} *M*; (*ii*), 1×10^{-4} *M*; (*iii*), 1×10^{-3} *M*; (*iv*), 1×10^{-5} *M*; (*v*), 1×10^{-4} *M*; (*vi*), 1×10^{-5} *M*; (*vii*), 1×10^{-4} *M*; and (*viii*), 1×10^{-3} *M*. * $P<0.05$; ** $P<0.01$; *** $P<0.001$. Basal Na, K-ATPase activity was 3.80 ± 0.08 (μmol Pi/mg protein/h)

simple detergent action of 15-HPAA was involved in its effect on the MV, because an ionic detergent such as SDS inhibited the ATPase activity at any concentrations used. Bearing in mind that lipid peroxides are required for the AA cascade to start [18], and that 15-HPAA enhances the eicosanoid synthetic capacity of the rat MV [15], the mechanism of action of 15-HPAA was examined with regard to the AA cascade. Pretreatment of the MV with either quinacrine or dexamethasone completely suppressed the enhancement of the ATPase activity by 15-HPAA (Fig. 2), indicating that liberation of free AA by phospholipase A_2 is an essential part in the action of 15-HPAA. That exogenous AA exerted an influence on the MV which was similar to that of 15-HPAA (Table 1) supports the above interpretation. Next, to find out which of lipoxygenase or cyclooxygenase pathway of the AA cascade within the MV participates in the stimulation of ATPase activity by 15-HPAA, the effects of pretreatments with ETYA (a dual inhibitor of cyclooxygenase and lipoxygenase) [12], indomethacin (a cyclooxygenase inhibitor), or caffeic acid (a lipoxygenase inhibitor) [16], were compared. The results (Fig. 3) clearly show that only the lipoxygenase pathway is relevant to the action of 15-HPAA. As the last step in the experiment, the effects of pretreatment with each of various radical scavengers were examined. This was done because it is known that the AA cascade per se leads to free radical formation [9]. Among the compounds tested, α-tocopherol, hydroquinone, and AVS showed significant suppressive effects on the enhancement of ATPase activity by 15-HPAA (Table 2). This result indicates that some radical species (possibly singlet oxygen or peroxy radical) participated in the action of 15-HPAA. However, since the above radical scavengers were shown also to suppress the 15-HPAA-induced enhancement of the eicosanoid synthetic capacity of the MV

[15], it remains to be seen at which reaction step within the AA cascade free radicals are generated, or what target they attack. Thus the present study unequivocally shows that the effects of AA and 15-HPAA on the Na, K-ATPase are completely different in the MV than in the synaptosomes [5]. The biological significance of such a mechanism needs to be pursued. In this respect, it may be pointed out that when cytotoxic edema occurs due to energy depletion, the extracellular space (ECS) shrinks and the sodium concentration in the extracellular fluid (ECF) decreases [13]. Since the BBB is freely permeable to water, but not to sodium [8], the drop in sodium concentration in the ECF would cause an immediate movement of water from the ECF to the blood, leading to further shrinkage of the ECS and a net loss of water from the brain. Then, if there were no mechanism supplying sodium from the blood to the ECF, the above process would proceed to the point where the cellular environment became incompatible with cell survival. As energy depletion simultaneously leads to release of free AA [24, 25], the mechanism in the MV, as revealed in the present study, would provide an adequate apparatus to pump sodium actively from the blood to the ECF. Therefore, the occurrence of edema, namely the net gain of water and sodium in the early phase of cerebral ischemia [11, 22; Asano et al., this volume], would be an active compensatory reaction of the brain, rather than an event succeeding cell death. It is not clear at present which of AA or its hydroperoxide(s) plays the major role in vivo. In the companion paper, we reported that the rat MV synthesizes a considerable amount of 11-HETE (hydroxyeicosatetraenoic acid) in the normal condition (Usui et al., this volume). Whether or not the precursor of 11-HETE, namely 11-HPETE (hydroperoxyeicosatetraenoic acid) possesses a similar action to 15-HPAA needs to be examined. Finally, the present findings could explain the hitherto paradoxical increase in the Na, K-ATPase activity in the reperfused brain [7].

Summary

Our earlier studies revealed that the capacity of the rat brain microvessel (MV) for eicosanoid synthesis is markedly enhanced by a lipid hydroperoxide, viz. 15-hydroperoxyarachidonic acid (15-HPAA). To obtain more detailed knowledge of the influence of arachidonic acid (AA) and its hydroperoxide on the function of the blood-brain barrier (BBB), the effect of AA or 15-HPAA on the Na, K-ATPase of the MV and brain synaptosomes was studied in rats. Even at a low concentration level (10^{-8} *M*), both AA and 15-HPAA significantly stimulated the Na, K-ATPase activity of the MV, while the synaptosomal ATPase activity was inhibited in a dose-dependent manner when the same concentration range was used (10^{-8} to 10^{-4} *M*). Results of experiments with different types of pharmacological agents indicated that activation of phospholipase A_2 and the generation of lipoxygenase product(s) and free radicals were involved in the enhancement of the Na, K-ATPase activity of the MV by 15-HPAA. On the basis of the above results, a hypothesis that AA and its hydroperoxide(s) modulate the activity of the Na, K-ATPase of the MV and control the sodium and water transport across the BBB is put forward.

References

1. Asano T, Gotoh O, Koide T, Takakura K (1985) Ischemic brain edema following occlusion of the middle cerebral artery in the rat. II: Alteration of the eicosanoid synthesis profile of brain microvessels. Stroke 16(1): (in press)
2. Betz L (1983) Sodium transport in capillaries isolated from rat brain. J Neurochem 41:1150–1157
3. Betz L, Firth A, Goldstein G (1980) Polarity of the blood-brain barrier: distribution of enzymes between the luminal and antiluminal membranes of brain capillary endothelial cells. Brain Res 192:17–28
4. Bradbury M (1979) The concept of a blood-brain barrier. Wiley, Chichester
5. Chan PH, Kerlan R, Fishman R (1983) Reductions of γ-aminobutyric acid and glutamate uptake and $(Na^+ + K^+)$-ATPase activity in brain slices and synaptosomes by arachidonic acid. J Neurochem 40:309–316
6. Djuričić BM, Rogac L, Spatz M, Rakić LM, Mršulja BB (1978) Brain microvessels. I: Enzymic activities. Adv Neurol 20:197–205
7. Enseleit W, Domer F, Jarrott D, Baricos W (1984) Cerebral phospholipid content and Na^+, K^+-ATPase activity during ischemia and postischemic reperfusion in the mongolian gerbil. J Neurochem 43:320–327
8. Fenstermacher JD, Patlak CS (1976) The movements of water and solutes in the brains of mammals. In: Pappius H, Feindel W (eds) Dynamics of brain edema. Springer, Berlin, pp 87–94
9. Gale P, Egan R (1984) Prostaglandin endoperoxide synthase-catalyzed oxidation reactions. In: Pryor WA (ed) Free radicals in biology, vol VI. Academic, Orlando, pp 1–38
10. Gotoh O, Koide T, Asano T, Takakura K, Tamura A, Sano K (1984) A model to study ischemic brain edema in rats and the influence of drugs. In: Go KG, Baethmann A (eds) Recent progress in the study and therapy of brain edema. Plenum, New York, pp 499–508
11. Gotoh O, Asano T, Koide T, Takakura K (1985) Ischemic cerebral edema following occlusion of the middle cerebral artery in the rat. I: The time courses of the brain water, sodium and potassium contents and blood-brain barrier permeability to ^{125}I-albumin. Stroke 16,(1): (in press)
12. Higgs G, Flower R, Vane J (1979) A new approach to anti-inflammatory drugs. Biochem Pharmacol 28:1959–1961
13. Hossmann KA, Sakaki S, Zimmermann V (1977) Cation activities in reversible ischemia of the cat brain. Stroke 8:77–81
14. Koide T, Neichi T, Takato M, Matsushita H, et al. (1982) Possible mechanisms of 15-hydroperoxyarachidonic acid-induced contraction of the canine basilar artery in vitro. J Pharmacol Exp Ther 22:481–488
15. Koide T, Gotoh O, Asano T, Takakura K (1985) Alterations of the eicosanoid synthetic capacity of the rat brain microvessel following ischemia: relevance to ischemic brain edema. J Neurochem (in press)
16. Koshihara Y, Niechi T, Murota S, et al. (1984) Caffeic acid is a selective inhibitor for leukotriene biosynthesis. Biochim Biophys Acta 792:92–97
17. Kovachich GB, Mishra OP (1981) Partial inactivation of Na, K-ATPase in cortical brain slices incubated in normal Krebs-Ringer phosphate medium at 1 and at 10 atm oxygen pressures. J Neurochem 36:333–335
18. Lands WEM, Kulmacz RJ, Marshall PJ (1984) Lipid peroxide actions in the regulation of prostaglandin biosynthesis. In: Pryor WA (ed) Free radicals in biology. Academic, Orlando, pp 39–61
19. Lowry OH, Rosebrough NJ, Farr AC, Randall RJ (1951) Protein measurement with the folin phenol reagent. J Biol Chem 193:265–275
20. Mršulja BB, Djuričić BM, Cvejić V, Mršulja BJ, Abe K, Spatz M, Klatzo I (1980) Biochemistry of experimental ischemic brain edema. Adv Neurol 28:217–230
21. Schuier FJ, Hossmann K-A (1980) Experimental brain infarcts in cats: II. Ischemic brain edema. Stroke 11:593–601
22. Spatz M, Mićić D, Mršulja BB, Klatzo I (1978) Cerebral microvessels as mediators of cerebral transport. Adv Neurol 20:189–195

23. Sun AY (1972) The effect of lipoxidation on synaptosomal $(Na^+ + K^+)$-ATPase isolated from the cerebral cortex of squirrel monkey. Biochim Biophys Acta 266: 350–360
24. Wolfe LS (1982) Eicosanoids: prostaglandins, thromboxanes, leukotrienes, and other derivatives of carbon-20 unsaturated fatty acids. J Neurochem 38: 1–14
25. Yoshida S, Inoh S, Asano T, Sano K, Kubota M, Shimazaki H, Ueta N (1980) Effect of transient ischemia on free fatty acids and phospholipids in the gerbil brain. J Neurosurg 53: 323–331

Na^+-K^+-Activated Adenosine Triphosphatase Activity and Lipoperoxide Metabolites in Microvessels and Parenchymas of the Ischemic Brain

Y. Fujita [1], T. Shingu, M. Kurihara, H. Miyake, T. Kono, and K. Mori

Key words: Ischemic brain edema, Na^+-K^+-ATPase, P-NPPase, lipoperoxide, prostaglandin

Introduction

To maintain electrolyte homeostasis in the brain, membrane-bound (Na + K)-ATPase is localized at the membranes of capillary endothelium, choroid plexus epithelium, and brain parenchymal cells (glia and neurons). This enzyme is susceptible to ischemic insults [16], and the different susceptibility of each membrane-bound (Na + K)ATPase to ischemic insults may modify the features of brain edema (cytotoxic or vasogenic edema). The precise mechanism of this susceptibility and inactivation of this enzyme in the ischemia is poorly understood.

Materials and Methods

Animal Preparation for Experimental Procedures

Male spontaneously hypertensive rats (SHRs) (15–17 weeks old) with a systolic blood pressure of 185 ± 2 mmHg were anesthetized with ethyl ether, and the bilateral common carotid arteries were clipped. Cerebral blood flow is reduced to 17% of the preischemic value in this model [9]. Ischemia was thus induced for 1, 3, and 5 h. In selected experiments the clips were removed from the rats in the 1-h or 5-h ischemia groups and recirculation was allowed for 15 min or 3 or 5 h before sacrifice. At the termination of ischemia and recirculation experiments the animals were decapitated and the brains rapidly removed.

Male Mongolian gerbils were subjected to ischemia for 15 min by bilateral common carotid ligation. These animals were decapitated during this period of ischemia and the brains were rapidly removed.

Preparation of Microvessels and Parenchyma

Microvessels were isolated by the method of Brendel et al. [4].

(Na + K)ATPase Measurements. (Na + K)ATPase was determined by the method of Proverbio et al. [24]. Inorganic phosphorus was determined by the method of Allen [1] as modified by Nakamura [17].

[1] Department of Neurosurgery, Kurashiki Central Hospital

P-NPPase Measurements. P-NPPase was measured by the method of Basu et al. [2]. Ouabain-sensitive (Na + K)ATPase and p-NPPase activities were expressed as the difference in the amount of Pi or phenol liberated in the presence and absence of ouabain. Protein was determined by the method of Lowry et al. [13].

Γ-GTP Measurements. Γ-GTP activity in the microvessels homogenates was estimated according to the method of Orlowski and Meister [20], L-γ-glutamyl nitroanilide being used as a substrate.

Measurement of Brain Edema

(a) Brain water content was estimated by a freeze-drying method. (b) Extravasation of HRP was observed under a light microscope and an electron microscope. HRP (50 mg/animal) was administered IV 30 min before induction of ischemia.

6-Keto-$PGF_{1\alpha}$ and Thromboxane B_2 Measurements. PG metabolites were extracted by the method of Spagnuolo et al. [27] and estimated by radioimmunoassay [10, 22].

TBA-RS Measurements. TBA-RS was determined by the method of Ohkawa et al. [19].

Results

Brain Water Content

Water content was not significantly altered during ischemia in the 1-h and 3-h occlusion groups of SHR, whereas it was markedly increased in the 5-h occlusion group (Fig. 1). The edema was significantly decreased during 3 h recirculation. In the 1-h occlusion group, preischemic values were recovered within 6 h of recirculation. In the 5-h occlusion group water content was slightly increased within 6 h of recirculation.

Histological Observation

Decreased extracellular spaces and swelling of perivascular astrocytes were observed in the electron microscope during ischemia in the 3-h occlusion group. Severe edema with extravasation of HRP was observed in the 5-h occlusion group following 3 h recirculation.

(Na + K)ATPase Activity

During Ischemia. (Na + K)ATPase activity was decreased in both microvessels and parenchyma in all groups (Fig. 2). The enzyme activity in the parenchyma in the 3-h

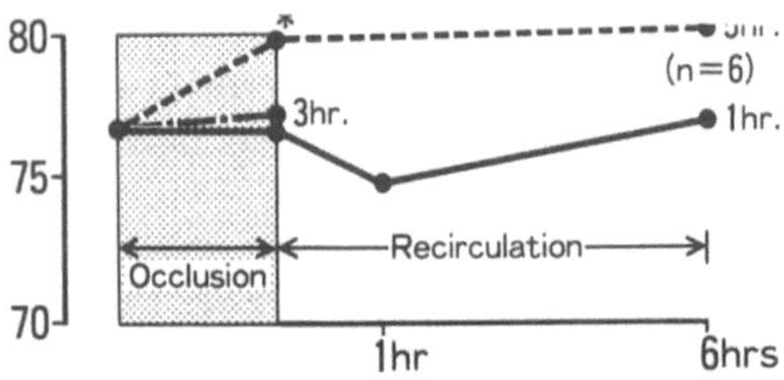

Fig. 1. Brain water content of SHRs with induced cerebral ischemia, expressed as percentages [(wet weight – dry weight) : wet weight]. Water content before ischemia 77.79 ± 0.09 (mean ± SD, 6 animals)

	Group with 1-h occlusion	Group with 5-h occlusion
During ischemia	77.88 ± 0.06 (6)	79.65 ± 0.09 (6)*
3 h after recirculation	78.75 ± 0.09 (6)	79.92 ± 0.06 (6)*
6 h after recirculation	78.15 ± 0.04 (6)	80.18 ± 0.05 (6)*

Figures in parentheses give number of animals in each case
* $P<0.001$

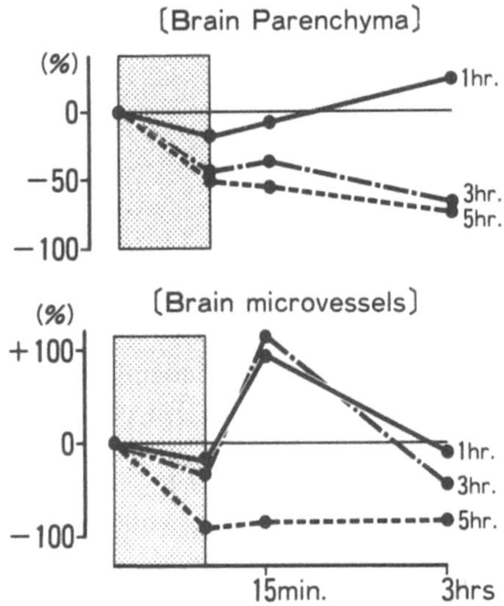

Fig. 2. Changes in SHR brain (Na + K)-ATPase activity during and after recirculation. Values for enzyme activity (μ*M*Pi/mg protein per min) are expressed as percentages of the preischemic values. Microvessels: 0.163 ± 0.018 (7); parenchyma: 0.314 ± 0.021 (7). There were seven to eight animals in each group

and 5-h occlusion groups and that in the microvessels in the 5-h occlusion group were particularly affected.

After Recirculation. In the 1-h occlusion group, the activity of the parenchyma gradually recovered preischemic values and there was no overshoot until 6 h after recirculation, but with over 3 h occlusion the activity did not recover its preischemic level at all. In the case of reduced activity of the microvessels following less than 3 h occlusion, recovery was rapid and activity exceeded the preischemic value immediately after reperfusion then fell slightly below the preischemic levels. Decreased activity in the microvessels following 5 h ischemia no longer reactivated on restoration of the cerebral circulation.

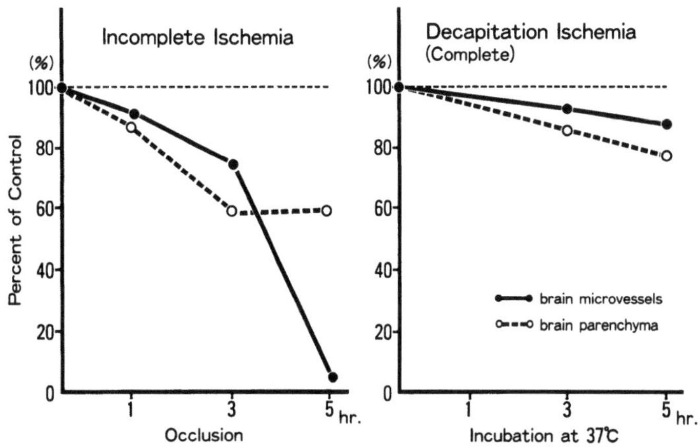

Fig. 3. Changes in microvessel and parenchyma (Na + K)ATPase in incomplete and complete ischemia. For all other explanations see legend to Fig. 2

(Na + K)ATPase in Complete or Incomplete Ischemia

Completely ischemic brains were obtained by incubation of the decapitated brain not removed from the skull at 37 °C for 3 or 5 h. (Na + K)ATPase in the microvessels and parenchyma were inactivated more extensively in cases of incomplete than of complete ischemia during 3- and 5-h ischemic periods (Fig. 3).

Γ-GTP Activity

Activity of Γ-GTP in the microvessels was inhibited in the groups subjected to 1 and 5 h ischemia and recovery was gradual following recirculation in the 1-h ischemia group. In the 5-h ischemia group the activity remained depressed until 6 h after the start of recirculation (Fig. 4).

Prostaglandin Metabolites

Changes During Ischemia. In the 1-h and 5-h occlusion groups, the concentrations of 6-keto-$PGF_{1\alpha}$ and thromboxane B_2 were decreased in both microvessels and parenchyma, except in the microvessels following 1-h occlusion, where it was increased.

Changes after Recirculation. The levels of these two metabolites rose during recirculation in all groups. There were various degrees of reactivity following recirculation (Fig. 5).

TBA-RS

The TBA-RS level was not elevated during ischemia but gradually increased after the initiation of recirculation in the 5-h occlusion group. Following 6 h of recircu-

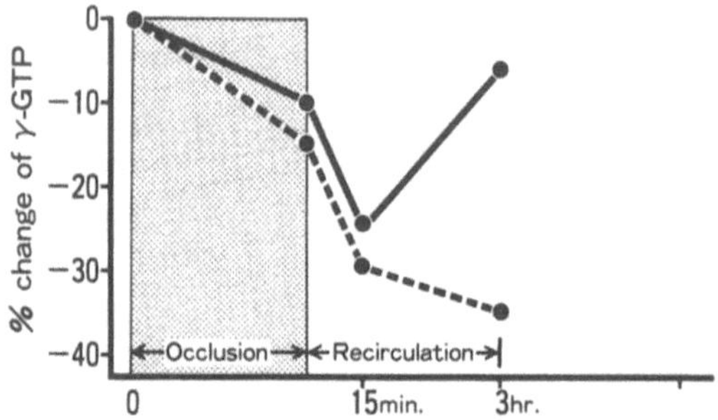

Fig. 4. Γ-GTP activity changes in microvessels during and after ischemia. The values are expressed as percentage changes from preischemic values

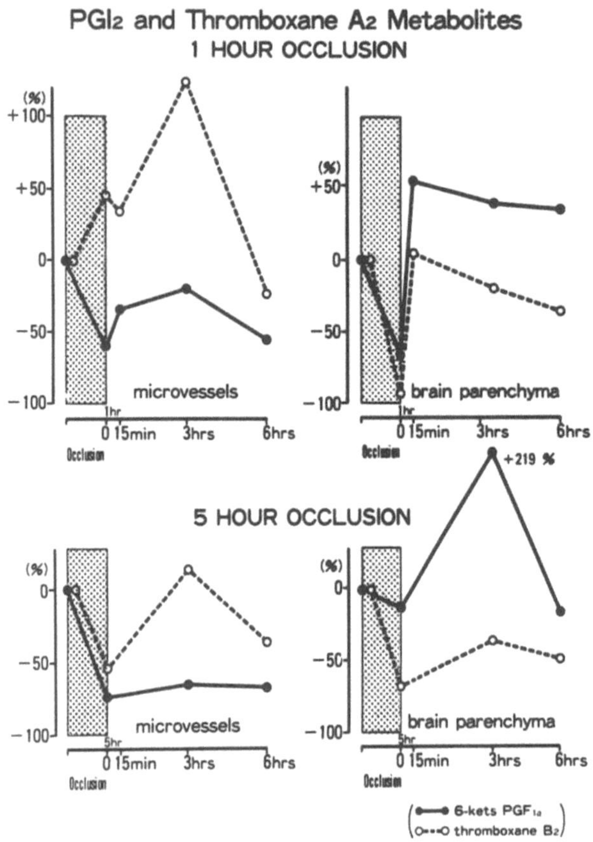

Fig. 5. Changes in 6-keto-$PGF_{1\alpha}$ and thromboxane B_2 in SHRs during and after ischemia. Preischemic values: 6-keto-$PGF_{1\alpha}$ 870 ± 123, 134 ± 15, thromboxane B_2 460 ± 56, 59 ± 8. The first values are for microvessels, and the second ones for parenchyma in each case. (Units are pg mg protein^{-1})

lation in this group, PG metabolites did not recover the preischemic level either in the microvessels or in the parenchyma. Thus PG metabolites do not seem to be linked to the increase in TBA-RS. Increased TBA-RS may reflect the presence of lipid peroxide metabolites, and do not necessarily arise via the cyclooxygenase pathway (Fig. 6).

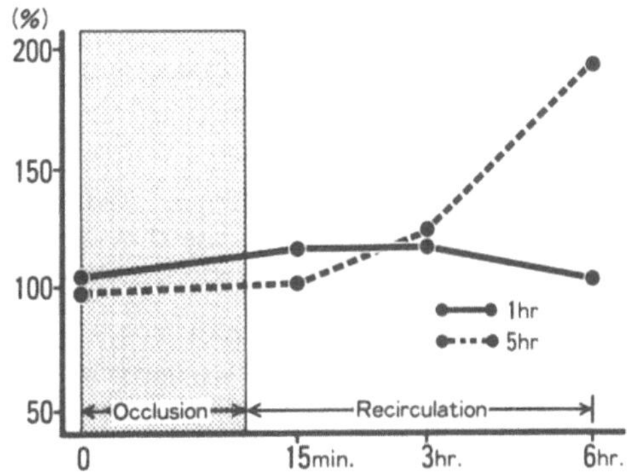

Fig. 6. Changes in TBA-RS in whole brains of SHRs during and after ischemia. The values are expressed as percentage changes from preischemic values

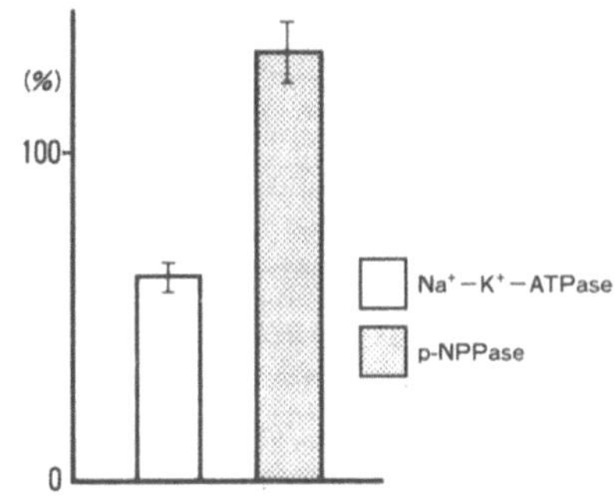

Fig. 7. (Na + K)ATPase and P-NPPase activity in gerbil brain parenchyma subjected to 15 min ischemia. Preischemic values of total p-NPPase activity: 40.9 ± 7.1 μ*M*/mg protein, ouabain-sensitive: 7.65 ± 0.15 μ*M*/mg protein. The values in the figure are percentages of the preischemic values

(Na + K)ATPase and P-NPPase Activity

In the gerbil brain parenchyma homogenates after removal of the microvessels, (Na + K)ATPase decreased to 62.4% ± 5% ($P<0.05$) of the preischemic values after 15 min of ischemia, while ouabain-sensitive p-NPPase activity was increased (though not to a statistically significant degree) (Fig. 7).

Discussion

Following ischemia for up to 3 h the water content was not significantly increased (Fig. 1), in contrast to the histological observations, while a significant increase was detected following a 5-h ischemic interval. These results indicate that cytotoxic edema induced within 3 h of the onset of ischemia is not associated with a water shift from the intravascular space, and in a longer ischemic interval than 3 h the water shift from the intravascular space was not associated with protein leakage. Extravasation of HRP was only observed after recirculation following a longer ischemic interval. It is suggested that intracapillary pressure and damaged endothelial cells may participate in HRP extravasation. The so-called vasogenic edema may be due to damage to the capillary endothelium induced by extended ischemia and by expansion of capillary walls following restoration of cerebral blood flow.

Changes in (Na + K)ATPase activity following ischemia and recirculation were of two kinds (Fig. 2): (a) Gradual or rapid reactivation after relatively slight inactivation, observed in 1-h ischemia of the parenchyma and 3-h or 5-h ischemia of the microvessels; (b) no recovery following pronounced inactivation, noted in the parenchyma following 3- and 5-h ischemia and in the microvessels following 5-h ischemia. These results indicate that there is a difference in susceptibility between the parenchyma and the microvessels. Mršulja et al. reported the same results [16]. Although (Na + K)ATPase was not inactivated further after recirculation either in the microvessels or in the parenchyma following a relatively short period of ischemia, marked reactivation in the microvessels was observed soon after recirculation (Fig. 2). The level of Γ-GTP, a marker enzyme for capillary endothelium [6, 28], declined further (Fig. 7), while (Na + K)ATPase activity was rapidly increased at the same time. Mršulja et al. suggested that 5-HT and cyclic AMP might be stimulants [16]. MacMillan suggested excessive lactoacidosis might be involved and did not think that damage to enzyme-associated membrane lipids would be concerned in inactivation of (Na + K)ATPase [14]. Enseleit et al. also reported that changes in this enzyme activity did not appear to be mediated by membrane phospholipid content [8]. In our experiment (Na + K)ATPase activity was more extensively inactivated in the microvessels and the parenchyma during incomplete than during complete ischemia (Fig. 4). Hossmann and Kleihues [12], Nordström et al. [18], and Rehncrona et al. [25] pointed out that the outcome in terms of mitochondrial respiratory function and certain neurophysiological parameters was paradoxically better after complete than after incomplete ischemia. Rehncrona et al. did not accept the hypothesis that peroxidation of membrane lipids caused brain cell damage, because of their experimental finding that both complete and severe but incomplete ischemia caused a similar increase in the tissue content of free fatty acids (FFAs) [26]. It is well known that ischemia, whether resulting from decapitation or from bilateral ligation of the common carotid arteries, leads to a rapid transient increase in the concentration of FFAs, particularly the polyunsaturated species [3, 30] by way of phospholipases activated following ischemic insults [3]. In spite of increased levels of precursors, the metabolites of PGs decrease during ischemia (Fig. 5), and it is suggested that increased quantities of FFAs were not sufficiently oxygenated by cyclooxygenase because of oxygen depletion. This speculation is supported by the results of TBA-RS measurements (Fig. 6). After recirculation levels of both the metabolites rose in the parenchyma and the microvessels following shorter ischemic periods. These results indicate that PGI_2 and thromboxane A_2 probably do not play a significant part in inactivation of (Na + K)ATPase during ischemia, but may be involved in reactivation of the enzyme after recirculation. Hexum and Fried [11] and Chan et al. [5] reported inactivation of this enzyme by superoxide anion and polyunsaturated fatty acids. PGI_2 synthesis is inhibited by hydroperoxide [15] or free radicals [7]. Polyunsaturated fatty acids and free radicals may induce inhibition of PGI_2 synthesis and inactivation of (Na + K)ATPase in the SHR brain subjected to ischemia.

In the gerbil ischemic brain, p-NPPase was preserved during ischemia, while (Na + K)ATPase was remarkably decreased (Fig. 7). (Na + K)ATPase is reversible from the E_1 to the E_2 state, and each state has different functions [23]. E_2 had a p-NPPase activity dependent on Mg^{2+} and K^+. Taniguchi and Tonomura reported that inactivated (Na + K)ATPase by phospholipase A_2 and C was recovered on incubation with pospholipids [29]. Ottolenghi demonstrated that this almost completely delipidated enzyme lost its activity as well as (Na + K)ATPase but that the activity was recovered, first as p-NPPase and then as (Na + K)ATPase by titration with phospholipids [21]. Post et al. called the active portion of p-NPPase (E_2) of (Na + K)ATPase the "occluded form"; this portion localized in the inside of the cell membrane, and was not exposed on both the surfaces of the membrane [23]. This location may explain why p-NPPase was resistant to phospholipases activated by ischemic insults. It is suggested that reversibility of the inactivation of (Na + K)-ATPase observed in our experiments in SHR may depend on the degree of delipidation of this enzyme lipid moiety.

Summary

Using a bilateral carotid artery occlusion technique in groups of male spontaneously hypertensive rats (SHRs) and male Mongolian gerbils, we examined the effects of ischemia on the following parameters: cerebral water content, extravasation of horseradish peroxidase (HRP), thiobarbituric acid-reactive substance (TBA-RS), Na^+- K^+-ATPase [(Na + K)ATPase] activity in the microvessels and parenchyma and gamma glutamyl transpeptidase (γ-GTP) activity in the microvessels in SHR. (Na + K)ATPase and potassium-dependent *p*-nitrophenyl phosphatase (p-NPPase) activities in gerbils were also studied.

Changes in water content and histological observations indicated that cytotoxic edema developed in the presence of ischemia induced by arterial occlusion for up to 3 h and was not necessarily associated with a water shift from the intravascular spaces. A significant water shift occurred with over 3 h occlusion: thus, vasogenic edema seemed to be induced only by recirculation when the capillary endothelium is damaged to the degree that a water shift occurs. (Na + K)ATPase in the parenchyma was substantially and irreversibly inactivated, while the enzyme activity in the microvessels was not virtually altered when water was shifted from the extra- to the intracellular spaces. During the 5-h ischemic period water shifted from the intravascular to the intra- and extracellular spaces, and the enzyme was severely and irreversibly inactivated in both the microvessels and the parenchyma. These results indicate that the wide variation in the features of brain edema may be due to the different susceptibility of (Na + K)ATPase. Changes in PG metabolites and TBA-RS suggest that the inactivation of (Na + K)ATPase during ischemia is not caused by lipoperoxide but rather by participation of free radicals during ischemia and lipoperoxides after recirculation. The activities of (Na + K)ATPase and p-NPPase in homogenates prepared from gerbil cerebral hemispheres subjected to 15 min ischemia were also determined. The former enzyme activity was reduced to 62.4% ± 5% of the preischemic value, while the latter remained almost unchanged. These findings indicate that partial delipidation from the lipid moiety of the enzyme by enhanced activity of phospholipases by ischemic insults may be responsible for the observed (Na + K)ATPase inactivation during ischemia.

References

1. Allen RJL (1940) The estimation of phosphorus. Biochem J 34:858–865
2. Basu MK, Colacicco G, Picciano PT, Rosenbaum RM, Wittner M (1979) Isolation and characterization of plasma membrane from monolayer cultures of epithelial type II lung cell. Arch Biochem Biophys 198:349–359
3. Bazan NG (1976) Free arachidonic and other lipids in nervous system during early ischemia and after electroshock. In: Porcellati G, Amaducci L, Galli C (eds) Central and peripheral nervous system. Plenum, New York, pp 317–335
4. Brendel K, Meezan E, Carson EC (1974) Isolated brain microvessels: A purified, metabolically active preparation from bovine cerebral cortex. Science 185:953–955
5. Chan PH, Quan SC, Fishmann RA (1980) Inhibition of rat brain (Na^+-K^+)ATPase by polyunsaturated fatty acids. Trans Am Soc Neurochem 11:120
6. De Bault LE (1982) Isolation and characterization of the cells of the cerebral microvessels. Adv Cell Neurobiol 3:339–371
7. Demopoulos HB, Flamm ES, Pietronigro DD, Seligman ML (1980) The free radical pathology and microcirculation in the major cerebral nervous system disorders. Acta Physiol Scand (Suppl) 492:91–119
8. Enseleit WH, Domer FR, Jarott DM, Baricos WH (1984) Cerebral phospholipid content and Na^+-K^+-ATPase activity during ischemia and postischemic reperfusion in the mongolian gerbils. J Neurochem 43:320–327
9. Fujishima M, Ishitsuka T, Nakatomi Y, Tamai K, Omae (1981) Changes in local cerebral blood flow following bilateral carotid occlusion in spontaneously hypertensive and normotensive rats. Stroke 12:874–876
10. Granström E, Kindahl H, Samuelsson B (1976) A method for measuring the unstable thromboxane A_2: radioimmunoassay of the derived mono-O-methyl-thromboxane B_2. Prostaglandins 12:929–941
11. Hexum TD, Fried R (1979) Effect of superoxide radicals on transport (Na + K) adenosine triphosphatase and protection by superoxide dismutase. Neurochem Res 4:73–82
12. Hossmann K-A, Kleinues (1973) Reversibility of ischemic brain damage. Arch Neurol 29:375–382
13. Lowry OH, Rosenbrough NJ, Farr AL, Randall PJ (1951) Protein measurement with the folin phenol reagent. J Biol Chem 193:265–275
14. MacMillan V (1982) Cerebral Na^+-K^+-ATPase activity during exposure to and recovery from acute ischemia. J Cereb Blood Flow Metab 2:457–465
15. Moncada S, Gryglewski RJ, Bunting S, Vane JR (1976) Lipid peroxide inhibits the enzyme in blood vessel microsomes that generates from prostaglandin endoperoxides the substance (Prostaglandin X) which prevents platelet aggregation. Prostaglandins 12:715–737
16. Mršulja BB, Djuričić BM, Cvejić V, Mršulja BJ, Abe K, Spats M, Klatzo I (1980) Biochemistry of experimental ischemic brain edema. Adv Neurol 28:217–230
17. Nakamura M, Mori K (1958) Calorimetric determination of inorganic phosphorus in the presence of glucose-1-phosphate and adenosine triphosphate. Nature 182:1441
18. Nordström C-H, Rehncrona S, Siesjö BK (1978) Effects of phenobarbital in cerebral ischemia. Part two: restitution of cerebral energy state, as well as glycolytic metabolites, citric acid cycle intermediates and associated amino acids after pronounced incomplete ischemia. Stroke 9:335–343
19. Ohkawa H, Ohnishi N, Yagi K (1979) Assay for lipid peroxides in animal tissue by thiobarbituric acid reaction. Anal Biochem 95:351–358
20. Orlowski M, Meister A (1965) Isolation of gamma-glutamyl transpeptidase from dog kidney. J Biol Chem 240:338–348
21. Ottolenghi P (1979) The relipidation of delipidated Na, K-ATPase. Eur J Biochem 99:113–131
22. Pong SS, Levine L (1977) Prostaglandin biosynthesis and metabolism as measured by radioimmunoassay. In: Ramwell PW (ed) The prostaglandins, vol 3. Plenum, New York, pp 41–76
23. Post RL, Hegyvery C, Kume S (1972) Activation by adenosine triphosphate in phosphorylation kinetics of sodium and potassium ion transport adenosine triphosphatase. J Biol Chem 247:6530–6540

24. Proverbio F, Condrescu-Guidi M, Whittembury G (1975) Ouabain sensitive Na^+ stimulation of an Mg^{+2}-dependent ATPase in kidney tissue. Biochem Biophys Acta 394:281–292
25. Rehncrona S, Mela L, Siesjö BK (1979) Recovery of brain mitochondrial function in the rat after complete and incomplete cerebral ischemia. Stroke 10:437–446
26. Rehncrona S, Westerberg E, Akesson B, Siesjö BK (1982) Brain cortical fatty acids and phospholipids during and following complete and severe incomplete ischemia. J Neurochem 38:84–93
27. Spagnuolo C, Sauterbin L, Galli G, Racagni G, Galli C, Massari S, Finesso M (1979) $PGF_{2\alpha}$, thromboxane B_2 and HETE levels in gerbil brain cortex after ligation of common carotid arteries and decapitation. Prostaglandins 18:53–61
28. Spatz M, Mršulja BB (1982) Progress in cerebral microvascular studies related to the function of the blood-brain barrier. Adv Cell Neurobiol 3:331–337
29. Taniguchi K, Tonomura Y (1971) Inactivation of Na^+-K^+-dependent ATPase by phospholipase treatment and its reactivation by phospholipids. J Biochem 69:543–557
30. Yoshida S, Inoh S, Asano T, Sano K, Kubota M, Shimazaki H, Ueda N (1980) Effect of transient ischemia on free fatty acids and possible cause of postischemic injury. J Neurosurg 53:323–331

PI-Specific Phospholipase C and Lipase Activity in Ischemic Rat Brain

Y. Hirashima [1], A. Moto, S. Endo, and A. Takaku

Introduction

A plasma membrane and an organelle are composed of almost identical substances, including phospholipid. The turnover of acyl groups of phospholipids in normal brain biomembrane is well known. Some types of enzymic system related to this turnover have been investigated. Phospholipase A1, A2, PI-specific phospholipase C, lipase, lysophospholipase, acylCoA ligase, and acylCoA: lysophospholipid acyltransferase are some of these enzymic systems.

In the ischemic brain, it has been reported that even in the early stage of ischemia, free fatty acids and diglycerols increase and phospholipids decrease [2, 12, 18]. Accordingly, it is assumed that in ischemia, phospholipase A1, A2, PI-specific phospholipase C, and lipase are activated and at the same time, acylCoA ligase and acylCoA: lysophospholipid acyltransferase are suppressed.

To investigate this hypothesis, we are conducting a study in which these enzyme activities are recorded. The present report gives the activity levels of PI-specific phospholipase C (PI-PLC) and lipase measured in ischemic rat brain.

Materials and Methods

Animals

Male Wistar rats weighing 250–280 g were decapitated at 9 weeks of age without anesthesia. The heads were incubated in artificial CSF at 37 °C for 0, 1, 5, 15, 30, 60, 120, 180, or 240 min. After the incubation the brains were quickly removed and immersed in liquid nitrogen. Each ischemic group consisted of six rats.

Enzyme Preparation

One gram of frozen brain was homogenized in 9 ml ice-cold 0.25 *M* sucrose solution with a homogenizer. A microsomal fraction was obtained by Webster's method [16]. The fraction was immediately resuspended in 0.5 ml ice-cold sucrose solution to make enzyme solution. Protein was measured by the method of Lowry et al. [7].

---

[1] Department of Neurosurgery, Toyama Medical and Pharmaceutical University, 2630 S gitani, Toyama 930-01, Japan

Enzyme Assays

PI-PLC

The substrate used was phosphatidylinositol. L-3-Phosphatidyl[U-^{14}C]inositol was mixed to obtain a specific activity of about 0.5 µCi/µmol. The assay was carried out at pH 7.0 in 0.02 *M* Tris-HCl buffer, 0.2 m*M* $CaCl_2$, and 0.02 mg/ml sodium deoxycholate. The final incubation medium contained approximately 200 nmol per assay tube of substrate. The reaction was stopped by adding 0.1 ml enzyme solution and was allowed to proceed at 37 °C in a shaking water bath for 1 h. The reaction was stopped by the addition of 1 ml chloroform-methanol (2:1, v/v). The radioactivities of the upper and lower phase were measured. The activity of PI-PLC was determined by using the following equation:

$$\frac{\text{Radioactivity of upper phase} \times 200}{\text{Total radioactivity} \times 1 \times \text{Protein}} \text{ (nmol/h/mg protein)}$$

Lipase

We measured monoacylglycerol lipase and diacylglycerol lipase together as α lipase. As the substrate for the assay of lipase, glycerol, 1,2-di[1-^{14}C]palmitate was produced from L-3-phosphatidylcholine, 1,2-di[1-^{14}C]palmitoyl along with PLC isolated from *Cl. perfringens.* Specific activity of substrate was about 2 µCi/µmol. The lipase assay was carried out at pH 7.0 in 0.04 *M* Tris-HCl buffer and 20 m*M* $CaCl_2$. The final incubation medium contained about 125 nmol per assay tube of substrate. The reaction was started by adding 0.1 ml enzyme solution and allowed to proceed at 37 °C in shaking water bath for 1 h. The reaction was stopped by the addition of 1 ml chloroform-methanol mixture. The lower phase was dried down and redissolved in a minimal amount of chloroform. Lipids were separated by TLC (silica gel) in the solvent system: petroleum ether/diethyl ether/acetic acid (60:40:1, v/v/v). The distribution of radioactivity was measured in a radio thin-layer chromatograph. The radioactivities of peaks were measured and the activity of lipase was determined by using the following equation:

$$\frac{\text{Radioactivity of palmitic acid} \times 125}{\text{Total radioactivity} \times 1 \times \text{Protein}} \text{ (nmol/h/mg protein)}$$

Results

General Properties of Enzymes

Substrate Specificity of PI-PLC

No activities were detected in phosphatidylcholine and phosphatidylethanolamine. The activity of phosphatidylserine was 7.8%, and that of phosphatidylinositol was 56.8% (Fig. 1).

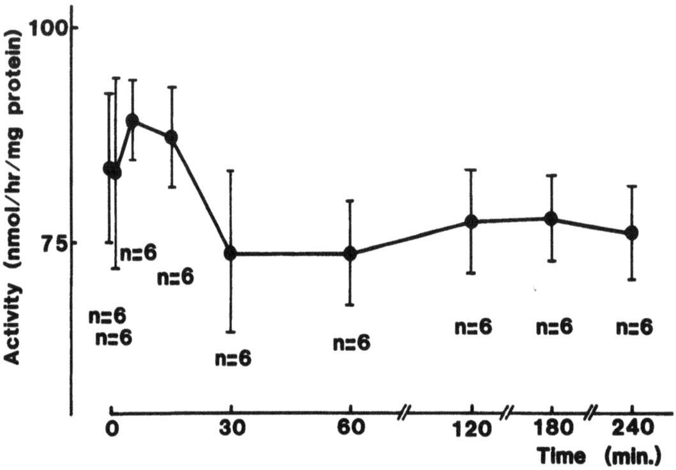

Fig. 1. Sequential changes in PI-PLC activity in ischemic rat brain

The Effect of pH

The optimum pH of PI-PLC was 4.5. Those of lipase were 5.5, 7.0, and 8.5.

The Effect of Ca^{2+} Ions

The optimum condition of PI-PLC was at 0.2 m*M*. That of lipase was at 20 m*M*.

Sequential Changes in Enzyme Activities

PI-PLC

Although there was no statistically significant difference, at the early stage of ischemia there was a tendency for increased activity (Fig. 2).

Lipase

After 5 min of ischemia the activity had already increased significantly ($P<0.05$). This high level was maintained until 30 min and thereafter decreased gradually (Fig. 2).

Discussion

Phospholipids are an important element of the biomembrane and are contained in brain in particularly large quantities.

According to Sun's report [12] (Fig. 3), acyl groups of phospholipid have a constant turnover, and the quantities of free fatty acids, lysophospholipids, and di-

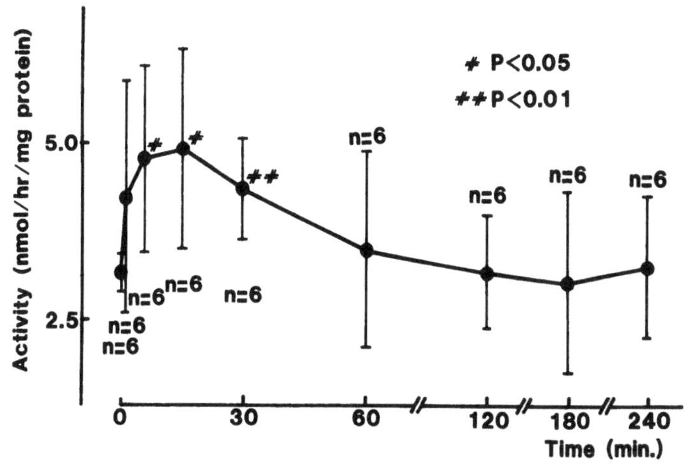

Fig. 2. Sequential changes in lipase activity in ischemic rat brain

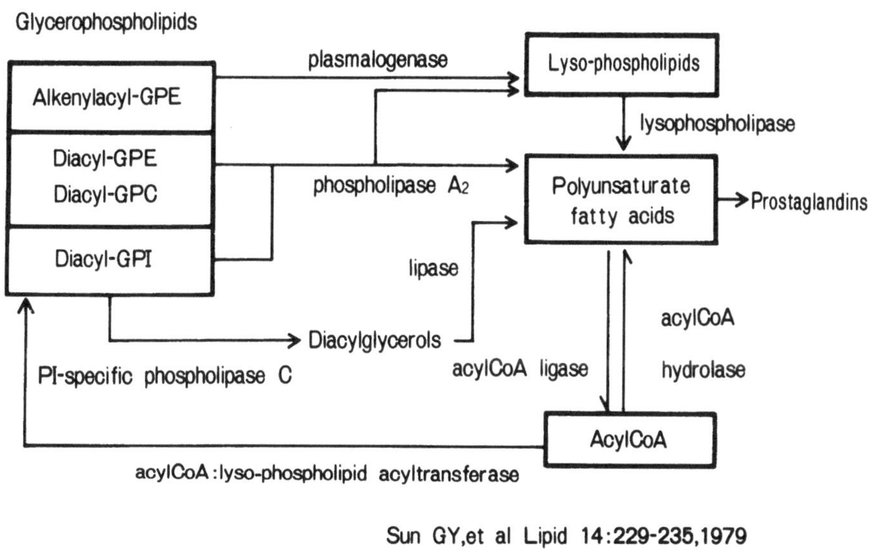

Fig. 3. Metabolic relationship between polyunsaturated fatty acids and membrane phospholipids in brain

Table 1. Substrate specificity of PI-PLC in rat brain microsomal fraction

	Activity of PLC (%)
PC	ND
PE	ND
PS	7.8
PI	56.8

Results are expressed as percentages of the initial substrate after 1 h incubation at 37 °C

acylglycerols are known to be extremely small in normal brain [8, 13, 15]. However, in the ischemic brain, Bazan [2] and Yoshida et al. [18] have reported that levels of free fatty acids increase and phospholipids decline even in the early stage of ischemia. Lysophospholipid and diacylglycerol also increase during the ischemic state [12, 17]. The changes in these metabolites reflect not only membrane destruction, but also additional injury to the brain. Free fatty acids are known to impair mitochondrial ATP production [6], to increase cerebral edema [14], and to suppress glycolysis [3]. Lysophospholipid has cytolytic and solubilizing activities to neural tissues [17]. Accordingly, it is considered that in ischemia, phospholipase A_1, A_2, PI-PLC, and lipase are activated while acylCoA : ligase and acylCoA : lysophospholipid acyltransferase are suppressed.

To elucidate this hypothesis, we are investigating the enzyme activities in the ischemic brain of rats.

Among the free fatty acids, most of the arachidonic acid released upon ischemia has been postulated to be formed at the expense of phosphatidylinositol, 80% of which has a 1-stearoyl-2-arachidonoyl acyl composition in the brain [11]. In this paper, we have reported the activities of PI-PLC and lipase in ischemic brain. The results showed that activities of both PI-PLC and lipase increased in the early ischemic stage and then decreased gradually.

Some hypotheses are described below in attempts to explain the activation of deacylation enzymes in ischemia.

First, it is well known that the level of cyclic AMP increases markedly when a brain becomes ischemic. Therefore it was postulated that this change in cyclic AMP activates phospholipase mediated by proteinkinase [1]. However, Yoshida et al. [19] reported that the increase in cyclic AMP levels is not paralleled by changes in free fatty acid levels in the brain of decapitated rat with unilateral lesion of the locus ceruleus. Secondly, it is generally accepted that intracellular calcium concentration increase in ischemia. There is some speculation [9, 10] that this phenomenon activates phospholipase. In the present study, PI-PLC and lipase were proved to be Ca^{2+} dependent. However, the activities of phospholipases in the brain are not always regulated by the Ca^{2+} ion. For example, phospholipase A_1 and A_2 activity reported by Edgar et al. [5] were not Ca^{2+} dependent. Thirdly, intracellular pH changes are also considered to be important for the activation of phospholipase. In ischemia, intracellular pH decreases rapidly, and then PI-PLC and lipase may be activated because their optimum pH is an acid one. Nonetheless, Edgar and Freusz [4] report that PLC has an alkaline pH optimum, and the activity of this enzyme decreases in an acid environment.

Although the enzyme activities were assayed during the same condition in the present study, the enzymes were found to be activated in the early stage of ischemia. Many kinds of phospholipases and lipases, which have different optimum pH values and optimum Ca^{2+} concentrations, have been reported from a number of institutions. The mechanism of the activation of enzymes is bound to be more complex, and it is impossible to explain these phenomena by any single theory.

Edgar et al. [5] suggested that an enzyme was activated by a covalent modification of its structure in ischemia. This question requires further study.

Summary

1. The optimum pH of PI-specific phospholipase C was 4.5. Those of lipase were 5.5, 7.0, and 8.5.
2. The optimum Ca^{2+} concentration of PI-specific phospholipase C was 0.2 mM. That of lipase was 20 mM.
3. The activities of PI-specific phospholipase C and lipase increased from the early stage of ischemia onward.

References

1. Bazan NG (1976) Free arachidonic acid and other lipids in the nervous system during early ischemia and after electroshock. In: Porcellati G, Amaducci L, Galli C (eds) Function and metabolism of phospholipids in central and peripheral nervous system. Plenum, New York, pp 317–335
2. Bazan NF Jr (1970) Effect of ischemia and electroconvulsive shock on free fatty acid pool in the brain. Biochim Biophys Acta 218:1–10
3. Broniszewska-Ardert B, Dabrowiecki Z (1976) Studies on the inhibition of brain phosphofructokinase by oleate and the determination of fatty acids in normal and hypoxic brain. J Neurochem 27:585–587
4. Edgar AD, Freysz L (1982) Phospholipase activities of rat brain. Cytosol occurrence of phospholipase C activity with phosphatidylcholine. Biochim Biophys Acta 711:224–228
5. Edgar AD, Strosznajder J, Horrocks LA (1982) Activation of ethanolamine phospholipase A2 in brain during ischemia. J Neurochem 39:1111–1116
6. Kuwashima J, Fujitani B, Nakamura K, Kadokawa T, Yoshida K, Shimizu M (1976) Biochemical changes in unilateral brain injury in the rat: a possible role of free fatty acid accumulation. Brain Res 110:547–557
7. Lowry OH, Rosebrough NJ, Farr AL, Randal RJ (1951) Protein measurement with the Folin phenol reagent. J Biol Chem 193:265–275
8. Lunt GG, Rowe CE (1968) The production of unesterified fatty acid in brain. Biochim Biophys Acta 152:681–693
9. Markelonis G, Garbus J (1975) Alterations of intracellular oxidative metabolism as stimuli evoking prostaglandin biosynthesis. Prostaglandins 10:1087–1106
10. Siesjö BK (1981) Cell damage in the brain: a speculative synthesis. J Cereb Blood Flow Metabol 1:155–185
11. Su KL, Sun GY (1978) Acyl group composition of metabolically active lipids in brain: variances among subcellular fractions and during post-natal development. J Neurochem 31:1043–1050
12. Sun GY, Su KL, Der OM, Tang W (1978) Enzymic regulation of arachidonate metabolism in brain membrane phosphoglycerides. Lipids 14:229–235
13. Thompson RHS, Niemiro R, Webster GR (1960) The identification of lysolecithin in lipid extracts of brain. Biochim Biophs Acta 43:142–144
14. Wakai S, Aritake K, Asano T, Takakura K (1982) Selective destruction of the outer leaflet of the capillary endothelial membrane after intracerebral injection of arachidonic acid in the rat. Acta Neuropathol 58:303–306
15. Webster GR, Thompson RHS (1962) Observations of the presence of lysolecithin in nervous tissues. Biochim Biophys Acta 63:38–45
16. Webster GR, Alpern RJ (1964) Studies on the acylation of lysolecithin by rat brain. Biochem J 90:35–42
17. Webster GR, Thompson RHS (1965) Accumulation of lysolecithin in rat brain on incubation in vitro. Nature 206:296–297
18. Yoshida S, Inoh S, Asano T, Sano K, Kubota M, Shimazaki H, Ueta N (1980) Effect of transient ischemia on free fatty acids and phospholipids in the gerbil brain: lipid peroxidation as a possible cause of postischemic injury. J Neurosurg 53:323–331
19. Yoshida S, Buso R, Ginsberg MD, Haric SI, Scheinberg P (1983) Brain ischemia, brain edema and free radicals. In: Sano K, Handa H, Takakura K, Kogure K, Asano T (eds) Brain edema and free radicals. Neuron (Tokyo) pp 67–87

Dynamics of Tissue Water Content, Free and Bound Components, Associated with Ischemic Brain Edema

S. INAO[1], H. KUCHIWAKI, N. HIRAI, S. TAKADA, N. KAGEYAMA, M. FURUSE, and T. GONDA

Key words: Ischemic brain edema, thermal analysis (DSC), water components, free water, bound water

Introduction

Analysis of tissue water in the brain is known to be of paramount importance for the understanding of the pathogenesis of brain edema. Recently NMR techniques have been applied to evaluate the status of biological water in both experimental and clinical studies. Despite the potential usefulness, however, it remains difficult to measure the absolute amounts of free and bound water by NMR techniques.

In the present study we attempted to quantitate the free and bound water components in ischemic brain edema by means of differential scanning calorimetry (DSC). Emphasis was laid upon the time course of changes in the ratio of free and bound water during the processes of formation and regression of brain edema.

Materials and Methods

Wistar rats weighing 150–220 g were anesthetized with pentobarbital sodium (50 mg/kg) IP, and the left middle cerebral artery (MCA) was microsurgically coagulated through a small subtemporal craniectomy [5]. Experimental animals were examined at 2, 4, 8, 16, and 24 h and 3 and 6 days after MCA occlusion. At the end of each experiment carbon black suspension was injected directly into the left ventricle exposed by thoracotomy to allow visualization of the site and spread of the infarcted area. After decapitation the brain was removed as rapidly as possible and sliced in coronal sections of 1–2 mm thickness. The outer appearance of the brain and the spread of nonfilling areas were recorded on the appropriate schemas. The nonfilling areas were localized mainly in the left lateral cortex. Small pieces of brain tissue (sampling weight 15–30 mg) were taken from the center of the ischemic area (infarcted area, I), the peripheral part of the ischemic area (marginal area, M), and the contralateral hemisphere (noninfarcted hemisphere, N).

The different components of total water in the tissue samples were measured with the aid of a DSC system (SSC/560 S, Seiko-Instruments & Electronics Ltd). Each

[1] Department of Neurosurgery, Nakatsugawa Municipal General Hospital, 1-33 Ebisu-Machi, Nakatsugawa 508, Japan

Table 1. Formulae for calculation of water components

Water component	Formula
Total water (mg)	Total weight (mg) – Dry weight (mg)
Water content (%)	$\frac{\text{Total weight (mg)} - \text{Dry weight (mg)}}{\text{Total weight (mg)}} \times 100$
Free water (mg)	$\frac{\text{Calorific value (cal) (estimated in DSC freezing)}}{\text{79.4 (cal/mg)}}$
Free water (%)	$\frac{\text{Free water (mg)}}{\text{Total water (mg)}} \times 100$
Bound water (mg)	Total water (mg) – Free water (mg)
Bound water (%)	100–Free water (%)
Water bonding to solid tissue component	$\frac{\text{Bound water (mg)}}{\text{Dry weight (mg)}}$

sample was encased in closed-type aluminum capsule and put into the cell (measuring part) of DSC equipment for programmed freezing (cooling rate –10 °C/min). The amount of free water was calculated from the area under the thermal curve, which corresponded to the calorific value of freezable water in the sample. The total tissue water was determined by exsiccation of the sample up to 200 °C, which was performed as the second step of the thermal procedure with the seal of the capsule opened. The amount of bound water was determined by subtracting free water from total water. The amount of bound water per unit of solid (dry) component was also estimated. The formulae used for calculation are shown in Table 1. Details of this method have already been described elsewhere [1, 2].

Results

Water Components in the Control Group

Mean values for the water components in both normal brain and serum are shown in Table 2. The water content in the brain was 80.3% ± 0.6% (SD). A constitutional analysis revealed that the free and bound water fractions were 89.5% ± 2.5% and 10.5% ± 2.5%, respectively. Water binding to solid tissue components (BW/SC) amounted to 0.43 ± 0.11 mg/mg. The corresponding amount of free water to tissue dry weight (FW/SC) was 3.64 ± 0.14 mg/mg. Since there was no significant difference in the ratio of the different water components between the animals with and without dye infusion the experimental group without dye infusion was used as the control group for comparison with the ischemic group.

In comparison with the values obtained in brain tissue the serum had a much higher water content of 94.4% ± 1.2%. Much higher values were found for BW/SC and FW/SC, averaging 1.61 mg/mg and 15.29 mg/mg, which were three- to four-

Table 2. Water components in normal brain and serum

	Brain Infusion of dye		Serum
	Without ($n = 15$)	With ($n = 12$)	($n = 11$)
Water content (%)	80.3±0.6	80 ±0.5	94.4±1.2
Free water (%)	89.5±2.5	90.0±2.2	90.7±2.6
Bound water (%)	10.5	9.1	9.3
Total water (%)	100	100	100
Free water/solid component (FW/SC) (mg/mg)	3.64±0.14	3.66±0.13	15.29
Bound water/solid component (BW/SC) (mg/mg)	0.43±0.11	0.37±0.09	1.61±0.44

Values given are means±SD

fold those in the brain. The fractions of free and bound water in normal serum were found to be 90.7%±2.6% and 9.3%±2.6%.

Changes in Water Components in the Ischemic Group

The time courses of changes in the various water components in the ischemic brain are shown in Fig. 1. After MCA occlusion the water content in the infarcted area increased as a function of time, showing a peak of around 90% at 16–24 h of the experiment. In the marginal area the water content reached 85% at its peak, while there were only minimal changes in the contralateral (noninfarcted) hemisphere and in rats subjected to sham operation performed after 24 h (Fig. 1A).

The free water fraction began to increase significantly in the infarcted area from the 8th hour of the experimental period, and higher values were maintained until the 6th day, with a peak at the 16th hour following MCA occlusion. In the marginal area the free water fraction increased significantly at 24 h (Fig. 1B).

Water binding to the solid component increased significantly in the ischemic brain during the period from 24 h to 3 days. Despite the increase in water content there were no significant changes in BW/SC during the earlier phase before 24 h (Fig. 1C).

The changes in water constitution in the infarcted area are summarized in Fig. 2. As shown in Fig. 2A, the fraction of free water did not increase in the initial phase in the first 4 h in spite of the consistent increase in total water content, which started at 2 h. From 8 h to 16 h the free water fraction then began to increase in parallel with the marked increment of water content, with a subsequent gradual decrease in

Fig. 1A–C. Time courses of water content (**A**), free water fraction (**B**), and BW/SC (**C**) measured in various parts of ischemic brain

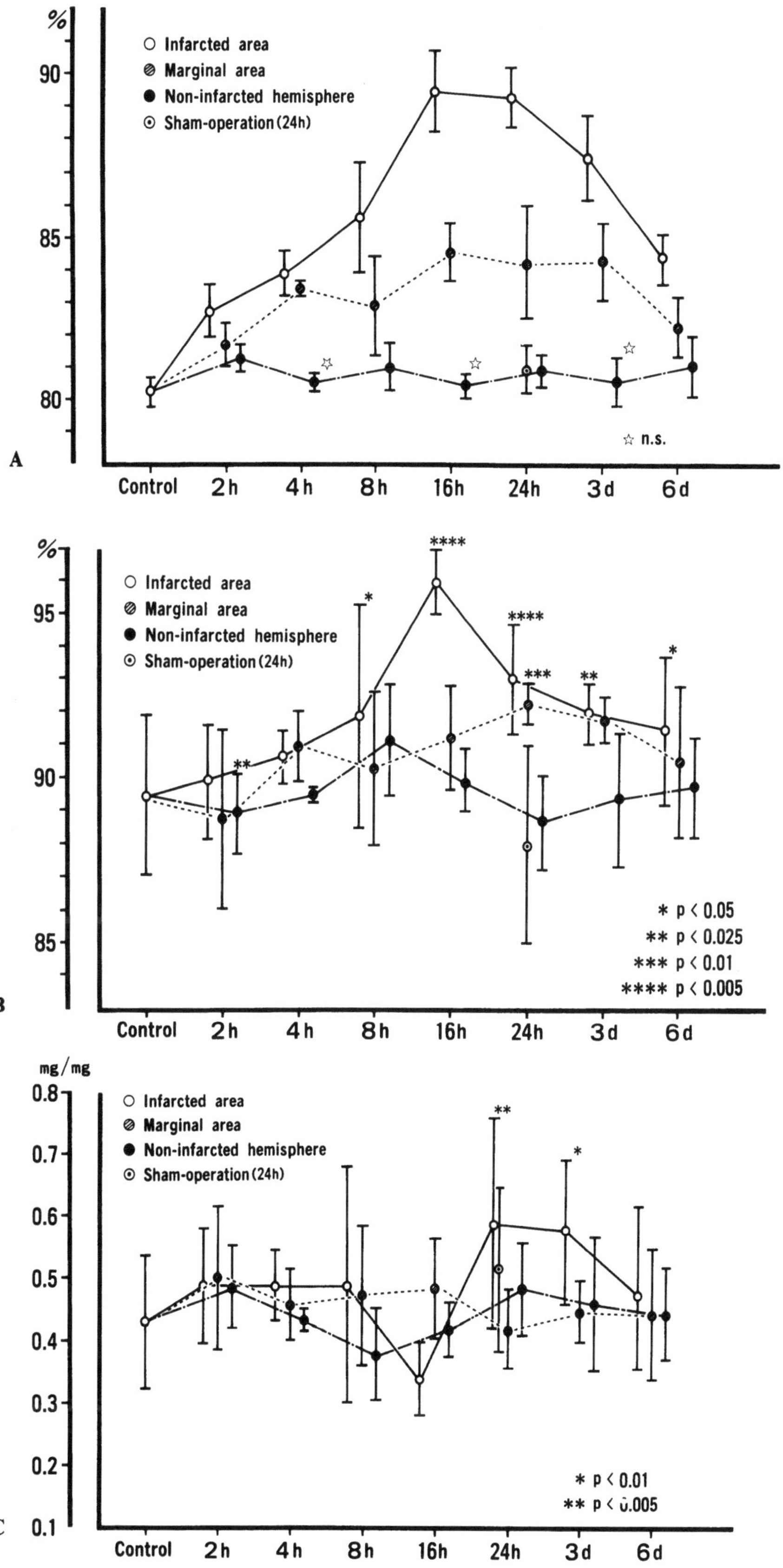
A
%
90
85
80
Infarcted area
Marginal area
Non-infarcted hemisphere
Sham-operation (24h)
☆ n.s.
Control
2h
4h
8h
16h
24h
3d
6d
B
%
95
90
85
Infarcted area
Marginal area
Non-infarcted hemisphere
Sham-operation (24h)
* p < 0.05
** p < 0.025
*** p < 0.01
**** p < 0.005
Control
2h
4h
8h
16h
24h
3d
6d
C
mg/mg
0.8
0.7
0.6
0.5
0.4
0.3
0.2
0.1
Infarcted area
Marginal area
Non-infarcted hemisphere
Sham-operation (24h)
* p < 0.01
** p < 0.005
Control
2h
4h
8h
16h
24h
3d
6d

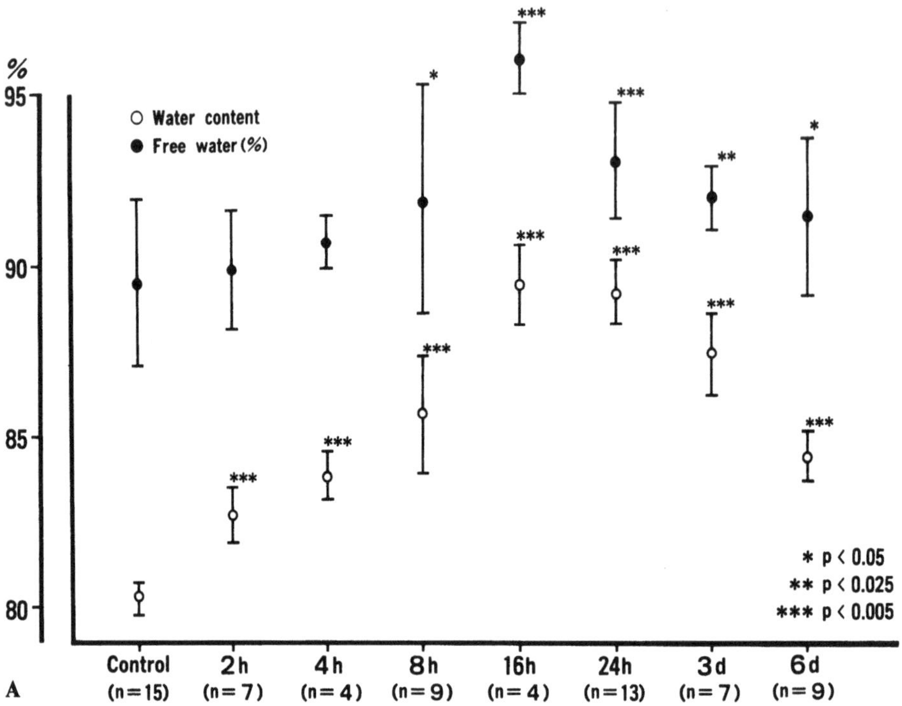

A

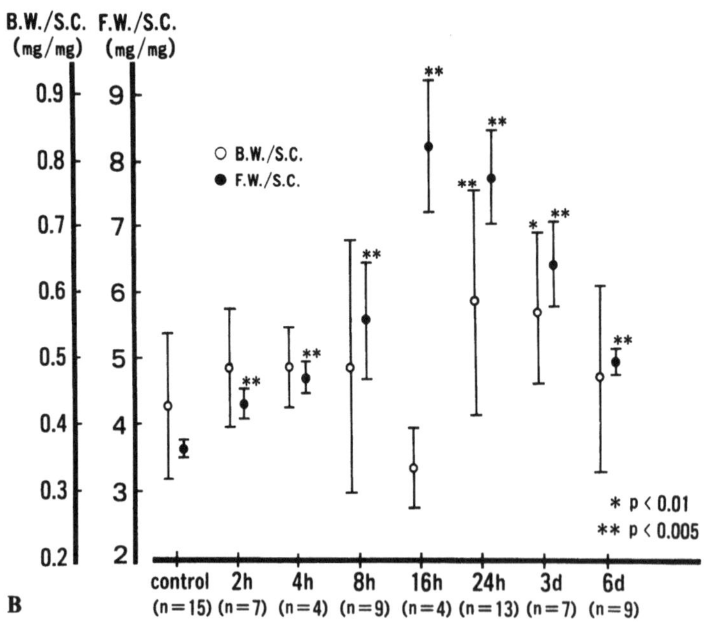

B

Fig. 2 A, B. Time courses of water components in infarcted area. Comparative changes in water content and free water ratio (**A**) and in BW/SC and FW/SC (**B**)

both water fractions. This time course of changes in the water constitution indicates that both free and bound water fractions increased in almost the same proportions in the initial phase of edema formation and that the increase in free water predominated in the period when brain edema was becoming established.

Figure 2B shows comparative changes in BW/SC and FW/SC in these infarcted areas. The value of FW/SC started to increase significantly even at 2 h of the experiment. In contrast, the value for BW/SC remained almost unchanged during the earlier stage up to 16 h. The value for BW/SC increased progressively in the late phase of edema formation from 24 h to 3 days.

Discussion

Our observations suggest that the movement of tissue water is biphasic during the process of edema formation following cerebral ischemia. In the early stage, within 2–4 h after arterial occlusion, the water content begins to increase without evidence of constitutional change in either the free or the bound water fraction. The second stage of ischemia begins at approximately 8 h and reaches its peak at 24 h or later. This period of edema establishment is characterized by a marked increase in the free water fraction, which coincides with the increase in total water content. The bound water fraction also increases at the end of this stage, this increase lasting from 24 h to 3 days.

With regard to these time courses it is assumed that the initial phase of edema formation is based not only on the shift of freely mobile water into the ischemic zone owing to an increased hydrostatic pressure gradient or involvement of the ion pump [3], but also on a change in the conformation of tissue proteins, which elevates the binding capacity to water. In contrast, the later stage of edema establishment seems to be strongly affected by disruption of the blood-brain barrier [4]. As a result of consistent impairment of the barrier function movement of free water into the infarcted area can be accelerated. Furthermore, diffusion of serum proteins into the ischemic region causes a considerable increase in both free and bound water components.

With reference to the pathophysiology of ischemic brain edema, the component of freely mobile water is a major factor in the increasing amount of tissue water in edema formation. At the same time, it is also very significant that the fraction of bound water increases at the period of established brain edema. It is reasonable to assume that the increase in the bound water component during brain edema contributes to the maintenance of ischemic cerebral edema.

Summary

The present study was designed to examine the time course of tissue water components such as free and bound water in experimental cerebral infarction induced by unilateral occlusion of the middle cerebral artery in Wistar rats. Water components in the brain tissue were measured by means of differential scanning calorimetry, each component of free and bound water and of total tissue water being refined.

In the ischemic cerebral lesion the water content began to increase in its earlier phase after arterial occlusion, showing no significant changes in the proportions of free and bound water fractions. In the later phase, however, the proportion of free water increased in keeping with the marked increment in tissue water content. The bound water fraction also increased in the final phase of edema formation. Freely mobile water accounts for most of the increased amount of tissue water in edema formation, and the increase in the bound water fraction may contribute to the maintenance of ischemic cerebral edema.

References

1. Furuse M, Kuchiwaki H, Gonda T, Kageyama N, Kawajiri H, Kontani J (1981) Thermoanalytical investigation on the state of free and bound water in normal and edematous brains. J Cereb Blood Flow Metab 1 [Suppl 1]: 154–155
2. Furuse M, Gonda T, Kuchiwaki H, Hirai N, Inao S, Kageyama N (1984) Thermal analysis on the state of free and bound water in normal and edematous brains. In: Go KG, Baethmann A (eds) Recent progress in the study and therapy of brain edema. Plenum, New York, pp 293–298
3. Kogure K, Busto R, Schenberg P (1981) The role of hydrostatic pressure in ischemic brain edema. Ann Neurol 9: 273–282
4. O'Brien MD, Waltz AG, Jordan MM (1974) Ischemic cerebral edema and the blood-brain barrier: distributions of pertechnetate, albumin, sodium and antipyrine in brains of cats after occlusion of the middle cerebral artery. Arch Neurol 30: 461–465
5. Tamura A, Graham DI, McCulloh J, Teasdale GM (1981) Focal cerebral ischemia in the rat: 1. description of technique and early neuropathological consequences following middle cerebral artery occlusion. J Cereb Blood Flow Metab 1: 53–60

The Pathophysiology of Ischemic Brain Swelling

K.-A. Hossmann [1]

Key words: Ischemic brain edema, postischemic brain edema, blood-brain barrier, treatment of edema

Introduction

Brain swelling associated with cerebral ischemia is a well-known phenomenon, which was identified long ago as one of the major complicating factors promoting the progression or impeding the reversal of circulatory impairment. Considerable attention has therefore been devoted to the elucidation of the pathophysiology of this process, and numerous studies have been carried out in which amelioration by therapeutic intervention has been attempted [29]. Despite these efforts no major breakthrough has been achieved in the therapy of ischemic brain swelling, and many of the various procedures proposed remain highly controversial.

There are several possible reasons for this situation. One is the complexity of the process, which involves fluid and electrolyte shifts among at least four compartments, i.e., blood, cerebrospinal fluid, extracellular space, and intracellular compartment. Other possible reasons are that differences exist between the factors promoting edema formation during or after ischemia and, finally, that the blood-brain barrier suffers differential permeability changes for large and small molecules, which may even vary in the course of the pathologic process. Hence, the extent, composition, and therapeutic susceptibility of ischemic brain edema may vary considerably depending on the type, degree, and timepoint of ischemia.

In the present paper an attempt is made to unravel some of the factors involved by differentiating between ischemic and postischemic edema and between the net changes in brain water and electrolytes, the intercompartmental shifts, and the changes in blood-brain barrier permeability. The data presented and the conclusions drawn are based mainly on our own experiments [15, 54, 18, 20, 45, 35], but reference will also be made to studies conducted in other laboratories and to a number of previous review articles [29, 30, 37, 36, 12].

Definitions

According to Klatzo [30], brain edema is defined as an abnormal accumulation of fluid, primarily of water, within the brain parenchyma, producing a volumetric en-

[1] Max Planck Institute for Neurological Research, Department of Experimental Neurology, Ostmerheimer Str. 200, D-5000 Köln 91

largement of the tissue. *Vasogenic edema* results from an increase in the permeability of the blood-brain barrier to serum constituents, and *cytotoxic edema* from a disturbance of cell metabolism. *Ischemic brain edema* is the increase of tissue water developing *during* a period of reduced cerebral blood flow. *Postischemic edema* is the accumulation of water during recirculation of the brain *after* a period of reduced flow. *Ischemic brain swelling* is the increase in brain volume during or after a period of circulatory impairment. It is the combined effect of ischemic or postischemic brain edema and an increase in blood volume. The *blood-brain* and *blood-CSF barriers* are the interfaces between the intravascular and extracellular and the extracellular and CSF compartments, respectively. Barrier disturbances are always expressed as changes in transport or permeability properties in respect of a particular molecule, e.g., sodium, albumin, etc., but never as global changes.

Ischemic Brain Edema

Net Changes in Water and Tissue Electrolyte Content

The classic experimental model for the study of ischemic brain edema is stroke induced by clipping of the middle cerebral artery (MCA). With sensitive volume gauges which allow monitoring of the displacement of the cortex in respect to the skull, incipient swelling can be detected after as little as 1–2 min following vascular occlusion (Fig. 1). This increase is initially due to the autoregulatory dilatation of the vascular bed within the ischemic territory (hypoperfusion hyperemia) but later to the progressing accumulation of fluid in the parenchyma.

The development of ischemic brain edema is flow dependent (Fig. 2). As long as flow stays above a critical threshold water and electrolyte content of brain tissue remain normal even if electrophysiological disturbances are already present (noncritical ischemia [17]). Below this threshold, the water and electrolyte homeostasis is disturbed (critical ischemia), the degree of disturbance being determined by the duration of ischemia. The threshold for edema development is about 20 ml/100 g/min in gerbil [9], 15–20 ml/100 g/min in monkey [50], and 10–15 ml/100 g/min in cats [17, 49]. Symon et al. [50] suggested that the threshold for water uptake is slightly higher than that for electrolyte disturbances, but this was not confirmed in later experiments in cats [17, 49].

The development of ischemic brain edema is progressive. In cats the cortical water content rises from 4.18 ± 0.10 to 4.90 ± 0.12 ml/g dry weight (d.w.) (means $\pm$ SE) within 4 h after MCA occlusion (Fig. 3), and to about 8 ml/g d.w. after 24 h (according to [38], Fig. 2). In monkeys, a maximum of 5.2 ml/g d.w. has been observed in the sylvian cortex 24 h after the onset of ischemia [7]. In the white matter of cat water rises from 2.12 ± 0.06 to 2.55 ± 0.3 ml/g d.w. within 4 h, and in the monkey from 2.09 to 2.94 ml/g d.w. within 48 h [7]. The accumulation of fluid is caused by or associated with an increase of tissue osmolality and tissue electrolyte content. In cats, tissue osmolality increases from 308 ± 3 to 317 ± 5 mosmol and remains at this level at least during the initial 4 h, thus creating a small but persisting osmotic gradient to the blood. Cortical sodium continuously rises from 262 ± 9 to 440 ± 22 μEq/g d.w. within 4 h (Fig. 3), and further to almost 700 μEq/g d.w. after 48 h [27]. Bremer et

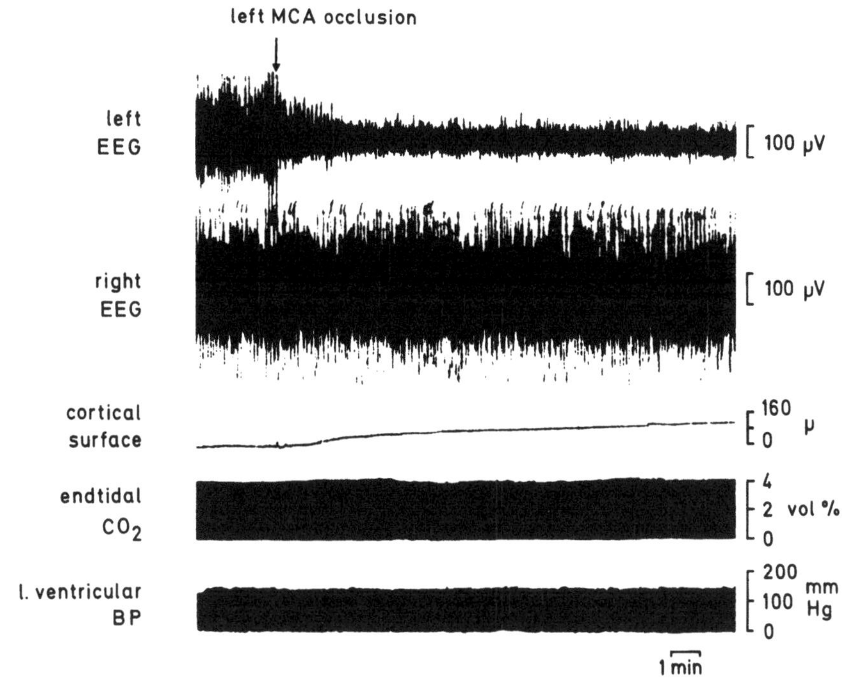

Fig. 1. Brain swelling after transorbital occlusion of the left middle cerebral artery in cat. Swelling of the cortex is recorded by measuring the displacement of the cortical surface in respect to the skull. Ischemia causes immediate reduction of EEG amplitude and incipient swelling of the ipsilateral hemisphere within 2 min after vascular occlusion. (Reproduced from Schuier and Hossmann [45] by permission of the American Heart Association, Inc.)

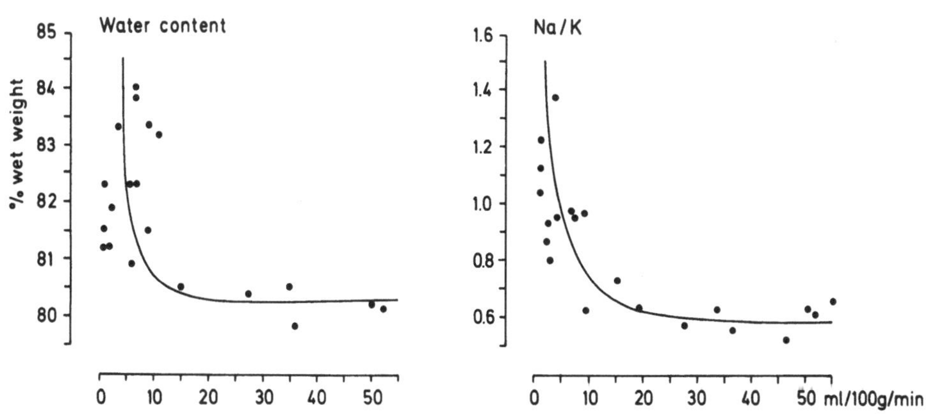

Fig. 2. Relationships among cerebral blood flow (measured with radioactive microspheres), water content of the cerebral cortex and the sodium : potassium content ratio after middle cerebral artery occlusion of cat. The threshold at which disturbances of water and ion homeostasis begin is 10–15 ml/100 g/min. (Modified from Hossmann and Schuier [17] by permission of the American Heart Association, Inc.)

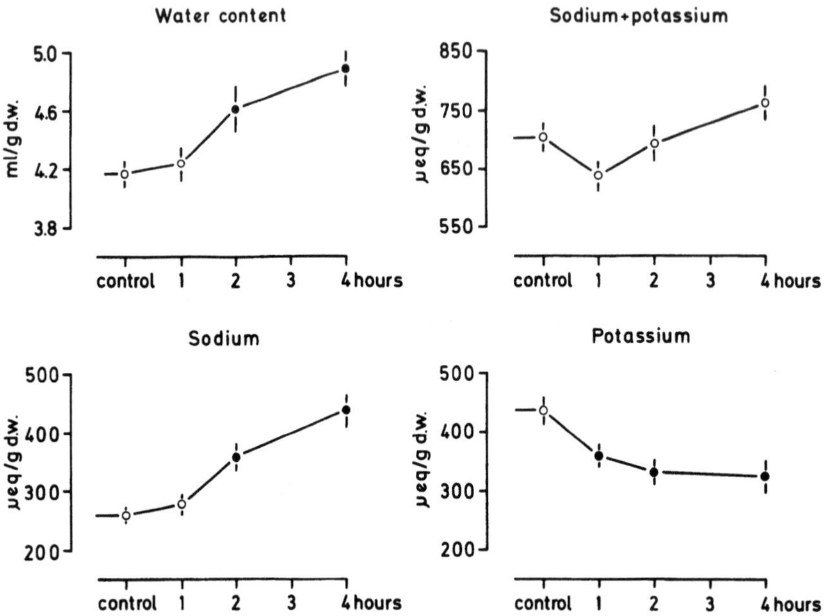

Fig. 3. Changes in the content of water, sodium, and potassium in cerebral cortex of cat following middle cerebral artery occlusion. Note the inverse changes of sodium and potassium content. Brain edema begins to develop before the sum of sodium and potassium content increases. Values are means ± SE; *filled circles* indicate statistically significant difference from control ($P<0.05$)

al. [7] also report a gradual increase in chloride, which almost doubles within 12 h after MCA occlusion in monkey. Cortical potassium, on the other hand, declines from 442 ± 20 to 328 ± 28 µEq/g d.w. within 4 h in cats (Fig. 3), and to 408 µEq/g d.w. after 24 h in monkeys [7]. Since sodium and potassium shift in different directions, the ratio of sodium to potassium is a sensitive indicator of early electrolyte disturbances. In cats, a significant increase in this ratio is observed in both gray and white matter after as little as 1 h.

Net fluid and electrolyte uptake of the ischemic brain are closely associated. When the increment of cortical cation content (the sum of sodium and potassium) is plotted against the increase of water (in respect of the means of control brains), a slope of 146 µEq/ml edema fluid is calculated (Fig. 4). Assuming that the loss of potassium is compensated by an equimolar uptake of sodium, and that this exchange does not result in a change in net water content, the cation content of edema fluid is mainly made up by sodium. The sodium content of cat plasma is about 140 µEq/ml; it is, therefore, reasonable to conclude that ischemic brain edema fluid is essentially an ultrafiltrate of blood serum. It should be noted, however, that the intercept of the calculated regression between water and cations is negative, i.e., a certain amount of water is taken up by the brain without any net cation changes. According to the correlation shown in Fig. 4, this amount is 0.35 ml/g d.w., or about 9% of the total brain water. In monkeys a similar calculation based on data published by Bremer et al. [7] reveals an increment of as much as 0.98 ml water/g d.w. before the net ion content begins to rise. It is likely that this amount of water is taken up by the brain

Fig. 4. Relationship between the increase in water and the increase in sodium and potassium content of cerebral cortex of cat 2–4 h after middle cerebral artery occlusion. Values are means of three groups with different duration of ischemia. Note the negative intercept of the calculated regression, indicating that brain edema develops before cation content increases. (Data taken from Schuier and Hossmann [45] by permission of the American Heart Association, Inc.)

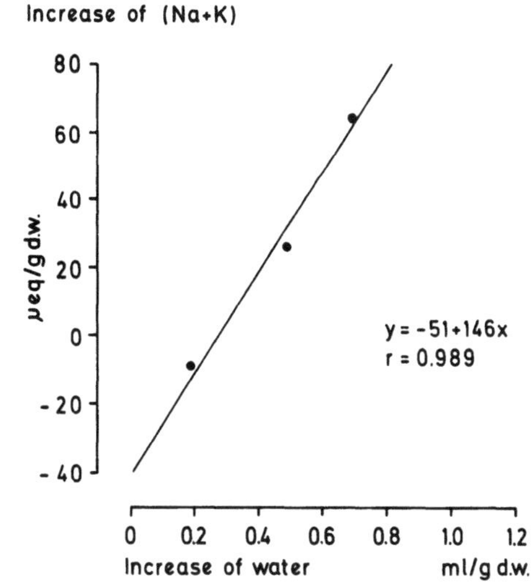

to maintain osmotic equilibrium with blood and cerebrospinal fluid. The brain, in consequence, generates "idiogenic," osmotically active particles which, in addition to extravasated electrolytes, contribute to the development of ischemic edema. Consideration of the time course of water and net cation changes may further lead to the conclusion that the generation of idiogenic osmols precedes ultrafiltration of plasma, because the net increase in cations follows that in water by about 1 h (Fig. 3).

The origin and nature of the idiogenic osmols is not clear. As discussed below, tissue osmolality increases by about 50 mosmol during 1 h of total cerebrocirculatory arrest, although the sum of major osmotically active solutes (including lactate) does not change. Bito and Myers [4] have suggested that the generation of NH_4 may release intracellular cations from their binding sites by glutamate-glutamine interconversion. However, the amount of NH_4 generated does not suffice to account for the increase measured. Another possible explanation is the presence of intracellular acidosis, which during ischemia may reach pH values as low as 6.1 and which may be directly or indirectly involved in the release of electrolytes from inactive binding sites.

There is some indirect evidence that most of the idiogenic osmols must be accounted for by cations. Data published by Bremer et al. [7] were used to plot the increment of water during edema formation against the increase in tissue chloride content. It turned out that the intercept of this regression was close to zero, indicating that in contrast to cations, the brain does not generate an excess of anions. In consequence, the brain imbibes a substantial amount of water and anions during the early development of ischemic brain edema in order to maintain both osmotic and electric neutrality.

Compartmentation of Fluid and Electrolytes

The net uptake of fluid and electrolytes by the ischemic brain is accompanied by or associated with considerable shifts of fluid and electrolytes between the intra- and

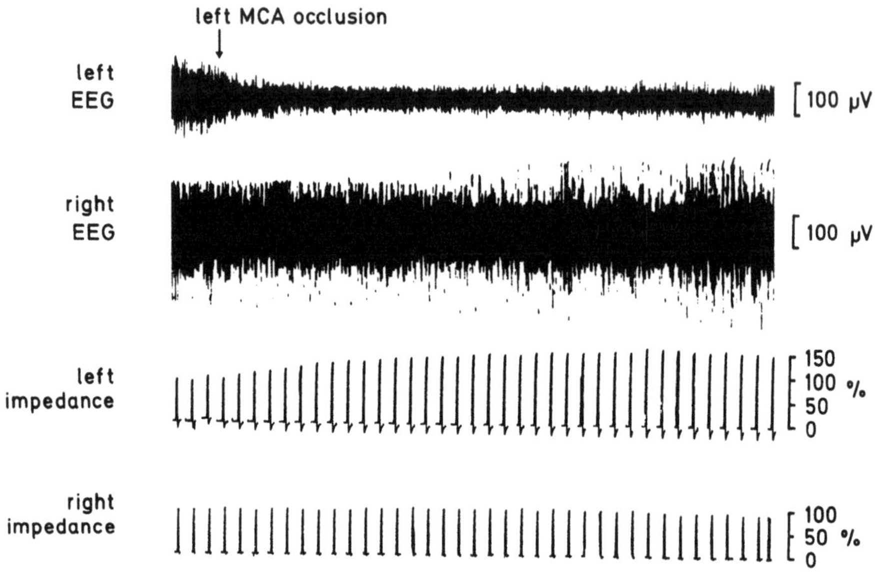

Fig. 5. Recording of electrical impedance of left and right parietal cortex of cat after occlusion of the left middle cerebral artery. In the ischemic territory cortical impedance increases shortly after vascular occlusion, indicating the beginning shrinkage of extracellular space. (Reproduced from Schuier and Hossmann [45] by permission of the American Heart Association, Inc.)

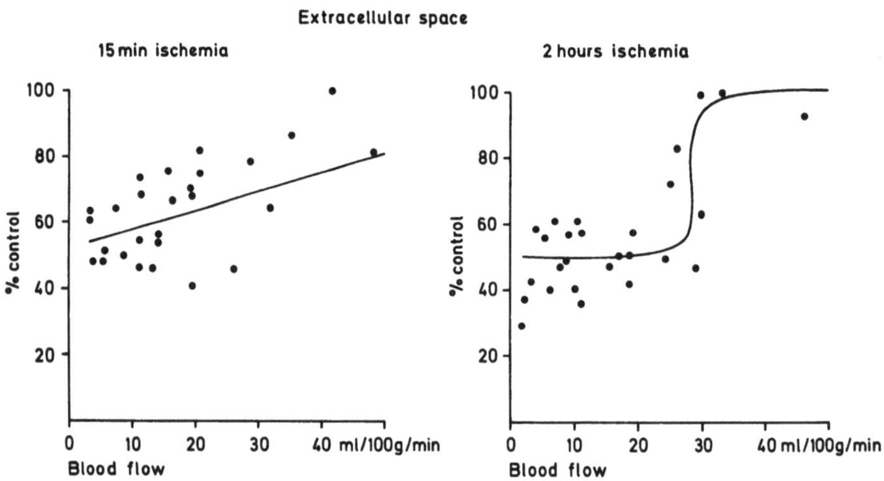

Fig. 6. Relationship between cerebral blood flow and extracellular space in parietal cortex at 15 min and at 2 h after occlusion of the ipsilateral middle cerebral artery of cat. After 15 min a linear, and after 2 h a threshold relationship is obtained. For explanation see text. Extracellular space was determined by the electrical impedance method. (Matsuoka and Hossmann [35])

extracellular compartments. Using electrical impedance measurements of cortex for continuous evaluation of the size of the extracellular compartment, incipient narrowing can be detected within 2 min after the onset of ischemia (Fig. 5). Quantitative evaluation of intracerebral fluid shifts with the aid of the Maxwell algorithm reveals a decrease in the relative extracellular volume from 19% to 14% within 5 min, and a leveling off at about 11% after 30 min. This finding is supported by electron microscopical estimates of extracellular space following freeze substitution [52] and by extracellular markers monitored with ion-sensitive electrodes [13].

Immediately after the onset of ischemia, the relationship between flow reduction and the narrowing of the extracellular space is linear; at later times, however, a threshold relationship at about 30 ml/100 g/min is observed (Fig. 6). Below this threshold, extracellular volume is reduced to about 50% of control, whereas at higher flow values it remains normal. The flow threshold for evoking intercompartmental fluid shifts, in consequence, is substantially higher than that for the net uptake of water or net changes of electrolyte content. It is also higher than the threshold for release of intracellular potassium ions into the extracellular space, which according to Branston et al. [5] is between 8 and 11 ml/100 g/min.

The reason for this phenomenon is presumably the accumulation of intracellular osmotically active particles, as described above. Another explanation, suggested by van Harreveld and Fifkova [51], is the opening of sodium channels by glutamate, evoking an influx of sodium along its electrochemical gradient from the extra- into the intracellular compartment which is followed passively by an influx of chloride and water. If this explanation is correct, the ischemic threshold for cation shifts across the cell membrane is biphasic: a higher threshold of about 30 ml/100 g/min for sodium, and a lower threshold of about 10 ml/100 g/min for the release of potassium. Correlations between flow and electrophysiological changes carried out in several laboratories suggest that this range is the so-called ischemic penumbra [2], in which functional changes evolve even though cell membranes are not yet depolarized.

At flow values below 10 ml/100 g/min, ion exchange pumps break down and equimolar amounts of sodium and potassium are exchanged across the cell membranes, causing a rise in potassium and a decrease in sodium activity in the extracellular compartment. Since this exchange does not lead to alterations of osmotic activity in either compartment, the size of the extracellular space does not decrease further (Fig. 6). However, the build-up of ionic gradients between extracellular compartment and blood causes corresponding electrolyte shifts across the blood-brain barrier, resulting in reciprocal concentration changes in net sodium and potassium content, as described above (Fig. 3).

After a few hours of severe ischemia, the blood-brain barrier becomes permeable to macromolecules and blood serum extravasates into the brain tissue (see below). As a consequence, the extracellular compartment again enlarges, as evidenced by a secondary decrease in electrical impedance. After about the same interval, electron microscopy reveals physical breaks of cell membranes and a release of cell organelles into the widely enlarged extracellular compartment [11]. Eventually, after digestion of cell debris by blood-borne cells, a cyst develops which is filled by protein-rich fluid [40]. The secondary enlargement of extracellular space, therefore, may be considered as one of the first signs of irreversible cell damage.

Blood-Brain Barrier Permeability

Ischemic brain edema is initially of the cytotoxic type, followed after a certain interval by a vasogenic component. This interval, however, is not clearly defined. During the initial 3–6 h of ischemia the blood-brain barrier remains impermeable to the passage of conventional barrier tracers such as Evans blue [39, 28]. With more sensitive methods the passage of macromolecules can be observed to be starting even after 1 h [33]. There are also indications that early and late mechanisms of increased vascular permeability may be present. As demonstrated by Petito [41], a transient (active) increase in permeability to horseradish peroxidase – but not to Evans blue – occurs during the first minutes after the ischemic insult, followed by a permanent (passive) leakage of both Evans blue and horseradish peroxidase after 1.5–2 h. As a result of this disturbance, serum proteins gradually accumulate in the ischemic territory and after several hours spread into the surrounding intact brain tissue. Klatzo et al. [31] have pointed out that development of edema is closely associated with protein extravasation because, according to the Starling hypothesis, the proteins acquire an important role as colloidal osmotic forces for water movement.

This is also suggested by the observation that edema is resolved when extravasated proteins are cleared from the extracellular compartment by cellular uptake [31]. However, it must also be considered that permeability changes of electrolytes are of equal importance for fluid shifts across the vascular wall. Under physiological conditions the osmotic reflection coefficient of electrolytes at the blood-brain barrier is close to unity, and fluid shifts are dominated mainly by hydrostatic and protein osmotic pressures [43]. An increase in electrolyte permeability, and hence a decrease in the reflection coefficient, during ischemia causes an efflux of solutes from the blood into the brain by hydraulic forces. Changes in the permeability of the blood-brain barrier to electrolytes, in consequence, may be sufficient to explain the observed accumulation of water and sodium in the brain tissue.

Treatment of Ischemic Brain Edema

The only causal approach to reducing ischemic brain edema is reversal of the ischemia itself. As has been described above, edema develops when blood flow decreases below a threshold of about 10 ml/100 g/min. Raising blood flow just above this threshold, however, does not necessarily reverse edema or the associated electrolyte disturbances. Branston et al. [6] reported that the average postischemic flow rate in regions with complete recovery of extracellular potassium activity was 65.4 ml/100 g/min, whereas in regions without recovery flow was 20.3 ml/100 g/min, i.e., distinctly above the threshold for initiating ischemic brain edema. They further observed that in some regions with secondary increase of extracellular potassium flow was almost normal, indicating that restoration of flow alone does not reverse electrolyte shifts. This is also supported by the recent finding that in the territory of a permanently occluded MCA focal areas with high flow rates may be present in which the energy-producing metabolism is impaired and the tissue content of potassium depleted [23]. It is obvious that reactivation of metabolic activity depends not only on the density but also on the duration of ischemia. The revival time of brain tissue after circulatory arrest is 1 h at the most at normal temperature; blood flow, in consequence, must be restored within this time limit to prevent persisting cell damage and to reverse ischemic brain edema [24, 46].

If metabolic activity cannot be reactivated, any treatment of edema is symptomatic. As long as the blood-brain barrier to macromolecules remains intact, i.e., during the cytotoxic phase of ischemic brain edema, dehydration by osmotherapy is the most direct approach. In fact, a reduction of tissue water by more than 0.4 ml/g d.w. was induced by 20% mannitol, 1.5 g/kg body weight, given during the initial 2 h after ischemia [21]. However, despite dehydration the blood flow did not improve and the electrolyte disturbances within the ischemic territory were not affected. Reduction of edema, in consequence, may reduce complicating side effects, such as mass shifts or intracranial hypertension, but does not reverse the ischemic process itself.

After several hours of ischemia the blood-brain barrier becomes permeable to serum proteins and a vasogenic type of edema supervenes. During this stage osmotherapy reduces water content only in the intact and not in damaged tissue [8], because the osmotic reflection coefficient of the dehydrating agent at the vessel wall breaks down. In this situation the use of corticosteroids may be of benefit. In fact, morphometric determinations of serum protein extravasation around chronic infarcts induced by permanent MCA occlusion in monkeys revealed a reduction in the spread of edema although the size of the infarcts did not change [3]. This differential effect on edema and ischemia may explain why previous reports about the effect of corticosteroids are highly controversial [14, 34, 10]. Similar divergent opinions have also been expressed about the role of barbiturates, which may [47] or may not [21] reduce ischemic brain edema.

Postischemic Brain Edema

The development of edema during ischemia, as described above, requires a certain amount of persisting blood flow, which functions as a reservoir of fluid and electrolytes taken up by the brain. During complete ischemia such as that induced by cardiac arrest, this reservoir is restricted to the cerebrospinal fluid compartment, and ischemic brain swelling, in consequence, is minor. However, as soon as recirculation is restored after a period of ischemia the brain swells abruptly, and remains swollen as long as metabolic activity is impaired (Fig. 7). This type of edema has been termed postischemic brain edema, and it has been identified as one of the major factors responsible for postischemic recirculation disturbances and hence for the irreversibility of ischemic brain damage. Prevention or reversal of postischemic edema, in consequence, is of considerable therapeutic importance. In an earlier Workshop on Brain Edema, the pathophysiology of this type of ischemic brain swelling has been discussed in detail elsewhere [16]. The general pathophysiological principles outlined in the article cited are still valid; only a brief survey will therefore be given below, updated by reference to more recent observations.

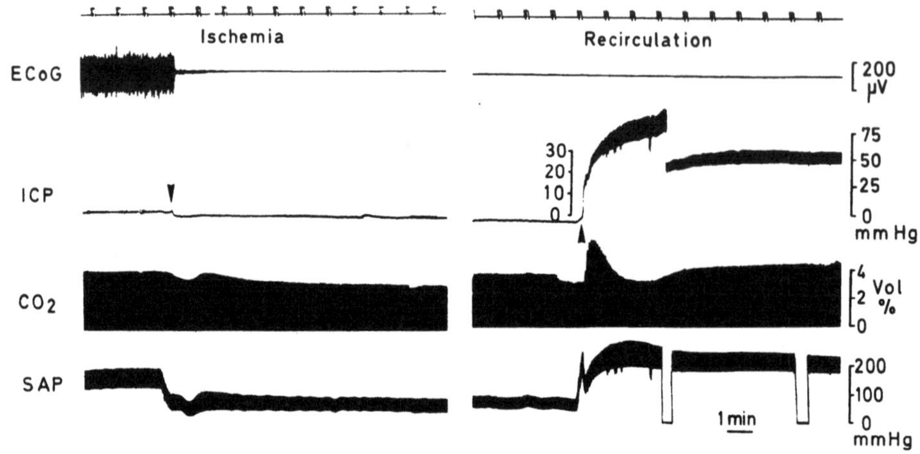

Fig. 7. Recording of the electrocorticogram, intracranial pressure, tidal CO_2, and systemic arterial pressure at the beginning and end of 1 h of complete ischemia in cat followed by recirculation at elevated blood pressure. Note the rapid increase in intracranial pressure, reaching a peak of 50 mmHg after 5 min of recirculation

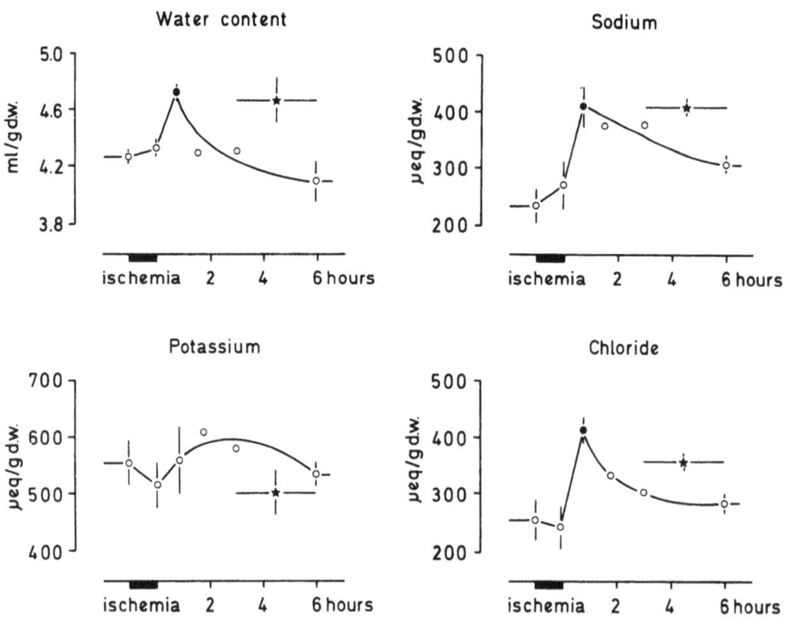

Fig. 8. Changes of cortical content of water, sodium, potassium, and chloride during and after 1 h of complete cerebrocirculatory arrest in monkeys. Immediately after the beginning of recirculation water, sodium, and chloride contents significantly increase, followed by a gradual decline in those animals in which metabolic activity is restored (*circles*). In a few animals without metabolic recovery (*stars*) postischemic brain edema is not reversible. Values are means ± SE. *Filled circles* indicate statistically significant difference from control ($P<0.05$)

Net Changes in Water and Tissue Electrolyte Content

During ischemia the net water content of the brain changes only slightly. In the cortex of monkeys an average increase by 0.05 ml/g d.w. has been observed during 1 h of ischemia, which is presumably due to an uptake of water from the cerebrospinal fluid compartment (Fig. 8). For the same reason, some electrolyte changes also occur: a loss of potassium by 44 μEq/g d.w., which is balanced by an equimolar increase of sodium. This is why the chloride content remains stable. When the ischemic brain is recirculated with blood, the water content increases sharply. After 45 min of recirculation following 1 h of ischemia, the cortical water uptake is about 0.4 ml/g d.w., or 10% of the total brain water. The maximum water increase presumably is even higher, because brain swelling reaches its peak within 30 min of recirculation.

Uptake of water is accompanied by marked increases in sodium and chloride, amounting to 171 μEq/g and 157 μEq/g d.w. after 45 min recirculation, respectively. Potassium, on the other hand, returns to normal during this interval. After longer recirculation times two different pathophysiological sequels can be distinguished (Fig. 8). In animals with restored metabolic activity the water content rapidly decreases to or even falls below the control level. Sodium and chloride also decrease, although they remain slightly above the control level for at least 6 h after ischemia. In animals without metabolic recovery brain edema is not resolved: the water, sodium, and chloride contents are distinctly above, and the content of potassium below, those observed in animals with restitution of the energy-producing metabolism (Fig. 8). In the white matter directional changes are similar to those in the cortex, although with greater individual variability.

In contrast to net water and electrolyte changes, osmolality of the brain tissue increases considerably during ischemia. The average rise amounts to about 50 mosmol, the steepest increase occurring during the initial 15 min of ischemia (Fig. 9). The increase is partly due to the accumulation of lactate, which during complete cerebrocirculatory arrest rises to about 15 μmol/g wet weight (w.w.). However, the sum of the major osmotically active solutes, i.e., glucose, lactate, pyruvate, sodium,

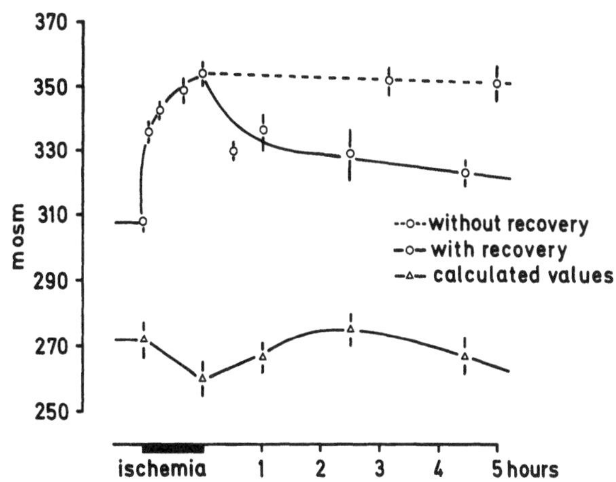

Fig. 9. Changes of brain tissue osmolality during and after 1 h complete ischemia of cats. *Solid line,* animals with metabolic recovery; *broken line,* animals without recovery. *Triangles* represent the calculated osmolarity of major brain solutes. Note the discrepancy between calculated and measured tissue osmolality, indicating the generation of iodiogenic osmols during ischemia. (Hossmann and Takagi [18])

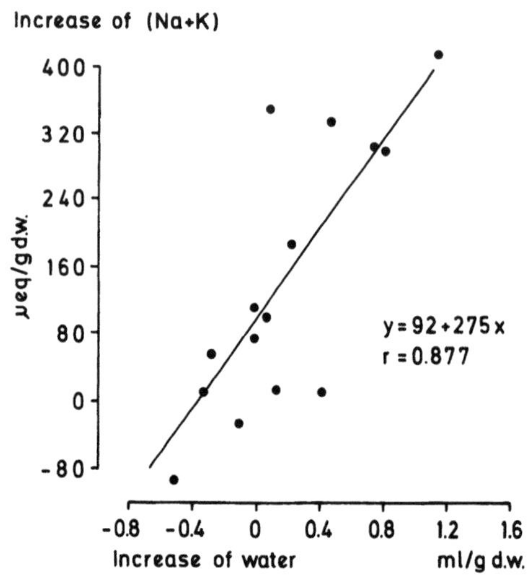

Fig. 10. Relationship between the increase in water and the increase in sodium and potassium in cerebral cortex of cats recirculated for 3–8 h after 1 h of complete cerebrocirculatory arrest. The intercept of the calculated regression line is positive, indicating the uptake of an excess of cations with respect to water content

potassium and their respective anions, does not increase significantly, indicating that a substantial amount of idiogenic osmols is created during ischemia. When the brain is recirculated after ischemia, osmolality rapidly decreases and stabilizes at approximately 20 mosmol above the preischemic level after 30 min. This level progresses in parallel to blood osmolality, which has to be raised to prevent fatal postischemic brain swelling (see below). In animals with recirculation disturbances osmolality remains elevated and functional or metabolic recovery does not occur.

When the increase in cations (the sum of sodium and potassium) is plotted against the increase in water, a correlation is obtained which is markedly different from that observed during ischemic brain edema (Fig. 10). The intercept of the regression line is positive, and the regression coefficient is much higher than the cation content of blood serum. The brain, in consequence, takes up much less water than expected from the increase in cation concentration. This is partly because the brain is osmotically dehydrated during the early recirculated period (see below). However, blood osmolality rises only by about 20 mosmol/liter, whereas the isovolemic increment of cations is 92 mEq/liter (i.e., the intercept of the regression line). This suggests that other factors are also involved, e.g., a release of idiogenic osmols into the blood, or an inactivation of ions by nuclear sequestration [25] or intracellular protein-binding sites [4]. Postischemic brain edema, in consequence, is characterized by changes which are just the opposite of those observed in ischemic edema (see above).

Compartmentation of Fluid and Electrolytes

During ischemia considerable shifts of fluids and electrolytes occur between the intra- and extracellular compartments (Fig. 11). The volume of the extracellular space shrinks by about 50%, extracellular potassium increases to 50–60 mEq, and extracellular sodium decreases to approximately the same level. Comparison of the time course of these changes with that of tissue osmolality and those of net water

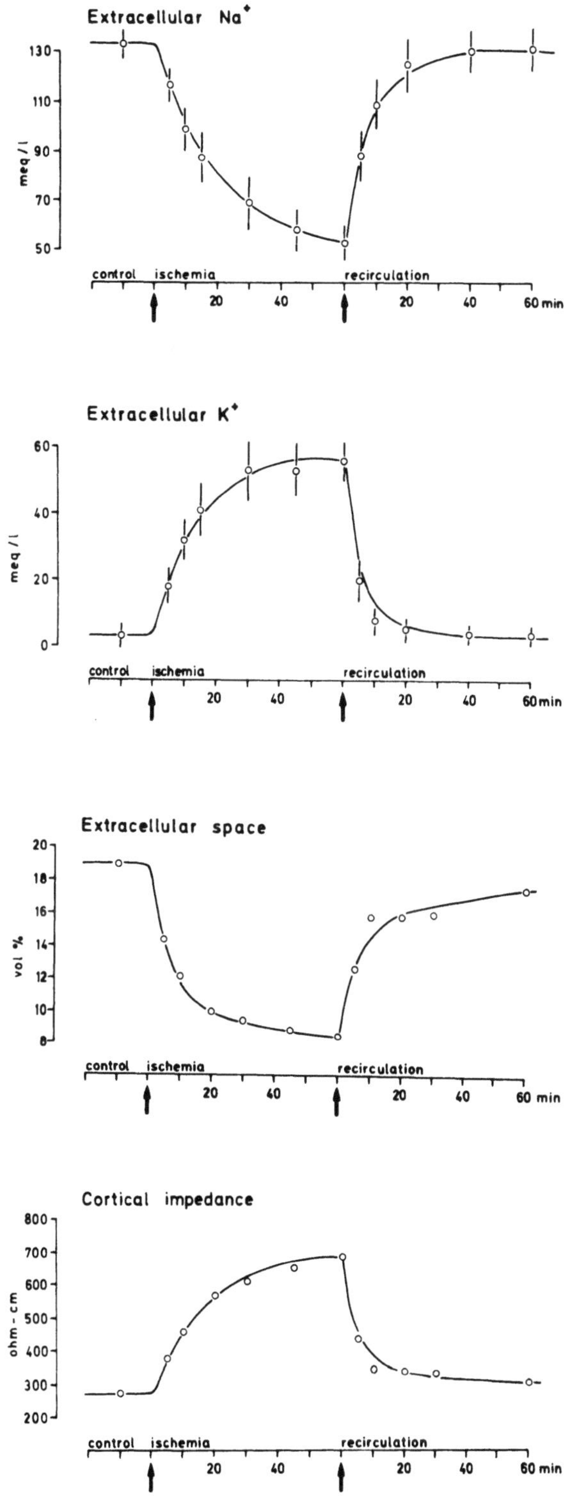

Fig. 11. Changes in the extracellular activity of sodium and potassium, of cortical electrical impedance, and calculated extracellular space (ECS) in parietal cortex of cat during and after 1 h of complete cerebrocirculatory arrest. Note the bidirectional changes of sodium and potassium and the close correlation between changes in sodium activity and the size of the extracellular space. (Modified from Hossmann [15], and from Hossmann et al. [20] by permission of the American Heart Association, Inc.)

and electrolyte content suggests the following interpretation. During ischemia accumulation of intracellular idiogenic osmols causes an osmotic shift of water from the extra- into the intracellular compartment. Simultaneously, the membrane channels for both potassium and sodium ions open, resulting in a passive equilibration of intra- and extracellular ion gradients. The shrinkage of extracellular space during equilibration of ion concentrations indicates that the net influx of sodium into the cells is much higher than the release of potassium; this can only be explained by the fact that the membranes are more permeable for sodium and potassium than for the idiogenic osmols accumulating intracellularly.

After the beginning of recirculation two groups of animals can be distinguished. In one group the flow rate is low and metabolic activity does not recover, or recovers only partially. In other animals reactive hyperemia is present, resulting in rapid restoration of the energy state of the brain. In the first group intracerebral ion and fluid shifts are irreversible, and the postischemic net uptake of fluid and electrolytes remains elevated (see above). In the other group, the observed changes rapidly normalize (Fig. 11). After a few hours of recirculation the total sodium content of brain tissue is nevertheless still higher than before ischemia (Fig. 8), although neither extracellular sodium activity nor the volume of the extracellular fluid compartment is increased. Excess sodium, in consequence, must be located intracellularly. Morphological studies demonstrate that during postischemic recirculation glial cells appear to be swollen whereas neurons tend to shrink [1]. It is therefore likely that excess sodium is mainly located in the glial compartment.

A process which is indirectly related to the changes in cell membrane permeability is intracellular accumulation of calcium. During postischemic recirculation the net calcium content of the brain gradually increases [53], but there is no correlation either with the tissue content of water and electrolytes, or with the energy state of the brain [22]. A causal relationship between calcium influx and edema formation, in consequence, does not exist.

Blood-Brain Barrier Permeability

During the early recirculation phase after prolonged ischemia, edema is of the cytotoxic type, i.e., the blood-brain barrier remains impermeable to serum proteins. In fact, there seems to be a tightening of the barrier, because additional lesions which usually result in an immediate breakdown of the barrier to serum proteins, such as induced hypertension or mercury chloride poisoning, have no effect [39]. This "tightening" seems to be a unique response of the brain vasculature after long-lasting ischemia, because 5-min bilateral carotid artery ligation in the gerbil resulted in a transient "first" opening of the barrier to horseradish peroxidase within 1 min of recirculation [48]. Between 1 and 6 h after ischemia, macromolecules do not cross the blood-brain barrier after either short- or long-lasting ischemia. This is why the brain can be dehydrated during this period by osmotherapy. After even longer periods of recirculation, a "second" opening of the blood-brain barrier may occur [48].

This phenomenon has been investigated most frequently in gerbils [26, 48]. In this species the latency of the opening is inversely proportional to the density and duration of ischemia: After 5 min of bilateral ischemia the barrier does not open until as

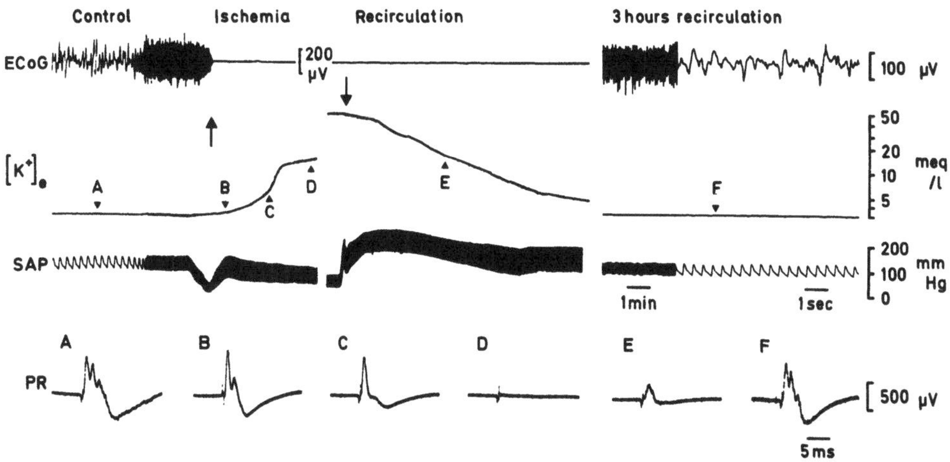

Fig. 12. Recording of the electrocorticogram (*ECoG*), extracellular potassium activity $[K^+]$ e, systemic arterial pressure (*SAP*), and the pyramidal response following electrical stimulation of the motor cortex (*RP*) during and after 1 h of complete ischemia in the normothermic cat brain. The PR was evoked at times indicated by (*A–F*). Note the return of electrical activity after normalization of extracellular ion homeostasis. (Reproduced from Hossmann et al. [20] by permission of the American Heart Association, Inc.)

much as 12 h later, whereas after 6 h of unilateral ischemia the latent period is only a few minutes. Most of the regions in which barrier lesions develop are in so-called selectively vulnerable areas of the brain, indicating that the second barrier disturbance accompanies irreversible cell damage similar to that observed following ischemic stroke. It is of interest that disturbances develop only when blood vessels and astrocytes become necrotic; neuronal damage alone is insufficient [42].

Independently of, and presumably prior to, these permeability changes of macromolecules, long-lasting and pronounced alterations of the permeability of small molecules occur. This is reflected by the massive uptake of sodium immediately after ischemia (see above), the postischemic increase of amino acid influx [32, 44], and the rapid postischemic accumulation of tissue glucose [19]. However, systematic investigations of permeability changes of these and other small molecules have not been carried out, and further work has to be done to obtain more precise information.

Therapy of Postischemic Brain Edema

As has been discussed above, postischemic brain edema is reversible after cerebrocirculatory arrest for as long as 1 h if the energy-producing metabolism is restored upon recirculation. A major problem, however, is the fact that edema develops so rapidly that the resulting increase in intracranial pressure may interfere with the recirculation and hence with the reoxygenation of the tissue. Spontaneous recovery can therefore only be expected if systemic blood pressure is high enough to overcome the increased intracranial pressure and if the latter is reduced by impeding the osmotic influx of fluid from the blood into the brain. This can be achieved by rapid systemic infusion of osmotically active substances such as sorbitol or mannitol. If recirculation of the brain succeeds, metabolic activity recovers within a few minutes, brain swelling and electrolyte disturbances dissipate shortly afterward, and electrophysiological recovery ensues (Fig. 12). In the case of insufficient or inhomogeneous reperfusion, on the other hand, swelling will progress to such a degree that even the buildup of very high blood perfusion pressure is not able to overcome the increased vascular resistance. In this situation the energy-producing metabolism does not recover and postischemic brain edema is irreversible.

Treatment of the delayed vasogenic type of edema is presumably of little relevance, because its appearance is a symptom of irreversible tissue damage and its amelioration is only of interest insofar as the spread into undamaged brain tissue or the buildup of intracranial pressure is concerned. However, in view of the severity of the ischemic damage, such an effect is probably an epiphenomenon and for this reason of little pathophysiological significance.

Summary

Both ischemic and postischemic brain edema are characterized by the initial uptake of water and electrolytes from blood and cerebrospinal fluid, followed by a breakdown of the blood-brain barrier making it permeable to serum proteins in the case of irreversible tissue changes. Edema, in consequence, is initially cytotoxic and later vasogenic in type. Postischemic brain edema is rapidly resolved if the metabolic activity of the brain is restored before the blood-brain barrier breaks down, but it progresses continuously if tissue damage becomes irreversible. Amelioration of edema, therefore, can be achieved during the early phase of development by restoration of metabolic activity, i.e., by adequate reoxygenation of the brain tissue, and by osmotherapy. Later, when cells are irreversibly damaged and the blood-brain barrier has become permeable to macromolecules, amelioration is no longer possible either by improvement of oxygenation or by osmotherapy. The strategy for treatment of ischemic brain edema therefore depends on the level of blood flow, metabolic activity, and the permeability of the blood-brain barrier, and therefore requires detailed knowledge of the pathophysiology of the individual condition.

References

1. Arsenio-Nunes ML, Hossmann KA, Farkas-Bargeton E (1973) Ultrastructural and histochemical investigation of the cerebral cortex of cat during and after complete ischemia. Acta Neuropathol 26:329–344
2. Astrup J, Siesjö BK, Symon L (1981) Thresholds in cerebral ischemia – The ischemic penumbra. Stroke 12:723–725
3. Barbosa-Coutinho LM, Hartmann A, Hossmann KA, Rommel TH (1984) Effect of dexamethasone on serum protein extravasation in experimental brain infarcts of monkeys: an immunohistochemical study. Acta Neuropathol (in press)
4. Bito LZ, Myers RE (1972) On the physiological response of the cerebral cortex to acute stress (reversible asphyxia). J Physiol (Lond) 221:349–370
5. Branston NM, Strong AJ, Symon L (1977) Extracellular potassium activity, evoked potential and tissue blood flow. J Neurol Sci 32:305–321

6. Branston NM, Symon L, Strong AJ (1978) Reversibility of ischemically induced changes in extracellular potassium in primate cortex. J Neurol Sci 37:37–49
7. Bremer AM, West CR, Yamada K (1978) Alterations in distribution of water, sodium, potassium, and chloride in brain during evolution of ischemic cerebral edema. Neurosurgery 3:187–195
8. Bremer AM, Yamada K, West CR (1980) Ischemic cerebral edema in primates: Effects of acetazolamide, phenytoin, sorbitol, dexamethasone, and methylprednisolone on brain water and electrolytes. Neurosurgery 6:149–154
9. Crockard A, Iannotti F, Hunstock AT, Smith RD, Harris RJ, Symon L (1980) Cerebral blood flow and edema following carotid occlusion in the gerbil. Stroke 11:494–498
10. Fenske A, Fischer M, Regli F, Hase U (1979) The response of focal ischemic cerebral edema to dexamethasone. J Neurol 220:199–209
11. Garcia JH, Kalimo H, Kamijyo Y, Trump BF (1977) Cellular events during partial cerebral ischemia. I. Electron microscopy of feline cerebral cortex after middle cerebral artery occlusion. Virchows Arch [Cell Pathol] 25:191–206
12. Garcia JH, Conger KA, Morawetz R, Halsey JH Jr (1980) Postischemic brain edema: Quantitation and evolution. Adv Neurol 28:147–169
13. Hansen AJ, Olsen CE (1980) Brain extracellular space during spreading depression and ischemia. Acta Physiol Scand 108:355–365
14. Harrison MJ, Brownbill D, Lewis PD, Ross Russell RW (1973) Cerebral edema following carotid artery ligation in the gerbil. Arch Neurol 28:389–391
15. Hossmann KA (1971) Cortical steady potential, impedance and excitability changes during and after total ischemia of cat brain. Exp Neurol 32:163–175
16. Hossmann KA (1976) Development and resolution of ischemic brain swelling. In: Pappius HM, Feindel W (eds) Dynamics of brain edema. Springer, Berlin Heidelberg New York, pp 219–227
17. Hossmann KA, Schuier FJ (1980) Experimental brain infarcts in cats. I. Pathophysiological observations. Stroke 11:583–592
18. Hossmann KA, Takagi S (1976) Osmolality of brain in cerebral ischemia. Exp Neurol 51:124–131
19. Hossmann KA, Sakaki S, Kimoto K (1976) Cerebral uptake of glucose and oxygen in the cat brain after prolonged ischemia. Stroke 7:301–305
20. Hossmann KA, Sakaki S, Zimmermann V (1977) Cation activities in reversible ischemia of the cat brain. Stroke 8:77–81
21. Hossmann KA, Matsuoka Y, Blöink M, Fitzgerald G, Hossmann V (1981) Treatment of experimental infarction of the cat brain. In Cahn J (ed) Drugs and methods in cerebrovascular diseases. Pergamon, Paris, pp 427–434
22. Hossmann KA, Paschen W, Csiba L (1983) Relationship between calcium accumulation and recovery of cat brain after prolonged cerebral ischemia. J Cereb Blood Flow Metab 3:346–353
23. Hossmann KA, Mies G, Paschen W, Csiba L, Bodsch W, Rapin JR, le Poncin-Lafitte M, Takahashi K (1984) Multiparametric imaging of blood flow and metabolism after middle cerebral artery occlusion in cats. J Cereb Blood Flow Metab (in press)
24. Iannotti F, Hoff JT, Crockard A (1981) Does reperfusion improve ischemic edema? J Cereb Blood Flow Metabol 1 [Suppl 1]:S168–S169
25. Ignelzi RJ, Kirsch WM (1978) Sodium sequestration in vertebrate glial nuclei: Implications in the pathogenesis of ischemic brain injury. Adv Neurol 20:231–236
26. Ito U, Go KG, Walker JT Jr, Spatz M, Klatzo I (1976) Experimental cerebral ischemia in mongolian gerbils. III. Behaviour of the blood-brain barrier. Acta Neuropathol 34:1–6
27. Ito U, Ohno K, Nakamura R, Suganuma F, Inaba Y (1979) Brain edema during ischemia and after restoration of blood flow. Measurement of water, sodium, potassium content and plasma protein permeability. Stroke 10:542–547
28. Kamijyo Y, Garcia JH, Cooper J (1977) Temporary regional cerebral ischemia in the cat. A model of hemorrhagic and subcortical infarction. J Neuropathol Exp Neurol 36:338–350
29. Katzman R, Clasen R, Klatzo I, Meyer JS, Pappius HM, Waltz AG (1977) Report of joint committee for stroke resources. IV. Brain edema in stroke. Study group of brain edema in stroke. Stroke 8:512–540

30. Klatzo I (1979) 2. Cerebral oedema and ischaemia. In: Smith WT, Cavanagh JB (eds) Recent advances in neuropathology. Churchill Livingstone, Edinburgh, pp 27–39
31. Klatzo I, Chui F, Fujiwara K, Spatz M (1980) Resolution of vasogenic brain edema. Adv Neurol 28:359–373
32. Kleihues P, Hossmann KA (1971) Protein synthesis in the cat brain after prolonged cerebral ischemia. Brain Res 35:409–418
33. Laursen H, Suzuki R, Kuroiwa T, Fenton I, Klatzo I (1983) Changes of cerebrovascular permeability in middle cerebral artery occlusion. In: Stefanovich V (ed) Stroke: animal models. Proceedings of an international symposium held at Wiesbaden, Germany, 1981. Pergamon, Oxford, pp 13–25
34. Lee MC, Mastri AR, Waltz AG, Loewenson RB (1974) Ineffectiveness of dexamethasone for treatment of experimental cerebral infarction. Stroke 5:216–218
35. Matsuoka Y, Hossmann KA (1982) Cortical impedance and extracellular volume changes following middle cerebral artery occlusion in cats. J Cereb Blood Flow Metab 2:466–474
36. Mršulja BB, Djuričić BM, Cvejić V, Mršulja BJ, Abe K, Spatz M, Klatzo I (1980) Biochemistry of experimental ischemic brain edema. Adv Neurol 28:217–230
37. O'Brien MD (1979) Ischemic cerebral edema. A review. Stroke 10:623–628
38. O'Brien MD, Waltz AG, Jordan MM (1974) Ischemic cerebral edema. Distribution of water in brains of cats after occlusion of the middle cerebral artery. Arch Neurol 30:456–460
39. Olsson Y, Crowell RM, Klatzo I (1971) The blood-brain barrier to protein tracers in focal cerebral ischemia and infarction caused by occlusion of the middle cerebral artery. Acta Neuropathol (Berl) 18:89–102
40. Paschen W, Mies G, Bodsch W, Yamori Y, Hossmann KA (1984) Regional cerebral blood flow and metabolism in stroke-prone spontaneously hypertensive rats. Stroke (in press)
41. Petito CK (1979) Early and late mechanisms of increased vascular permeability following experimental cerebral infarction. J Neuropathol 38:222–234
42. Petito CK, Pulsinelli WA, Jacobson G, Plum F (1982) Edema and vascular permeability in cerebral ischemia: comparison between ischemic neuronal damage and infarction. J Neuropathol Exp Neurol 41:423–436
43. Rapoport SI (1976) Blood-brain barrier in physiology and medicine. Raven, New York
44. Sage JI, Van Uitert RL, Duffy TE (1984) Early changes in blood barrier permeability to small molecules after transient cerebral ischemia. Stroke 15:46–50
45. Schuier FJ, Hossmann KA (1980) Experimental brain infarcts in cats. II. Ischemic brain edema. Stroke 11:593–601
46. Shigeno T, Teasdale GM, McCulloch J, Mandelow D, Graham DI (1984) Brain edema following focal cerebral ischemia in the rat. In: Go KG, Baethmann A (eds) Recent progress in the study and therapy of brain edema. Plenum, New York, pp 449–458
47. Simeone FA, Frazer G, Lawner P (1979) Ischemic brain edema: Comparative effects of barbiturates and hypothermia. Stroke 10:8–12
48. Suzuki R, Yamaguchi T, Kirino T, Orzi F, Klatzo I (1983) The effects of 5-minute ischemia in Mongolian gerbils: I. Blood-brain barrier, cerebral blood flow, and local cerebral glucose utilization. Acta Neuropathol (Berl) 60:207–216
49. Strong AJ, Tomlinson BE, Venables GS, Gibson G, Hardy JA (1983) The cortical ischaemic penumbra associated with occlusion of the middle cerebral artery in the cat: 2. Studies of histopathology, water content, and in vitro neurotransmitter uptake. J Cereb Blood Flow Metab 3:97–108
50. Symon L, Branston NM, Chikovani O (1979) Ischemic brain edema following middle cerebral artery occlusion in baboons: relationship between regional cerebral water content and blood flow at 1 to 2 hours. Stroke 10:184–191
51. van Harreveld A, Fifkova E (1971) Light- and electron-microscopic changes in central nervous tissue after electrophoretic injection of glutamate. Exp Mol Pathol 15:61–81
52. van Harreveld A, Fifkova E (1975) Rapid freezing of deep cerebral structures for electron-microscopy. Anat Rec 182:377–385
53. Yanagihara T, McCall JT (1982) Ionic shift in cerebral ischemia. Life Sci 30:1921–1925
54. Zimmermann V, Hossmann KA (1975) Resuscitation of the monkey brain after one hour's complete ischemia: II. Brain water and electrolytes. Brain Res 85:1–11

Experimental Study of Ischemic Brain Edema by Differential Scanning Calorimetry and NMR Spin Analysis

T. KAYAMA [1], Y. SAKURAI, S. FUJIMOTO, T. YOSHIMOTO, and J. SUZUKI

Introduction

Clinically, it is important to treat brain edema resulting from brain ischemia, which is the final cause of death in cerebral infarction. However, although there are many kinds of treatment for ischemic brain edema, they are still unsatisfactory (e.g., steroid medication, osmotherapy, hyperbaric therapy). An analysis of the composition of water in ischemic brain edema is an advantage for its treatment, since if the nature of the water in the tissues is known it might be possible to remove the water from the edematous brain cells by physical or chemical means. However, previous reports [1, 3, 7] have not provided details of the nature of water in the tissues.

Furthermore, a comparison of the nature of the water and of the electrolytes in brain tissue is very helpful in the treatment of patients who have suffered a cerebral infarction.

In this study, highly sensitive differential scanning calorimetry (DSC) was used in an attempt to record thermoanalytic and quantitative measurements of the water in normal brains and in brains affected by ischemic edema. Tissue electrolytes were analyzed to determine the origin of the restored water. The amount of water measured by the calorimetric method was compared with the nature of electrolytes measured with an NMR spin analyzer.

Materials and Methods

Analysis of the Water in Normal Rat Brain

Adult Wistar rats weighing 150–200 g were used in this study. The brain was removed immediately after cardiac arrest caused by injecting a KCl solution IV. About 20 mg brain tissue was weighed out and put into a silver pellet. To analyze the state of tissue water, highly sensitive differential scanning calorimetry (DSC; Daini Seikosha, SSC-560U) was used. The total water content was measured by the drying method. The estimated water present in the free and other states was calculated by using the formula in Table 1.

[1] Stroke Center National Sendai Hospital, 2-8-8, Miyagino, Sendai, 983 Japan

Table 1. Calculation of water components

Free water (mg)	$\frac{\text{Calorific value (cal): approx. } -4\,^{\circ}\text{C} - 6\,^{\circ}\text{C}}{79.6 \text{ (mcal/mg)}}$
Half-bound water (mg)	$\frac{\text{Calorific value (cal): approx. } -58\,^{\circ}\text{C} - 60\,^{\circ}\text{C}}{79.6 \text{ (mcal/mg)}}$

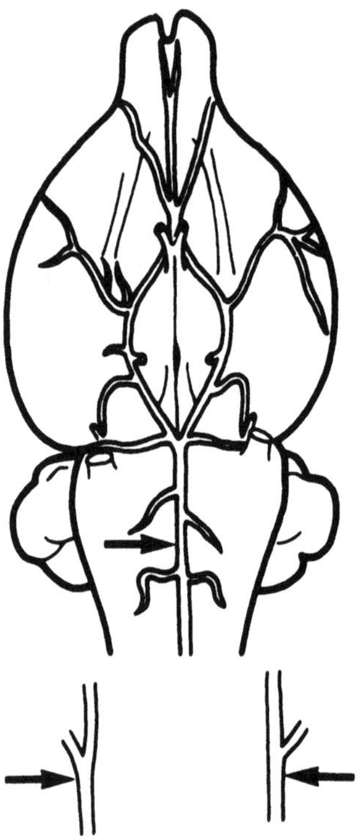

Fig. 1. Sites of occlusion of vessels: basilar and both common carotid arteries

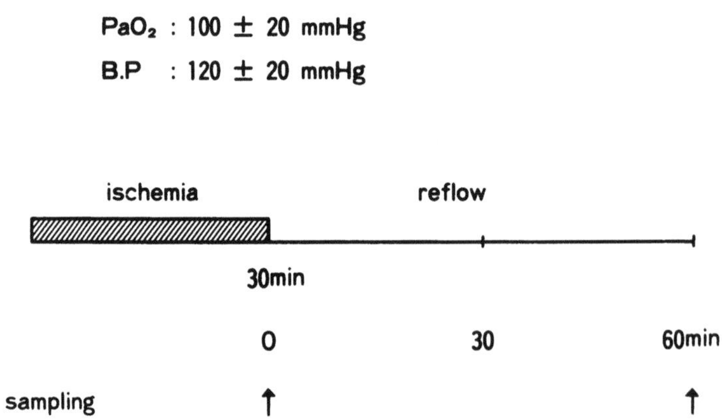

Fig. 2. Experimental program

Analysis of the Water in Ischemic Brain Edema

The model used was that of bilateral hemispheric ischemia produced in the rat by three-vessel occlusion [6]. Cerebral blood flow was consistently and severely impaired. The details of how this model is produced are not given here, but the occlusion sites of the vessels are shown (Fig. 1). The experimental program was as shown in Fig. 2. To analyze the composition of the water the DSC method mentioned above was applied. The various components of the water were estimated as above. Sodium and potassium in the brain tissue were measured by the flame photometric method.

Comparison of the Nature of the Water and the Electrolytes Present in Brain Tissue

To analyze the state of proton in the tissue, an NMR Spin Analyzer (Radx, NMR spin analyzer) was used, in which excitation frequencies around 10 MHz and a magnetic field of 2.3 kG was used. Samples were removed from normal and edematous brain tissue. The results obtained by the DSC method and those yielded by the NMR spin analyzer were compared for each sample.

Results

Water in the Normal Rat Brain

The first peak was seen at about −4 °C to −10 °C and indicated the free water content. The second peak was seen at about −50 °C to −60 °C and indicated the half-bound water content (Figs. 3 and 4). These two peaks were seen with a high degree

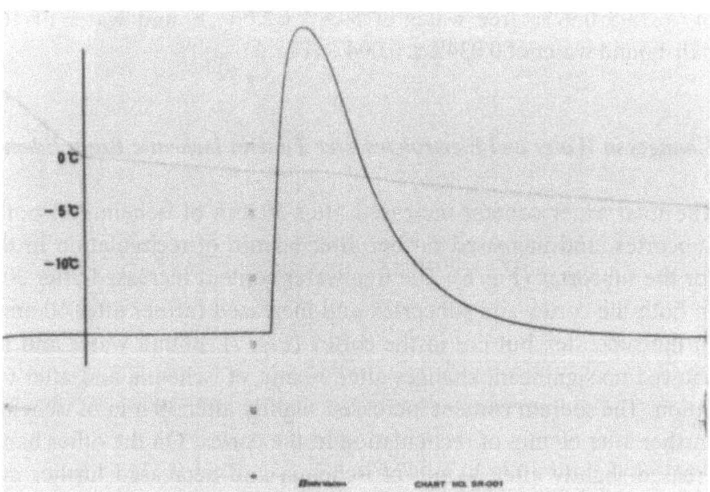

Fig. 3. First peak at about −4 °C to −10 °C

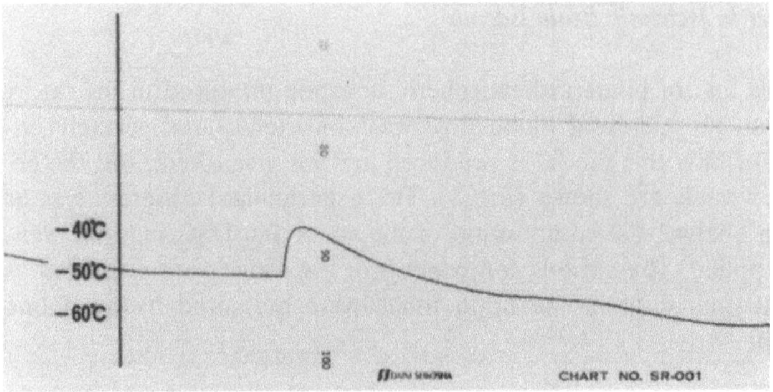

Fig. 4. Second peak at −50 °C to −60 °C

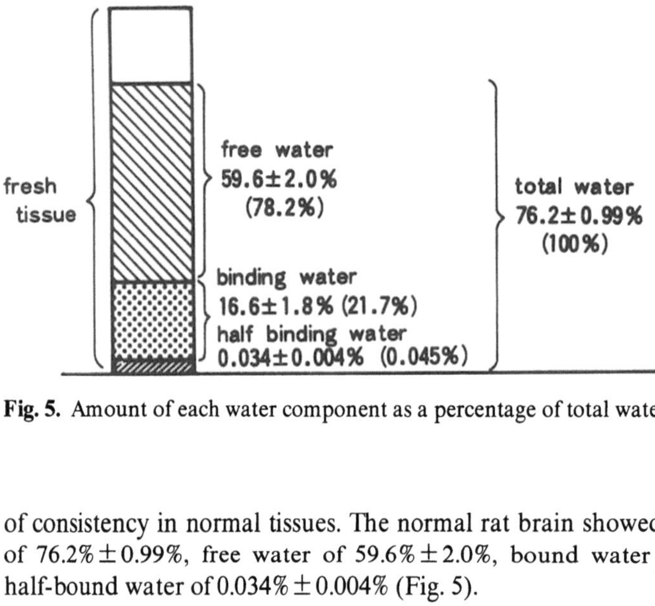

Fig. 5. Amount of each water component as a percentage of total water in normal rat brain

of consistency in normal tissues. The normal rat brain showed a total water content of 76.2% ± 0.99%, free water of 59.6% ± 2.0%, bound water of 16.1% ± 1.8%, and half-bound water of 0.034% ± 0.004% (Fig. 5).

Changes in Water and Electrolytes over Time in Ischemic Brain Edema

The total water content increased after 30 min of ischemia in both the cortex and subcortex, and increased further after 60 min of recirculation in the cortex, except for the subcortex (Fig. 6). The free water content increased after 30 min of ischemia in both the cortex and subcortex and increased further after 60 min of recirculation in the subcortex but not in the cortex (Fig. 7). Bound water and half-bound water showed no significant changes after 30 min of ischemia and after 60 min of recirculation. The sodium content increased slightly after 30 min of ischemia and increased further after 60 min of recirculation in the cortex. On the other hand, potassium decreased slightly after 30 min of ischemia and decreased further in both the cortex and the subcortex (Figs. 8 and 9).

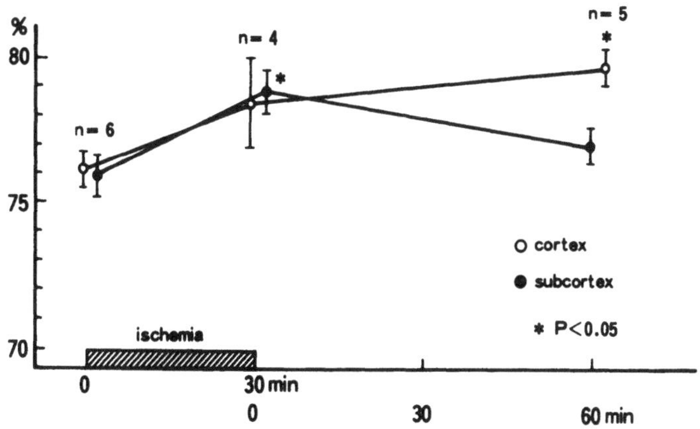

Fig. 6. Changes in total water content over time

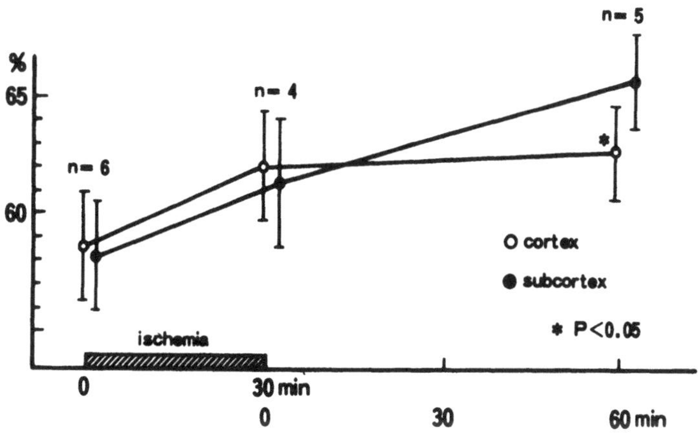

Fig. 7. Changes in free water content over time

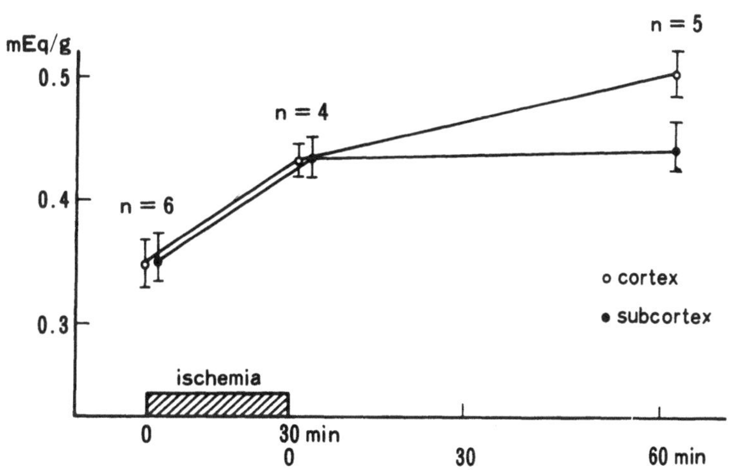

Fig. 8. Changes in tissue sodium content over time

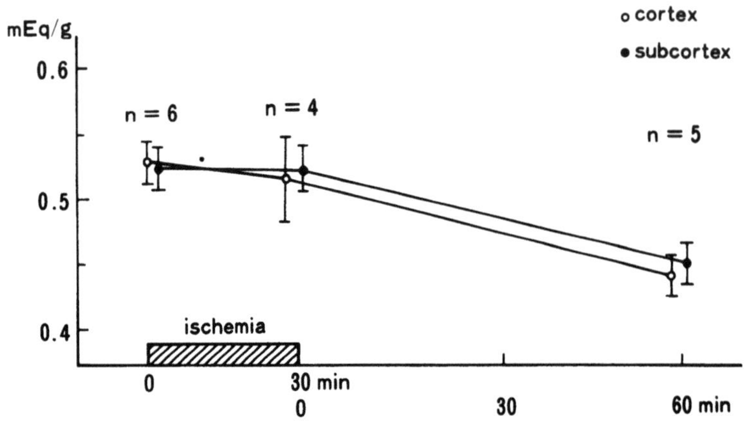

Fig. 9. Changes in tissue potassium content over time

Comparison of Composition of Water and Proton Content, and Relaxation Values

A significant correlation was shown only between the free water content and the proton content in normal and pathologic brain tissues.

Discussion

Some researchers have analyzed the composition of water by the DSC method [2], but the sensitivity of the calorimetric method they used was not high and did not allow differentiation of free, half-bound, and bound water in the brain tissue. In our study, half-bound water was detected at –50 °C to –60 °C in normal brain tissue by using highly sensitive DSC. According to some reports half-bound water has been detected in collagen and not in the brain tissue by the calorimetric method [4, 7] and by the induced electricity method, but no report of half-bound water detected in brain tissue has been found in the literature. The amount of half-bound water was very small, but the reliability of detection in normal tissue is 100%. On the other hand, low detection reliability was shown in the pathologic brain. This might suggest that the half-bound water transferred into either the free water zone or the bound water zone of pathologic brain tissue.

Examination of the changes in the composition of the water over time in the brain affected by ischemic edema shows that during ischemia the total water and free water contents increase in both the cortex and the subcortex. In this model, the cerebral blood flow might be very low during ischemia, so that these facts suggest that in the early stage of brain edema in this model of severe ischemia the water restored during ischemia might be produced by means of anaerobic metabolism.

After recirculation, a significant increase in the total and free water contents is seen in the cortex. This suggests that even 30 min of ischemia in this model causes hyperpermeability of the blood-brain barrier and recovery of water from the serum, accompanied by sequential changes of sodium and potassium [5].

When the composition of water measured by the calorimetric method and the protons analyzed by the NMR spin analyzer are compared, a significant correlation is revealed between the free water content and proton content. It seems that the problems with measurement were caused by the NMR spin analyzer, which is still under development.

Summary

Clinically, it is important to treat brain edema resulting from brain ischemia. However, though there are many kinds of treatment for ischemic brain edema, they are still unsatisfactory. Analysis of the state of water in ischemic brain edema is helpful in the treatment of ischemic brain edema, since if the status of water in the tissue is known it might be possible to remove the water from the edema brain cells by physical or chemical means.

In this study highly sensitive differential scanning calorimetry was applied in an attempt to record thermoanalytic measurements of the different water components in fresh normal brains and ischemic edematous brains. The water status measured by the calorimetric method and the proton status measured by the handy NMR spin analyzer were also compared.

The total water content in the normal rat brain was 76.2% ± 0.99%, free water accounting for 59.6% ± 2.0%, bound water for 16.1% ± 1.8%, and half-bound water for 0.034% ± 0.004%.

The bilateral hemispheric ischemia model in the rat (three-vessel occlusion) was used to analyze changes in the composition of the total water content in the brain over time. The total water content increased by the end of 30 min of ischemia in both the cortex and the subcortex, and increased further after 60 min of recirculation in the cortex except for the subcortex. The free water content increased after 30 min of ischemia in both cortex and subcortex, and increased further after 60 min of recirculation in the subcortex but not in the cortex. Bound water and half-bound water showed no significant changes after 30 min of ischemia or 60 min of recirculation.

References

1. Fujimoto T, Walker JT, Spatz M, Klatzo I (1976) Pathophysiologic aspects of ischemic edema. In: Pappius HM, Feindel W (eds) Dynamics of brain edema. Springer. Berlin Heidelberg New York, p 171
2. Furuse M, Gonda T, Kuchiwaki H, Hirai N, Inao S, Kageyama N (1984) Thermal analysis on the state of free and bound water in normal and edematous brains. In: Go KG, Baethmann A (eds) Brain edema. Plenum, New York, p 293
3. Go KG, Edzes HT (1975) Water in brain edema. Observations by the pulsed nuclear magnetic resonance technique. Arch Neurol 32:462
4. Haly AR, Snaith JW (1971) Thermal analysis of the water in collagen absorption model. Biopolymers 10:1681
5. Hossmann KA (1976) Development and resolution of ischemic brain swelling. In: Pappius HM, Feindel W (eds) Dynamics of brain edema. Springer, Berlin Heidelberg New York, p 219
6. Kameyama M, Suzuki J, Shirane R, Ogawa A (in press) A new model of bilateral hemispheric ischemia in the rat. Three vessel occlusion model. Stroke
7. Kunz ID, Kauzmann W (1974) Hydration of proteins and polypeptides. Adv Protein Chem 38:239

Role of Prostaglandins in Experimental Ischemic Brain Edema in Hypertensive Rats: TXA_2 Priority in Hypertensive Rats

S. SUGIMOTO[1], A. TERASHI, Y. KATAYAMA, M. MIZOGUCHI, T. SOEDA, K. INAMURA, S. SUZUKI, J. SHIMIZU, H. MEMEZAWA, and H. MINAMIZAWA

Introduction

Hypertensive rats are known to be more susceptible to ischemic insults than normotensive rats [1, 2], but the reason for this is still obscure.

The aim of this study is to clarify the reason with reference to the assumption that prostaglandins (PGs) or the response to PGs may play a role in aggravating ischemic brain damage in hypertensive rats.

Materials and Methods

Male stroke-prone spontaneously hypertensive rats (SHRSP), stroke-resistant spontaneously hypertensive rats (SHRSR) and normotensive Wistar Kyoto rats (WKY) were used at the age of 16 weeks. The blood pressure range in SHRSP was around 200–250 mmHg, while that in SHRSR was 170–240 mmHg and that in WKY, around 120–150 mmHg.

Bilateral common carotid artery ligation (BLCL) was performed in the rats to induce experimental cerebral ischemia in SHRSP, SHRSR, and WKY. Regional cerebral blood flow (rCBF), energy metabolism (ATP, lactate, cAMP), cerebral edema production and serum PGs (TXA_2 and PGI_2) were measured in each group of rats (SHRSP, SHRSR, and WKY) before and after 3 h of ischemia induced by BLCL and compared with each other. The ischemic focus was examined by colloidal carbon perfusion methods. Cerebral tissue ATP levels were determined by the luciferin-luciferase method. Tissue lactate levels were determined by an enzymatic method using lactate hydrogenase. cAMP levels were determined by radioimmunoassay. Cerebral blood flow was determined by a hydrogen clearance method. The electrode for CBF measurement was inserted in the parietal cortex. The cerebral water content, which is an index for cerebral edema, was measured by a freeze-dry method.

Serum TXB_2 and 6-keto-$PGF_{1\alpha}$, which are the stable metabolites of TXA_2 and PGI_2, respectively, were measured by radioimmunoassay. The blood samples for PG assay were collected from the abdominal aorta, care being taken not to stimulate coagulation, and swiftly placed in the tube containing indomethacin and EDTA. Plasma was collected after centrifugation at 4 °C 3000 rpm for 10 min.

---

[1] 2nd Dept. of Internal Medicine, Nippon Medical School, 3-5-5, Iidabashi, Chiyoda-ku, Tokyo 102, Japan

The differences in cerebral water content and the PG changes before and after ischemia was achieved by performing BLCL in SHRSR were thoroughly investigated.

Results

The ischemic focus was most prominent in the SHRSP, while SHRSR had moderately sized ischemic focuses. But no ischemic focus was observed in WKY. The cerebral energy metabolism was severely impaired in SHRSP and SHRSR, and at the same time a decrease was noted in CBF 3 h after BLCL (Fig. 1). The water content was also increased 3 h after BLCL (Fig. 2).

CBF decrease, metabolic impairment, and production of brain edema were more prominent in the hypertensive groups (SHRSP and SHRSR) than in normotensive WKY after subjection to the same procedure of BLCL.

There were no statistical differences in the plasma TSB_2 and 6-keto-$PGF_{1\alpha}$ levels between SHRSP, SHRSR, and WKY in the untreated rats before the induction of ischemia. But at 3 h after BLCL, serum TXB_2 was elevated in the hypertensive groups (SHRSP and SHRSR), the difference from control being statistically significant, while no elevation was observed in WKY. On the other hand, 6-keto-$PGF_{1\alpha}$ levels were elevated to a similar degree in all three groups of rats.

With reference to the TXA_2-PGI_2 balance, the TXB_2/6-keto $PGF_{1\alpha}$ ratio was calculated before and after ischemia. The ratio rose significantly in the hypertensive groups but there was no change in the ratio in the normotensive WKY group (Fig. 3).

In the series of experiments with SHRSR, the changes in PGs over time were examined. Plasma TXB_2 showed a continuous and significant elevation after 1 h of BLCL, but the increase was slight after 3 h of BLCL (Fig. 4). There was no increase in water content up to 1 h of BLCL, but it was elevated significantly after 3 h of BLCL.

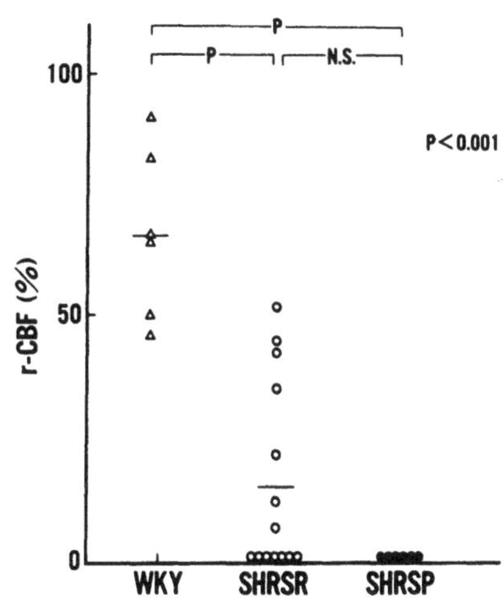

Fig. 1. Differences in rCBF 3 h after performance of BLCL (parietal cortex)

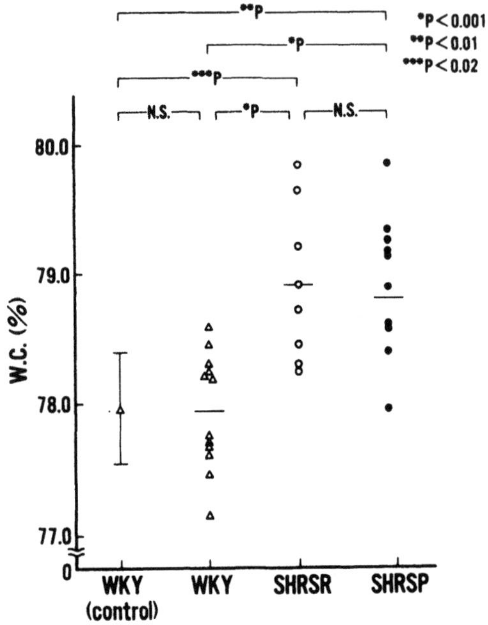

Fig. 2. Differences in brain water content 3 h after performance of BLCL

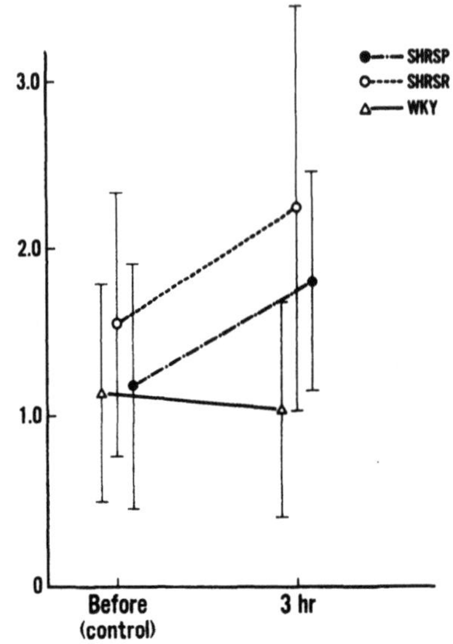

Fig. 3. Ratio of TXB_2 to 6-keto-$PGF_{1\alpha}$ before and 3 h after performance of BLCL

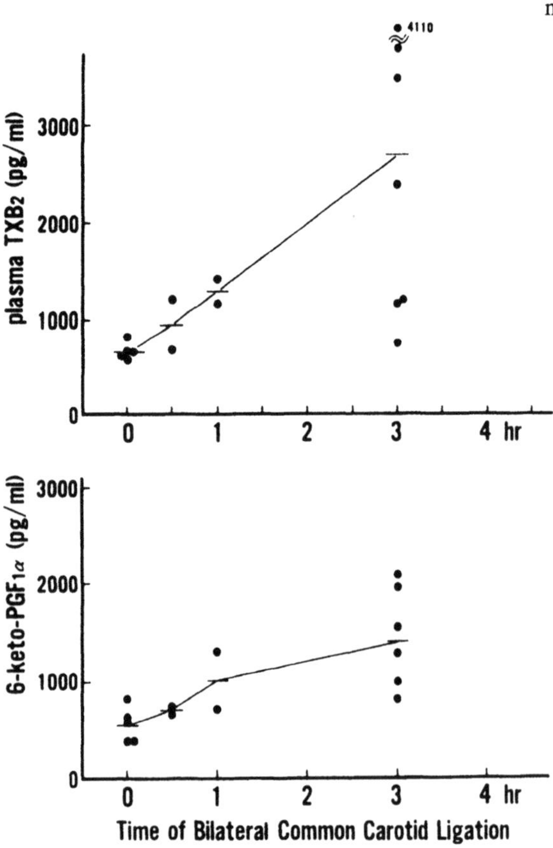

Fig. 4. Changes in plasma levels of TXB_2 (*above*) and 6-keto-$PGF_{1\alpha}$ (*below*) over time after BLCL in SHRSR

Discussion

Hypertensive rats (SHRSP and SHRSR) demonstrated a high susceptibility to ischemia, as confirmed by severe impairment of cerebral energy metabolism and aggravation of cerebral edema compared with the normotensive WKY after 3 h of ischemia following BLCL. The metabolic impairment and aggravation of edema may be attributable to the decrease in cerebral blood flow in the SHRSP and SHRSR groups. The high susceptibility to ischemia in the hypertensive groups might also be attributed to a relative disposition to reduced cerebral blood flow, the mechanisms of which are not fully understood.

In our study, the vasoconstrictive TXA_2 [3] was shown to be significantly elevated in the plasma of hypertensive SHRSP and SHRSR following BLCL. The elevation of vascular resistance [4] due to vasoconstriction by this elevated TXA_2 may be one factor contributing to hypoperfusion in the hypertensive groups. The vascular arteriosclerotic changes induced by persistent hypertension may also contribute to this hypoperfusion [5].

In a series of experiments examining the time course of TXA_2 and PGI_2, the enhanced elevation of TXA_2 was observed 3 h after BLCL in SHRSR, whereas PGI_2 was only slightly increased. In view of the TXA_2 and PGI_2 balance hypothesis, this priority of TXA_2 over PGI_2 may enhance vasoconstriction, platelet aggregation, and ischemia.

Summary

Plasma prostaglandins (TXB_2 and 6-keto $PGF_{1\alpha}$) were measured before and after bilateral carotid ligation (BLCL) in hypertensive rats (SHRSP, SHRSR) and normotensive rats (WKY). After BLCL, the elevation of plasma TXA_2 and superiority of TXA_2 over PGI_2 were shown in hypertensive rats, which may be one of the major factors in the aggravation of cerebral ischemia.

References

1. Fujishima M, Tamaki K, Nakatomi Y, Ishithuka T, Nakagawara K, Omae T (1980) Experimental cerebral ischemia in spontaneously hypertensive rats (SHR); importance of degree of hypertension. Stroke 11:612–616
2. Katayama Y, Terashi A, Sugimoto S, Inamura K, Suzuki S, Sekiguchi F, Akashi A (1984) Experimental cerebral ischemia after bilateral common carotid artery ligation in SHRSP, SHRSR and Wistar rats. Brain Nerve 36:1069–1075
3. Needleman P, Wyche A, Raz A (1979) Platelet and blood vessel arachidonate metabolism and interactions. J Clin Invest 63:345–349
4. Fujishima M, Omae T (1976) Carotid back pressure following bilateral carotid occlusion in normotensive and spontaneously hypertensive rats. Experimentia 32:1021–1022
5. Terashi A, Katayama Y, Sugimoto S, Soeda T, Inamura K, Shimizu J, Suzuki S, Mizoguchi M, Okamoto A, Nagazumi A (1983) Pathogenesis and treatment of cerebral edema. Prog Med 3:507–516

Identification of a Lipoxygenase Product (11-HETE) in Rat Brain Microvessel, and Its Relevance to Ischemic Brain Edema

M. Usui[1], T. Asano, S. Terao, and K. Takakura

Key words: Lipid hydroperoxide, lipoxygenase, microvessel, brain edema, cerebral ischemia

Introduction

Great progress has been made in the study of polyunsaturated fatty acids comprising membrane lipids and their metabolites in the biological field. It has been shown that eicosanoids are involved in a variety of pathologic conditions such as inflammation and asthma. In the brain, an ischemic insult stimulates the liberation of free fatty acids from membranes [10, 14]. Among these fatty acids, arachidonic acid was shown to cause brain edema when directly injected into the brain [1]. Although the exact mechanism is unknown, its conversion to various eicosanoids by the arachidonate cascade appears to be involved. Our earlier study revealed that the activities of both lipoxygenase and cyclooxygenase in the brain microvessel were significantly enhanced after ischemia [5]. The administration of the cyclooxygenase inhibitor indomethacin did not alleviate ischemic brain edema, but a lipoxygenase-inhibiting radical scavenger, i.e., AVS, did [1, 5, 7]. Therefore, it was speculated that lipoxygenase products rather than cyclooxygenase products might be the causative factors of ischemic brain edema, if eicosanoids are at all responsible for its occurrence. However, little is known about the lipoxygenase pathway in the central nervous system. The aim of the present study was to identify the lipoxygenase products in the rat brain and clarify their relation to the ischemic brain edema.

Materials and Methods

Male Sprague-Dawley rats weighing about 200 g were anesthetized with 2% halothane. According to the method reported elsewhere [12], the left middle cerebral artery (MCA) was occluded in the proximal portion. After surgery, these rats were returned to cages and fed ad libitum. These rats were again anesthetized 24 and 72 h after MCA occlusion. They were put on artificial respiration, and their brains were fixed in situ by funnel freezing with liquid nitrogen. The left hemispheres were chiseled out and weighed. They were stored at –80 °C for later analysis.

[1] Department of Neurosurgery, University of Tokyo, 7-3-1 Hongo, Bunkyo-ku, Tokyo 113, Japan

HPLC and GC-MS Analysis

The cerebral hemisphere was homogenized in 60% methanol. The homogenate was centrifuged at 1000 *g*, and the supernatant was passed through Sep-Pak. The material eluted in ethyl acetate was studied by reversed-phase high-performance liquid chromatography (HPLC). Hydroxy acids were identified by retention times compared with those of standard hydroxy-eicosatetraenoic acids (HETEs), and quantitative analysis was performed with reference to the peak height.

The material in the peak on HPLC was fractionated and transformed into trimethylsilyl ester. Then gas chromatography-mass spectrometry (GC-MS) analysis was carried out for further confirmation.

Preparation of the Microvessel Fraction and the Other Fraction of Rat Brain

The MV fraction was obtained according to the method of Gecse [2]. Rats weighing about 200 g were anesthetized with ether, and their brains were perfused with 0.9% (w/v) saline. The brains were removed and chopped in Tris-HCl buffer. The suspension was passed through nylon meshes with pore sizes of 670 μm and 335 μm in turn. The filtrate was centrifuged at 3500 *g* for 10 min, and the precipitate was resuspended in the same buffer. It was layered on a discontinuous density gradient, and centrifuged at 58 000 *g* for 60 min. The MV fraction was collected from the bottom of the tube. The other layers were collected together into one fraction.

The same HPLC analysis was performed in the MV and the other fractions. The protein contents of the both fractions were determined by Bio-Rad Protein Assay Kit.

Results

Identification of Lipoxygenase Metabolite

The brain sample had only one peak on HPLC, and its retention time was the same as that of 11-HETE (Fig. 1). Mass fragmentographic analysis of this peak showed ions of high intensity at m/e 225 (base peak), 73, 93, 155, 368, 391. The MS pattern of the brain sample was identical with that of 11-HETE (Fig. 2). Both HPLC and GC-MS analyses revealed that the normal and ischemic rat brains contained 11-HETE as the only lipoxygenase product.

Table 1. 11-HETE content in MV and other fractions

Fraction	11-HETE content
MV fraction	653 ng/mg protein
Other fractions	64 ng/mg protein

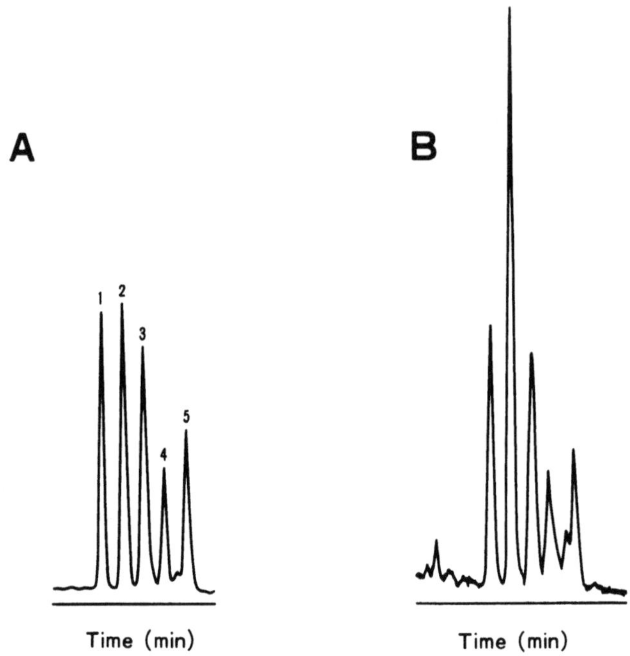

Fig. 1. A Reversed-phase HPLC of standard six HETEs: peak *1*, 15-HETE; peak *2*, 11-HETE; peak *3*, 8- and 12-HETE; peak *4*, 9-HETE; peak *5*, 5-HETE; **B** reversed-phase HPLC of the mixture of the rat brain sample and the same standard six HETEs. The peak corresponding to 11-HETE was increased by adding the brain sample to the standard HETEs

Distribution of 11-HETE

The contents of 11-HETE in the MV and the other fractions were 653 ng/mg protein and 64 ng/mg protein, respectively. The MV fraction contained 10 times as much 11-HETE as the other fraction (Table 1).

Change in Quantity of 11-HETE After Ischemia

Quantitative analysis by HPLC revealed that the content of 11-HETE was 1288 ± 66 (mean ± SE) ng/g wet weight in the control sham-operated rat brain hemispheres (n = 18). On the other hand, the brains rendered ischemic for 24 h (n = 10) and 72 h (n = 18) contained 1101 ± 48 and 1663 ± 147 ng/g wet weight, respectively. The content of 11-HETE was significantly increased 72 h after MCA occlusion. The wet weight of rat brain was progressively increased until 72 h after MCA occlusion because of the edema formation, which distorted the amount of the hydroxy acid per gram of wet weight of brain by the excess water. As the mean values for excess water 24 and 72 h after MCA occlusion were known in this model [3] the corrected amounts could be calculated. They were 1245 and 2104 ng/g wet weight in the 24- and 72-h ischemia groups, respectively (Fig. 3).

Discussion

The recent discovery of lipoxygenase pathway of the arachidonate cascade has attracted renewed interest in the possible role of eicosanoids in a variety of pathologic

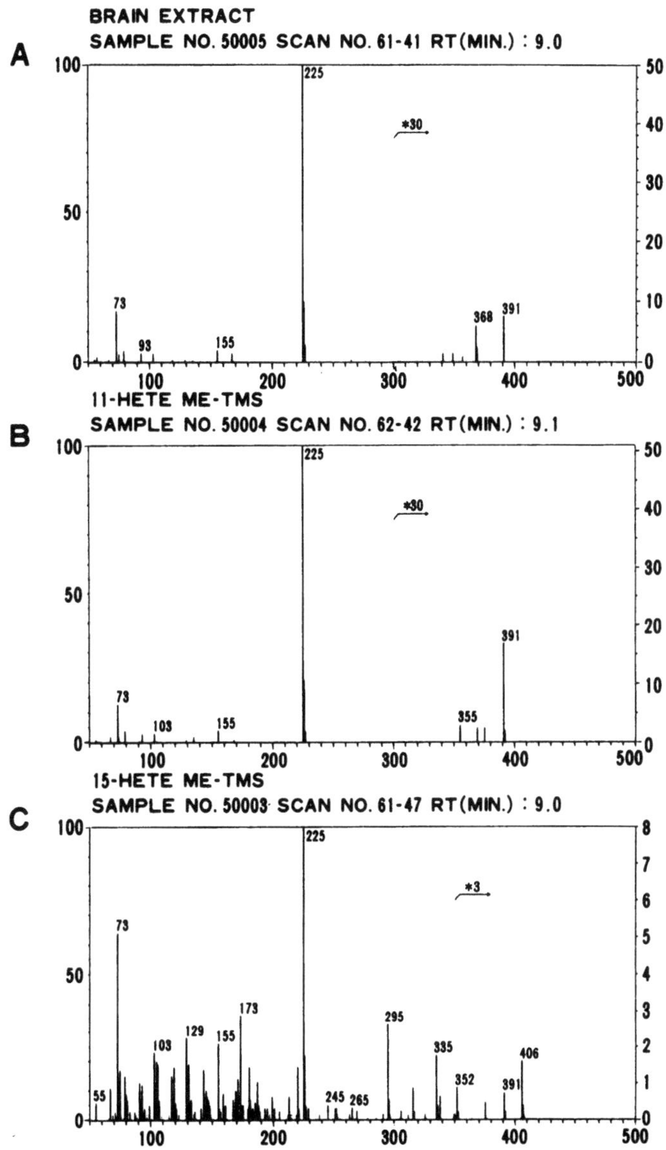

Fig. 2A–C. Mass spectra of trimethylsilyl ethers of brain sample (**A**) standard 11-HETE (**B**) and standard 15-HETE methyl esters (**C**)

conditions. For example, the inhibition of lipoxygenase reduced the size of cardiac infarction [9]. It was also shown that lipoxygenase metabolites are involved in the increased vascular permeability or vasoconstriction in inflammatory reactions. As lipoxygenase products modulate the peripheral circulation and vascular permeability in various tissues [11], it might be anticipated that they are somehow involved in the pathomechanism of brain edema ensuing from ischemic or traumatic insult. Presently, however, few data are available about lipoxygenase metabolism in the brain. Leukotrienes and 12-HETE were detected in the gerbil brain after isch-

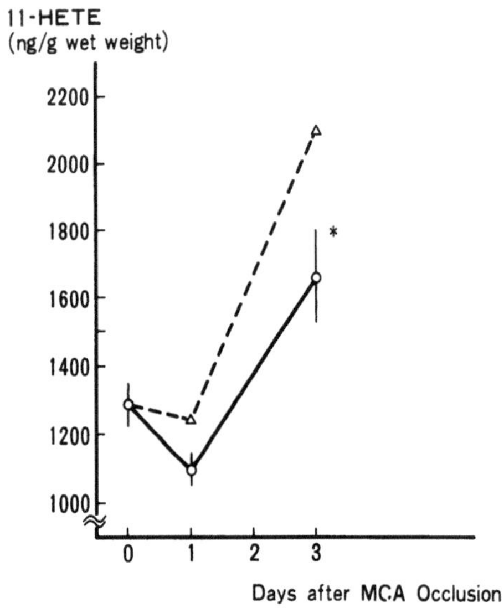

Fig. 3. Content of 11-HETE in the rat brain before ischemia (day 0) and after ischemia (1 and 3 days) (*solid line*). *Dotted line,* corrected values calculated with reference to the excess water in brain edema. Significantly different from the control at $P<0.05$ (Student's *t*-test)

emia by radioimmunoassay [8]. In the present study, we identified 11-HETE as the major lipoxygenase product in the rat brain. Although 11-HETE was found in the sheep vesicular gland and the rat neutrophil, its physiologic properties are not known. Our study revealed that the microvessel of rat brain contained 10 times as much 11-HETE as the rest of the brain. Previous data suggest that the brain microvessel synthesizes PGI_2, which possesses a regulatory function on the peripheral circulation. By the same token, 11-HETE or its precursor 11-HPETE synthesized within the microvessel may play a regulatory role on the cerebral microcirculation. It also seems possible that 11-HPETE might exert an indirect influence on the cerebral circulation through modulation of the eicosanoid synthesis within the microvessel, because hydroperoxides are known to influence the enzyme activities of the arachidonate cascade [4, 5]. In addition, the microvessel is an important structural and functional component of the blood-brain barrier (BBB). Thus, the lipoxygenase products synthesized within the microvessel could potentially affect the BBB function.

We used the rat MCA occlusion model to clarify the relation between the lipoxygenase pathway and ischemic brain edema. In this model, both the changes in the local blood flow and the extent of cerebral infarction are well known [12, 13]. Also, the time course of edema development in the affected hemisphere has been delineated [3]. Hence, the analysis of HETEs was performed 24 h after ischemia, when the edema was progressing most rapidly, and at 72 h, when the edema reached its peak. The significant increase in the 11-HETE content in the affected hemisphere was therefore considered to be an important piece of evidence linking lipoxygenase products with ischemic brain edema.

The biological activities of 11-HETE on the human neutrophils or the airway mucous membrane are much less than those of other eicosanoids [6]. On the other hand, the lipid hydroperoxides such as 12-HPETE and 15-HPETE are potent bioactive substances. They cause marked vasoconstriction and inhibit the synthesis of

PGI_2. Further, we have shown that a lipid hydroperoxide, i.e., 15-HPAA, acts to enhance the lipoxygenase activity of the rat brain microvessel [5]. This seems to imply that the lipoxygenase of the brain microvessel is stimulated by its own products, leading to accelerated production of hydroperoxides in some pathologic conditions. Thus, accumulated hydroperoxides may exert significant influences on the cerebral microcirculation or the function of the BBB. Although the bioactivity of 11-HPETE is not clear, it may be more relevant to the pathogenetic mechanism of ischemic brain edema than the presently discovered 11-HETE.

Summary

Eicosanoids are thought to contribute to the pathogenesis of ischemic brain damage. But little is known about lipoxygenase products and their roles in brain. The present study aimed to detect the lipoxygenase products in the rat brain using high-performance liquid chromatography (HPLC) and gas chromatography-mass spectrometry (GC-MS) and clarify their possible roles in the pathomechanism of ischemic brain edema. The rat middle cerebral artery (MCA) occlusion model was used because the time course of edema development in the affected hemisphere has been well analyzed. The fixation of rat brain was carried out by in situ freezing 24 and 72 h after MCA occlusion. Identification and quantitative analysis of hydroxyeicosatetraenoic acids (HETEs) in normal and ischemic brain homogenates was performed by HPLC and GC-MS. The same analysis was carried out in the microvessel (MV) fraction and the remaining fraction obtained from the normal rat brain. With the method used only 11-HETE was detected in the normal and ischemic brain. Quantitatively, normal brains contained 1288 ± 66 (mean $\pm$ SE) ng/g wet weight 11-HETE, while the hemispheres rendered ischemic for 24 and 72 h after MCA occlusion contained 1101 ± 48 and 1663 ± 147 ng/g wet weight, respectively. The 11-HETE content was significantly increased 72 h after MCA occlusion ($P<0.05$). The MV fraction of rat brain contained 10 times as much 11-HETE (653 ng/mg protein) as the other fraction.

The present study revealed that 11-HETE was produced mainly in the brain MC and its synthesis was activated simultaneously with edema formation. The above results indicate the possibility that the lipoxygenase products are involved in the pathogenesis of ischemic brain edema.

References

1. Chan PH, Fishman RA, Caronna J, Schmidley JW, Prioleau G, Lee J (1983) Induction of brain edema following intracerebral injection of arachidonic acid. Ann Neurol 13:625–632
2. Gecse A, Ottlecz A, Mezei Z, Telegdy G, Joo F, Dux E, Karnushina I (1982) Prostacyclin and prostaglandin synthesis in isolated brain capillaries. Prostaglandins 23:287–297
3. Gotoh O, Koide T, Asano T, Takakura K, Tamura A, Sano K (1984) A model to study ischemic brain edema in rats and the influence of drugs. In: Go KG, Baethmann A (eds) Recent progress in the study and therapy of brain edema. Plenum, New York, pp 499–508
4. Hemler ME, Cook HW, Lands WE (1979) Prostaglandin biosynthesis can be triggered by lipid peroxides. Arch Biochem Biophys 193:340–345

5. Koide T, Gotoh O, Asano T, Takakura K (in press) Alterations of the eicosanoid synthetic capacity of the rat brain microvessel following ischemia: its relevance to ischemic brain edema. J Neurochem
6. Marom Z, Shelhamer JH, Sun F, Kaliner M (1983) Human airway monohydroxyeicosatetraenoic acid generation and mucus release. J Clin Invest 72: 122–127
7. Matsui T, Basugi N, Asano T, Takakura K (1984) The effect of indomethacin on ischemic brain edema. Neurol Med Chir (Tokyo) 24:5–12
8. Moskowitz MA, Kiwak KJ, Hekimian K, Levine L (1984) Synthesis of compounds with properties of leukotrienes C4 and D4 in gerbil brains after ischemia and reperfusion. Science 224:886–889
9. Mullane KM, Moncada S (1982) The salvage of ischemic myocardium by BW755C in anesthetized dogs. Prostaglandins 24:255–265
10. Rehncrona S, Westerberg E, Akesson B, Siesjö BK (1982) Brain cortical fatty acids and phospholipids during and following complete and severe incomplete ischemia. J Neurochem 38:83–93
11. Seeger W, Wolf H, Staehler G, Neuhof H, Roeka L (1982) Increased pulmonary vascular resistance and permeability due to arachidonate metabolism in isolated rabbit lungs. Prostaglandins 23:157–173
12. Tamura A, Graham DI, McCulloch J, Teasdale GM (1981) Focal cerebral ischemia in the rat: 1. Description of technique and early neuropathological consequences following middle cerebral artery occlusion. J Cereb Blood Flow Metab 1:53–60
13. Tamura A, Graham DI, McCulloch J, Teasdale GM (1981) Focal cerebral ischemia in the rat: 2. Regional cerebral blood flow determined by (14C)-iodoantipyrine autoradiography following middle cerebral artery occlusion. J Cereb Blood Flow Metab 1:61–69
14. Yoshida S, Inoh S, Asano T, Sano K, Kubota M, Shimazaki H, Ueta N (1980) Effect of transient ischemia on free fatty acids and phospholipids in the gerbil brain. J Neurosurg 53:323–331

Cerebrovascular Permeability and Ischemic Brain Damage Following MCA Occlusion in the Rat:

A Comparative Study with ^{14}C-AIB Transfer, Enzyme Histochemistry, and Neuropathology

T. SHIGENO [1], D. I. GRAHAM, J. McCULLOCH, and G. M. TEASDALE

Key words: Rat MCA occlusion, ischemic brain edema, microvascular permeability, ischemic brain damage

Introduction

Focal cerebral ischemia produces heterogeneous alterations in the cerebral circulation and metabolism, which eventually lead to the development of ischemic brain damage. It is not, however, in the period after irreversible brain damage is established that brain water is increased. Early ischemic oedema seems rather to be a reversible functional event, in which a change in the permeability of the blood-brain barrier (BBB) to cations is involved through unknown mechanisms of brain capillary function. In the later stage, however, when gross changes in the BBB are induced, the development of brain oedema may well be linked with that of ischemic brain damage. Therefore, an important question at this stage is whether brain oedema itself has neuropathologic consequences. Since no correlative investigations have so far been published, we report here topographical alterations and the correlation between IBD and oedema formation following occlusion of the middle cerebral artery (MCA) in the rat.

Materials and Methods

Focal cerebral ischemia was produced by occluding the MCA of anaesthetised (halothane 1–2% and nitrous oxide: oxygen mixture) and physiologically monitored adult Sprague Dawley rats. The vessel was occluded at its stem proximal to the lenticulostriate branches in order to ensure IBD in both striatum and cortex [10]. Anaesthesia was discontinued immediately after surgery. For measurement of oedema, tissue-specific gravity was determined by column gravimetry [7] in both the acute and chronic stages: estimations were made at 4 h, 1 day, 2 days, 3 days, 5 days, 1 week and 3 weeks after MCA occlusion. Five animals from each group were used at each time point. Topographic determination of specific gravity was carried out in the cortex and caudate nucleus of both hemispheres. In the cortex the area was divided into the lateral cortex, where cerebral blood flow was greatly reduced to

[1] Department of Neurosurgery, University of Tokyo, 7-3-1 Hongo, Bunkyo-ku, Tokyo 113, Japan

the extent that this area was defined as the ischemic core, and into the dorsal cortex surrounding this core, which was defined as the penumbra.

Correlations between oedema formation (as determined by [^{14}C]AIB) and cerebral blood flow (as determined by [^{14}C]iodoantipyrine) were determined in animals killed 30 min, 4 h, 2 days and 3 weeks after occlusion of the MCA.

Changes in cerebrovascular permeability were studied by autoradiography using [^{14}C]AIB. Since we did not observe any changes in permeability to AIB in the acute stage of ischemia, that is, 4 h after occlusion of the MCA [12], the present investigation was carried out on the second day when oedema formation was most pronounced according to specific gravity measurements. [^{14}C]AIB 50 μCi was injected IV, and timed arterial blood samples were collected until 20 min later, when the animal was sacrificed. The brain was immediately frozen and cut into 20-μm-thick sections for autoradiography, for histological study, and for the histochemical staining of glycogen phosphorylase. We have previously found that glycogen phosphorylase staining can delineate IBD and identify heterogeneous metabolic changes [8]. Microvascular permeability of AIB was determined in terms of the blood tissue transfer ratio K_i [1] in the region of interest as seen by neuropathological and enzyme histochemical mapping of the disturbances. Eight rats were subjected to occlusion of the MCA, and four rats (controls) underwent sham operation with exposure of MCA only and without occlusion.

Results

Chronological Changes in Specific Gravity

The reduction in specific gravity (SG) was most pronounced between 1 and 2 days after the onset of ischemia and recovered, reaching values close to control, within 3 weeks (Fig. 1). A definite tendency was noted for the greatest reduction in SG to be found in the most profoundly ischemic area, that is, in the caudate nucleus. In the cortex, oedema was most marked in the ischemic area, whereas in the penumbra the reduction in specific gravity was small and not significant.

Brain Swelling

Autoradiography showed profound ischaemia in the caudate nucleus and moderate ischemia in the lateral cortex ipsilateral to the occlusion (Fig. 2). Hemispheric brain swelling with a midline shift was marked 2 days after the onset of ischemia, in parallel with changes in specific gravity.

Microvascular Permeability and Ischemic Brain Damage

There was extensive ischemic damage in the caudate nucleus of all the animals studied. Diffuse leakage of AIB was observed in the caudate nucleus, and a markedly enhanced rim surrounded this lesion. A similar rim was also noted in sections

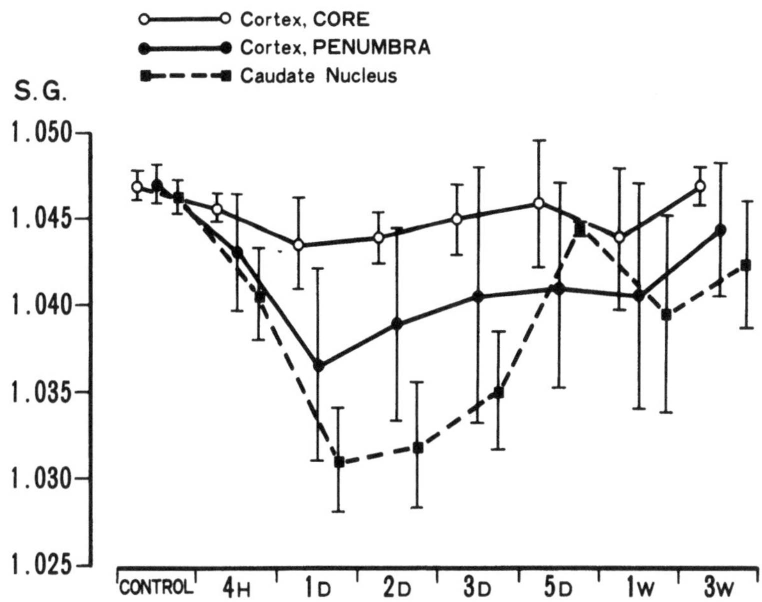

Fig. 1. Chronological changes in specific gravity

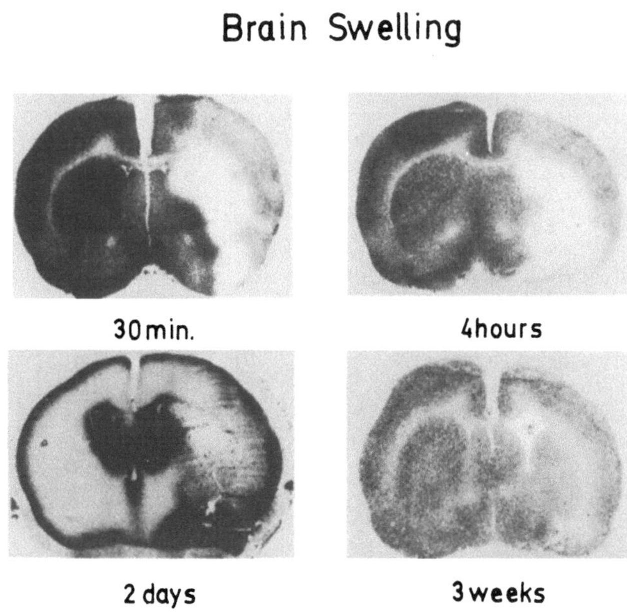

Fig. 2. Coronal autoradiographic sections at the level of the caudate nucleus following MCA occlusion. Autoradiograms at 30 min, 4 h, and 3 weeks are of CBF, performed with [^{14}C]iodoantipyrine, and that at 2 days was performed with [^{14}C]aminoisobutyric acid. Note marked hemispheric swelling 2 days after onset of ischemia

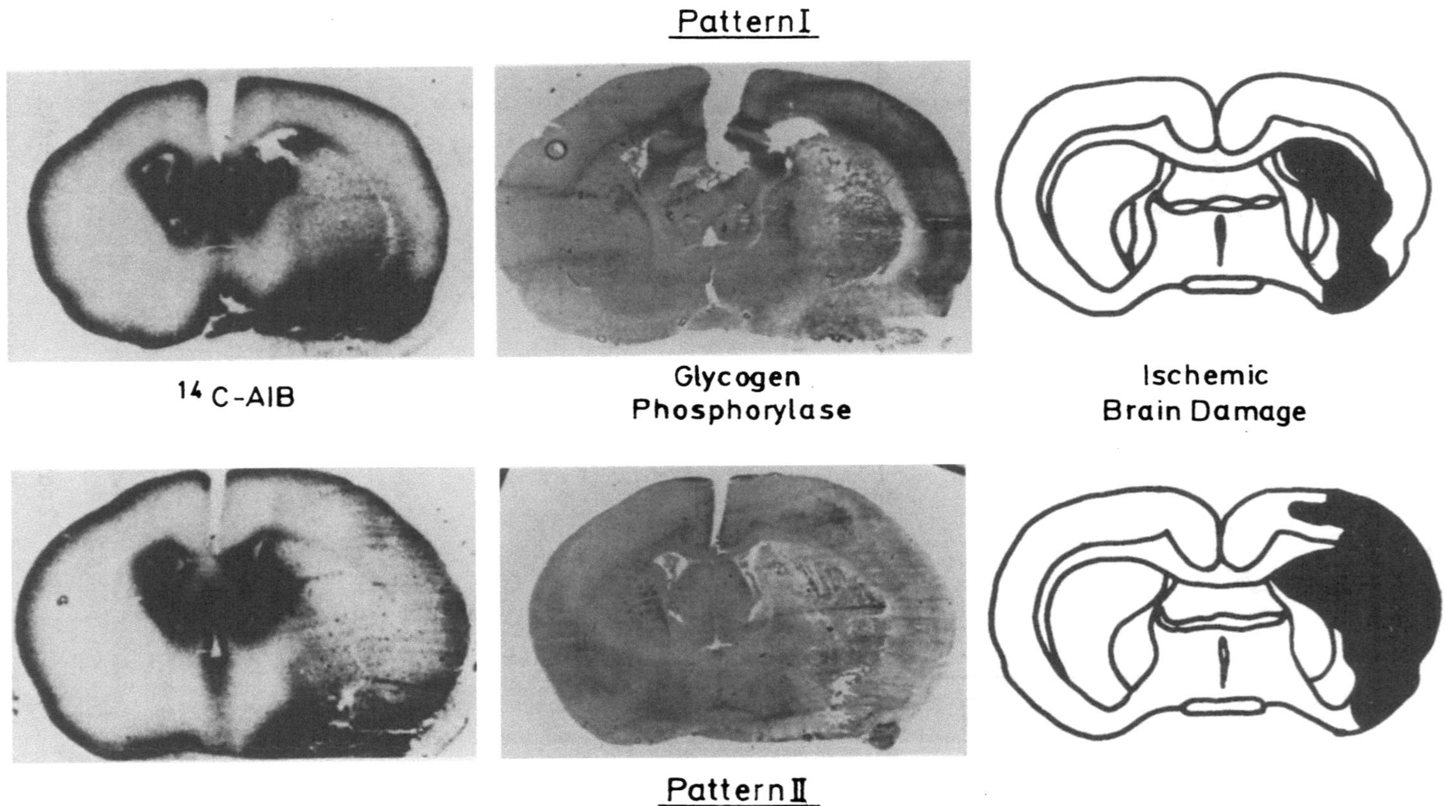

Fig. 3. Correlative patterns for microvascular permeability for [^{14}C]AIB, enzyme-histochemistry for glycogen phosphorylase, and ischemic brain damage. Note enhanced AIB leakage surrounding ischemic lesion in both caudate nucleus (patterns I and II) and cortex (pattern II). Cortical AIB leakage is absent when there is no ischemic brain damage as seen in pattern I

Table 1. AIB transfer and glycogen phosphorylase activity in the cortex ipsilateral to occlusion

		AIB (K_i mg^{-1} $min^{-1} \times 10^3$)		Glycogen phosphorylase (%)	
	(*n*)	Core	Penumbra	Core	Penumbra
Sham control	(4)	2.1±0.6	2.2±0.6	100± 3	103±10
Infarction (+)	(4)	4.1±1.3*	4.4±1.4*	78±32	294±50**
Infarction (−)	(4)	2.6±0.7	3.1±1.4	159±67	245±34**

Values are means±SD
* $P<0.05$; ** $P<0.01$

stained for glycogen phosphorylase, and the border of the ischemic damage was clearly demonstrable at this rim. However, there were two patterns in the cortex according to the presence or absence of IBD (Fig. 3). In rats without IBD (pattern I, $n=4$), there were no changes in cortical AIB radioactivity and glycogen phosphorylase was diffusely enhanced. In the other rats, which developed IBD in the cortex (pattern II, $n=4$), AIB leaked at the periphery of the ischemic damage and there was also increased glycogen phosphorylase activity. When the values for AIB transfer (K_i) and glycogen phosphorylase activity measured as percentages of the contralateral values in optical density (Quantimet 720) were compared in the cortex, a significant increase in both K_i and glycogen phosphorylase activity was noted at the periphery of the ischemic area (Table 1).

Discussion

In spite of a rather homogeneous reduction in cerebral blood flow in the cortex and striatum following occlusion of the MCA in the rat, the resulting events in metabolism and ischemic damage were highly heterogeneous and subject to inter-animal variability, as has been reported previously [8, 10]. This is because the ischemic core is influenced by its environment, viz. the collateral circulation and the metabolic state of the core/penumbra interface. Identification of these heterogeneous and topographically variable disturbances was made easier by examining the enzyme-histochemical preparations and the autoradiograms simultaneously. In particular, glycogen phosphorylase was found to match the pattern seen on [^{14}C]2-deoxyglucose autoradiography exactly as it appeared in both reduced and enhanced regions [8]. We therefore used this technique for the study of microvascular permeability, in the hope of seeing whether permeability changes might be linked with metabolic and neuropathological changes.

[^{14}C]AIB is a low-molecular-weight tracer suited for the study of microvascular permeability. Having crossed the BBB, AIB is quickly taken up and trapped by brain cells for a long time without diffusion, so that the oedema front can be visualized [1]. In a previous study when it was used in rats 4 h after MCA occlusion, there was no increase in blood tissue transfer, K_i, unless brief hypotension was induced with halothane [12]. Similarly, even after recirculation in the acute state, it was not possible to identify the early stages of brain oedema using AIB as an index of permeability [9].

Oedema formation was maximal at 1–2 days after the induction of ischemia in terms of both reduction in SG and brain swelling. At this stage, the increase in permeability of the BBB to AIB was always sufficiently marked to indicate the presence of ischemic brain damage and to localize the origin of the oedema to the edge of the ischemic area. Glycogen phosphorylase activity was also increased at this edge, which in the past has been considered to be a state of enhanced anaerobic glycolysis, that is, an area where cells are probably deranged functionally but still viable [8]. Although it is clear that an increase in permeability does not necessarily indicate an increase in water movement, it might be surmised that water has passed through the disturbed BBB, and the following are possible mechanisms. First, hydrostatic pressure might be involved [5]. It has been hypothesized that the difference in hydrostatic pressure may be greatest at the boundary zone of ischemia between perfused and nonperfused vessels, and Starling's law allows movement of water into the interstitial space in the presence of BBB dysfunction such as may occur in peripheral organs and tissues without a blood-tissue barrier. Second, an increase in colloidal osmotic pressure [4] in the ischemic core produces a force that drives cations and water towards the core in the sense of increased "osmotic potential", a term coined by Tomita et al. [11]. Third, although the energy-dependent ionic pump within the ischemic core is no longer working, brain capillary function in the penumbra may be enhanced for pumping out sodium from blood into the extracellular space by way of possible activation of capillary sodium potassium ATPase channel [2]. Recent reports on the enhanced activity of sodium potassium ATPase, probably of capillary origin [Asano et al. and Shigeno et al., this volume; 3], in early ischemia when the tissue is not yet necrotic might indicate a similar situation in the penumbral tissue even in the chronic stage.

It has been suggested that changes in the permeability to large molecules and brain oedema develop only when vessel and glial elements are damaged in models of transient global ischemia [6]. In the present study with focal cerebral ischemia, however, although precise histopathological analysis was not possible since frozen sections were used, the distribution of neuronal death was well matched with that of permeability changes. It is therefore of interest to speculate on the relationship between neuronal death and oedema and whether or not they can be influenced.

Summary

A link between ischemic brain damage, changes in blood-brain barrier permeability and oedema formation was investigated in rats after middle cerebral artery occlusion. Since oedema formation is maximal between 1 and 2 days after the induction of ischemia, studies were undertaken to determine microvascular permeability using [^{14}C]aminoisobutyric acid (AIB), structural alterations and the pattern of enzyme histochemistry for glycogen phosphorylase 2 days after occlusion of the middle cerebral artery. It was found that there was no leakage of AIB in the absence of ischemic brain damage. Marked AIB leakage was observed at the periphery of the ischemic area, at which site glycogen phosphorylase activity was also increased. Thus, it has become apparent that the oedema front is located at the periphery of the ischemic area. Such a penumbral region is of significance in determining consequences of oedema formation and neuronal damage.

References

1. Blasberg RG, Fenstermacher JD, Patlak CS (1983) Transport of aminoisobutyric acid across brain capillary and cellular membranes. J Cereb Blood Flow Metab 3:8–32
2. Enseleit WH, Domer FR, Jarrott DM, Baricos WH (1984) Cerebral phospholipid content and Na^+, K^+-ATPase activity during ischemia and postischemic reperfusion in the Mongolian gerbil. J Neurochem 43:320–327
3. Goldstein GW, Betz AL (1983) Recent advances in understanding brain capillary function. Ann Neurol 14:389–395
4. Hossmann KA, Takagi S (1976) Osmolarity of brain in cerebral ischemia. Exp Neurol 51:124–131
5. Kogure K, Busto R, Scheinberg P (1981) The role of hydrostatic pressure in ischemic brain edema. Ann Neurol 9:273–282
6. Petito CK, Pulsinelli WA, Jacobson G, Plum F (1982) Edema and vascular permeability in cerebral ischemia: comparison between ischemic neuronal damage and infarction. J Neuropathol Exp Neurol 41:423–436
7. Shigeno T, Brock M, Shigeno S, Fritschka E, Cervos-Navarro J (1982) The determination of brain water content: microgravimetry versus drying-weighing method. J Neurosurg 57:99–107
8. Shigeno T, McCulloch J, Graham DI, Kirkham D, Teasdale GM (1983) Ischaemic core and penumbra: a multifactorial analysis of the metabolic consequences. J Cereb Blood Flow Metab 3 [Suppl 1]: S403–S404
9. Shigeno T, Teasdale GM, McCulloch J, Mendelow D, Graham DI (1984) Brain edema following focal cerebral ischemia in the rat. In: Go KG, Baethmann A (eds) Recent progress in the study and therapy of brain edema. Plenum Press, New York, pp 449–458
10. Shigeno T, McCulloch J, Graham DI, Mendelow D (1985) Pure cortical ischaemia versus striatal ischaemia: circulatory metabolic and neuropathological consequences. Surg Neurol 24:47–51
11. Tomita M, Gotoh F, Sato T, Yamamoto M, Amano T, Tanahashi N, Tanaka K (1979) Determination of the osmotic potential for swelling of cat brain in vitro. Exp Neurol 65:66–77
12. Tyson GW, Teasdale GM, Graham DI, McCulloch J (1982) Cerebrovascular permeability following MCA occlusion in the rat. The effect of halothane-induced hypotension. J Neurosurg 57:186–196

The Duration of Ischemia Influences Ischemic and Postischemic Brain Edema

N. V. TODD[1], P. PICOZZI, H. A. CROCKARD, and R. R. RUSSELL

Introduction

The development and resolution of ischemic brain edema is a complex problem. During ischemia the failure of cellular metabolism leads to a failure of ionic homeostasis and an increase in brain osmolality, and water tends to move into the brain to balance this. The amount of water accumulating during ischemia depends upon the level of flow during ischemia [3, 17], its duration [10, 12], and whether the ischemia is complete or incomplete [16]. Reestablishment of blood flow to an ischemic region may lead to an increase in brain water, occurring either immediately [2, 9] or later, in association with breakdown of the blood-brain barrier (BBB) [10].

In this study we report on the changes in brain water, as reflected by changes in specific gravity (SG), following ischemia and reperfusion. We chose to vary the duration of ischemia whilst maintaining a fixed ischemic flow, to determine whether the duration of ischemia influenced the postischemic change in brain water.

Temporary global hemispheric ischemia was produced in rats. Cerebral blood flow (CBF) was measured by hydrogen clearance and SG was measured on a regional basis at sacrifice.

Methods

Animal Preparation

Adult, male Sprague-Dawley rats were paralyzed (2 mg/kg *d*-tubocurarine IP) and ventilated via a tracheostomy with 70% nitrous oxide, 30% oxygen, and 1.5% halothane delivered by a small-animal ventilator. The carotid arteries were isolated to facilitate later clipping. The left femoral vein and left and right femoral arteries were cannulated. The animal was then turned prone and the vertebral arteries were coagulated as they lay in the foramina transversaria of the first cervical vertebra (C 1). Burr holes were made in the skull and platinum electrodes placed into the frontal, parietal, and occipital cortical regions on each side and held fixed in place with cold-setting methylmethacrylate cement. A silver/silver chloride reference electrode was placed subcutaneously in the back. Following surgery the animal was

[1] The National Hospitals for Nervous Diseases, Institute of Neurology, Queen Square, London W.C.1., 3BG, Great Brain

placed in lateral decubitus and the halothane reduced to 0.5%. With the vertebral arteries occluded cerebral ischemia was produced by bilateral carotid artery occlusion with Scoville-Lewis aneurysm clips. This is a modification of the four-vessel occlusion model of Pulsinelli and Brierly [15], and it is a one-stage procedure with a very high reliability.

Regional CBF

CBF was measured by hydrogen clearance and the flow calculated by the initial slope technique between 30 and 90 s.

Brain Edema

Brain water was measured by the SG method in all animals at sacrifice. Six brain samples 1 mm in thickness were taken from each cortical region and inserted into the bromobenzene/kerosene gradient column. The position of six samples was read 3 min after insertion of the sample into the column, and the regional SG was taken as the mean of the six samples. Columns were calibrated with potassium sulfate solutions of known SG and columns were used only where the coefficient of linearity was greater than 0.9950 [14].

Experimental Protocol

Control Group. Under anesthesia 12 animals were decapitated and their brains sampled for assessment of the SG before ischemia.

Experimental Groups. A further 48 rats were divided into three experimental groups:

Group A ($n=16$, ischemia for 15 min)
Group B ($n=16$, ischemia for 30 min)
Group C ($n=16$, ischemia for 60 min)

In groups A, B, and C animals were made ischemic for the stated period and were sacrificed immediately after ischemia (i.e. without reperfusion), at 30 min after reperfusion, at 60 min after reperfusion, and at 180 min after reperfusion.

Systemic blood pressure was measured continuously; $PaCO_2$, pH, and PaO_2 were measured before each flow. rCBF was measured at rest, throughout ischemia, and in reperfusion.

Statistical Analysis

The data were analysed by analysis of variance and covariance with repeated measures and data compared using a modified *t*-test.

Results

General Physiological Parameters

Systemic arterial blood pressure, $PaCO_2$, PaO_2, and systemic pH remained stable throughout the experiment. On reperfusion there was a slight reduction in systemic pH, which was greater following 60 min of ischemia, and this was corrected by IV infusion of bicarbonate. The whole-blood hematocrit lay between 0.45 and 0.40.

Cerebral Blood Flow

Four-vessel occlusion produced severe forebrain ischemia, with cortical blood flow reduced to 5.8 ± 0.4 ml/100 g/min. The cortical regions did not differ in ischemic flow, nor did the three experimental groups. On reperfusion there was immediate hyperemia followed by a reduction in CBF, delayed hypoperfusion (Fig. 1).

Brain Water

The SG of rat cortex was 1.0484 ± 0.0001 (mean $\pm$ SEM). There was no significant difference in specific gravity between the frontal, parietal, or occipital cortical regions.

During ischemia there was a significant fall in SG (increase in brain water; Table 1). There was no regional difference in SG within any one group, but the end-

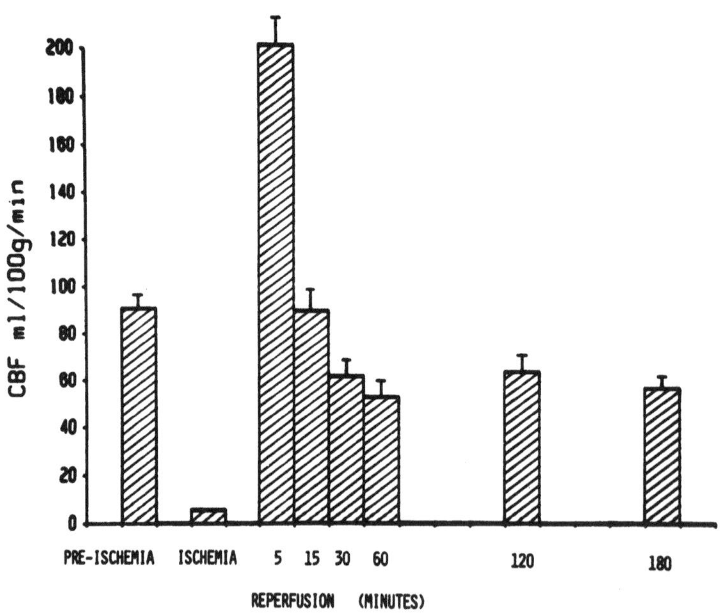

Fig. 1. Cortical CBF (mean $\pm$ SEM, ml/g/min) after 15 min of ischemia. On reperfusion there is an immediate increase in flow (hyperemia) followed by a reduction (hypoperfusion)

Table 1. Specific gravity of rat cortex at various times after initiation of reperfusion

Region	Duration of ischemia (min)	Reperfusion time (min) 0	30	60	180
Frontal	15	1.0470±0.00024	1.0455±0.00032	1.0462±0.00010	1.0474±0.00013
	30	1.0463±0.00032	1.0453±0.00019	1.0459±0.00014	1.0459±0.00033
	60	1.0442±0.00025	1.0446±0.00073	1.0449±0.00032	1.0452±0.00037
Parietal	15	1.0469±0.00036	1.0462±0.00031	1.0468±0.00027	1.0476±0.00016
	30	1.0465±0.00030	1.0457±0.00041	1.0460±0.00020	1.0459±0.00022
	60	1.0448±0.00023	1.0449±0.00043	1.0450±0.00036	1.0451±0.00034
Occipital	15	1.0469±0.00031	1.0461±0.00031	1.0464±0.00045	1.0469±0.00013
	30	1.0457±0.00039	1.0454±0.00039	1.0454±0.00086	1.0459±0.00034
	60	1.0448±0.00040	1.0450±0.00020	1.0440±0.00066	1.0449±0.00089

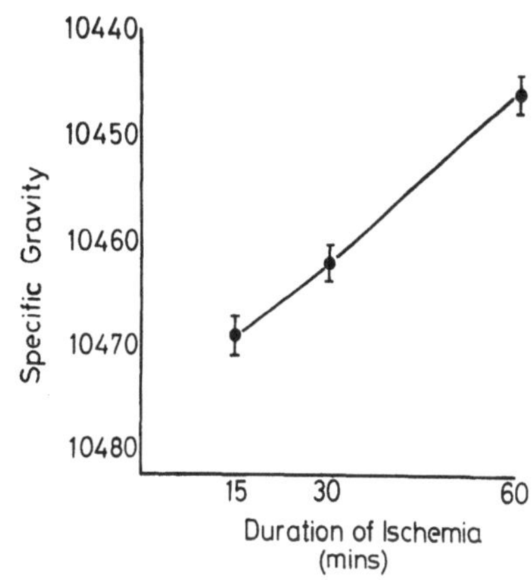

Fig. 2. Mean cortical SG (*bars*, standard error) measured after 15, 30, or 60 min of ischemia with no subsequent reperfusion. There is a linear increase in brain water with increasing duration of ischemia

ischemic (no reperfusion) SG was significantly reduced with increasing duration of ischemia. Indeed, taking the mean cortical SG at the end of ischemia in the three groups, there was a linear reduction in SG with increasing duration of ischemia (Fig. 2).

On reperfusion there were marked differences in the pattern of SG change in the three groups (Fig. 3).

Group A. There was a further marked decrease in SG in the first 30 min of reperfusion, which was most marked in the frontal cortex, and the change in SG at this time was greater than the change occurring on the induction of ischemia. Further reperfusion from 30 to 180 min led to a significant resolution of water in all three regions ($P<0.05$).

Group B. There was a similar though less marked decrease in SG in the first 30 min of reperfusion. From 30 to 60 min there was a trend toward resolution of this peak of brain edema, but further reperfusion up to 180 min was not associated with any significant change in SG.

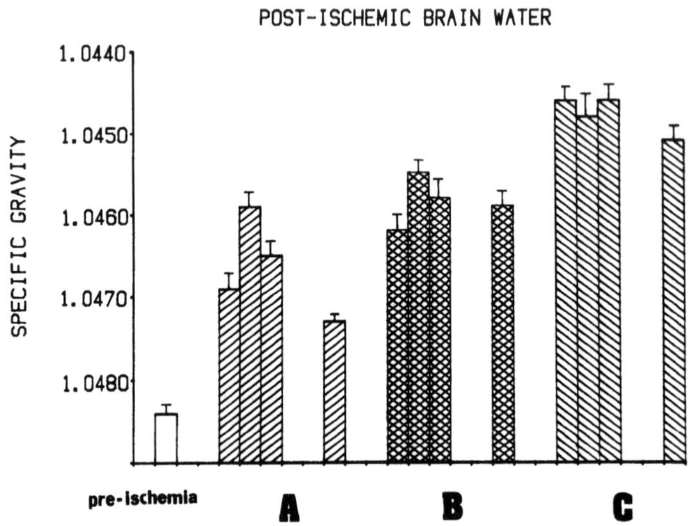

Fig. 3. Postischemic brain edema. For each group the *histogram bars* represent the times at which SG was measured (left to right):
End-ischemia (no reperfusion); 30 min reperfusion; 60 min reperfusion; 180 min reperfusion. In groups A and B reperfusion is associated with an immediate increase in brain edema. Further reperfusion to 180 min leads to resolution of brain edema in group A but not in groups B or C. ▭, control SG; ▨, group A (15 min of ischemia); ▩, group B (30 min of ischemia); ▧, group C (60 min of ischemia). Results are mean cortical specific gravity with standard error bars for each group

Group C. The SG values were very low on reperfusion; there was a trend toward resolution of brain water in the frontal cortex and toward worsening of brain water in the occipital cortex. These changes were not significant, however, and the overall pattern in this group was of severe brain edema with no improvement on reperfusion.

Discussion

This modification of the four-vessel occlusion model of cerebral ischemia in the rat [14] allows the preparation to be completed as a single-stage procedure. The global nature of the insult allows a large volume of mammalian brain to be rendered uniformly ischemic, and a mean ischemic flow of 5.8 ± 0.4 ml/100 g/min was achieved in this study.

During ischemia we found an increase in cortical water in all brain regions and in all three groups. Within each group there was no regional difference in the level of SG at the end of ischemia, and this reflects the uniform reduction of flow in the cortex in this model. This decrease in SG was most pronounced in group C and least in group A. Any increase in brain water occurring during ischemia must depend on an increase in brain osmolality together with some residual flow during ischemia. The failure of cellular metabolism during brain ischemia leads to an increase in intracellular osmolality (Na^+/Ca^{2+} and Cl^-) [4, 8]. There is also an increase in total brain osmolality because of the increase in small molecules (H^+, pyruvate and lactate) produced by anaerobic metabolism [6, 7]. Our results suggest that this increase in brain osmolality and the consequent increase in brain water content are directly proportional to the duration of ischemia.

Reduction in SG on reperfusion could theoretically reflect a water movement into the brain secondary either to a change that has occurred during ischemia or to a change precipitated specificially by reperfusion. A sudden increase in brain water on reperfusion has been shown [5, 9], but in both cases this followed complete cerebral ischemia and represents a balancing of the osmolality gradients built up at this time. The presence of a residual flow in our experiments and the linear reduction in SG with increasing duration of ischemia suggests to us that there is sufficient water present during incomplete ischemia to balance the increase in osmolality. Thus, the observed changes in SG in early reperfusion (groups A and B) are probably specific to reperfusion. The water movement may be generated by an increase in either hydrostatic or osmotic forces across the endothelium. There is a sudden increase in blood flow on reperfusion, with the systemic arterial pressure transmitted directly to the capillaries. Some argue that this increase in hydrostatic pressure will drive water from the vascular compartment into the brain [1, 13]. Others suggest that with an intact BBB hydrostatic pressure, differences between brain tissue and blood contribute very little to volume flow across the capillary wall [11]. The observed increase in water could also be secondary to a change in brain osmolality specific to reperfusion. On reperfusion there is a burst of energy production, which may be associated with an increase in tissue osmolality. The low extracellular Na^+ and Cl^- leads to a gain of these ions from the blood. There is increasing evidence that reperfusion also leads to a massive shift of Ca^{2+} into cells and into intracellular organelles, especially mitochondria, and this may be linked to the burst of cAMP production at this time. We are unable to decide whether the increase in brain water in early reperfusion (groups A and B) has a predominantly hydrostatic or osmolal basis.

Further reperfusion from 30 to 180 min was associated with a significant resolution of brain water in group A. It has been stated that there is a flow threshold of 10 ml/100 g/min for resolution of ischemic brain water, and that if CBF during ischemia falls below this level there is no resolution of brain edema on reperfusion [9]. This study shows that resolution of brain edema is possible even if the ischemic flow is 5.8 ml/100 g/min, provided the duration of ischemia is relatively short. This resolution of water occurs at a time when there is a reduction in CBF, hypoperfusion. In all three experimental groups CBF was reduced to similar levels (approximately 65% of control values) from 30 to 180 min of reperfusion.

In groups B and C there was an indolent course with no significant change in SG from 30 to 180 min of reperfusion. This may reflect the death of a significant proportion of cells so that ischemic water can no longer be cleared, or it may reflect the dynamic nature of edema formation and resolution, with a secondary worsening of brain edema (perhaps in association with BBB breakdown) running in parallel with some resolution of the early cytotoxic water.

In conclusion, we have demonstrated in a rat model of global hemispheric ischemia that the SG change occurring during ischemia is proportional to the duration of ischemia provided the ischemic flow is kept constant. On reperfusion there is a marked further decrease in SG in the first 30 min of reperfusion. Further reperfusion up to 2–3 h is associated with resolution of ischemic brain edema after 15 min of ischemia, but not after 30 or 60 min of ischemia.

Summary

In a rat model of global forebrain ischemia we have measured the change in brain water (specific gravity method) that occurs during ischemia and reperfusion. We have shown that the volume of edema formed during ischemia is proportional to the duration of ischemia. On reperfusion there is a sharp increase in brain water after 15 and 30 min of ischemia. Resolution of brain edema occurs after 15 min of ischemia but not after 30 or 60 min of ischemia.

The formation and resolution of brain edema is dependent upon the duration of ischemia.

Acknowledgements. We wish to thank the following for their generous support: The British Council (Dr. P. Picozzi), The Medical Research Council (Mr. N. V. Todd), and Action Research for Crippling Diseases.

References

1. Auer L (1977) The role of cerebral perfusion pressure as origin of brain edema in acute arterial hypertension. Eur Neurol 15:153–156
2. Avery S, Crockard HA, Ross-Russell R (1984) Evolution and resolution of oedema following severe temporary cerebral ischaemia in the gerbil. J Neurol Neurosurg Psychiatry 47:604–610
3. Crockard A, Iannotti F, Hunstock AT, Smith RD, Harris RJ, Symon L (1980) Cerebral blood flow and edema following cortical occlusion in the gerbil. Stroke 2:494–498
4. Harris RJ, Symon J, Branston NM, Bayhan M (1981) Changes in extracellular cation activity in cerebral ischaemia. J Cereb Blood Flow Metab 1:203–209
5. Hossmann KA (1976) Development and resolution of ischemic brain swelling: In: Pappius HM, Feindel W (eds) Dynamics of brain edema. Springer, Berlin Heidelberg New York, pp 219–227
6. Hossmann KA (1977) Total ischemia of the brain. In: Zulch KJ, Kaufmann W, Hossmann KA, Hossmann V (eds) Brain and heart infarct. Springer, Berlin Heidelberg New York, pp 219–227
7. Hossmann KA, Matsucka Y (1982) Brain tissue osmolality following middle cerebral artery occlusion in cats. J Cereb Blood flow Metab 2:262–263
8. Hossmann KA, Sakahi S, Zimmerman V (1977) Cation activities in reversible ischemia of the cat brain. Stroke 8:77–81
9. Iannotti F, Hoff JT (1983) Ischemic brain edema with and without reperfusion: an experimental study in gerbils. Stroke 14:562–567
10. Ito U, Ohno K, Nakamura R, Suganuma F, Inaba Y (1979) Brain edema during ischemia and after restoration of blood flow. Measurement of water, sodium, potassium content and plasma protein permeability. Stroke 10:542–547
11. Ito U, Kito K, Okada K, Ohno K, Tomita H, Inaba Y (1984) Brain edema and E.E.G. during ischemia and after restoration of blood flow. In: Go KG, Baethmann A (eds) Recent progress in the study and therapy of brain edema. Plenum, New York, pp 429–440
12. Klatzo I, Schuier F, Orzi F, Wilmes F, Chui E, Suzuki R, Fujiwara K, Nitsch C, Laursen H, Fenton I, Goping G (1981) Interrelationships between cerebral blood flow (CBF) and brain edema (BE). In: Minderhond JM (ed) Cerebral blood flow: basic knowledge and clinical implications. Excerpta Medica, Amsterdam, pp 160–173

13. Kogure K, Busto R, Scheinberg P (1981) The role of hydrostatic pressure in ischemic brain edema. Ann Neurol 9:273–282
14. Nelson SR, Mantz ML, Maxwell JA (1971) Use of specific gravity in the measurement of cerebral edema. J Appl Physiol 30:268–271
15. Pulsinelli WA, Brierly JB (1979) A new model of bilateral hemispheric ischemia in the unanesthetized rat. Stroke 10:267–271
16. Schuier FJ, Hossmann KA (1980) Experimental brain infarcts in cats: II. Ischemic brain edema. Stroke 2:593–601
17. Symon L, Branston NM, Chikovani O (1979) Ischemic brain edema following middle cerebral artery occlusion in baboons: relationship between regional cerebral water content and blood flow at 1 to 2 hours. Stroke 10:184–191

Selective Inhibition of Protein Synthesis After Severe Forebrain Ischemia of Gerbil Brain

K. TAKAHASHI[1] and W. BODSCH

Key words: Cerebral protein synthesis, 5-min ischemia, gerbil brain

Introduction

The occurrence of selective vulnerability of distinct neuronal structures has been described in gerbil and rat brain [3, 4] following transient forebrain ischemia. Neither cerebral blood flow nor glucose utilization limits the metabolic requirements of central nervous system cells throughout the first day of recirculation after 5-min ischemia induced by bilateral occlusion of common carotid arteries in the gerbil [5]. Two separate openings of the blood-brain barrier (BBB) have been reported [6], one occurring immediately after reperfusion in the CA4 sector, and a second one after several days in the CA1 structure. However, we have recently observed different intrinsic biochemical properties of CA1 neurons in this model of ischemia with respect to cerebral protein synthesis [2]. Although RNA synthesis was unaffected, CA1 neurons suddenly failed to reactivate their protein synthesis machinery to maintain normal protein turnover. Furthermore, susceptibility to protein synthesis reductions in the hippocampus was absent in infant animals at the age of 15–17 days [7], while it started to appear at around 20–22 days of life.

The present investigation establishes the time course of protein synthesis changes between the first visible reduction in the pyramidal layer of CA1 neurons in the hippocampus and the appearance of irreversible neuronal death by morphological criteria.

Materials and Methods

Mongolian gerbils (50–70 g body weight) were loosely immobilized and anesthetized with a mixture of 30% oxygen, 70% nitrogen and 1%–2% halothane. Femoral veins and arteries were cannulated with polyethylene catheters. Common carotid arteries were exposed bilaterally through a midline cervical incision and clips were applied as the anesthesia was reduced to 0.5% halothane. After 5 min, circulation was restored by releasing the clips and halothane was increased to 1%. Recirculation periods were 1, 2, and 4 h and 4 days. For measurement of [^{14}C]protein synthesis 70 μCi [^{14}C]carboxyl amino acids (phenylalanine, tyrosine, isoleucine, leucine and

[1] Juntendo Izunagaoka Hospital, Izunagaoka, Tugata-yn, Shizuoka-ken, Japan

methionine) were administered at time zero as a bolus and a period of 45 min was allowed for incorporation. Systemic circulation was stopped by intraarterial injection of saturated potassium chloride solution, and the animals were then decapitated. Brains were quickly removed, frozen in methylbutane at −50° C for 3 min, and maintained at −20° C in a cryostat until sectioning. Coronal sections (20 and 200 μm thick) were cut at −20 °C, and 20-μm sections were dried at 45 °C. Five days later these sections were incubated for 12 h in a solution containing 10% TCA, 70% ethanol, and 2% polyvinylpropolidone to remove nonincorporated ^{14}C radioactivity from the tissue. Dried sections were placed into X-ray cassettes along with calibrated [^{14}C] methyl methacrylate standards.

Timed plasma samples obtained from the blood collected throughout the in vivo labeling were analyzed for amino acid content and counted by liquid scintillation. ^{14}C-Labeled free amino acids of brain tissue and aminoacyl tRNAs and proteins were measured biochemically in microsamples obtained from 200-μm sections [1].

Separate cryostat sections of the same brains were counterstained for histology by the Klüver-Barrera procedure with luxol fast blue and cresyl violet.

Results

^{14}C-Autoradiograms of amino acid incorporation into proteins and recirculation periods of 1, 2, 4, and 96 h are illustrated in Fig. 1. Compared with the control images no changes in protein synthesis had occurred by 1 h after ischemia. A slight reduction in CA1 neurons was visible at the level of the anterior but not of the posterior hippocampus. Most animals recirculated for 1 h show protein synthesis changes at neither hippocampal levels. Instead, severe decreases in amino acid incorporation were obvious in the anterior and posterior parts of hippocampal CA1 neurons at 2 h after ischemia. A small depression in the outer layer of the frontal cortex had also occurred at this stage, which, however, had diminished at this level at 4 h. Progression of the reduction in protein synthesis of CA1 neurons was observed in the entire CA1 subfield, leading to total absence of incorporated label at 4 h. Only after longer recirculation times did additional influences on other structures than CA1 become visible. At 4 days, pronounced changes had also occurred in

Table 1. Quantitative data relating to cerebral protein synthesis in vivo in the hippocampal CA 1 region of the gerbil brain

	Brain amino acids (nCi/nmol)	Aminoacyl tRNA (nCi/nmol)	Proteins (nCi/nmol)	Brain amino acids[a] (nmol/g)
Control ($n=6$)	5.82±0.72	1.27±0.16	20.13±1.24	586±46
1 h ($n=4$)	5.42±0.86	1.36±0.18	19.40±1.06	602±34
2 h ($n=4$)	6.02±0.25	1.42±0.21	1.78±0.23	612±38
4 h ($n=3$)	5.86±0.61	1.28±0.20	0.50±0.07	597±44
4 days ($n=3$)	2.51±0.36	0.82±0.10	0.12±0.02	4273±59

[a] Phenylalanine, tyrosine, isoleucine, leucine, and methionine combined

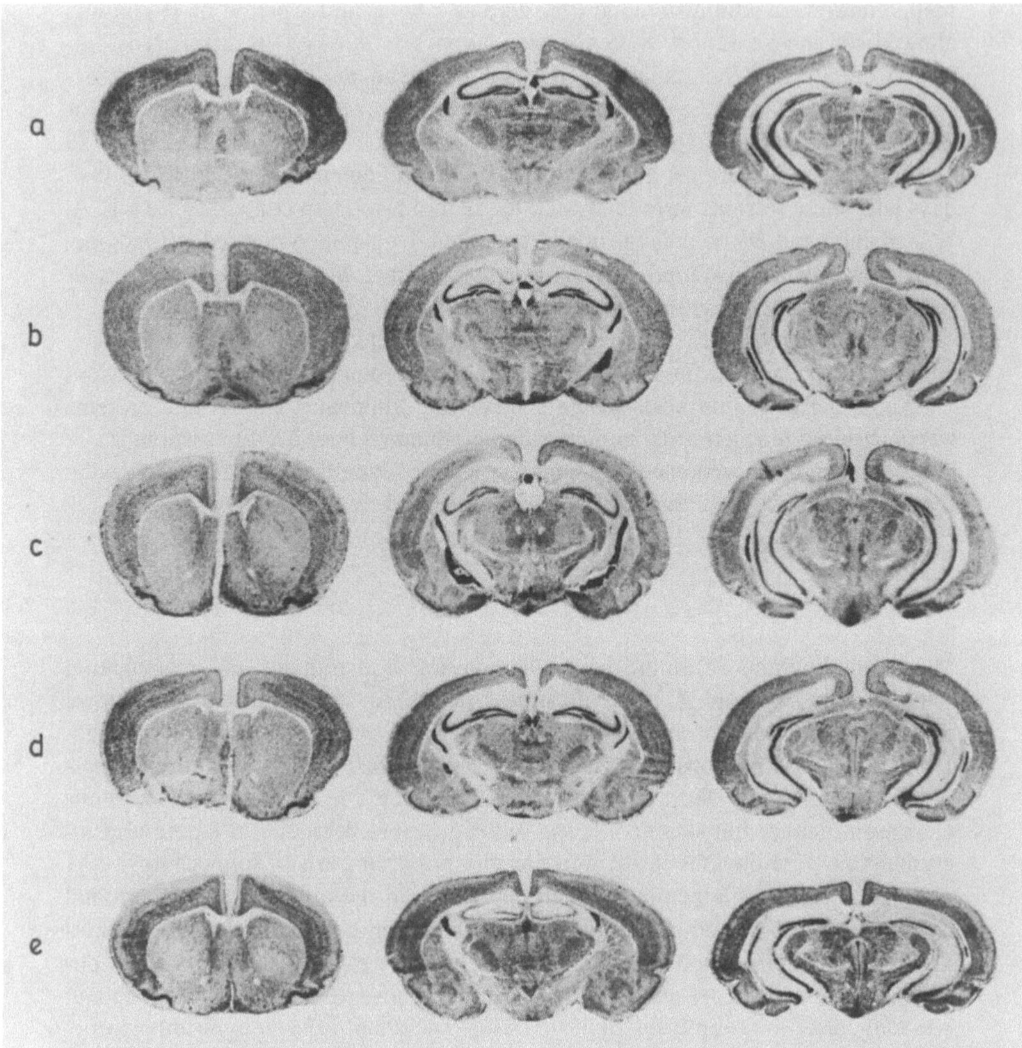

Fig. 1a–e. Cerebral protein synthesis in the gerbil brain of (**a**) control animal and (**b–e**) of animals subjected to 5-min bilateral occlusion of common carotid arteries and postischemic recirculation for 1 h (**b**), 2 h (**c**), 4 h (**d**), and 4 days (**e**). ^{14}C-Autoradiograms of amino acid incorporation are illustrated at the levels of the frontal cortex and the anterior and posterior hippocampus, respectively

the caudate nucleus, in the outer layers of the frontal and parietal cortex, and in CA3 and CA4 of the hippocampus. The last observations are illustrated in the enlarged autoradiograms (Fig. 2). Protein synthesis is totally absent in CA1 and CA4, though neuronal cell loss only affects the CA1 pyramidal cell layer. However, incorporation into CA3 is reduced in addition, more so in CA3b than in CA3a and CA3c. The dentate gyrus seems to be the hippocampal structure least influenced in the sense of protein synthesis reduction. No difference in the cellular density of the

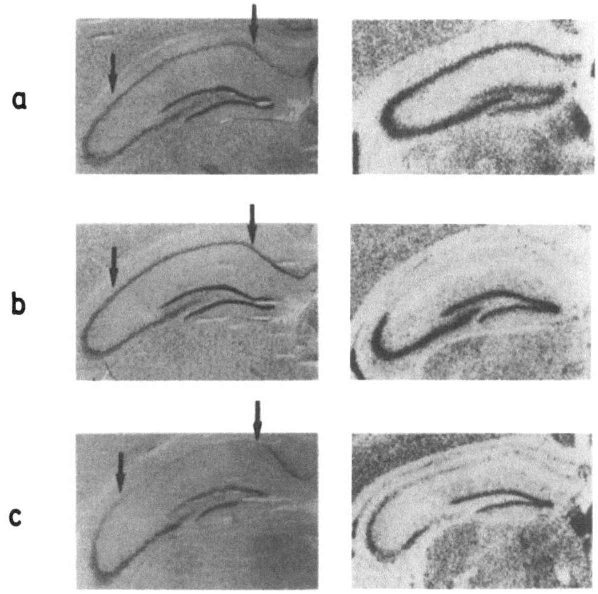

Fig. 2a–c. Hippocampal protein synthesis and histology in the gerbil brain (**a**) of control animal and (**b, c**) of animals subjected to 5-min forebrain ischemia and reperfusion for 4 h (**b**) and 4 days (**c**). ^{14}C-Autoradiograms of the hippocampus (*right*) have been enlarged for comparison with histological preparations (*left*) stained according to the Klüver-Barrera technique. *Arrows* indicate the extension of the CA1 pyramidal cell layer

CA1 pyramidal cell layer was detected at 4 h, while amino acid incorporation was absent throughout the CA1 layer.

Amino acid content and specific activities in the precursor pools and proteins of the CA1 structure (Table 1) indicate that significant precursor pool changes do not occur for up to 4 h after ischemia. A tremendous increase in the amino acid content at 4 days was not accompanied by a simultaneous decrease in specific activity in the precursor pool to the same extent. We therefore surmise that proteolysis increases the free amino acid level from protein breakdown, while BBB leakage increases the net influx of labeled amino acids.

Discussion

The present work on protein synthesis changes following brief transient forebrain ischemia in gerbils established the time course of events during reperfusion on the regional level. The most significant result is the early reduction in the activity of the protein machinery in CA1 neurons at a time when there is neither neuronal cell loss nor pronounced destruction of the cytoplasm of these neurons, as reported before [3]. Apart from reversible changes in the frontal cortex occurring at 2 h after ischemia, the overall depression of hippocampal CA1 persists until 4 days after ischemia, when pronounced neuronal death can be observed in this area. However, at this stage several other regions of the brain previously also reported to have been rendered selectively vulnerable after 30-min ischemia of the rat brain [4], i.e., cerebral cortex and caudate nucleus, stopped protein synthesis. If the observed BBB opening immediately after the start of recirculation [5] influenced the protein synthesis machinery, changes would have to be expected in the CA4 region of the hippocampus, which obviously was not the case in this study. Moreover, CA4 and CA1 protein synthesis were already depressed several days after recirculation, indicating that BBB openings in the hippocampus were not responsible for altered amino acid incorporations. The irreversibility of protein synthesis destruction in CA1 may indicate that in the absence of this fundamental cellular requirement neurons must die as a consequence of total failure to start cytoplasmic repair processes. However, not all the animals with the described reductions in amino acid incorporation of the hippocampus at 4 days also had total neuronal cell loss in the CA1 sector. Instead, protein synthesis destructions were observed in 100% of these animals subjected to ischemia followed by recirculation periods longer than 2 h.

For cytoplasmic repair processes to be initiated there may be a requirement for proteins that allow neurons to survive for a certain period of absence to synthesize new proteins. Since in normal conditions the half-life of proteins is synchronized in each cell according to a programmed biological clock, the synchrony of protein synthesis may be destroyed after ischemia. This interruption of the biological half-life cannot always be achieved at the same time in each animal subjected to ischemia. Therefore, although the protein synthesis machinery becomes affected in each case, the significance for survival or neuronal death may not always be the same for the same neuronal cell population. The outcome may be decided as a result of persistence in the level of those proteins with long half-lives. The fractional half-lives of protein in the brain vary from several minutes to several days. In most cases those with long half-lives are present at much lower concentrations, are unique to the brain, and may therefore play a key role in cellular survival.

Summary

Incorporation of radioactive amino acids into proteins in vivo was studied in the gerbil brain with reperfusions between 1 h and 4 days after bilateral common carotid artery ligation for 5 min. The degree of cerebral protein synthesis was determined by autoradiography and biochemical data that verify the autoradiographic comparison between animals with different recirculation periods.

No disturbances of amino acid incorporation were observed until 1 h after ischemia, indicating that the 5-min ischemia itself did not cause the onset of protein synthesis changes in the gerbil brain. However, sudden reductions in the activity of the synthesis machinery occurred between 1 and 2 h after ischemia in CA1 pyramidal cells of the dorsal hippocampus. Further destruction of protein synthesis became visible in CA3, cerebral cortex, and caudate nucleus by 4 days after the initiation of recirculation, while complete disappearance was observed in hippocampal CA1 and CA4 cells. Although neuronal cell loss in CA1 neurons was obvious at 4 days, the reduction of protein synthesis was already completed at 4 h with no accompanying cell loss in CA1 at this stage. Inhibition of protein synthesis, in consequence, occurs much earlier than the opening of the blood-brain barrier for macromolecules, indicating that the metabolic disturbance is not directly related to the development of postischemic edema.

References

1. Bodsch W, Hossmann KA (1983) A quantitative regional analysis of amino acids involved in rat brain protein synthesis by HPLC. J Neurochem 40:371–382
2. Bodsch W, Takahashi K (1984) Selective neuronal vulnerability to cerebral protein- and RNA-synthesis in the hippocampus of the gerbil brain. In: Bes A, Braquet P, Paoletti R, Siesjö BK (eds) Cerebral ischemia. Elsevier, New York, pp 197–208
3. Kirino T (1982) Delayed neuronal death in the gerbil hippocampus following ischemia. Brain Res 239:57–69
4. Pulsinelli WA, Brierley JB, Plum F (1982) Temporal profile of neuronal damage in a model of transient forebrain ischemia. Ann Neurol 11:491–498
5. Suzuki R, Yamaguchi T, Kirino T, Orzi F, Klatzo I (1983 a) The effects of 5-minute ischemia in mongolian gerbils: I. Blood-brain barrier, cerebral blood flow, and local cerebral glucose utilization changes. Acta Neuropathol 60:207–216
6. Suzuki R, Yamaguchi T, Li CL, Klatzo I (1983 b) The effect of 5-minute ischemia in mongolian gerbils: II. Changes of spontaneous neuronal activity in cerebral cortex and CA1 sector of hippocampus. Acta Neuropathol 60:217–222
7. Takahashi K, Bodsch W, Hossmann KA (1984) Susceptibility of hippocampal protein synthesis to transient forebrain ischemia of adult and infant gerbil brain. In: Lassen Na, Cahn J (eds) Drugs and diseases, vol 1. Libbey Eurotext, Paris, pp 72–78

Ischemic Brain Edema: Influence of Ischemia Duration on Edema Formation

K. ARITAKE [1] and M. BROCK

Key words: Brain edema, ischemia, blood-brain barrier, cerebral blood flow

Introduction

Brain edema secondary to focal ischemia is not uncommon in stroke, where death is often due to transtentorial herniation. However, the factors initiating development of brain edema associated with ischemic lesion or changes in vascular permeability are still not completely understood. Some authors have repeatedly confirmed a threshold for ischemic edema [2, 3, 5, 6, 12]. Most studies have been performed during permanent ischemia without subsequent reperfusion. Only models of temporary ischemia can really permit the identification of factors limiting recovery from ischemic insults or the evaluation of development and regression of focal ischemia. However, there have so far been few papers reporting on ischemic edema and/or alterations in blood flow examined in temporary focal ischemia [2, 6, 10, 13].

The present experiment was designed to assess the effects of various factors, such as the severity of ischemia and its duration, and reperfusion flow, on the occurrence of brain edema and changes in blood-brain barrier (BBB) function, using a stroke model of temporary ischemia.

Materials and Methods

Regional tissue water content and cerebral blood flow (CBF) were determined in the same areas following middle cerebral artery (MCA) occlusion in cats, which were mechanically ventilated with nitrous oxide/oxygen. Occlusion lasted for either 1 h (11 animals) or 2 h (20 animals), followed by recirculation (194 ± 21 min, 218 ± 42 min, respectively; means $\pm$ SD). The CBF was measured by the hydrogen clearance method, six different electrodes being implanted in cortical areas. One electrode was used as a control in the nonischemic hemisphere. Flow was measured 10 and 45 min after MCA occlusion in 1-h ischemia, and additionally at 105 min in 2-h ischemia. Blood flow values were measured 10 min after reopening of the occluded MCA (initial postocclusion flow values) and every 30 min thereafter. The regional water content of the cortical area surrounding the hydrogen electrode was de-

[1] Department of Neurosurgery, Universitätsklinikum Steglitz, Free University of Berlin, Hindenburgdamm 30, D-1000 Berlin 45

termined by the vacuum freeze-drying method. A solution of 2% Evans blue (EB) was administered IV within 30 or 60 min after reperfusion, as an indicator for BBB changes.

Results

Reperfusion following 1-h ischemia usually led to hyperperfusion in the formerly ischemic MCA territory, whereas that following 2-h ischemia led to a pronounced diversity of postischemic blood flow values, rapidly followed by subsequent hypoperfusion (Table 1). This evolution of hypoperfusion during the reperfusion period seemed to be related to the duration of MCA occlusion. On the other hand, blood flow was not altered at any period in the nonischemic hemispheres.

The mean water content in the nonischemic hemisphere was 78.91% ± 1.41% in 1-h ischemia and 78.74% ± 1.51% in 2-h ischemia (means ± SD). In neither group was the development of brain edema correlated with the different postischemic flow

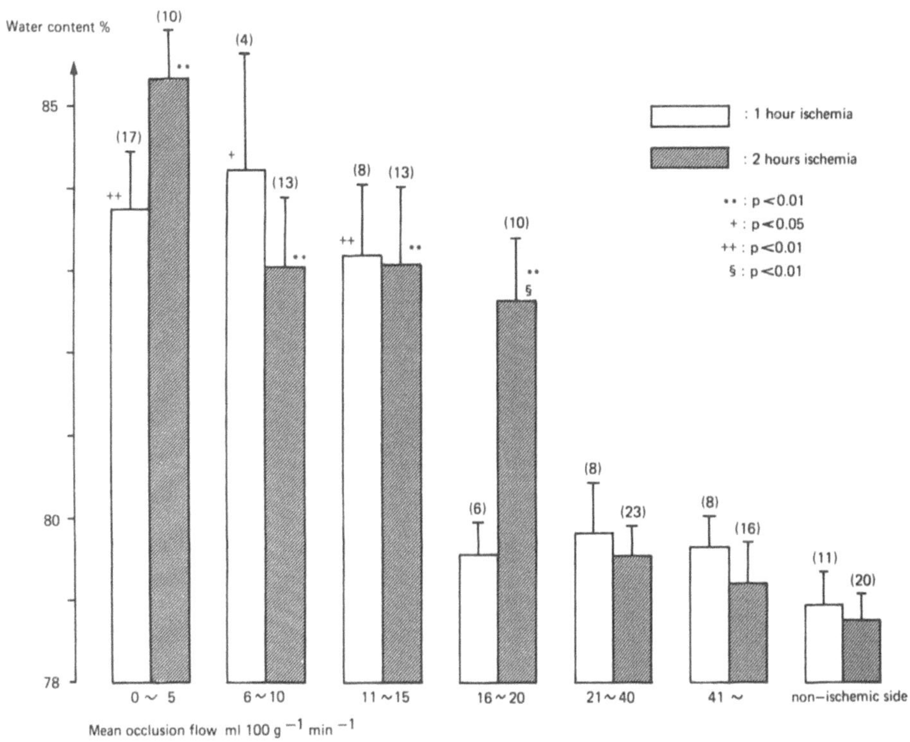

Fig. 1. Correlation between water content and occlusion flow. Cortical water content for the group with 1-h ischemia and the group with 2-h ischemia is related to the corresponding blood flow rate during the period of MCA occlusion. Mean water content (± SEM) was obtained for each 5 ml/100 g/min blood flow interval in both groups. ( ): number of cases considered. **, significantly different from mean water content on the nonischemic side in 1-h ischemia; +, + +, significantly different from mean water content on the nonischemic side in 2-h ischemia; §, significantly different from mean water content for each corresponding 5 ml/100 g/min blood flow interval in the group with 1 h ischemia

Table 1. Mean values (± SD) of blood flow before, during and after MCA occlusion, based on EB leakage (ml/100 g/min)

Duration of ischemia	Ischemic level[a]	Leakage of EB	Basal values	Occlusion values	Initial post-occlusion values	Maximum post-occlusion values	Final values
1 h	Critical	+ (11)	61±10	5± 4**	131±49**§	140±46**§	111±53*§
		− (18)	57±16	8± 4**	95±37**	105±36**§	74±39
	Noncritical	− (22)	61±14	36±16**	59±38	76±54	56±41
	Control	− (11)	67±18	66±20	67±18	77±25	59±21
2 h	Critical	+ (25)	67±27	10± 6**	79±35§§	115±66**§§	57±46§§
		− (21)	57±13	10± 5**	36±16**	44±17**	25±18**
	Noncritical	− (39)	61±18	38±13**	54±33	67±33	35±20**
	Control	− (20)	59±14	59±22	58±20	63±25	35±20**

[a] Critical, mean occlusion flow values of less than 15 ml/100 g/min in 1-h ischemia or 20 ml/100 g/min in 2-h ischemia. Noncritical, mean occlusion flow values of more than the critical flow values; control, nonischemic side. ( ): number of cases considered
* $P<0.05$; ** $P<0.01$ (significant differences from corresponding basal values); § $P<0.05$; §§ $P<0.01$ (significant differences from mean blood flow values during the corresponding periods in the critical group without EB leakage)

values; it correlated only with the residual flow rates during the MCA occlusion period. The cortical water content began to increase when occlusion flow values fell below 15 ml/100 g/min in 1-h ischemia or below 20 ml/100 g/min in 2-h ischemia (Fig. 1): the correlation thus appeared to be threshold dependent. Probably edema required lower ischemic flow rates in ischemia of shorter duration.

Extravasation of EB occurred at occlusion flow values of less than 12 ml/100 g/min in 1-h ischemia or less than 19 ml/100 g/min in 2-h ischemia. These critical thresholds for leakage of EB corresponded closely to those for edema formation. As described above, the duration of ischemia seemed to influence the hemodynamic pattern of postischemic flow. However, in both groups there were clear-cut differences between areas with and without EB leakage (Table 1). Mean postocclusion flow values in areas with EB leakage were significantly higher than those in areas without it. Moreover, the development of hyperperfusion following critical ischemia was concomitant with the disruption of the BBB as indicated by EB. Therefore, alterations in vascular permeability to EB were dependent on both the intensity of ischemia and the postischemic hemodynamics during the recirculation period.

Discussion

Our present study revealed that the duration of MCA occlusion played an important role not only in the temporal pattern of postischemic flow changes, but also in the critical threshold for the occurrence of ischemic edema [5, 6, 7, 11, 13]. The development of brain edema with temporary ischemia was correlated to the residual flow values during the period of ischemia, and its critical threshold was also time dependent. Cell survival and functional recovery are reported to be dependent on the severity of ischemia, that is, the combined influence of the severity of ischemia and its duration [4, 10]. Reported critical blood flow values for the evolution of such irreversibility seem to correspond closely to those of edema formation in our experiment [4]. It is, therefore, probable that critical blood flow values for progression of ischemic brain edema, defined as a function of the severity of ischemia and its duration, are similar to those for ischemic neuronal injuries.

On the other hand, it is likely that the breakdown of the BBB to EB is dependent on the intensity of ischemia and the subsequent postischemic perfusion. In other words, these data may indicate that ischemic damage of brain tissue and adequacy of reperfusion are both responsible for the appearance of the BBB dysfunction. Alterations in vascular permeability take place or are accelerated following restoration of blood supply to the ischemic brain [7, 8]. An opening of the BBB associated with a marked increase in regional perfusion after the reestablishment of blood flow to the critically ischemic regions may in some respects resemble the BBB disruption experimentally demonstrated in induced hypertension [8, 9]. Some compounds released from ischemically damaged brain tissue, or their metabolites produced in the reperfusion period, can be considered to contribute to the altered vascular permeability [1, 12, 14]. Moreover, the similarity of critical flow rates in the presence of edema formation, BBB dysfunction, functional irreversibility, and morphological changes suggests that ischemic neuronal injury and altered BBB function of the cerebral vessels are both necessary for edema formation.

Summary

Depth and duration of ischemia and the reperfusion flow were assessed as factors initiating either the development of ischemic brain edema or alterations in blood-brain barrier (BBB) function in a temporary focal ischemia model with two different durations. Cortical water content and regional cerebral blood flow (CBF) were determined in the same areas following middle cerebral artery (MCA) occlusion in a total of 31 cats. Occlusion lasted for either 1 or 2 h and was subsequently followed by reperfusion. CBF was determined by the hydrogen clearance method. Evans blue was employed to evaluate changes in the BBB function. Residual blood flow values during the ischemia period were correlated with edema formation in both groups. The critical thresholds for edema formation were 15 ml/100 g/min in 1-h ischemia and 20 ml/100 g/min in 2-h ischemia. The duration of MCA occlusion was related not only to the critical threshold for the development of brain edema but also to the temporal pattern of postischemic flow changes. The breakdown of the BBB was related to both critical occlusion flow (similar to that in edema formation) and post-occlusion blood flow. It seems likely that the development of ischemic edema is dependent on the combined influence of both the severity of ischemia and its duration (the intensity of ischemia). The similarity of the critical flow rates for edema formation to either those for altered BBB function or those for ischemic irreversibility may indicate that ischemic brain edema arises only when both ischemic tissue injuries and alterations in the BBB function are present.

References

1. Aritake K, Wakai S, Asano T, Takakura K (1983) Peroxidation of arachidonic acid and brain edema. Brain Nerve 35:965–973
2. Branston NM, Bell BA, Hunstock A, Symon L (1980) Time and flow as factors in the formation of postischemic edema in primate cortex. In: Cervós-Navarro J, Ferszt R (eds) Brain edema. Raven, New York, pp 291–298 (Advances in neurology, vol 28)
3. Crockard A, Iannotti F, Hunstock A, Smith RD, Harris RJ, Symon L (1980) Cerebral blood flow and edema following carotid occlusion in the gerbil. Stroke 11:494–498
4. Heiss WD, Rosner G (1983) Functional recovery of cortical neurons as related to degree and duration of ischemia. Ann Neurol 14:294–301
5. Hossmann KA, Schuier FJ (1980) Experimental brain infarcts in cats. I. Pathophysiological observation. Stroke 11:583–591
6. Iannotti F, Hoff J (1983) Ischemic brain edema with and without reperfusion: an experimental study in gerbils. Stroke 14:562–567
7. Ito U, Ohno K, Nakamura R, Suganuma F, Inaba Y (1979) Brain edema during ischemia and after restoration of blood flow. Stroke 10:542–547
8. Ito U, Ohno K, Yamaguchi T, Takei H, Tomita H, Inaba Y (1980) Effect of hypertension on blood-brain barrier changes after restoration of blood flow in post-ischemic gerbil brains. Stroke 11:606–611
9. Johansson BB (1976) Water content of rat brain in acute arterial hypertension. In: Pappius HM, Feindel W (eds) Dynamics of brain edema. Springer, Berlin Heidelberg New York, pp 28–31
10. Jones TH, Morawetz RB, Crowell RM, Carcoux FW, Fitzgibbon SJ, Degirolami U, Ojemann G (1981) Thresholds of focal cerebral ischemia in awake monkeys. J Neurosurg 54:773–782

11. O'Brien MD (1979) Ischemic cerebral edema. A review. Stroke 10:623–628
12. Symon L, Branston NM, Chikavani O (1979) Ischemic brain edema following middle cerebral artery occlusion in baboons: relationship between regional cerebral water content and blood flow at 1 and 2 hours. Stroke 10:184–191
13. Traupe H, Kruse E, Heiss WD (1982) Reperfusion of focal ischemia of varying duration: Postischemic hyper- and hypoperfusion. Stroke 13:615–622
14. Wakai S, Aritake K, Asano T, Takakura K (1982) Selective destruction of the outer leaflet of the capillary endothelial membrane after intercerebral injection of arachidonic acid. Acta Neuropathol 58:303–306

Changes in Specific Gravity of Discrete Brain Regions and Postischemic Morbidity Following Reversible and Irreversible Cerebral Ischemia in Mongolian Gerbil

A. Fujisawa [1], M. Matsumoto, T. Matsuyama, S. Yoneda, and K. Kimura

Key words: Cerebral ischemia, Mongolian gerbil, cerebral edema, postischemic morbidity, stroke index

Introduction

The occlusion of the bilateral common carotid arteries (CCA) in Mongolian gerbil causes severe telencephalic ischemia [4, 5], and the temporary occlusion of bilateral CCA has been used as a good model for reversible and/or irreversible global cerebral ischemia [2]. There have been no studies on the changes in water content of brain in association with the duration of ischemic period or on the relationship between the changes and neurologic deficits following transient global cerebral ischemia in this animal. In the present study we evaluated the changes in water content of four brain regions and the neurologic deficits in the same animals, and investigated the relationship between these two variables.

Materials and Methods

A total of 96 adult gerbils were used in this study, 10 of which were used as sham-operated controls while 86 were divided into three groups (10-, 15-, 20-min ischemia groups) according to the duration of bilateral CCA occlusion because, as reported by Jarrott and Domer [2], our preliminary study showed that under light ketamine anesthesia no gerbils died when the ischemic period was less than 10 min, while all gerbils died within 24 h after reperfusion when it was longer than 20 min. The animals were anesthetized with ketamine hydrochloride and both CCAs were exposed and then occluded with clips in each. The animals in the nonreperfusion group were sacrificed 10, 15, and 20 min after bilateral CCA occlusion. The other animals were returned to their cages for recovery and observation after removal of the clips. The neurologic status was evaluated for stroke index [6] every 1 h up to just before sacrifice at 1, 3, or 6 h of reperfusion by a rater who was blind as to the duration of cerebral ischemia. The cerebral water content was measured by the specific gravity (SG) method essentially described by Marmarou et al. [1, 3, 5]. Animals were sacrificed by decapitation, and the brain was rapidly removed and placed in a water-treated

[1] The First Department of Internal Medicine, Osaka University, 1-1-50 Fukushima, Fukushima-ku, Osaka 553, Japan

kerosene [1] filled petri dish. Four pieces 1 mm³ in size were cut from each region (cerebral cortex, basal ganglia, hippocampus, cerebellum). Care was taken to obtain tissue samples from the same regions in each animal.

Results

The changes in the SG of each region during or after telencephalic ischemia are presented in Fig. 1. No significant changes were seen in the SG of cerebellum. On the other hand, the SG of the other regions (telencephalic regions) in each group of animals showed a significant decrease at 1–3 h of reperfusion. Significant differences in the SG among the three ischemia groups were observed only at 3 h of reperfusion. Figure 2 shows the changes in the stroke index. All animals showed neurologic improvement at least up to 2 h after clip removal, but all animals in the 20-min ischemia group and two of the six gerbils in the 15-min ischemia group relapsed into the

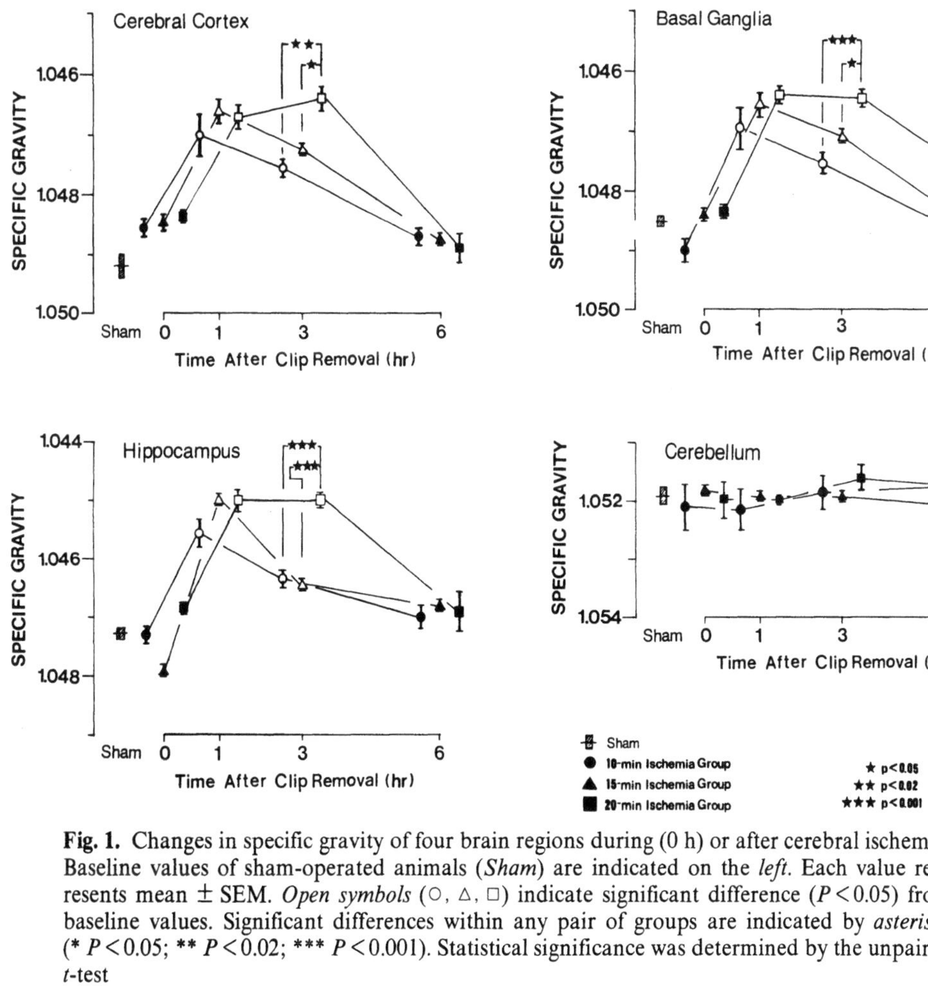

Fig. 1. Changes in specific gravity of four brain regions during (0 h) or after cerebral ischemia. Baseline values of sham-operated animals (*Sham*) are indicated on the *left*. Each value represents mean ± SEM. *Open symbols* (○, △, □) indicate significant difference ($P<0.05$) from baseline values. Significant differences within any pair of groups are indicated by *asterisks* (* $P<0.05$; ** $P<0.02$; *** $P<0.001$). Statistical significance was determined by the unpaired *t*-test

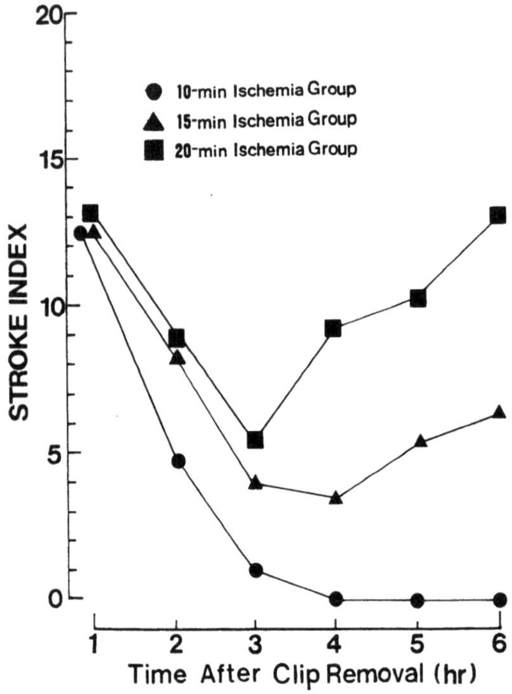

Fig. 2. Sequential changes in stroke index score of animals sacrificed 6 h after clip removal. Each *point* represents the average for a group of six animals

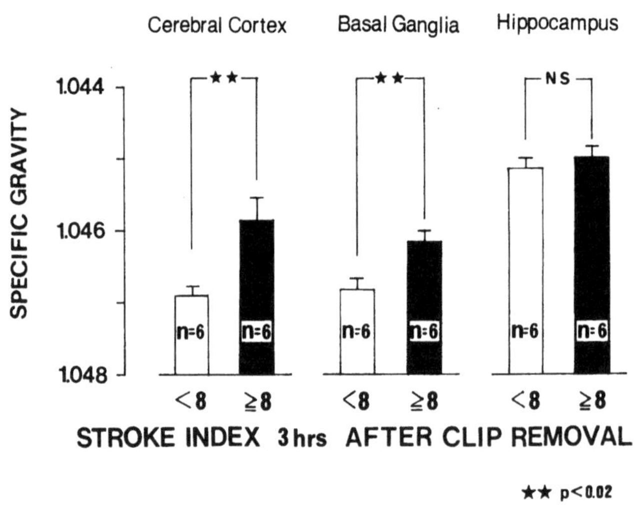

Fig. 3. Difference in specific gravity after 3 h of reperfusion of the telencephalic regions in the 20-min ischemia group, between animals in relapse (*black column*) and not in relapse (*white column*). In our preliminary study, animals which relapsed and had a stroke index in excess of 8 died within 24 h after clip removal. Statistical significance was determined by the unpaired *t*-test

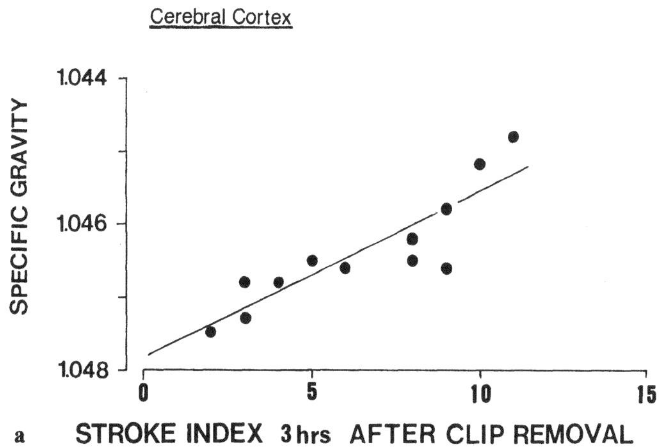

a

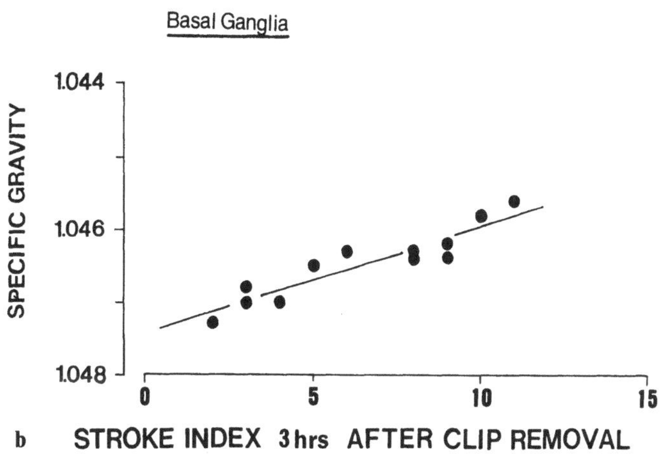

b

Fig. 4. a, b. Correlation between specific gravity of cerebral cortex (**a**) or basal ganglia (**b**) and stroke index in 20-min ischemia animals at 3 h after clip removal. Significant negative correlations were obtained in the cerebral cortex ($r = -0.878$, $P < 0.001$) and basal ganglia ($r = -0.928$, $P < 0.001$) between the specific gravity and the stroke index. The correlation coefficient was calculated by a conventional method and the regression line by the method of least squares

deteriorated state (elapsing phenomenon). In these animals, signs of severe cerebral damage began to appear after 3–5 h of reperfusion. In the 20-min ischemia group, the differences between the animals in relapse and the others in the SG of telencephalic regions were investigated after 3 h of reperfusion. As shown in Fig. 3, there was a significant difference in the SG in the cerebral cortex and the basal ganglia between the two groups. We also investigated the relationship between the SG in the 20-min ischemia group and the stroke index at 3 h after clip removal. A significant negative correlation was noted between the two (Fig. 4a, b).

Discussion

These results clearly show that the accumulation of cerebral edema following severe ischemia are closely associated with ischemic injury of the brain, and in the present study this association was noted at 3 h into the reperfusion period (Fig. 1). Since the elapsing phenomenon usually occurred 3–5 h after clip removal (Fig. 2) and the maximum accumulation of cerebral edema was observed after 1–3 h of reperfusion (Fig. 1), it is speculated that relapse is related to the accumulation of cerebral edema. The significant differences between the SG of cerebral cortex or basal ganglia in the animals in relapse and the others (Fig. 3) may support this view. With respect to the interrelationship between postischemic morbidity and the SG after 3 h of reperfusion, significant negative correlations were found between the stroke index and the SG of cerebral cortex or basal ganglia (Fig. 4). On the basis of these results, an interrelationship is postulated between the SG of these regions after 3 h of reperfusion and the degree of ischemic insult to the brain, and it is considered that the stroke index [6] is a useful indicator for observation of these ischemic insults.

The results of the present study indicate that the accumulation of cerebral edema is associated with the duration of cerebral ischemia and postischemic morbidity and that cerebral edema may play an important role in the pathophysiology of cerebral ischemia itself.

Summary

The changes in specific gravity (SG) of four brain regions (cerebral cortex, basal ganglia, hippocampus, cerebellum), during or at 1, 3, 6 h after bilateral cerebral ischemia for 10, 15, or 20 min, were evaluated in gerbils. Neurologic deficits were also recorded as a stroke index every 1 h up to just before the measurement of SG to investigate the relationship between the SG of brain and postischemic morbidity. Changes in SG of the cerebellum were very small, but in the other regions (telencephalic regions) the SG showed a significant decrease at 1–3 h after clip removal. At 3 h into the reperfusion period the SG values for telencephalic regions were significantly lower in the 20-min group than in the other groups. All animals in the 20-min group relapsed into the deteriorated state within 3–5 h of reperfusion. After 3 h of reperfusion, in cerebral cortex and basal ganglia significant differences in SG were detected between the relapsed animals and the others. Furthermore, significant negative correlations were also obtained between the SG of these regions and the stroke index. Changes in the SG of brain may represent the development of ischemic insults to the brain.

References

1. Fujiwara K, Nitsch C, Suzuki R, Klatzo I (1981) Factors in the reproducibility of the gravimetric method for evaluation of edematous changes in the brain. Neurol Res 3:345–361
2. Jarrott DM, Domer FR (1980) A gerbil model of cerebral ischemia suitable for drug evaluation. Stroke 11:203–209

3. Marmarou A, Poll W, Shulman K, Bhagavan H (1978) A simple gravimetric technique for measurement of cerebral edema. J Neurosurg 49:530–537
4. Matsumoto M, Kimura K, Fujisawa A, Matsuyama T, Fukunaga R, Yoneda S, Wada H, Abe H (1984) Differential effect of cerebral ischemia on monoamine content of discrete brain regions of the Mongolian gerbil (*Meriones unguiculatus*). J Neurochem 42:647–651
5. Matsuyama T, Matsumoto M, Fujisawa A, Handa N, Tanaka K, Yoneda S, Kimura K, Abe H (1983) Why are infant gerbils more resistant than adults to cerebral infarction after carotid ligation? J Cereb Blood Flow Metab 3:381–385
6. McGraw CP (1977) Experimental cerebral infarction effects of pentobarbital in Mongolian gerbils. Arch Neurol 34:334–336
7. Nelson SR, Mantz ML, Maxwell JA (1971) Use of specific gravity in the measurement of cerebral edema. J Appl Physiol 30:268–271

Relationship of Ischemic Brain Edema to Electrical Impedance and Intracranial Pressure Changes

H. G. WAGNER [1], P. TING, K. KITO, and T. YAMAGUCHI

Key words: Ischemic brain edema, cerebral electrical impedance, cerebral extracellular space, intracranial pressure, regional cerebral blood flow

Introduction

Brain edema has been defined as an abnormal accumulation of a fluid within the brain parenchyma, producing a volumetric enlargement of the tissue [1]. This enlargement may cause compression of the brain and the vasculature. Compression could restrict the regional cerebral blood flow (rCBF) to ischemic levels, which if protracted would lead to lasting damage to the brain. The CEI is sensitive to the presence of ischemia and may be a useful indicator of the pathophysiology of ischemia. Since the CEI is considered to be a measure of the extracellular space [2], it was of interest to consider whether direct compression of the brain parenchyma by surrounding edematous brain would directly reduce extracellular space as determined by measurement of cerebral electrical impedance (CEI). We studied the effects of artificially induced intracranial brain compression by balloon inflation and compared this with the effects of focal and global cerebral ischemia produced by restricting CBF.

Methods and Materials

Adult cats weighing 2.5–3.5 kg (either sex) were anesthetized with ketamine HCl (30 mg/kg, IM) for intubation, catheterization of femoral artery and vein, craniotomy, and other surgical procedures. The cats were artificially ventilated and maintained with alpha chloralose (60 mg/kg IV).

CEI was measured by means of a coplanar four-pole platinum-iridium alloy microelectrode array [3] inserted stereotaxically into the region of the caudate nucleus which is supplied by the middle cerebral artery (MCA). Constant-current (1 μA) square pulses of 1 ms duration were passed through the outer electrode pair of the array, while a voltage drop across the inner pair of electrodes was sensed, amplified, and displayed oscillographically. Using the hydrogen clearance method, rCBF was measured by means of a fifth platinum-iridium alloy microelectrode close

[1] Laboratory of Neuropathology, NINCDS, National Institutes of Health, Bldg. 36, Rm 4 DO4, Bethesda, MD 20205, USA

to the array in the caudate nucleus. ICP was measured by means of a miniature strain gauge transducer (Gaeltec ICT/b) placed into a parietal epidural space ipsilateral to the electrode array. Arterial pressure and rectal temperature were monitored continuously and arterial blood sampled intermittently to determine pH, pO_2, pCO_2, and base excess. Every craniotomy, including incision of the orbit opened to reach the MCA [4], was sealed with silicone rubber cement to prevent CSF leakage.

Results

The effect of occluding the left MCA on the CEI of the caudate nucleus can be seen in Fig. 1.

Within 1–2 min MCA occlusion a rapid rise in impedance was observed, which reached over 140% of the control baseline value within 10 min. Subsequently, the rise was more gradual but the impedance continued to rise, reaching 185% at the end of 1 h. Upon release of the occlusion the CEI dropped immediately and precipitously, reaching the baseline in an asymptotic fashion within about 30 min of recirculation. Although manifest at different times following the release of the MCAO, a second rise in CEI was recognized in five of seven cats (see Table 1) which were monitored for periods of up to 15 h. The values during the recirculation period were measured at the time point when the CEI showed its lowest value after recirculation before the secondary rise.

The values for the secondary rise in CEI were measured at the time when the CEI reached the peak of the secondary rise. The secondary rise was more gradual and

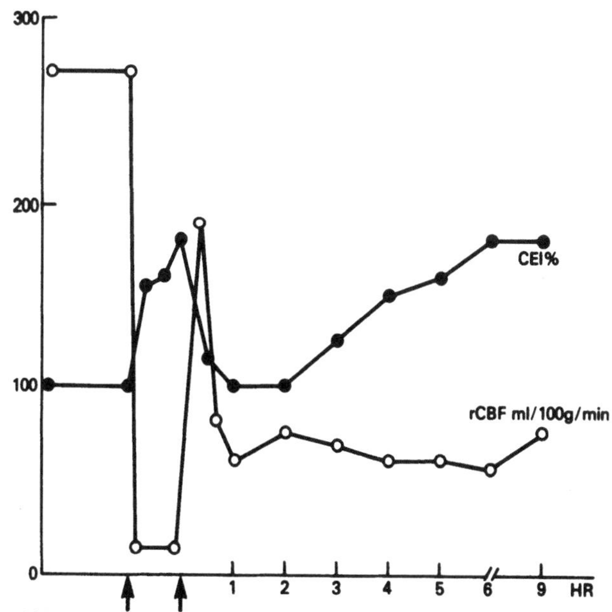

Fig. 1. Change in CEI and rCBF of the left caudate nucleus of a cat subjected to 1-h MCAO. The CEI was measured as a percentage of initial preischemic values. Note the second rise of CEI about 2 h after release of the MCAO

variable in time than the primary rise during the ischemia. When the occlusion was released at the end of 1 h, the rCBF became hyperemic momentarily but then settled down to a relatively stable value. The first rise in CEI seemed to require that the drop in rCBF reach levels of less than about 12 ml/100 g/min. The secondary rise in impedance was not necessarily accompanied by a fall in rCBF, particularly to the values that were present in the initial reduction in rCBF associated with a rise in CEI. The rCBF still had a value of 53 ± 5 ml/100 g/min at the peak of the secondary rise. This suggested that some other factor than ischemia was responsible for the secondary rise in CEI.

We then monitored the ICP simultaneously with CEI to ascertain whether the ICP was related to the secondary rise in CEI (see Fig. 2). We found that the ICP did not rise during the MCAO period, but did rise significantly at approximately the

Table 1. Comparison of CEI and rCBF values for the phase identified in a series of five cats subjected to 1-h MCAO, in which a secondary rise in CEI was seen

	Baseline	Ischemia	Recirculation	Secondary rise in CEI
CEI ± SEM (%)	100.0	220.0 ± 20.8	111.1 ± 12.1	176.4 ± 11.9
4CBF ± SEM (ml/100 g/min)	75.8 ± 39.3	8.4 ± 1.4	65.2 ± 8.7	52.8 ± 5.2

Standard errors of the mean are shown for each mean value except for the baseline CEI. See text for further detail

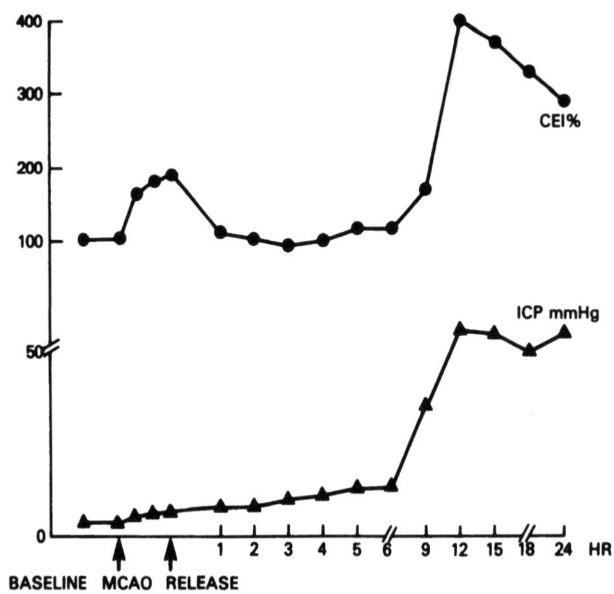

Fig. 2. Rise of ICP coincident with secondary rise of CEI in a cat subjected to 1-h MCAO. Note that no significant rise in ICP was observed related to the MCAO phase, but a definite rise at the time of the second rise in CEI

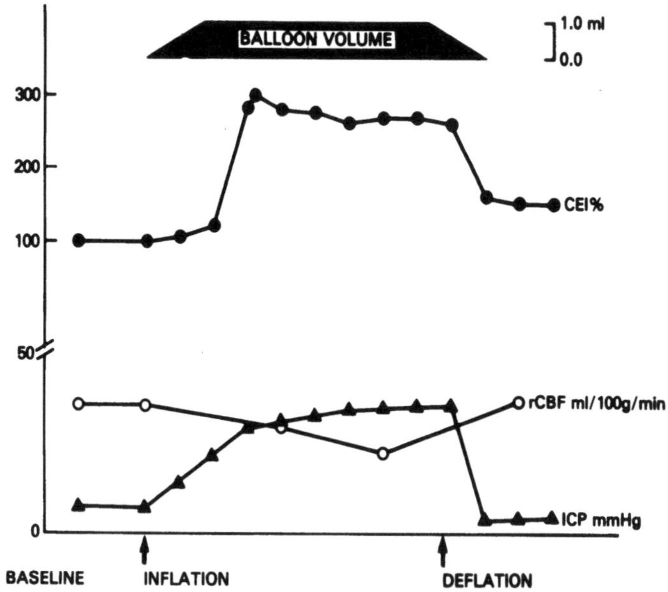

Fig. 3. The effect of inflating an epidurally placed balloon upon CEI, rCBF, and ICP. The placement of the balloon was in a location that would compress the left caudate nucleus where CEI and rCBF were measured. The ICP device was placed on the contralateral side in these experiments so that the ICP values reflected the ICP less reliably in the caudate nucleus

time of secondary rise in the CEI. Discrepancies in exact correspondence were not unexpected and were assumed to be due to the extradural location of the ICP device.

The effect of compression of the caudate nucleus on the CEI was studied in an experimental model with ipsilateral epidural placement of a balloon which could be inflated under controlled conditions (see Fig. 3). In this model, it was necessary that the ICP device be placed on the controlateral side of the brain opposite the electrode array. The balloon was inflated at a rate of 0.05 ml/min. The rise in ICP corresponded well with the increase in balloon volume, but the rise in CEI lagged behind the rise in ICP until the balloon volume reached about 1 ml, when it rapidly increased to almost 300% of the baseline value. The rCBF was reduced slightly in this instance, but remained well above the threshold of ischemia associated with a rise in CEI.

The relationship between the rise in CEI and the volume of the balloon was explored further in a series of nine cats (see Fig. 4). It will be noted that up to about 0.9 ml there was only a slight rise in CEI, but above that value the CEI for each cat began rising rapidly. We have interpreted this finding as an indication that within the fixed volume of the cranial space the expanding balloon initially displaces cerebrospinal fluid. Once this reserve is substantially displaced further expansion of the balloon causes compression of the brain extracellular space and of the volume that the vascular system occupies.

For further examination of the possibility that an elevated ICP can also be the cause of a rise in the CEI by way of direct compression of the extracellular space of

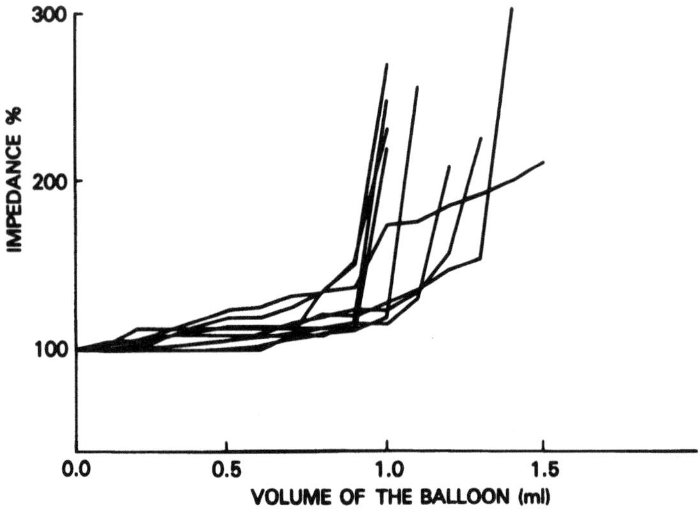

Fig. 4. The relationship between the volume of the balloon and the CEI in a series of cats. Each *solid line* plotted represents a separate and different experiment. The CEI was measured in the caudate nucleus ipsilateral to the balloon

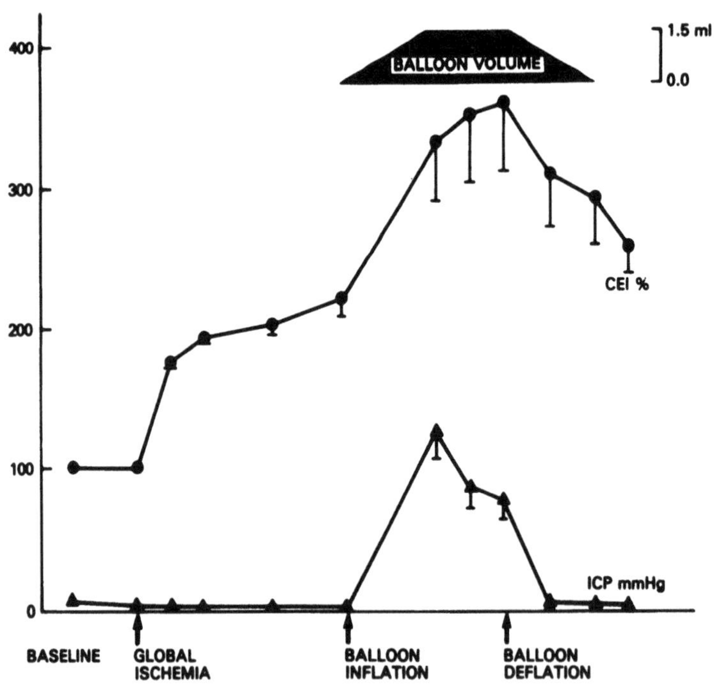

Fig. 5. The relationship observed between balloon volume, CEI, and ICP 30 min after exsanguination of the cat sufficient to lower the rCBF to no measurable H_2 clearance

the brain parenchyma, we ran another set of experiments (see Fig. 5). In these, the epidural balloon was inflated 30 min after global ischemia had been instituted by rapid exsanguination sufficient to drop the rCBF to zero, where it remained throughout the experiment. After the anticipated rise in CEI due to the global ischemia, balloon inflation caused the CEI to rise still further, reaching almost 400% of the control value. It will be noted that the CEI rose concordantly with the ICP, but fell rapidly when the balloon volume was stabilized. The fall-off of the CEI with the reduction in balloon volume was further evidence that the CEI rise was the direct result of compression and not due to ischemia per se.

Conclusions

Cerebral edema of sufficient severity to increase the brain volume beyond the capacity of the intracranial space to accept it can compress the extracellular space. This would result in a rise in the cerebral electrical impedance, resembling in many ways the rise in CEI associated with ischemia produced by a severe restriction of CBF to the same tissue. These two mechanisms for producing reduced extracellular space may coexist and be indistinguishable unless the cause can be determined. Indeed, they may reinforce each other, causing more severe tissue damage. Relief would depend upon recognition of the causes of each and the implementation of appropriate measures to correct these causes.

Summary

This study was undertaken to evaluate the effects of focal ischemic brain edema upon cerebral extracellular space in cats subjected to 1 h of middle cerebral artery occlusion (MCAO). The extracellular space was determined by the measurement of cerebral electrical impedance (CEI), whereas regional cerebral blood flow (rCBF) was recorded simultaneously by the hydrogen clearance method.

During MCAO, the CEI rose to 220% ± 21% of the preischemic baseline value while rCBF dropped to 8 ± 1.5 ml/100 g/min from 76 ± 39 ml/100 g/min (baseline value). Immediately after release of MCAO, the CEI decreased almost to the baseline value, but only in five of seven cases. There followed a second rise to 176% ± 12% at different times, but usually not beyond 15 h after recirculation. At the peak of this secondary rise, the rCBF was well above the ischemic level (53 ± 5 ml/100 g/min).

These findings suggested to us that there was another factor that could reduce extracellular space in addition to ischemia. We explored this possibility by means of a model with epidural balloon inflation and simultaneous recording of intracranial pressure (ICP), CEI, and rCBF. This model indicated that this other factor was probably direct mechanical compression of the brain extracellular space by postischemic edema.

References

1. Klatzo I (1967) Neuropathological aspects of brain edema. J Neuropathol Exp Neurol 26:1–14
2. Van Harreveld A, Ochs S (1956) Cerebral impedance changes after circulatory arrest. Am J Physiol 187:180–192
3. Li C, Bak AF, Parker LO (1968) Specific resistivity of the cerebral cortex and white matter. Exp Neurol 20:544–557
4. O'Brien MD, Waltz AG (1973) Transorbital approach for occluding the middle cerebral artery without craniectomy. Stroke 4:201–206

Effect of Lowering Blood Pressure on Two Different Types of Experimental Ischemic Brain Edema

Y. KATAYAMA[1], A. TERASHI, A. NAGAZUMI, S. SUGIMOTO, M. MIZOGUCHI, K. INAMURA, T. SOEDA, J. SHIMIZU, S. SUZUKI, H. MINAMISAWA, and H. MEMEZAWA

Key words: Lowering blood pressure, ischemia, brain edema, brain metabolites

Introduction

It is a difficult clinical problem whether to treat hypertension during the acute phase of cerebral ischemic diseases.

Cerebral ischemia was produced in two different ways and the effects of lowering blood pressure on cerebral metabolism and the production of cerebral edema were investigated.

Materials and Methods

Stroke-resistant spontaneously hypertensive (SHRSR) male rats aged 16 weeks and with blood pressure of 170–240 mmHg were used. The ischemic models used were (a) the infarction model, induced by bilateral carotid artery ligation (BLCL), and (b) the thromboembolic model, induced by retrograde infusion of arachidonic acid (AA) into the left internal carotid through the external carotid artery. Blood pressure was lowered to 120–160 mmHg after the induction of ischemia, by IP administration of reserpine. Blood pressure was monitored through the femoral artery. Cerebral blood flow (CBF) was measured by the hydrogen clearance method. Cerebral energy metabolites (ATP, lactate, cAMP) were measured 3 h after the induction of cerebral ischemia. The cerebral edema was expressed as the water content, which was measured by the freeze-dry method.

Results

Cerebral Infarction Model

In the BLCL model the ischemic damage was most prominent in the frontal region, where the main supplying arteries are the internal carotids. The occipital region supplied by the vertebral arteries sustained moderate ischemic damage. Lowering of blood pressure after the induction of ischemia resulted in a deterioration in cerebral

[1] Second Department of Internal Medicine, Nippon Medical School, 3-5-5 Iidabashi, Chiyoda-ku, Tokyo 102, Japan

blood flow, metabolism, and edema in both the frontal and the occipital region, but the effect was more prominent in the occipital region. The lowered blood pressure at 3 h after BLCL was in linear relation to the augmentation of cerebral water content, decrease in ATP, and increase in lactate level in the occipital region. As the blood pressure decrease became more pronounced the increase in water content and accumulation of lactate rose and the decrease in ATP also progressed (Table 1).

In the AA-infused model, ischemic damage and infarction were noted in the ipsilateral frontal and lateral portion of the brain and the extravasation of Evans blue was observed in the same region.

Table 1. Effect of lowered blood pressure on brain metabolites and water content in SHRSR after BLCL

		Frontal	Occipital
ATP	Treated	0.21±0.14 (12)	0.38±0.17 (12)*
	Untreated	0.25±0.07 (8)	0.61±0.19 (8)*
Lactate	Treated	36.76±3.83 (12)	31.61±4.01 (12)*
	Untreated	36.59±3.23 (8)	27.17±2.78 (8)*
cAMP	Treated	0.95±0.57 (12)	1.02±0.46 (12)
	Untreated	1.19±0.45 (8)	1.27±0.39 (8)
Water content	Treated	79.02±0.61 (10)**	78.29±0.64 (10)**
	Untreated	78.42±0.48 (12)**	77.77±0.46 (12)**

ATP and lacate expressed in nmol/mg wet wt. tissue, cAMP as pmol/mg wet wt. tissue, and water content as percentage
( ): Number of hemispheres
Statistical differences: * $P<0.02$; ** $P<0.05$

Table 2. Effect of lowered blood pressure on brain metabolites and water content in SHRSR after arachidonic acid infusion

		Infused hemisphere		Contralateral hemisphere	
		Frontal	Occipital	Frontal	Occipital
ATP	Treated (5)	0.62±0.13	1.24±0.40	0.96±0.43	1.53±0.56
	Untreated (5)	0.71±0.10	1.04±0.23	1.05±0.43	1.65±0.88
Lactate	Treated (5)	12.11±5.69*	7.06±3.33	3.11±1.50	1.65±0.49
	Untreated (6)	5.24±2.84*	3.92±2.88	3.48±1.74	2.01±0.57
cAMP	Treated (5)	0.48±0.19	0.52±0.11	0.48±0.13	0.56±0.13
	Untreated (6)	0.58±0.22	0.55±0.19	0.45±0.21	0.54±0.19
Water content	Treated (5)	80.36±1.15*		78.72±0.53	
	Untreated (10)	79.22±0.54*		78.52±0.27	

Statistical difference: * $P<0.05$
( ): Number of animals

Lowering of blood pressure resulted in an increase in the water content of the infused hemisphere, which showed a negative correlation with the lowered blood pressure at 3 h after AA infusion. The ATP levels showed no difference between the untreated and the lowered-pressure group in either hemisphere. The lactate level was increased in the AA-infused hemisphere, and this increase showed a negative correlation with the lowering of blood pressure.

Reduction of blood pressure aggravated brain edema and metabolism in the AA-infused hemisphere, but had no effect on the contralateral hemisphere (Table 2).

Discussion

The effect of lowering blood pressure was investigated in two ischemic models in SHRSR.

The BLCL model can be considered as a global form of ischemia, with near-complete ischemia in the frontal region and incomplete ischemia in the occipital region [1]. A severe infarction was produced in the frontal region, which was supplied by the occluded carotid arteries. The occipital region supplied mainly by the vertebral arteries sustained moderate ischemic damage.

Lowering of blood pressure resulted in a further decrease in cerebral blood flow in the occipital region, and aggravated edema and metabolism. This may be because the residual blood flow which was somewhat near the threshold level for ischemic damage [2, 3], is reduced below the threshold level in the occipital region, thereby extending the metabolically impaired area.

The AA infusion model can be considered as a thromboembolic model induced by plateled aggregation and endothelial damage. This model demonstrated infarction in the frontal and lateral portions of the infused hemisphere and there was Evans blue extravasation in the same area, indicating that this edema may be vasogenic in nature, in contrast to the BLCL model. Severe edema was observed in the infused hemisphere.

Lowering the blood pressure in this model aggravated the cerebral metabolism and edema in the infused hemisphere, but there was no effect on the contralateral hemisphere.

These results indicate that in the acute phase of cerebral ischemia the cerebral circulation may be in the so-called dysautoregulative [4] state and the lowering of blood pressure can aggravate ischemic damage by way of a further reduction in residual flow.

Therefore, hypertension in acute cardiovascular disease must be carefully managed.

Summary

Cerebral ischemia was induced by two different methods, and the effects of lowering the blood pressure were investigated. Male stroke-resistant, spontaneously hypertensive rats (SHRSR) aged 16 weeks and with blood pressure of 170–240 mmHg were used throughout. For the first model, cerebral infarction was induced by bilateral carotid artery ligation (BLCL). For the second, thromboembolism was induced by infusion of arachidonic acid (AA) into the internal carotid artery. Blood pressure was lowered to about 120–160 mmHg by IP injection of reserpine. Brain energy metabolites (ATP, lactate, cAMP), CBF, and brain water content were investigated 3 h after ischemia in both models.

Brain edema, CBF, and metabolites were aggravated by reduction in blood pressure in both these models.

References

1. Katayama Y, Terashi A, Sugimoto S, et al. (1984) Experimental cerebral ischemia after bilateral common carotid artery ligation in SHRSP, SHRSR and Wistar rats. Brain Nerve 36:1069–1075
2. Astrup J, Symon L, Branston NM, et al. (1977) Cortical evoked potential and extracellular K^+ and H^+ at critical levels of brain ischemia. Stroke 8:51–57
3. Hossmann KA, Schuier FJ (1980) Experimental brain infarcts in cats: pathophysiological observations. Stroke 11:583–592
4. Symon L, Branston NM, Strong AJ (1976) Autoregulation in acute focal ischemia. Stroke 7:547–554

Quantification of Blood-Brain-Barrier Permeability Following Varying Periods of Severe Temporary Cerebral Ischemia *

P. PICOZZI[1], N. V. TODD, H. A. CROCKARD, and R. R. RUSSELL

Introduction

Ischemic brain edema follows a complex pattern: water begins to accumulate early after an ischemic insult without major disruption of the blood-brain barrier (BBB), but with time a vasogenic component is added [4, 7]. Alteration in BBB permeability is known to be faster after restoration of blood flow than in permanent ischemia [4]. This causes an extravasation of plasma protein into the tissue and a further accumulation of water in the brain. The damage to the cerebral vessels following recirculation, as reflected by the BBB disruption, is related to the duration of the ischemic period [4, 6]. We have used an experimental model of reversible cerebral ischemia to investigate and quantify the changes in brain water and BBB permeability at the end of a fixed interval of reperfusion following different periods of ischemia.

Materials and Methods

Adult, male Sprague-Dawley rats (200–300 g) were anesthetized, paralyzed, and ventilated with *d*-tubocurarine 2 mg/kg, halothane 0.5%, and a nitrous oxide/oxygen mixture (70% : 30%). Arterial blood pressure, blood gases, and pH were measured throughout the experiment. Hematocrit was assessed at the end of the procedure. Body temperature was maintained at 37 ± 1 °C. The vertebral arteries were coagulated and divided as they lay in the foramina transversaria [9]. Burr holes were made in the skull and platinum electrodes were inserted bilaterally into the frontal, parietal, and occipital cortex on each side and fixed with dental cement. Regional cerebral blood flow (rCBF) was measured by hydrogen clearance technique [3]. Cerebral ischemia was produced by bilateral carotid artery occlusion with Scoville-Lewis clips. Reperfusion of the ischemic brain followed removal of the clips.

Brain Edema

Brain water was measured at the end of the procedure by the specific gravity (SG) method using linearly inhomogeneous bromobenzene-kerosene columns [3, 8]. Six

* Generous support was received for this work from the British Council (Dr. P. Picozzi); the Medical Research Council (Mr. N. V. Todd); and Action Research for Crippling Diseases

[1] Institute of Neurosurgery, First Medical School, University of Naples, Naples, Italy

1-mm samples were dissected from each brain area and placed in the columns; regional SG was taken as the mean of the six samples.

Blood-Brain-Barrier Permeability

The BBB was assessed qualitatively with the aid of a macromolecular tracer, and quantitatively using a low-molecular-weight tracer.

Evans' blue in 0.2 ml of a 2% buffered saline solution was injected IV before the induction of ischemia. The dye binds to albumin (mol. wt. 70 000) immediately after its injection into the blood-stream. Its presence in the brain, indicating a BBB breakdown, was scored simply as either present (EB positive) or absent (EB negative).

We used a quantitative radioisotopic technique to evaluate cerebrovascular permeability [1]. ^{14}C-Alpha aminoisobutyric acid ([^{14}C]AIB), a small (mol. wt. 103), metabolically inert amino acid, was used as tracer. In the normal animal this compound crosses the brain capillary endothelium slowly. However, once in the extracellular space, it is rapidly transported and trapped in the cells [1, 2]. It is possible in the experimental condition to derive a blood-to-brain transfer constant (K_i), according to the following equation:

$$K_i = \frac{C_i(T)}{\int_0^T C_p \, dt}$$

where C_i is the isotope concentration in the brain at the end of the experimental period, and the denominator is the integral of the tracer activity in the plasma (C_p) calculated over the experimental period. A suitable correction was evaluated for the amount of tracer in the vascular compartment at the end of the procedure. The calculated value for K_i may be expressed in terms of clearance (ml/g/min), and under the experimental conditions provides a good approximation of the permeability surface area product (PS) [1].

After the injection of 10 μCi [^{14}C]AIB, ten arterial blood samples were collected over a 10-min interval, and the plasma tracer concentration was measured by liquid scintillation counting. Ten minutes after administration of the tracer the animals were sacrificed, the brain was dissected under kerosene, and samples from each cortical area were used for SG measurement, while 70–100 mg of the remaining part was used for isotope counting.

Experimental Protocol

Control Group ($n=6$). Animals were sham-operated and decapitated up to 3 h after the preparation to assess the SG and K_i for AIB before ischemia.

Experimental Groups. The experimental animals were divided into three groups and subjected to ischemia for different periods of time:

Group A – 15 min ischemia ($n=4$)
Group B – 30 min ischemia ($n=4$)
Group C – 60 min ischemia ($n=4$)

Animals groups A, B, and C were made ischemic for the stated period and were sacrificed at 180 min after the initiation of reperfusion. Blood gases and pH were measured before each flow. rCBF was measured at rest, throughout ischemia, and at specific intervals in reperfusion.

Evans blue was administered prior to the induction of ischemia. AIB was injected 10 min before sacrifice.

Results

General Physiological Parameters

In all animals physiological parameters were kept constant (MABP = 124 ± 3; $PaCO_2 = 38.4 \pm 6$; pH = 7.389 ± 0.011). The whole-blood hematocrit was between 0.40 and 0.45.

Regional Cerebral Blood Flow

Before occlusion the rCBF was 91 ± 6 ml/100 g/min (mean $\pm$ SEM) in the frontal cortex. Severe incomplete ischemia (5.8 ± 0.4 ml/100 g/min) was produced in all animals. A marked reduction of flows to 60%–70% of the preischemic values was present after 180 min of reperfusion, with no significant difference related either to the brain region or to the duration of ischemia.

Brain Edema

Results from SG measurements are shown in Fig. 1. In the reperfused animals, SG cortical values were significantly lower than control in all the areas. There were significant differences in SG between the groups related with the length of ischemia. The most severe decrease in cortical SG was found in group C, while group A was least affected.

Blood-Brain-Barrier Permeability

The K_i for AIB was assessed in the gross brain samples in the same regions as were used for SG measurement. There was no statistically significant increase in K_i for AIB in group A or B, while the values in group C were significantly different from those in the control group, as shown in Fig. 2. There was a trend toward rising values for K_i with increasing duration of ischemia.

EB staining was present in 7 of 24 cortical areas sampled in group B and in 9 of 24 in group C. No animal in group A had EB staining in the cortex. In groups B and C there were statistically significant differences in K_i between the EB-positive and -negative areas (Fig. 3). The role of a BBB breakdown in the accumulation of water in the brain has been evaluated. We found no correlation between K_i for AIB and

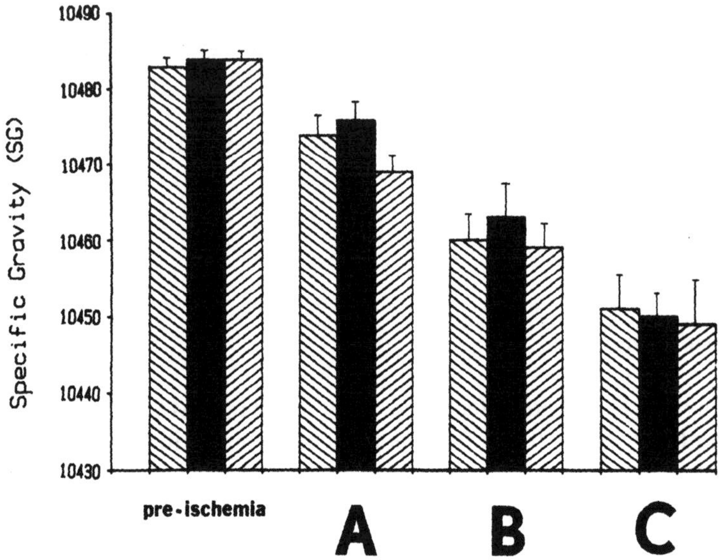

Fig. 1. Brain edema (mean SG) after 180 min of reperfusion following cerebral ischemia for 15 min (*A*), 30 min (*B*), or 60 min (*C*), ▧, frontal cortex; ■, parietal cortex; ▨, occipital cortex; *bars*, SEM

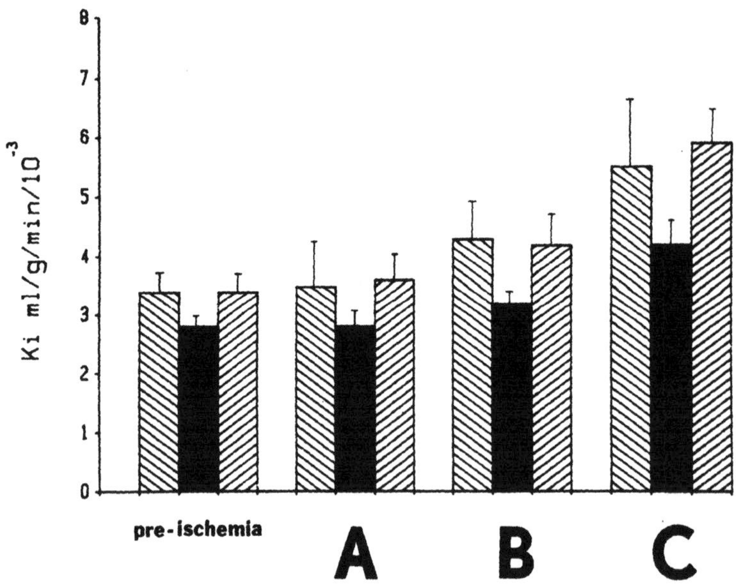

Fig. 2. Mean blood-brain barrier permeability (K_i ml/g/min/10^{-3}) to ^{14}C-AIB after 180 min of reperfusion following cerebral ischemia for 15 min (*A*), 30 min (*B*) or 60 min (*C*). ▧, frontal cortex; ■, parietal cortex; ▨, occipital cortex; *bars*, SEM

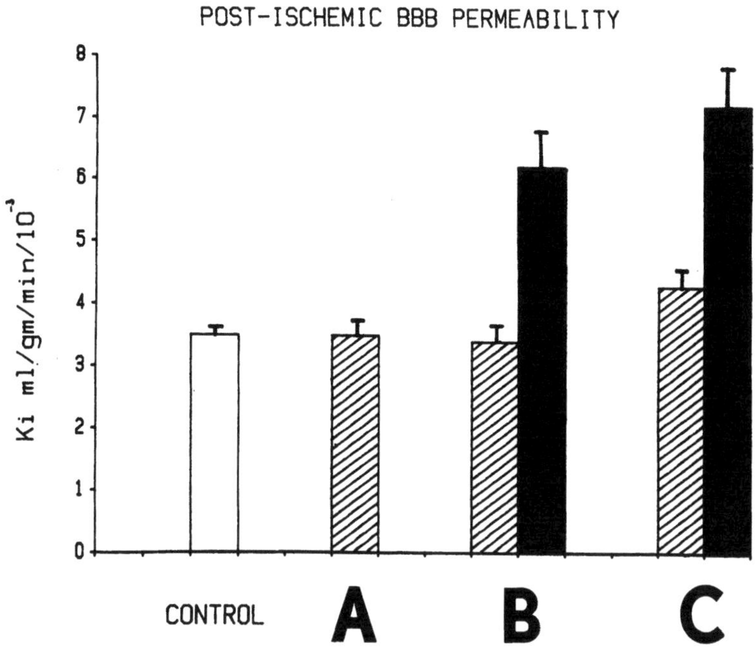

Fig. 3. Mean correlation between ^{14}C-AIB and EB permeability after 180 min of reperfusion following cerebral ischemia for 15 min (*A*), 30 min (*B*), or 60 min (*C*). ▨, EB negative; ■, EB positive; *bars*, SEM

water, as judged by SG, in groups A and B. In Group C, where more pronounced EB extravasation was also present, there was a correlation between K_i values and the SG measured in the same area.

Discussion

To study the influence of the duration of ischemia on the postischemic brain water and BBB damage, it is important to control the levels of the ischemic rCBF to produce comparable and uniform damage in all the animals. The rat four-vessel occlusion model used in this study is a stable and reproducible preparation, producing global forebrain ischemia [9] and allowing full physiological monitoring. We were able to measure cerebral blood flow, brain edema, and BBB permeability simultaneously and in the same cortical region in each preparation on a regional quantitative basis.

At 180 min after the reestablishment of blood flow to ischemic brains we found that both the water content and the degree of BBB breakdown were related to the length of the ischemic period. In permanent ischemia there is known to be a delay of 6–9 h before EB leakage is detected [6], but reperfusion through an ischemic area will accelerate this event [4, 6]. Our findings confirm these results, but in addition they define specifically the simultaneous changes in water and BBB permeability which depend on the duration of ischemia rather than on events during reperfusion.

There have been separate studies on BBB permeability to large molecules [4] and small proteins [10]. In this study we measured permeability to both simultaneously and found no difference in the permeability to large and small tracers following ischemic insult. In mild ischemia (group A) there was no EB staining and no change in K_i for AIB, while in group C there were marked changes in both. Within the same brain we found areas free of EB staining adjacent to areas that were deeply stained. In the latter areas there was a significantly higher K_i for AIB and a marked increase in water as judged by SG measurement. This relationship has also been suggested by Hossmann et al. [5]. The exact relationship between water content and degree of BBB permeability at microregional level, however, will be a complicated mathematical, physiochemical and pathophysiological relationship. The leakage of protein into the brain extracellular space will also produce an error in the water estimation by SG, as pointed out by Marmarou, who has devised a correction factor. The "correction," however, is at best empirical, and caution should be exercised in the interpretation of data so expressed.

Our combined results from three differing periods of ischemia illustrate the complexity of such a relationship. We suggest that with an ischemic insult which is insufficient to damage the BBB, cellular water accumulates during the reperfusion period. A more severe insult (group C) will produce increased BBB permeability with a further increase in brain water, which is probably underestimated with the SG method. It is the edema associated with BBB breakdown that is related to the animals' demise during reperfusion after an ischemic insult.

Conclusions

At 180 min of reperfusion:

1. The amount of water in the brain and the BBB damage are dependent on the duration of ischemia.
2. When BBB impairment is present the damage involves the movement of both small and large tracers across the barrier.
3. Within a group the amount of water in the brain appears to be higher in these regions where BBB damage has occurred.
4. There is a limit to the amount of water that accumulates in the brain when the BBB is intact; damage to the latter results in a further major increase in water accumulation.

Summary

Using the four-vessel occlusion model in rats we have measured simultaneously rCBF, brain water as judged by SG, and BBB permeability to large and small molecules. By varying the length of the ischemic period we have shown that the amount of water accumulation and BBB breakdown depends on the duration of ischemia. The blood flow 180 min after the ischemic period is identical. The water and protein accumulation therefore depend solely on the events in ischemia.

References

1. Blasberg RG, Gazedam J, Patlak CS, Fenstermacher JD (1980) Quantitative autoradiographic studies of brain edema and a comparison of multi-isotope autoradiographic technique. In: Cervós-Navarro J, Ferszt R (eds) Brain edema. Raven, New York, pp 255–270 (Advances in neurology, vol 28)
2. Blasberg RG, Fenstermacher JD, Patlak CS (1983) Transport of alpha-aminoisobutyric acid across brain capillary and cellular membranes. J Cereb Blood Flow Metab 3:8–32
3. Crockard A, Iannotti F, Hunstock AT, Smith RD, Harris RJ, Symon L (1980) Cerebral blood flow and edema following carotid occlusion in the gerbil. Stroke 11:494–498
4. Fujimoto T, Walker JT, Spatz M, Klatzo I (1976) Pathophysiologic aspects of ischemic edema. In: Pappius HM, Feindel W (eds) Dynamics of brain edema. Springer, Berlin Heidelberg New York, pp 171–180
5. Hossmann KA, Bothe HW, Bodsch W, Paschen W (1983) Pathophysiological aspects of blood-brain barrier disturbances in experimental brain tumours and brain abscesses. In: Hossmann KA, Klatzo I (eds) Cerebrovascular transport mechanisms. Springer, Berlin Heidelberg New York, pp 89–102 (Acta Neuropathol, suppl 8).
6. Ito U, Ohno K, Nakamura R, Suganuma F, Inaba Y (1979) Brain edema during ischemia and after restoration of blood flow. Stroke 10:542–547
7. Klatzo I (1967) Neuropathological aspects of brain edema: Presidential address. J Neuropathol Exp Neurol 26:1–14
8. Marmarou A, Poll W, Shulman K, Bhagavan H (1978) A simple gravimetric technique for measurement of cerebral edema. J Neurosurg 49:530–537
9. Todd NV, Crockard HA, Ross Russell RW, Picozzi P (1984) Cerebral blood flow in the four-vessel occlusion model. Stroke 15:579 (letter)
10. Tyson GW, Teasdale GM, Graham DI, McCulloch J (1982) Cerebrovascular permeability following MCA occlusion in the rat. The effect of halothane-induced hypotension. J Neurosurg 57:186–196

Changes in Water Status of Rat Brain Tissue After Cardiocirculatory Arrest Measured by Nuclear Magnetic Resonance

M. YAMAMOTO[1], M. HAIDA, H. MATSUMURA, H. OHSUGA, and Y. SHINOHARA

Key words: Brain tissue, albumin solution, proteolysis, osmolality, proton relaxation times (T_1, T_2)

Introduction

It is speculated that the autolysis or physicochemical changes of protein in the brain tissue after brain damage such as trauma or stroke play an important role in the development of brain edema through the increase of tissue osmotic potential [1–3]. Many factors, including conformational or catabolic changes in macromolecules, are considered to contribute to the autolysis or physiochemical changes in protein. The contribution of hydrolytic changes in macromolecules to the increase in osmotic potential of brain tissue in permanent complete ischemia remains to be elucidated.

Recently, it has become possible to apply nuclear magnetic resonance (NMR) in the investigation of brain tissue. We have shown [4] that the transverse relaxation time (T_2) of protons of water molecules measured by NMR reflects the changes induced in the environment around water molecules by the alteration of macromolecules such as proteins.

The purpose of this study was to investigate the changes in longitudinal relaxation time (T_1) and transverse relaxation time (T_2) measured by NMR in the rat brain after cardiocirculatory arrest (CCA), and to estimate the importance of proteolysis, one of the factors involved in autolysis, in the increase in osmotic potential that occurs after brain damage.

Materials and Methods

Materials

Preparation of Rat Brain

Wistar rats (16–20 weeks old) were sacrificed by the injection of KCl solution into the heart. A hole (3 mm × 3 mm) was drilled in the frontoparietal region of the skull

[1] Department of Neurology, School of Medicine, Tokai University, Isehara, Kanagawa 259-11, Japan

at the following times after sacrifice; 30 min ($n=8$), 1 h ($n=8$), 5 h ($n=9$), 24 h ($n=5$), and 48 h ($n=7$).

A brain sample 2 mm thick measured from the brain surface was punched out through the hole by means of a sharp-edged Pyrex glass tube (i. d. = 2 mm) for NMR measurement. The biopsied sample in the tube was sealed tightly with waterproof Hematoseal, a compound for hematocrit measurement, which does not affect the NMR signals [4].

Preparation of Albumine Solutions

To investigate the effects of an increase in albumin concentration on the relaxation times and osmolality of albumin solution, albumin solutions of various concentrations were prepared from human albumin (Fraction V, Sigma). Furthermore, to study the influence of enzymatic proteolysis on the relaxation times and osmolality of albumin solutions, 2 mg trypsin (15 000 units/mg, Sigma) or 2 mg of trypsin and 2 mg trypsin inhibitor (Sigma) were added to test tubes containing 2 ml albumin solution (30 g/dl), and the mixtures were incubated in a water bath at 37 °C.

Aliquots of the albumin solutions made by the above preparation method were sealed in Pyrex tubes by the same procedure as was used in the case of brain tissue.

Methods

The relaxation times (T_1 and T_2) were measured on 100 MHz NMR equipment (Nihon Denshi, JNR-100). The sample tube containing brain tissue or albumin solution was coaxially placed in an outer tube containing D_2O to stabilize the magnetic field. The T_1 was measured by the inversion-recovery method ($180°-\tau-90°$ pulse sequence) and T_2 by the spin-echo method ($90°-\tau-180°$). The values of T_1 and T_2 were calculated by fitting the amplitude (τ) curve as reported previously [4].

Osmolality of the albumin solution was measured by the vapor-pressure method with an OSM-1 instrument (Shimadzu Co.) and expressed as milliosmols per kilogram. The water content of brain tissue was measured by the vacuum drying method.

Results

Values for T_1, T_2, and Osmotic Potential of Albumin Solution

As the concentration of albumin was increased the osmotic potential of the solutions rose (Fig. 1) and the values of T_1 and T_2 decreased as follows: water, $T_1 = 3.6$ s, $T_2 = 1.7$ s; 20 g/dl albumin, $T_1 = 1.7$ s, $T_2 = 230$ ms; 30 g/dl, $T_1 = 1.3$ s, $T_2 = 135$ ms; 50 g/dl, $T_1 = 0.78$ s, $T_2 = 53$ ms.

The relaxation rates ($1/T_1$, $1/T_2$) correlated well with the osmotic potential in the albumin solutions (Fig. 2). The enzymatic proteolysis of albumin by trypsin increased the osmotic potential compared with those of solutions of albumin alone

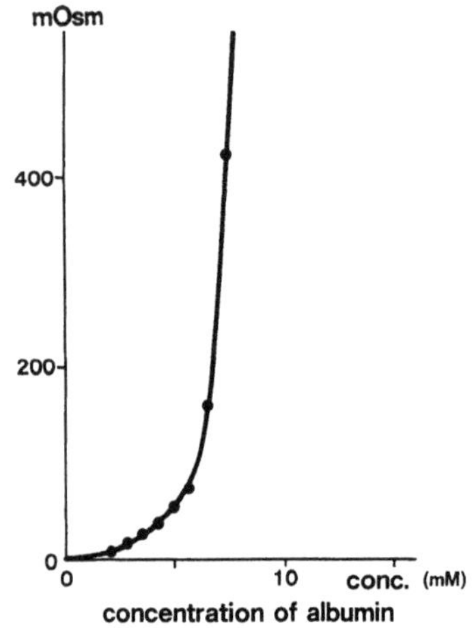

Fig. 1. Relationship between osmotic potential and concentration of albumin

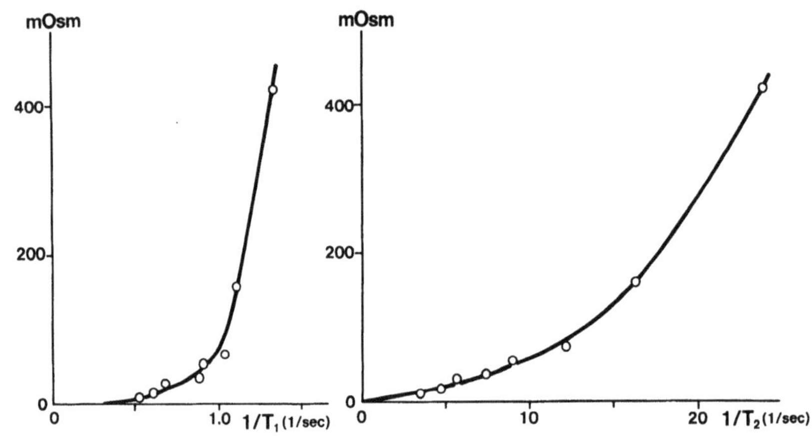

Fig. 2. Relationship between the relaxation rates ($1/T_1$, $1/T_2$) and the osmotic potential of albumin solutions

and the solution of albumin with trypsin and trypsin inhibitor (Fig. 3). The time courses of T_1 and T_2 in the proteolytic study showed gradual decreases of the T_1 and T_2 values up to at least 8 h after the start of incubation (Fig. 4). The values of T_1 and T_2 of albumin with trypsin were 1.34 s and 132 ms, respectively, at the start of incubation. After 8 h of incubation the T_1 value had decreased to 1.27 s, and the T_2 value, to 108 ms. The values of T_1 and T_2 for solutions of albumin alone were 1.32 s and 154 ms at the start of incubation and 1.33 s and 153 ms after 8 h of incubation.

Values for T_1, T_2, and Water Content of Rat Brain After Cardiocirculatory Arrest (CCA)

Figure 5 shows the changes in T_1, T_2 and water content of rat brain tissue after CCA. The value of T_2 (70.9 ± 1.6 ms) in the rat brain was increased significantly 30 min after CCA, compared with that of the normal control (63.5 ± 2.5 ms). At 1 h

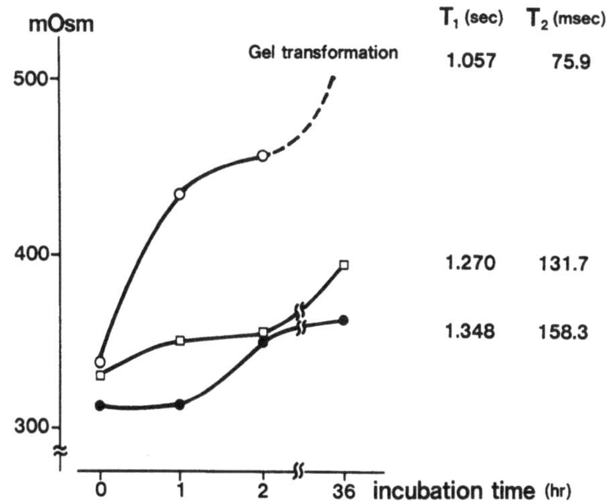

Fig. 3. Effects of enzymatic proteolysis of albumin using trypsin on the osmotic potential in albumin solutions (30 g/dl). The consistency of the albumin solution containing trypsin was changed to that of a gel 38 h after the start of incubation. In the albumin solution with trypsin the osmotic potential was higher than in the solutions of albumin alone or in albumin solution containing trypsin and trypsin inhibitor. The values for T_1 and T_2 measured in albumin solutions with trypsin at 36 h after incubation were markedly lower than in control solutions

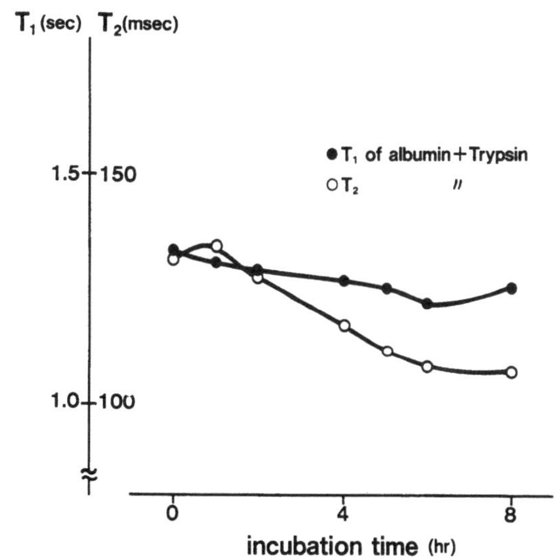

Fig. 4. Effects of enzymatic proteolysis on the proton relaxation times of albumin solutions. Proteolysis by trypsin gradually decreased the values for T_1 and T_2

after CCA the T_2 value was slightly decreased, but still above the normal value. Thereafter, T_2 values remained at a plateau level until 24 h after CCA, then decreasing to the control level by 48 h after CCA. The T_1 values showed similar changes to the T_2 values, but were not significantly increased over the normal control value. Water content was significantly higher than the normal control value from 1 h to 48 h after CCA.

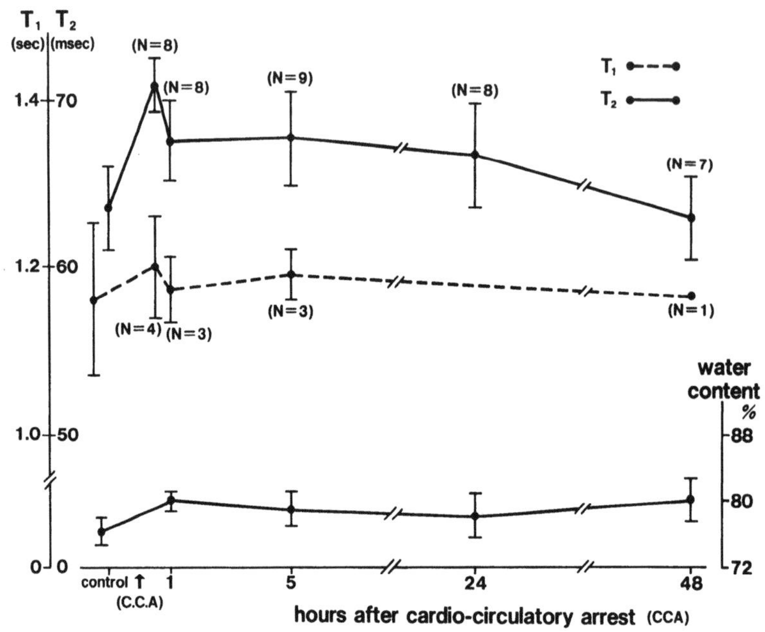

Fig. 5. The changes in T_1, T_2, and water content of rat brain tissue after cardiocirculatory arrest (CCA)

Discussion

The results of our present studies with albumin solutions can be summarized as follows:

1. Increases in albumin concentration decreased the proton relaxation times (T_1 and T_2) of water molecules, as reported by Daskiewicz [5], and the relaxation rates ($1/T_1$ and $1/T_2$) correlated well with the osmotic potential in albumin solutions of various concentrations.

2. Enzymatic proteolysis of albumin by trypsin decreased the relaxation times and increased the osmotic potential of albumin solutions up to 8 h after the start of incubation.

These findings suggest that changes of concentration or the occurrence of proteolysis can affect the relaxation times and osmotic potentials of protein solutions. In albumin solutions, T_2 was a more sensitive indicator of the changes in protein solutions than T_1, as reported previously [5].

As far as the changes in T_2 values of rat brain tissue after cardiocirculatory arrest are concerned, it seems likely that there are two phases. In the "early" phase (within 1 h after CCA) the values for T_2 first increased and then decreased. The value for T_2 was still above the normal control value at 1 h after CCA, and the water content was increased. In the "late" phase (from 1 h to 24 h after CCA) the T_2 values remained at a plateau level similar to that at 1 h, and the water content also changed little from that at the end of the early phase. In the early phase, the increase in T_2 values is considered to reflect the increase in water influx suggested by the increase in water content. After CCA, the rapid accumulation of intermediate metabolites such as lactic acid, release of electrolytes from macromolecules [6–8], and changes in membrane potential [9] promote water influx into extra- and intracellular spaces from CSF or blood. The water influx was limited, however, because there was no further supply of CSF or blood. The decrease in T_2 value following the increase in T_2 at 30 min after CCA could be accounted for by conformational changes of protein or lipid in the absence of a further supply of water. This decrease in the T_2 value indicated that the osmotic potential of rat brain tissue was increased, since we found a good correlation between increase in osmolality and decrease in relaxation rate of albumin solutions.

In the late phase, our study showed no definite changes in T_2 value and water content. If the activity of proteinase, which has been reported to be activated by a fall in pH [10], is high in the brain tissue, changes in T_2 would be expected in the late phase, as we observed a gradual decrease in the T_2 of albumin solutions treated with trypsin. Therefore, these findings suggested that there were no further changes of protein, such as conformational alterations or proteolysis, which might affect the state of water molecules in the rat brain tissue in the late phase. Since it has been reported that the activity of proteinase is decreased by the inhibition of protein synthesis or autophagocytosis [11, 12], enzymatic proteolysis was probably inhibited after CCA in our study. The activity of proteinase in the rat brain tissue may be low in any case. It is thus likely that proteolysis also makes relatively little contribution to the decrease in T_2 of rat brain either in the early phase or in the late phase.

Since a decrease in T_2 was reported in the cold injury model [13], further study in the incomplete ischemia model is needed to evaluate the effects of conformational or catabolic changes of macromolecules on the increase in tissue osmolality.

Summary

To evaluate the conformational or catabolic changes of macromolecules such as protein in the brain tissue after cardiocirculatory arrest (CCA), we measured the proton relaxation times (T_1 and T_2) by NMR and determined the water content of rat brain tissue after CCA. In addition, the effects of increasing albumin concentration and proteolysis of albumin by trypsin on T_1, T_2, and osmolality of albumin solutions were investigated by NMR and vapor pressure methods.

Increasing albumin concentrations led to a decline in T_1 and T_2 and an increase in the osmotic potential of albumin solutions. The increase of osmotic potential correlated well with the relaxation rates in the albumin solutions. The proteolysis of albumin increased the osmotic potential and decreased T_1 and T_2 of albumin solutions.

The values for T_2 of rat brain tissue increased significantly 30 min after CCA and decreased 1 h after CCA. From 1 h to 24 h after CCA the T_2 value remained at a plateau level, which was prolonged compared with that of the normal control. The T_1 values showed changes similar to those in T_2, but the changes were not significant compared with the normal control. Water content was increased from 1 h to 24 h after CCA.

Our findings indicate that conformational or hydrolytic changes of protein might contribute to the increase in osmotic potential of brain tissue (suggested by the decrease in T_2) within 1 h after CCA, but do not play a major role in the increased osmotic potential from 1 h to 24 h after CCA.

References

1. Hossmann KA, Takagi S (1976) Osmolality of brain in cerebral ischemia. Exp Neurol 51:124–131
2. Stern W, Coxon RV (1964) Osmolality of brain tissue and its relation to brain bulk. Am J Physiol 206:1–7
3. Tomita M, Gotoh F, Sato T, Yamamoto M, Amano T, Tanahashi N, Tanaka K (1979) Determination of the osmotic potential swelling of cat brain in vitro. Exp Neurol 65:66–77
4. Haida M, Yamamoto M, Matsumura H, Yoshii F, Shinohara Y, Fukuzaki M (1983) Two different states of water in normal adult rat brain based on the transverse relaxation time (T_2) of NMR. J Cereb Blood Flow Metab 3 (Suppl 1):S83–S84
5. Daszkiewicz OK, Hennel JW, Lubas BL, Szczepkowski TW (1982) Proton magnetic relaxation and proton hydration. Nature 200:1006–1007
6. Foilbergrova J, Ljunggsen KB, Norberg K, Siesjö BK (1974) Influence of complete ischemia on glycolytic metabolites, citric acid cycle intermediates and associated amino acids in the rat cerebral cortex. Brain Res 80:265–279
7. Kleihues P, Kobayashi K, Hossmann KA (1971) Purine nucleotide metabolism in the cat brain after one hour of complete ischemia. J Neurochem 23:417–425
8. Bito LZ, Myers RE (1973) On the physiological response of the cerebral cortex to acute stress (reversible asphyxia). J Physiol (Lond) 221:349–370
9. Matsuoka Y, Hossmann KA (1982) Cortical impedance and extracellular volume changes following middle cerebral artery occlusion in cats. J Cereb Blood Flow Metab 2:466–474
10. Koenig H (1984) Lysosomes. In: Laitha A (ed) Handbook of neurochemistry, vol 7. Plenum, New York, pp 177–203
11. Baccino FM, Tessitore L, Cecchini G, Messiner M et al. (1982) Control of cell protein catabolism in rat liver. Effects of starvation and administration of cycloheximide. Biochem J 206:395–405
12. Kovacs A, Seglen PO (1981) Inhibition of hepatocytic protein degradation by methylaminopurines and inhibitors of protein synthesis. Biochem Biophys Acta 676:213–220
13. Hirokawa K, Naruse S, Horikawa Y, Tanaka C, Nishikawa H (1984) Proton NMR study on brain edema. In: Go KG, Baethmann A (eds) Recent process in the study and therapy of brain edema. Plenum, New York, pp 271–282

Does Capillary Na, K-ATPase Play a Role in the Development of Ischemic Brain Edema?

T. SHIGENO [1], T. ASANO, E. WATANABE, H. JOHSHITA, and K. TAKAKURA

Key words: Ischemic edema, brain capillary function, Na, K-ATPase

Introduction

It is generally accepted that one effect of ouabain in the brain is the induction of swelling of brain cells through inhibition of Na, K-ATPase located at neuronal membranes. In the situation where ATP is depleted, as in cerebral ischemia, the swelling of brain cells is an early event, representing a cytotoxic aspect of ischemic edema formation. In this context, previous workers have already seen reduced neuronal Na, K-ATPase activity in experimental cerebral ischemia. Recently, however, another site of Na, K-ATPase activity has been found in the brain, viz. the capillaries. Goldstein and Betz [2] suggested that capillary Na, K-ATPase is present only on the abluminal side, pumping out Na^+ from blood into the brain as a unidirectional active transport mechanism. Furthermore, evidence has arisen that the capillary Na, K-ATPase activity may be increased at certain stages of cerebral ischemia [1, 5]. Should this be the case, it might be postulated that capillary Na, K-ATPase enhances pumping out of Na^+ and the associated H_2O shift in the presence of ion-pump failure in the neuronal membranes so that the total net result is an increase in brain Na^+ and H_2O in both intracellular and extracellular environments. Therefore, ischemic brain edema involves both cytotoxic and vasogenic factors in nature.

Along with the above concepts, we have observed an enhancement of capillary Na, K-ATPase activity in vitro by hydroperoxide of arachidonic acid (15-HPAA) which has been shown to act as a modulator of the arachidonic cascade in the brain microvessel [Asano et al. 1984, paper presented in this symposium; 4]. Thus, as the first step toward verification of the above hypothesis, it would be worthwhile to check whether or not inhibition of capillarly Na, K-ATPase mitigates ischemia-induced Na^+ influx into the brain, leading to the suppression of brain edema. Since the brain microvessel is exposed to an elevated tissue level of free arachidonic acid in ischemia, it is tempting to assume that some hydroperoxides of arachidonic acid such as 15-HPAA stimulate both the arachidonic cascade within the microvessel and the Na, K-ATPase activity. For this purpose, we established a new model for selective inhibition of capillary Na, K-ATPase via direct arterial infusion of ouabain into the ischemic area, and found that edema was indeed reduced in some situations.

---

[1] Department of Neurosurgery, University of Tokyo, 7-3-1 Hongo, Bunkyo-ku, Tokyo 113, Japan

Materials and Methods

In cats anesthetized with N_2O/O_2 a catheter was introduced directly into the occluded middle cerebral artery (MCA) just distal to the occlusion. Oxygenated solutions [either Krebs-Ringer or ouabain (10^{-5} *M*)] were then perfused in the ischemic area at a hydrostatic pressure exceeding the MCA stump pressure by enough to perfuse the entire territory of the MCA. Perfusion was done intermittently either every 5 min or every 2 min until 4 h after the induction of ischemia. CBF was measured every 30 min by the hydrogen clearance technique, and the topographic correlation between ischemic flow and specific gravity was investigated by means of column gravimetry [6]. The cats were divided into three main experimental groups: (a) no perfusion ($n = 11$), (b) Krebs-Ringer ($n = 7$), (c) ouabain every 5 min ($n = 6$) or every 2 min ($n = 4$).

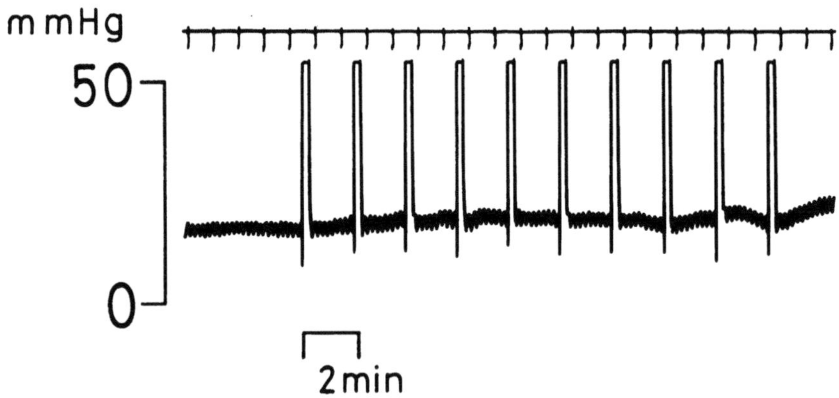

Fig. 1. Polygraph chart of MCA stump pressure following occlusion, with intermittent perfusion performed for 15 s every 2 min

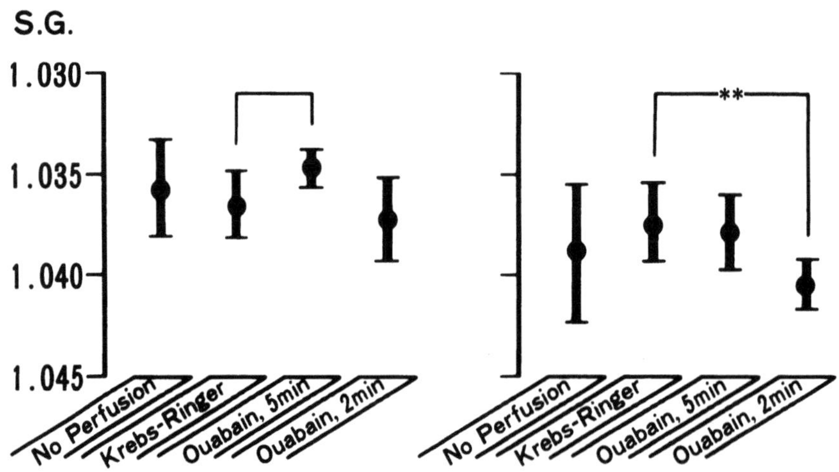

Fig. 2. Correlation between ischemic flow and changes in specific gravity in severe ischemia (*left*) and moderate ischemia (*right*). Note the increase in SG in ouabain perfusion every 2 min in the moderately ischemic area compared with the Krebs-Ringer perfusion control

Results

The MCA stump pressure was around 20 mmHg, and perfusion was successfully performed (Fig. 1). Mean ischemic flow did not differ significantly between groups. Ouabain significantly suppressed the reduction in specific gravity in the area with moderate ischemia ($15 < CBF < 30$), particularly when perfused every 2 min (Fig. 2).

Discussion

Our previous observation that the increase in water content following focal cerebral ischemia was in parallel with that in Na^+ [3] suggests that an active transport mechanism of Na^+ across the blood-brain barrier (BBB) is involved in ischemic edema formation at some stage. It is also starting to appear more likely that the arachidonic cascade, in particular that affecting the lipoxygenase pathway, may play a pivotal role in ischemic cell injury and edema formation. In fact, we recently found ischemia or 15-HPAA-induced enhancement of eicosanoid synthesis, particularly of hydroxy acids (possible lipoxygenase products) in brain microvessels [4; Usui et al. 1974, paper presented in this symposium]. Furthermore, 15-HPAA indeed enhanced Na, K-ATPase activity in the brain microvessels [Asano et al., this volume], whereas it suppressed the activity in the synaptosomes. Therefore, it is surmised that the lipoxygenase cascade is involved in the regulation of ion movements and the water shift through the BBB, by modifying the activity of Na, K-ATPase located at the endothelium.

A unique observation in the present study was that ouabain did not aggravate but ameliorated edema formation within the ischemic tissue. In considering the above working hypothesis, it is concluded that capillary Na, K-ATPase plays a role not only in normal cell volume regulation but also in cerebral ischemia as one of the causative factors of ischemic edema formation.

Summary

Previously accumulated evidence that capillary Na, K-ATPase activity was enhanced in cerebral ischemia, possibly via the lipoxygenase cascade, led to the present investigation designed to find whether inhibition of capillary Na, K-ATPase could suppress unidirectional transport of Na^+ across the BBB and thus ameliorate edema formation within the ischemic brain. For this purpose, ouabain was intermittently infused directly into the middle cerebral artery in cats immediately after occlusion. The result showed that edema which developed within 4 h of ischemia induction was suppressed in the moderately ischemic zone. Therefore, we suggest that activation of brain capillary function plays a role in ischemic pathophysiology and edema formation.

References

1. Enseleit WH, Domer FR, Jarrott DM, Baricos WH (1984) Cerebral phospholipid content and Na^+, K^+-ATPase activity during ischemia and postischemic reperfusion in the Mongolian gerbil. J Neurochem 43:320–327
2. Goldstein GW, Betz AL (1983) Recent advances in understanding brain capillary function. Ann Neurol 14:389–395
3. Gotoh O, Asano T, Koide T, Takakura K (1984) Ischemic cerebral edema following occlusion of the middle cerebral artery in the rat. I: The time courses of brain water, sodium and potassium contents and blood-brain barrier permeability to ^{125}I-albumin. Stroke (in press)
4. Koide T, Gotoh O, Asano T, Takakura K (1984) Alterations of the eicosanoid synthetic capacity of the rat brain microvessel following ischemia: relevance to ischemic brain edema. J Neurochem (in press)
5. MacMillan V (1982) Cerebral Na^+, K^+-ATPase activity during exposure to and recovery from acute ischemia. J Cereb Blood Flow Metab 2:457–465
6. Shigeno T, Brock M, Shigeno S, Fritschka E, Cervós-Navarro J (1982) The determination of brain water content: microgravimetry versus drying-weighing method. J Neurosurg 57:99–107

Investigation of Pathophysiology in Ischemic Brain Edema with ^{1}H-NMR and ^{31}P-NMR *

C. Tanaka [1], S. Naruse, Y. Horikawa, T. Higuchi, K. Hirakawa, and H. Nishikawa

Key words: Cerebral infarction, ischemic brain edema, energy metabolism, proton relaxation time, multinuclear NMR

Introduction

The NMR method is a powerful tool to investigate the pathophysiology of various cerebral diseases. In vivo ^{31}P-NMR is useful to investigate the energy metabolism of normal and pathologic brains. The ^{1}H-NMR is suitable to analyze the quality and behavior of water molecules in tissue through the proton relaxation time measurements. In this experiment, the pathophysiology of cerebral ischemia and ischemic brain edema was therefore investigated by using multinuclear magnetic resonance. The nonuniformity of the ischemic model using Mongolian gerbils is also discussed.

Materials and Methods

Materials

In this study 162 Mongolian gerbils weighing 80 g each were used. Cerebral ischemia was induced in each gerbil by ligating the unilateral common carotid artery under ether anesthesia.

In Vitro ^{1}H-NMR Study

Of the 150 gerbils used for the in vitro proton relaxation time measurement, 60% demonstrated symptoms of ischemia, viz. rotational movement and marked suppression of activity [5]. These gerbils were killed by decapitation at 1, 3, 5, and 7 h after ligation and each hemisphere was measured with the NMR equipment. The control group consisted of four gerbils which received the same treatment as the

---

* This work was supported in part by Grant-in-Aid for Scientific Research 58440059, 58570597 and 59570623 from the Ministry of Education, Science and Culture, Japan.

[1] Department of Neurosurgery, Kyoto Prefectural University of Medicine, Kawaramachi-Hirokoji, Kamigyo-Ku, Kyoto 602, Japan

ischemic group except that the carotid silk thread was not tied. After decapitation the brain was removed quickly, and the samples, weighing about 200 mg at wet weight, were put into an NMR tube 10 mm in diameter.

In Vivo ^{31}P-NMR Study

Twelve gerbils were anesthetized by IP injection of pentobarbital (35 mg/kg). A silk thread was placed at the right common carotid artery with operative microscopic monitoring. After a control ^{31}P-NMR spectrum of the right cerebral hemisphere had been taken in this condition, the right carotid was ligated and the change in the ^{31}P-NMR spectrum was observed. Five of the twelve gerbils showed changes in the NMR spectrum and the left hemisphere of these gerbils was also measured. After these measurements, three of the five gerbils had the cerebral circulation restored by release of the silk ligating thread under microscopy. Changes in the energy metabolism after recirculation were measured successively.

NMR Measurements

Two different NMR apparati were used in this study.

In Vitro ^{1}H-NMR Measurements

The in vitro study was performed with a PFT-100 NMR spectrometer (JEOL, Japan) at 2.4 Tesla. T_1 was measured by the inversion recovery method using 13 different τ and T_2 was measured by the Carr-Purcell-Meiboom-Gill pulse sequence using 80 spin echos [2]. The detail of these measurements and the calculation method for relaxation times have been reported in a previous paper [6].

In Vivo ^{31}P-NMR Measurements

A FX-270 NMR spectrometer (JEOL, Japan) at 6.5 Tesla was used. The measurement was carried out repetitively every 2 s for 400 times with a 15-ms pulse width. The chemical shift was expressed as parts per million, phosphocreatine being used as the internal reference. The surface coil, 8 mm in diameter, was placed on the scalp of the unilateral hemisphere of the gerbils.

Measurement of Water Content

Immediately after NMR measurements in vitro, the wet weight of the brain was measured. After 3 days' drying at 100 °C the dry weight of the brain was measured. The water content of the brain was calculated by the wet-dry method [6].

Results

Time Course of In Vitro Proton Relaxation Time Values

The T_1 value of the normal control brain was 1107 ± 63.1 ms (mean $\pm$ SD). After cerebral ischemia was induced, the T_1 value of the ligated hemisphere began to become longer more than that of the control (Fig. 1). The maximum value of T_1 was

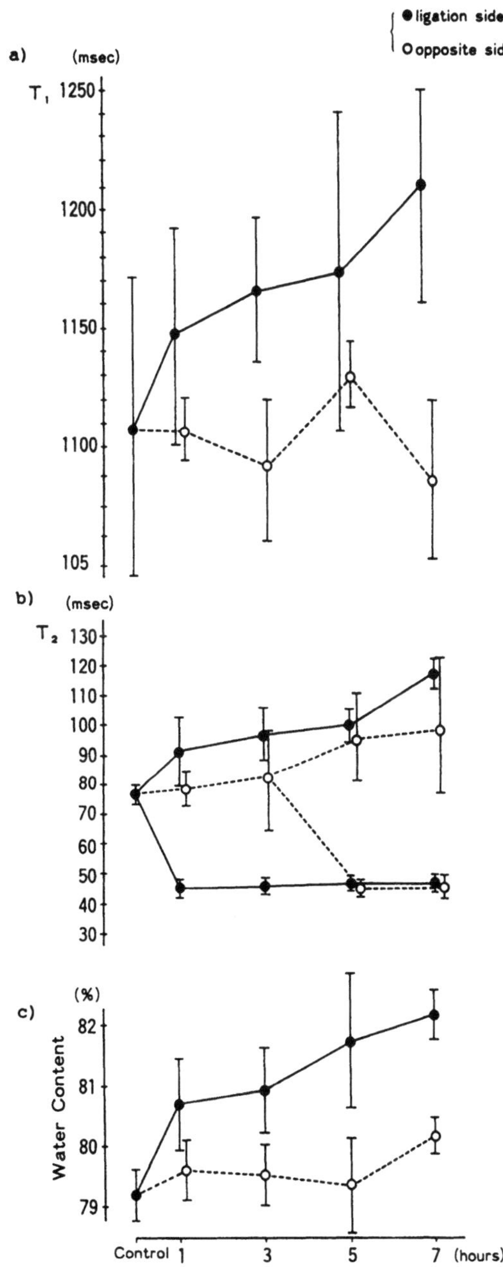

Fig. 1. a–c. Time courses of T_1, T_2, and water content in cerebral ischemia. ($n=4$–6) **a** Time course of T_1 in cerebral ischemia. **b** Time course of T_2 in cerebral ischemia. Separation into two components of T_2 was observed from 1 h after ligation up to 7 h after in the ligated hemisphere and from 5 h until 7 h after on the opposite side. **c** Time course of water content in cerebral ischemia

1210±39.9 ms at 7 h after ligation. The T_1 value of the opposite hemisphere showed a tendency to prolongation, but these changes were minimal, as shown in Fig. 1a.

The T_2 value of the normal control group was 76.2±2.2 ms and showed a single component. The change in T_2 during cerebral ischemia consisted of two phenomena: separation into two components, and prolongation of the slow component (Fig. 1b). The maximum T_2 value of the slow component was 117.7±6.1 ms at 7 h after ligation. The change in T_2 for the opposite side of the brain was observed at 5 and 7 h after ligation as separation into two components and prolongation of the slow component. However, these changes were smaller than those on the ligated side (Fig. 1b).

Time Course of Water Content

The water content of the normal brain was 79.2%±0.3% (mean ± SD). After ligation the water content on the ligated side gradually increased, reaching a maximum value of 82.1%±0.4% at 7 h after ligation (Fig. 1c). The changes in water content on the opposite side were minimal, as seen in Fig. 1c.

In Vivo ^{31}P-NMR Spectrum

The ^{31}P-NMR spectrum of the normal gerbil brain is shown in Fig. 2a. This spectrum consists of seven peaks (I–VII). Peak I was assigned as β-ATP; II as α-ATP and α-ADP, with NAD^+/NADH; III as γ-ATP and β-ADP; IV as phosphocreatine (PCr); V as phosphodiester; VI as inorganic phosphate (Pi); and VII as phosphomonoester (PME). After carotid ligation the Pi peak increased and the PCr and ATP peaks decreased markedly in the NMR spectrum (Fig. 2b–d). Cerebral ischemia in the ^{31}P-NMR spectrum was observed only as a large resonance of Pi in all cases. Four of five cases required two or three scans, requiring 26 or 39 min, for the complete ischemic patterns to be determined (Figs. 2b, c and 3b, c). Only one case in five showed the complete ischemic spectrum within 13 min after ligation. On the other hand, in the contralateral hemisphere no changes occurred in the ^{31}P-NMR spectrum during the measurements.

In the cases with restoration of the cerebral circulation, the ^{31}P-NMR spectrum gradually recovered, from a Pi-dominant spectrum to the normal spectrum of the control pattern (Fig. 3). Three cases, with different ischemic durations of 45, 70, and 90 min, showed full recovery of the ^{31}P-NMR spectra.

Discussion

For the quantitative analysis of ischemic brain edema, it is necessary to compare the relaxation rates R_1 and R_2 (reciprocal values of relaxation times) with the water content [3, 6]. The relationship between R_1, R_2, and the water content in the ischemic hemisphere is shown in Fig. 4. This figure includes previous data collected in other types of brain edema (vasogenic and cytotoxic types) to allow a comparison of

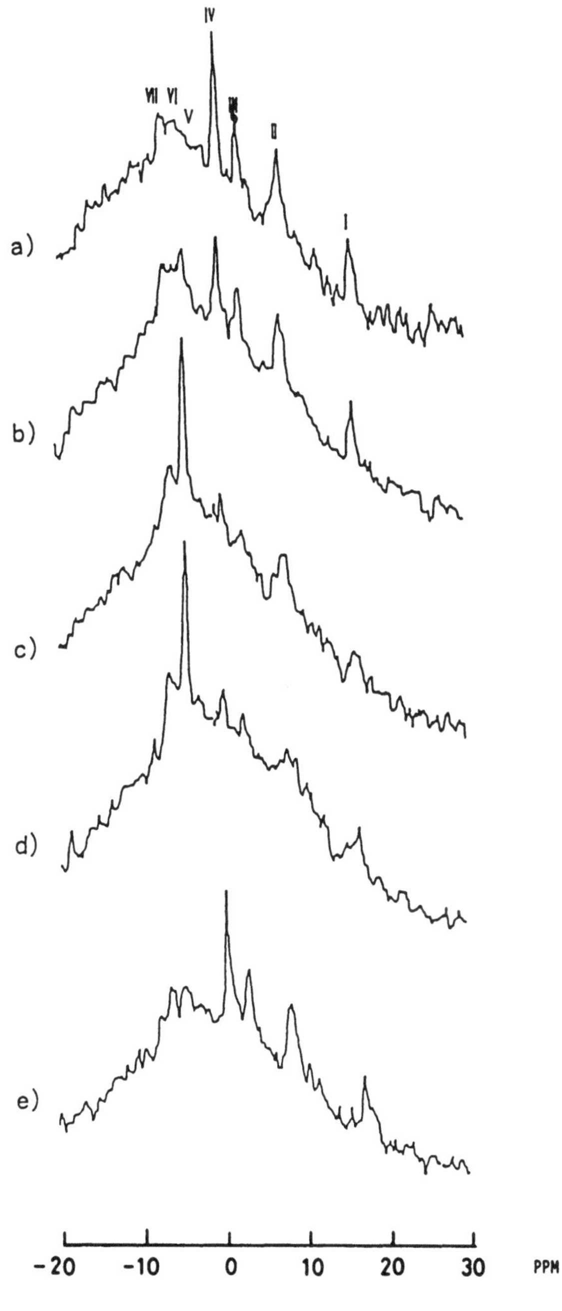

Fig. 2. In vivo ^{31}P-NMR spectra in brain before and after ischemia. Peak *I*, β-ATP; *II*, α-ATP and α-ADP, with NAD$^+$/NADH; *III*, γ-ATP and β-ADP; *IV*, phosphocreatine (PCr); *V*, phosphodiester (PDE); *VI*, inorganic phosphate (Pi); and *VII*, phosphomonoester (PME). *a*, ^{31}P-NMR spectrum of right hemisphere in Mongolian gerbil; *b*, ^{31}P-NMR spectrum immediately after carotid ligation of right hemisphere; *c*, ^{31}P-NMR spectrum during cerebral ischemia 25 min after ligation; *d*, ^{31}P-NMR spectrum 3 h after ligation; *e*, ^{31}P-NMR spectrum in left hemisphere (opposite side) 3 h after ligation

ischemic edema with other types of brain edema [3, 6]. There was a linear correlation between R_1 and the water content in all three types of brain edema. There were also linear correlations between R_2 and the water content in both cytotoxic and ischemic brain edema. However, the slope of these straight lines differed in these two types of brain edema. On the other hand, there was no linear correlation between R_2 and the water content in vasogenic brain edema. These analyses of R_2 ver-

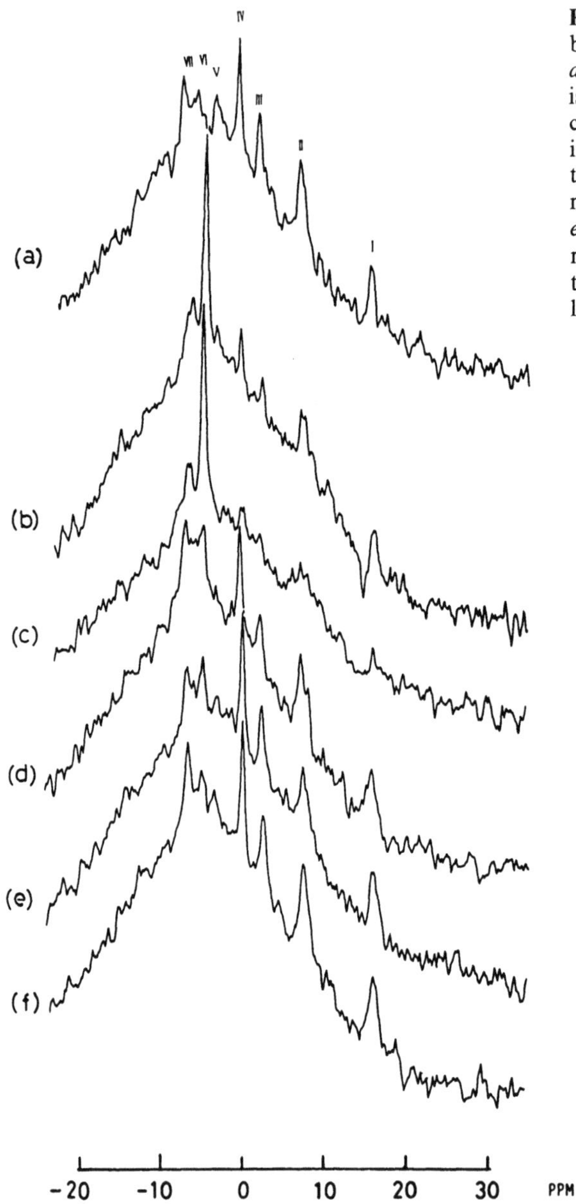

Fig. 3. ^{31}P-NMR spectra of cerebral ischemia and recirculation. *a*, ^{31}P-NMR spectrum in preischemic period; *b*, *c*, sequential changes of ^{31}P-NMR spectra during ischemia (45 min after ligation); *d*, ^{31}P-NMR spectrum immediately after recirculation; *e*, ^{31}P-NMR spectrum 45 min after recirculation; *f*, ^{31}P-NMR spectrum 70 min after recirculation following 45 min ischemia

sus water content suggested that ischemic brain edema possessed elements of both vasogenic and cytotoxic brain edema [3, 4].

In the ^{31}P-NMR studies, the changes in the energy metabolism in cerebral ischemia were measured successively. The measuring field of this method was fitted to the ischemic region of the ipsilateral hemisphere, because no changes in the energy metabolism had been observed in the opposite hemisphere for 3 h after ligation.

When recirculation was initiated 45–90 min after the induction of ischemia, the ^{31}P-NMR spectrum returned to the preischemic state within 1 h. Our preliminary

Fig. 4. Relaxation rates versus water content in three kinds of brain edema: cold-induced edema in rats; triethyl-tin (TET)-induced edema in rats; and ischemic brain edema in Mongolian gerbils

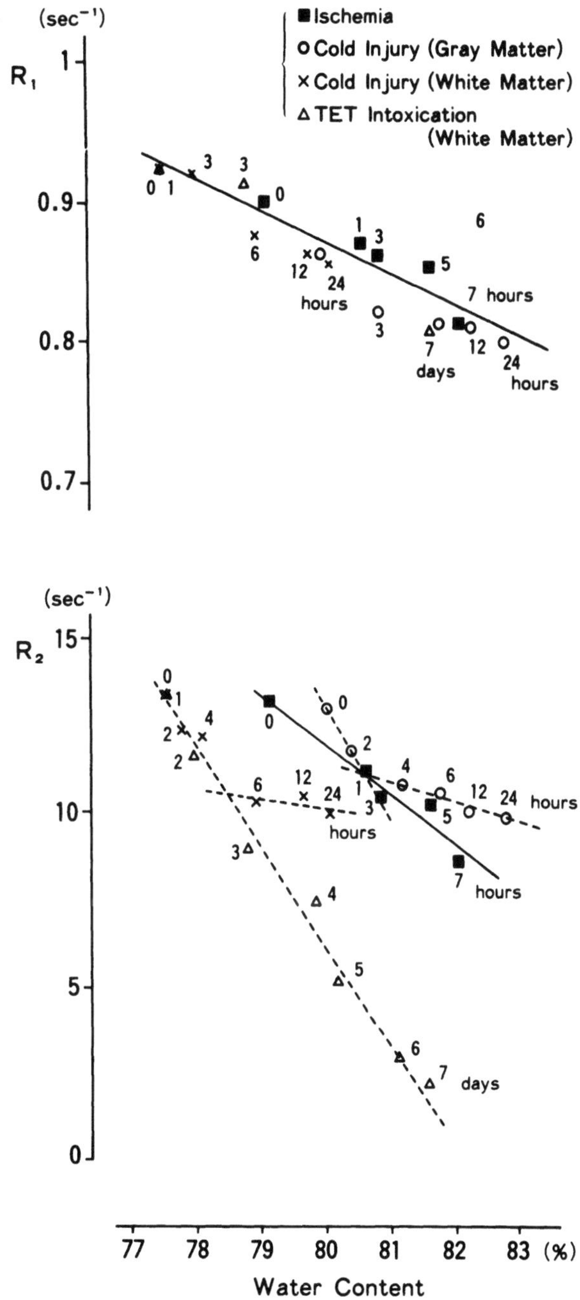

examination showed recovery of the ³¹P-NMR spectrum even after a 3-h period of ischemia. Thus, the reversibility of the energy metabolism was better in this model than in the diffuse ischemic model [7, 8].

In this model, there were also variations in the time course of the ³¹P-NMR spectrum changes during the early ischemic period (Fig. 2b, Fig. 3b). However, it reached a Pi-dominant pattern (Fig. 2c, Fig. 3c), the one reflecting the most pronounced changes in the spectrum, within 40 min after ligation in all cases examined. The lack of uniformity in this model was also demonstrated by the proton relaxation times measured [1]. The T_1 and T_2 values after carotid ligation showed a wide standard deviation in comparison with other brain edema models previously reported [3, 6]. In the time course of T_2 values, all cases showed prolongation 1 h after ligation, when the changes in the ^{31}P-NMR spectrum had already occurred. On the basis of this NMR experiment with two nuclei, the following mechanism was postulated for the occurrence of ischemic brain edema: When cerebral ischemia was induced the cerebral energy metabolism was initially disturbed; then cell damage occurred; and finally ischemic brain edema arose due to a change in cell permeability.

We were thus able to prove that the NMR method with two nuclei is useful for investigation of the changes in the state of water molecules and in the energy metabolism throughout the course of cerebral ischemia.

Summary

The pathophysiology of cerebral ischemia and ischemic brain edema was investigated by using multinuclear magnetic resonance. The state of water molecules in the ischemic brain was studied by measuring the proton relaxation times with ^{1}H-NMR, and the in vivo energy metabolism in the ischemic and recirculated brain was studied with the aid of ^{31}P-NMR. Experimental cerebral ischemia was induced in 162 Mongolian gerbils by ligation of the unilateral common carotid artery. In vitro longitudinal relaxation time (T_1) and transverse relaxation time (T_2) in the ischemic brain were measured sequentially with a pulse FT-NMR spectrometer (PFT-100. JEOL). In the normal brain, T_1 and T_2 were about 1107 ms and 76.2 ms respectively. Within 1 h after ischemia was induced, both T_1 and T_2 began to become prolonged, and they had maximum values of 1210 ms and 117.7 ms, respectively, after 7 h. T_2 had two components from an early stage of ischemia. The in vivo ^{31}P-NMR spectrum was measured sequentially in the ischemic and recirculated brain in the living gerbil by the surface coil method (FX-270, JEOL). After ischemia was induced, ATP and PCr decreased and Pi increased rapidly on the ischemic hemisphere. When recirculation was initiated 45–90 min after ischemia the ^{31}P-NMR spectrum returned to the preischemic state within 1 h. There were no changes in the spectrum in the opposite hemisphere.

We were thus able to demonstrate the changes in the state of water molecules and the energy metabolism throughout the course of cerebral ischemia by both ^{1}H-NMR and ^{31}P-NMR. These methods give us a new view of the pathophysiology of ischemic brain edema.

References

1. Buonanno FS, Pykett IL, Brady TJ, Vielma J, Burt CT, Goldman MR, Hinshaw WS, Pohost GM, Kistler JP (1983) Proton NMR imaging in experimental ischemic infarction. Stroke 14:178–184
2. Farrar TC, Becker ED (1971) Pulse and Fourier transform NMR: Induction to theory and methods. Academic, New York, pp 18–33

3. Hirakawa K, Naruse S, Horikawa Y, Tanaka C, Nishikawa H (1983) Proton NMR study on brain edema. In: Go KG, Baethmann A (eds) Recent progress in the study and therapy of brain edema. Plenum, New York
4. Ito U, Ohno K, Nakamura R, Suganuma R, Inaba Y (1979) Brain edema during ischemia and after restoration of blood flow. Measurement of water, sodium, potassium content and plasma protein permeability. Stroke 10:542–547
5. McGraw CP (1977) Experimental cerebral infarction. Effects of pentobarbital in Mongolian gerbils. Arch Neurol 34:334–336
6. Naruse S, Horikawa Y, Tanaka C, Hirakawa K, Nishikawa H, Yoshizaki K (1982) Proton nuclear magnetic resonance studies on brain edema. J Neurosurg 56:747–752
7. Naruse S, Takada S, Koizuka I, Watari H (1983) In vivo ^{31}P-NMR studies on experimental cerebral infarction. Jpn J Physiol 23:19–24
8. Naruse S, Horikawa Y, Tanaka C, Hirakawa K, Nishikawa H, Watari H (1984) In vivo measurement of energy metabolism and the concomitant monitoring of electroencephalogram in experimental cerebral ischemia. Brain Res 296:370–372

An Experimental Model of Cerebral Infarction Produced by Silicone Cylinder Embolization in Normotensive and Hypertensive Rat

K. OHTA [1], Y. OKADA, T. SHIMA, and T. UOZUMI

Key words: Cerebral infarction, embolization, spontaneously hypertensive rat

Introduction

We have produced a new experimental model of cerebral infarction in the rat by a silicone cylinder embolization method. The purpose of this report is to present the clinicopathologic changes in normotensive rat (NTR) and spontaneously hypertensive rat (SHR) [6] subjected to main cerebrovascular occlusion effected by silicone cylinder embolization.

Materials and Methods

Fifty-seven male NTRs and 38 male SHRs aged 20–23 weeks were used. The mean systolic blood pressure recorded by the tail pulse method was approximately 100 mmHg in NTRs and 200 mmHg in SHRs. The embolus was made by molding the silicone rubber (Xanthropren Plus, Bayer) with a catalyst into an elastic tube and cutting it into 1-mm lengths. Three types of emboluses, 300, 400, and 500 μm in diameter, were made. Under halothane anesthesia, the left common, internal, and external carotid arteries and the pterygopalatine artery were exposed. The pterygopalatine artery was clipped at its origin. Elastic tubing containing a silicone cylinder was inserted into the internal carotid artery from the external carotid artery. The silicone cylinder was injected into the internal carotid artery with 0.05 ml saline. The short- and long-term neurologic deficits and histological and microangiographic changes were observed. The neurologic deficits were evaluated with reference to our neurologic evaluation scores. After death or sacrifice of the animals the occluded sites were checked. The brain was fixed in 10% formalin solution. Coronal sections were prepared for macroscopic examination. They were embedded in paraffin and sectioned for H & E staining. Contact microangiograms were prepared according to the method reported by Okada [5].

[1] Department of Neurosurgery, Chugoku Rosai Hospital, Hiro 1477, Kure, Japan

Results

Segmental occlusion of the main cerebral arterial trunk was produced in more than 90% (53 of 57 NTRs and 35 of 38 SHRs) of animals (Fig. 1).

The occluded sites could be classified into four groups: proximal portion of the internal carotid artery (ICp), internal carotid bifurcation (ICb), main trunk of the anterior cerebral artery (A_1), and main trunk of the middle cerebral artery (M_1) (Fig. 2). The occluded site was determined by the diameter of the embolus used in each case.

The animals with emboli in the intracranial artery were found to have some neurologic deficits, such as hemiparesis and forced circling. Those with emboli in the ICb had the most serious neurologic deficits, which became progressively worse. Comparison of NTRs and SHRs revealed that the morbidity and mortality were higher in SHRs than in NTRs.

The coronal sections of brains taken from SHRs with emboli in the ICb at 2 days after embolization are shown in Fig. 3.

The cortex of the middle cerebral artery territory and the basal ganglia were affected. Trypan blue exudation was observed both at an earlier stage and in larger

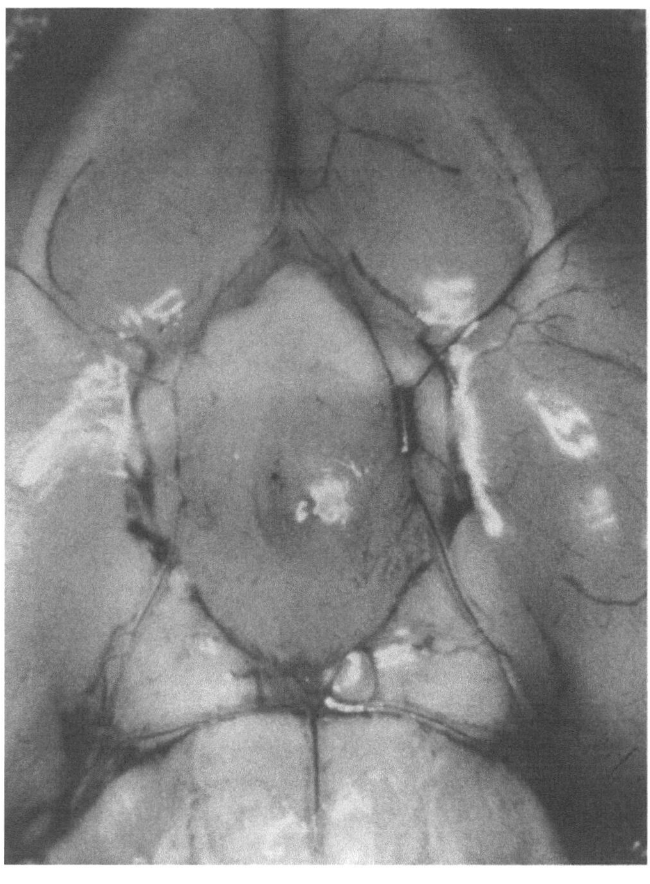

Fig. 1. The ventral surface of rat brain at 2 h after embolization: the embolus lodged in the internal carotid artery (*arrow*)

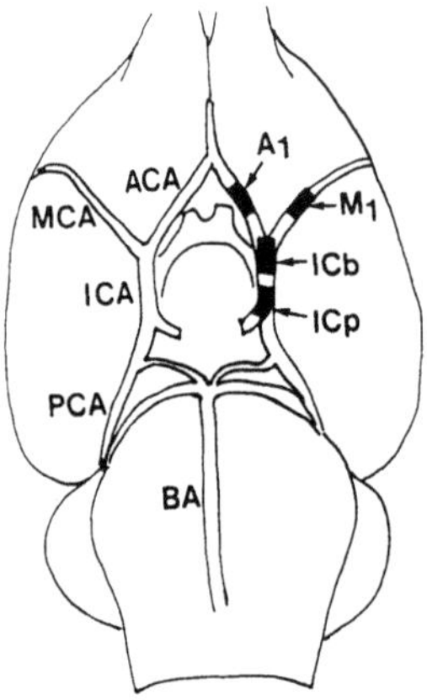

NTR

occluded site \ embolus size	400μ × 1mm	500μ × 1mm
ICp	1 (2%)	0
ICb	10 (25%)	13 (100%)
A1	26 (65%)	0
M1	3 (8%)	0

SHR

occluded site \ embolus size	300μ × 1mm	400μ × 1mm
ICp	2 (14%)	7 (33%)
ICb	12 (86%)	14 (67%)
A1	0	0
M1	0	0

Fig. 2. Relationship between size of embolus and occluded site: *ICA*, internal carotid artery; *ACA*, anterior cerebral artery; *MCA*, middle cerebral artery; *PCA*, posterior cerebral artery; *BA*, basilar artery; *TCp*, proximal portion of internal carotid artery; *ICb*, internal carotid bifurcation; A_1, main trunk of anterior cerebral artery; M_1, main trunk of middle cerebral artery

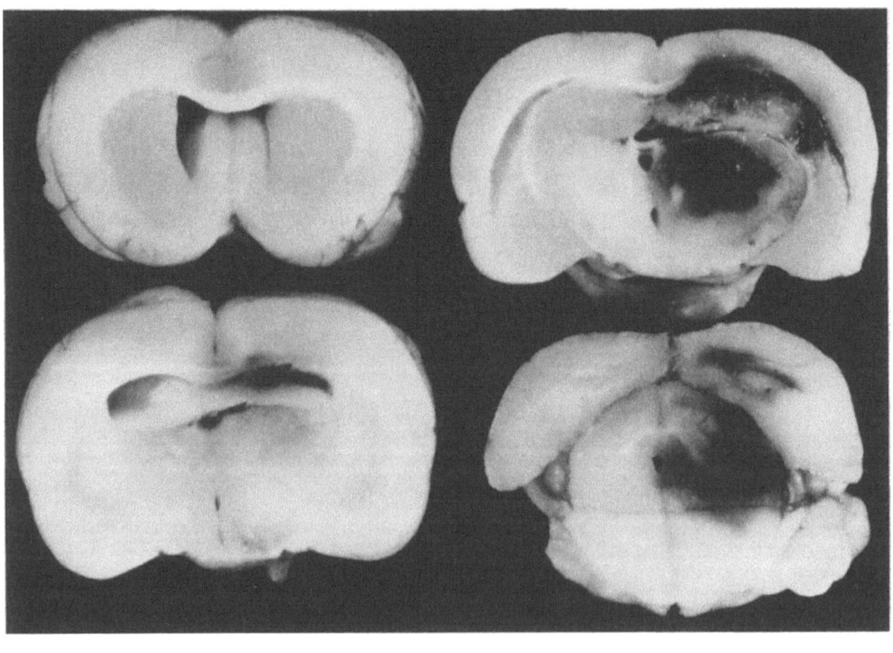

Fig. 3. Coronal sections of SHR brain with embolus in ICb at 2 days after embolization. Infarctions were produced deep in the cerebrum. Note trypan blue exudation

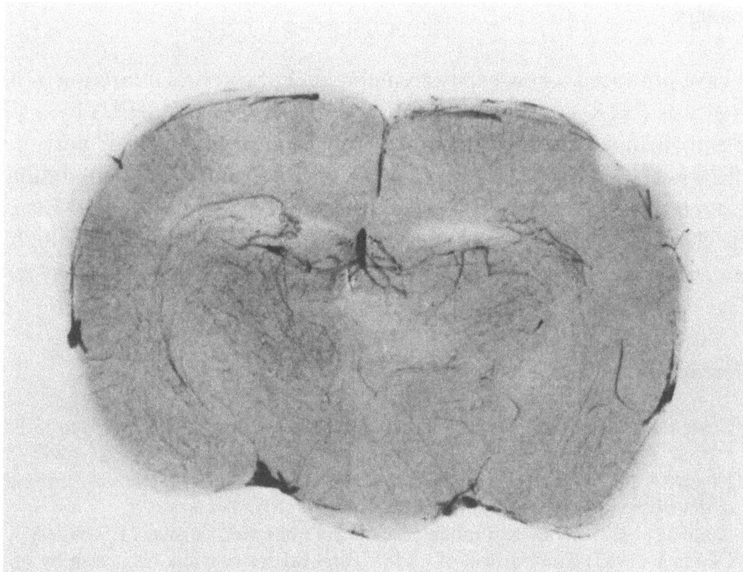

Fig. 4. Microangiogram of SHR with embolus in ICb at 2 h after embolization. Perceptible brain swelling with midline shift and poor filling areas deep in the affected cerebrum

areas in SHRs than in NTRs. The hypothalamus, thalamus, hippocampus, and parietotemporal cortex were involved in animals with emboli in the ICb. The anterior hypothalamus and caudate putamen were involved when emboli occluded the A_1.

The microangiogram demonstrated poor filling of the deep cerebrum, with a midline shift in the acute stage (Fig. 4). These findings were more prominent in SHR than in NTR.

Discussion

Many experimental rat models of cerebral ischemia and infarction have been reported [1–4, 7–9], such as MCA ligation [9] and blood clot embolization [4]. But these models have several disadvantages. For example, MCA ligation requires craniotomy, and blood clot microembolization [3] produces multifocal occlusion, and not necessarily occlusion of a preselected artery. With our method, occlusion was confined to definite arterial sections dependent on the size of embolus, without craniotomy.

The SHR, originally bred by Okamoto [6], is well known as a reliable experimental model of hypertension. The results of our experiment suggest that hypertensive insults in the rat brain lead to greater susceptibility to cerebral ischemia and to more severe sequelae of the ischemic period [8, 10].

Our highly reproducible embolization method yields a model that would be useful for studies of cerebral infarction and ischemia closely related to hypertension [10].

Summary

We have produced a new experimental model of cerebral infarction in normotensive Wistar rats (NTRs) and spontaneously hypertensive rat (SHRs) by a silicone cylinder embolization method. Segmental occlusion of the anterior part of the circle of Willis was achieved in a high proportion of cases, which led to infarction deep inside the cerebrum with major neurologic deficits in both strains of rats. The clinicopathologic changes in SHRs were more serious than those in NTR. Our highly reproducible method yields a model of cerebral infarction closely related to hypertension.

References

1. Coyle P (1982) Middle cerebral artery occlusion in the young rat. Stroke 13:855–859
2. Furlow T (1982) Experimental air embolism of the rat brain. Stroke 13:847–852
3. Kogure K (1974) Energy metabolism and water content in rat brain during the early stage of development of cerebral infarction. Brain 97:103–114
4. Kudo M (1982) An animal model of cerebral infarction. Stroke 13:505–508
5. Okada Y (1983) Comparison of middle cerebral artery trunk occlusion by silicone cylinder embolization and trapping. J Neurosurg 58:492–499
6. Okamoto K (1963) Development of a strain of spontaneously hypertensive rats. Jap Circ J 27:282–293
7. Pulsinelli WA (1979) A new model of bilateral hemispheric ischemia in the unanesthetized rat. Stroke 10:267–272
8. Shima T (1979) Cerebral ischemia due to bilateral common carotid artery ligation in SHR. Brain Nerve 31:1235–1243
9. Tamura A (1981) Focal cerebral ischemia in the rat. J Cereb Blood Flow Metab 1:53–60
10. Yamori Y (1976) Hypertension as an important factor for cerebrovascular atherogenesis in rats. Stroke 7:120–125

Peritumoral Edema: Analysis of CT Scan and Dynamic CT Scan *

Y. Ikeda [1] and S. Nakazawa

Key words: Brain tumor, cerebral edema, CT scan, dynamic CT scan, biogenic amines

Introduction

Peritumoral edema, a common occurrence in patients with malignant gliomas and meningiomas, is a major cause of mortality [9]. However, the causative mechanism of peritumoral edema has yet to be clarified. Peritumoral hypodense areas on CT scan have generally been interpreted as cerebral edema [1]. The purpose of this study was to assess clinical features of peritumoral edemas by CT scan and dynamic CT scan. It is possible that the tumors create some biochemical factors that increase the production of peritumoral edema [8]. We also used high-performance liquid chromatography with electrochemical detection to examine the tissue concentrations of biogenic amines in brain tumors.

Materials and Methods

Seventy patients with brain tumors (34 glioblastomas, 21 meningiomas, and 15 metastatic tumors) were examined by CT scan with and without contrast medium infusion, followed by postoperative histological verification in all cases. Peritumoral edema as seen in the CT scan was classified into four grades according to the ratio of the largest diameter of tumor to the size of the zone of edema [5]. Regional circulation and the extent of peritumoral edema were evaluated by dynamic CT scan. Dynamic CT consisted of performing several rapid sequential scans after a bolus IV injection of 50 ml contrast medium (65% Angiografin) using a GE CT/T 8800 scanner [4]. Serial fluorescein (0.5%, 10 ml) microangiography was performed after blood-brain barrier disruption by intracarotid infusion of mannitol (4 ml/kg, 1–1.5 ml/s) [6, 7]. The tissue concentrations of biogenic amines in brain tumors were measured by high-performance liquid chromatography (YANACO L-2000) with electrochemical detection (YANACO VMD 101) [3].

---

* This study has already been published in *Brain and Nerve* 36(11):1055–1062 (1984) and appears here by permission of Igaku-Shoin Ltd., Tokyo.

[1] Dept. of Neurosurgery, Nippon Medical School, 1-1-5 Sendagi, Bunkyo-ku, Tokyo 113, Japan

Results

Moderate or severe peritumoral edema (grade II or III) was seen with 25 of 34 glioblastomas and with all 15 metastatic tumors. However, 16 of 21 meningiomas demonstrated mild peritumoral edema (grade 0 or I). The grade of peritumoral edema was closely related to the degree of malignancy of the brain tumors. Of 9 glioblastomas that were surrounded by mild edema (grade I), 8 incorporated large cystic formations, which seemed to serve as buffers against exertion of a compression mechanism by brain tumors. The grade of peritumoral edema was also related to the location of the tumor and to venous involvement [2] (Table 1).

Intracarotid mannitol infusions produced a definite increase in contrast enhancement in one glioblastoma. Whether this phenomenon reflects an extravasation of contrast medium or the invasion of the tumor is not clear (Fig. 1).

In the case of glioblastoma, after mannitol infusion fluorescein sodium perfusion was increased with the enlargement of the venules and extravasation of fluorescein sodium (Fig. 2).

Table 1. Peritumoral edema in the three different types of tumor

Tumor type	Grade				Total cases
	0	I	II	III	
Glioblastoma	0	9	14	11	34
Meningioma	6	10	2	3	21
Metastatic tumor	0	0	5	10	15

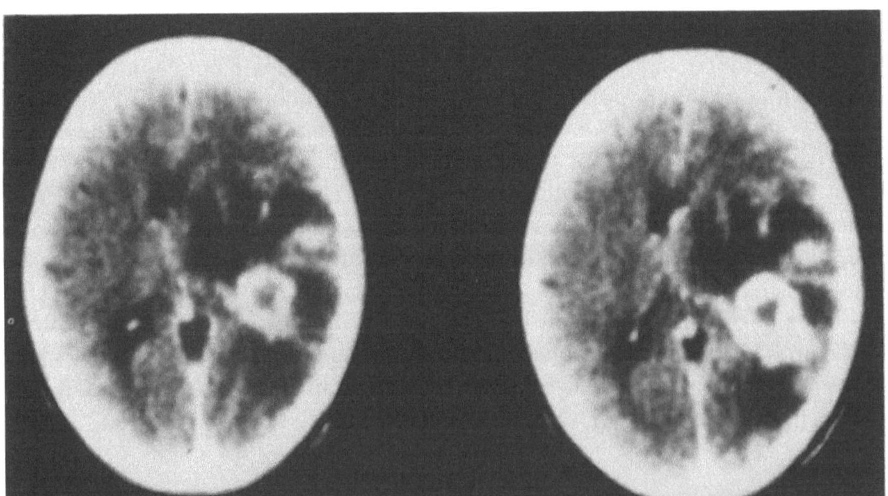

Fig. 1. CT scan of a glioblastoma before (*left*) and after (*right*) infusion of mannitol into the right internal carotid artery

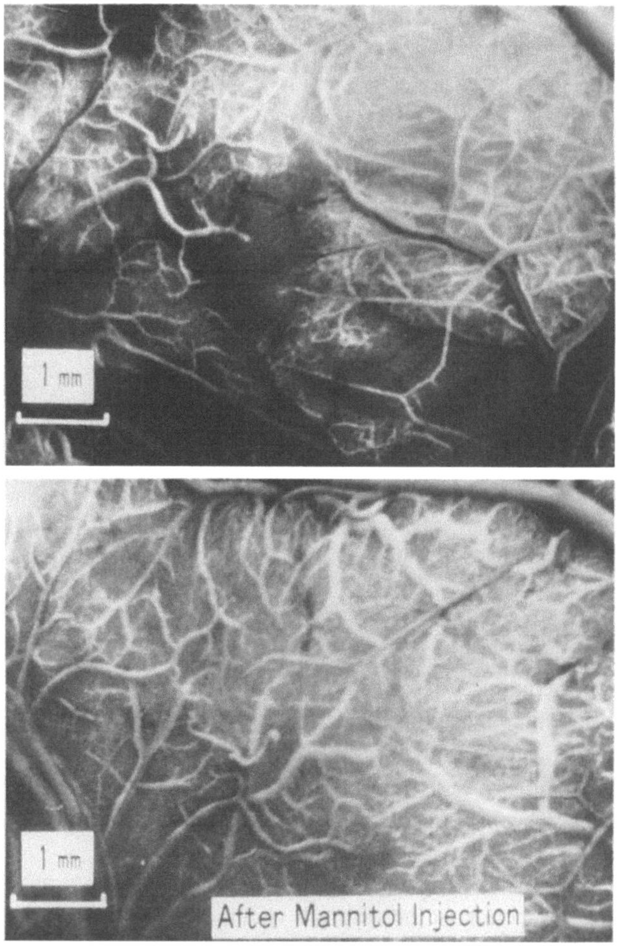

Fig. 2. Serial fluorescein microangiography of tumor surface (glioblastoma) before and after administration of mannitol

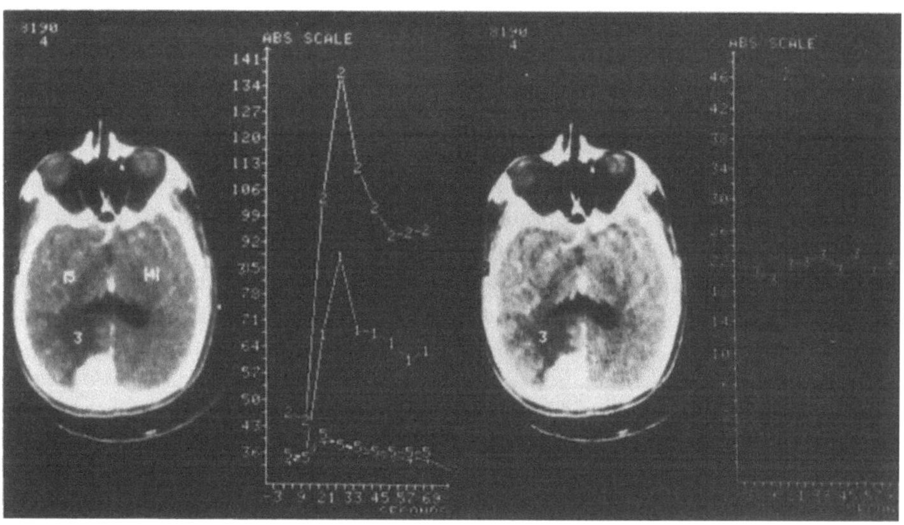

Fig. 3. Dynamic CT scan in a case of convexity meningioma (grade II)

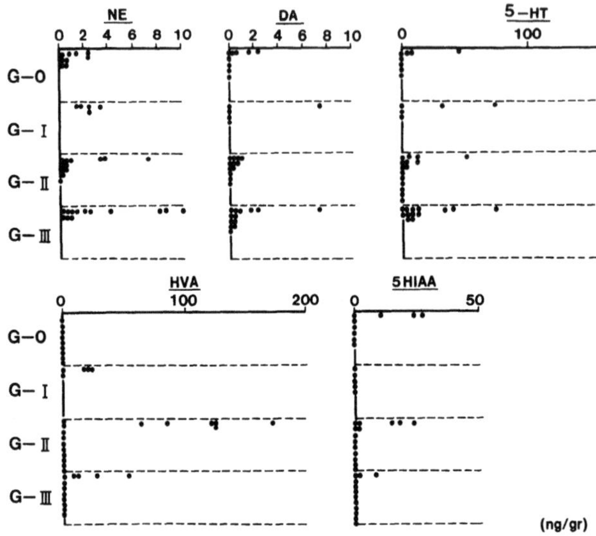

Fig. 4. Degree of peritumoral edema and biogenic amines in brain tumor tissue. *G*, grade

In dynamic CT scan, the CT number-time curve yielded several parameters. The peak value was considered to be related to the blood volume of the region of interest. A common finding was that the peak value was lower in the peritumoral edematous area than in the tumor and the normal region of the brain (Fig. 3). Clinical application of dynamic CT scan may be useful to evaluate the regional circulation and the extent of peritumoral edema.

Some studies [6, 10] have provided evidence that monoamines might play a role during the formation of brain edema. This study has provided no clear indications that biogenic amines as neurotransmitters are closely associated with the production of peritumoral edema (Fig. 4).

Summary

The clinical features of peritumoral edema were assessed by CT scan and dynamic CT scan in 70 patients with supratentorial brain tumors. Peritumoral edema was classified into four types by grade, and the grade was closely related to degree of malignancy, site, presence and extent of cystic formation, and venous involvement of the tumors. Serial fluorescein microangiography was performed after blood-brain barrier disruption by intracarotid infusion of mannitol in the patients with malignant gliomas. Regional circulation and the extent of peritumoral edema were evaluated by dynamic CT scan. Very low peak values were obtained in each case with peritumoral edema. Tissue concentration of biogenic amines in brain tumors were measured by high-performance liquid chromatography with electrochemical detection. This study has provided no clear evidence that biogenic amines as neurotransmitters are closely associated with the production of peritumoral edema.

References

1. Drayer BP, Rosenbaum AE (1979) Brain edema defined by cranial computed tomography. J Comput Assist Tomogr 3:317–323
2. Fine M, Brazis P, Palacios E, Neri G (1980) CT of sphenoid wing meningiomas: tumor location related to distal edema. Surg Neurol 13:385–390
3. Ikeda Y, Nakazawa S (1984) Tissue concentrations of biogenic amines in brain tumors and their distribution. Neurol Surg 12:787–793
4. Nakagomi T, Takakura K (1984) Dynamic computed tomography of brain tumor. Brain Nerve 36:1031–1040
5. Oi S, Wetzel N, Kim KS (1979) Gliomas in computerized axial tomography – Correlation with tumor malignancy in 100 cases. Neurol Surg 7:759–763
6. Osterholm JL, Bell J, Meyer R, Pyenson J (1969) Experimental effects of free serotonin on the brain and its relation to brain injury: III. Serotonin-induced cerebral edema. J Neurosurg 31:408–421
7. Rapoport SI (1970) Effect of concentrated solution on blood-brain barrier. Am J Physiol 219:270–274
8. Smith HP, Challa VR, Moody DA, Kelly DL (1981) Biological features of meningiomas that determine the production of cerebral edema. Neurosurgery 8:428–433
9. Tchang S, Scotti G, Terbrugge K, Melançon D, Belanger G, Milner G, Ethier R (1977) Computerized tomography as a possible aid to histological grading of supratentorial gliomas. J Neurosurg 46:735–739
10. Welch KMA, Meyer JS, Teraura T, Hashi K, Shinmaru S (1972) Ischemic anoxia and cerebral serotonin levels. J Neurol Sci 16:85–92

Influence of Peritumoral Edema on rCBF and on Cerebral Function: Analysis by Xenon-Enhanced CT and EEG Topography

T. Kawase[1], T. Ohira, H. Murakami, S. Toya, and H. Shiga

Key words: Brain tumor, cerebral edema, cerebral blood flow, electro-encephalography

Introduction

It is well known that perifocal edema is frequently associated with such brain tumors as meningiomas or metastatic tumors. However, it has not been definitively decided whether peritumoral edema affects the regional cerebral blood flow (rCBF) and/or the brain function. The aim of this study was to clarify these points by EEG topography and by tomographc measurements of rCBF.

Cases and Methods

This study included 12 patients with brain tumors (9 meningiomas and 3 metastatic tumors). There were six men and six women, with an age range of 27–67 years, and the diagnosis was by means of computed tomography (CT) and by surgery. Half of the patients were found to have marked peritumoral edema on CT, while the edema was minimal in the other six (Table 1). There was no significant difference in tumor size between the two groups. All patients were studied with EEG topography (Nissei Sangyo Co., Ltd). This system incorporates a microcomputer producing a two-dimensional display of equivalent potentials of EEG activities, which are defined as the square roots of the average power spectra over a given frequency band [2]. In six patients (cases 5–7, 9–11) the tomographic rCBF was measured by the xenon-enhanced CT method with GE CT/T 8800 scanners equipped with dynamic imaging capabilities. To ensure a reliable arterial enhancement curve, Teflon catheters were inserted into the cubital artery and vein and an arteriovenous shunt route was made through a phantom placed over the patient's head. Multiple CT slices of brain and of arterial blood in the phantom were thus obtained alternately by Shuttle's method [1] during 50% xenon inhalation.

---

[1] Department of Neurosurgery, School of Medicin, Keio University, 35 Shinanomachi, Shinjuku-ku, Tokyo 160, Japan

Table 1. Clinical data and EEG findings

Case no.	Patient	Site	Diagnosis	Tumor size (dia. in cm)	Edema	EEG	Clinical signs
1	K. N. (27 ♀)	Lt-F	Meningioma (meningotheliomatous)	1.0	–	Normal	None
2	K. I. (62 ♀)	Lt-P	Meningioma (transitional)	2.5	±	Normal	None
3	S. I. (46 ♀)	Rt-P	Meningioma (meningotheliomatous)	5.0	–	Normal	None (convulsive seizure)
4	M. H. (45 ♂)	Lt-P	Meningioma (fibroblastic)	5.0	±	Borderline	Rt sensory dist. (transient)
5	H. S. (44 ♂)	Lt-F	Meningioma (meningotheliomatous)	6.0	–	Normal	Rt-mild hpr
6	N. M. (42 ♂)	Bil-F	Meningioma (transitional)	8.0	±	Abnormal	Calculation ↓
7	M. S. (59 ♀)	Rt-F	Meningioma (vascular)	3.0	++	Abnormal	Lt-hpr Lt-hemianopsia
8	N. I. (67 ♀)	Rt-F · P	Meningioma (meningotheliomatous)	5.0	+	Abnormal	Lt-hpr
9	M. S. (55 ♀)	Lt-P	Meningioma (fibroblastic)	5.0	++	Abnormal	Calculation ↓
10	K. O. (56 ♂)	Lt-F	Metastatic (rectal cancer)	3.0	++	Abnormal	Aphasia, disorientation
11	M. E. (43 ♂)	Rt-F · P	Metastatic (lung cancer)	3.0	++	Abnormal	Lt-hpr (convulsive seizure)
12	K. I. (51 ♂)	Rt-T	Metastatic (lung cancer)	5.5	++	Abnormal	Lt-hpr hemianopsia

F, frontal; P, parietal; T, temporal; hpr, hemiparesis

Results

In patients with minimal peritumoral edema or none at all (cases 1–6), EEG changes were not conspicuous except in patient 6, who had a large meningioma. Regional CBF values around the tumor were not significantly altered by the tumor (Fig. 1), whereas EEG abnormality was conspicuous in all patients with peritumoral edema, in whom marked slowing was observed in the EEG (cases 7–12). Even in

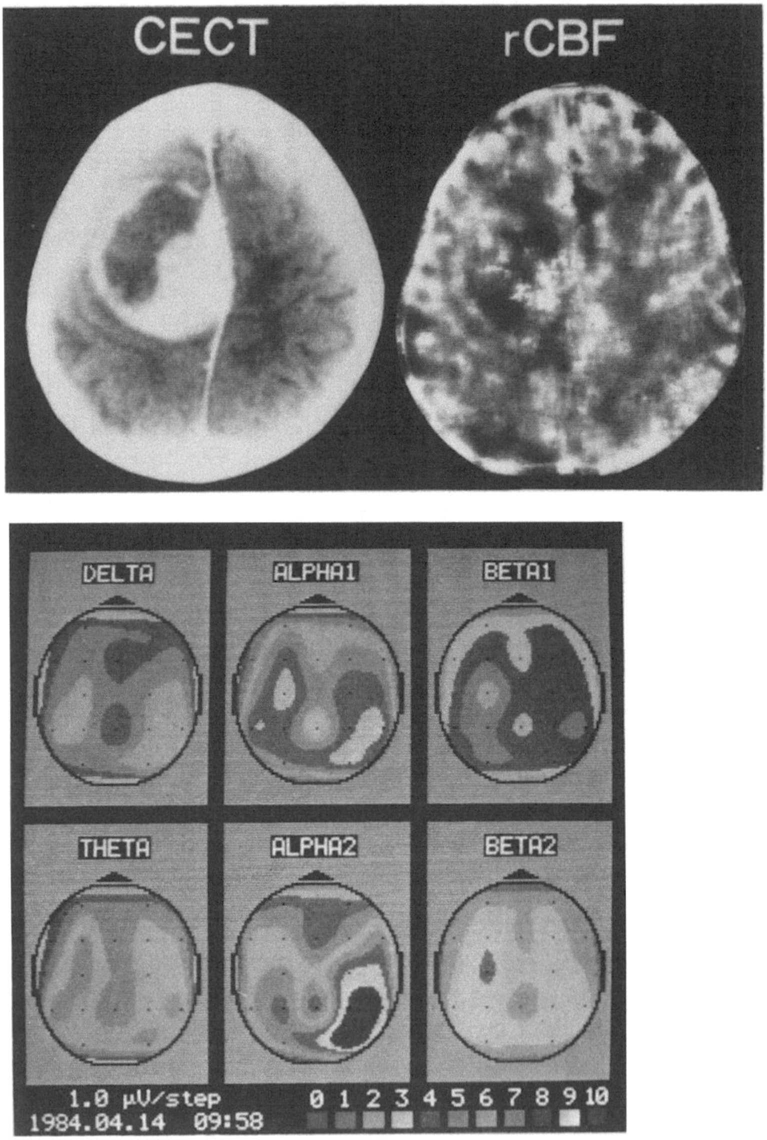

Fig. 1. Case 5: meningioma without peritumoral edema (after embolization). Changes in CBF and EEG were minimal

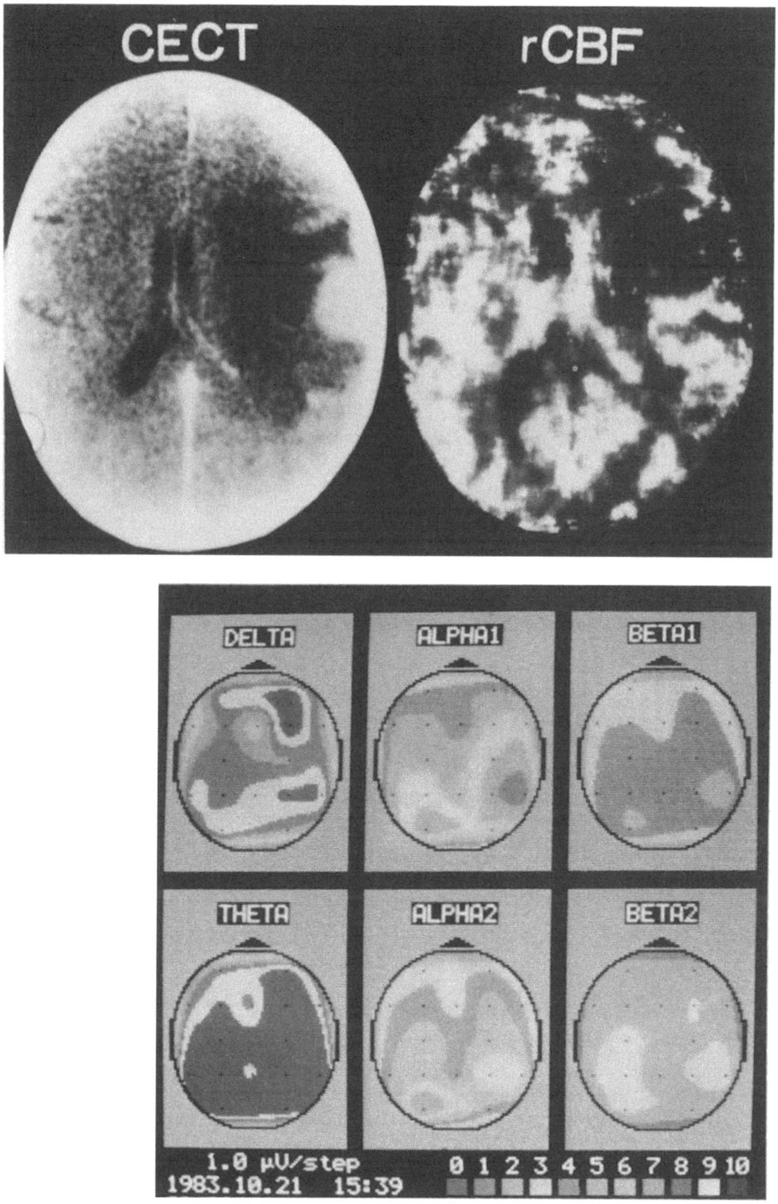

Fig. 2. Case 7: Meningioma with marked peritumoral edema. Values for CBF in the edematous zone are markedly lower than elsewhere, and hyperemic areas are present in the surrounding gray matter

the patient with a small meningioma, rCBF values were markedly reduced in the white matter, where the edema was present (Fig. 2). In contrast, hyperemic areas were observed in the gray matter around the perifocal edema. After removal of the tumor, these abnormalities of EEG and rCBF improved as the edema abated (Fig. 3).

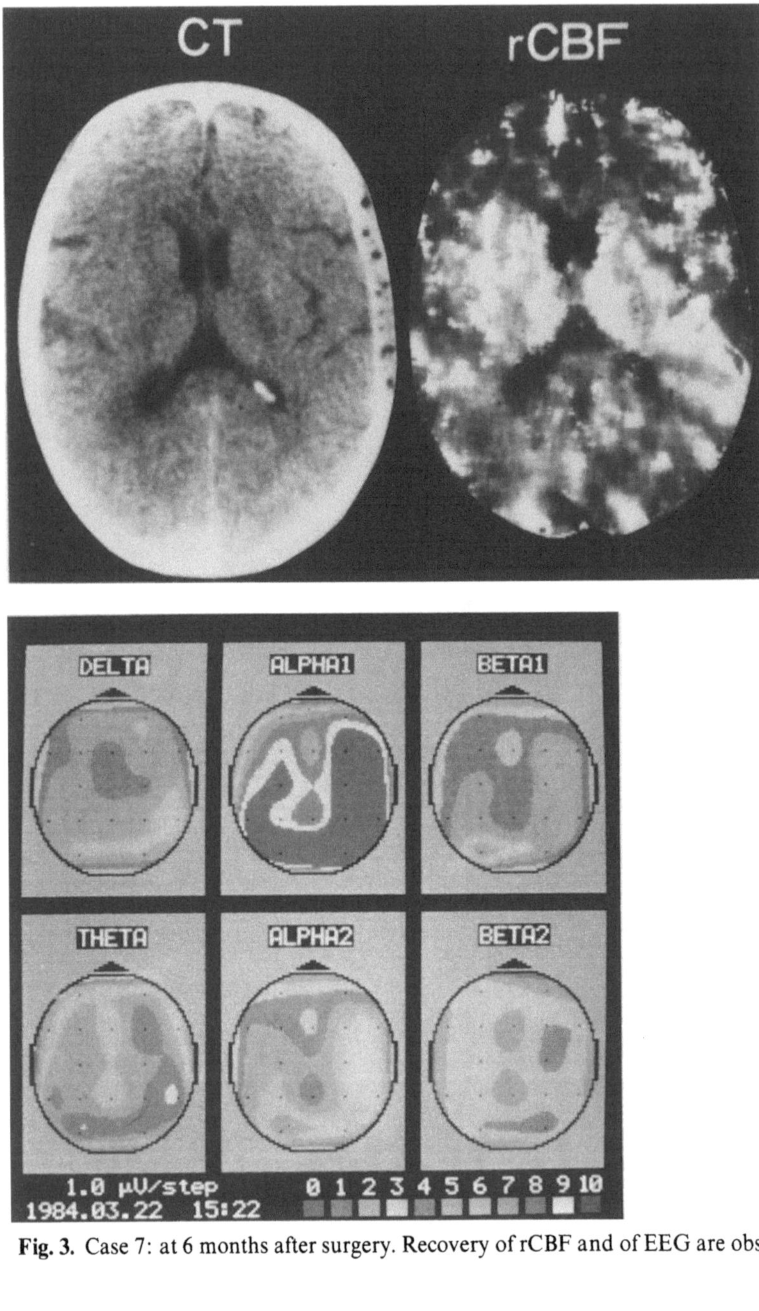

Fig. 3. Case 7: at 6 months after surgery. Recovery of rCBF and of EEG are observed

Discussion

The genetic mechanism of the perifocal edema has so far remained a mystery, but recent papers have speculated on the causation of the edema [4], and cerebral interstitial accumulation of water from the tumor has been suggested. Local reduction of rCBF corresponding to the spatial distribution of the edematous tissue was observed in our own tomographic rCBF study. It is presumed that the increase in interstitial pressure may cause a reduction of rCBF in the edematous tissue.

In functional observation of the patient with peritumoral edema, the size of the tumor may be another factor that influences the brain activity. When the tumor is large brain function may be reduced by direct compression from the tumor, as in case 6. However, overall the patients with peritumoral edema showed marked EEG abnormality even when the tumor was not so large, in contrast to the patients without edema. This observation may support the notion that the perifocal edema itself can reduce brain function. However, apparently perifocal edema itself does not always lead to a clinical neurologic deficit [3]. In our study, all the patients with edema had some neurologic deficits, but it was very difficult to estimate a relation between the degree of peritumoral edema and the neurologic symptoms, because quantitation of the symptoms is difficult. We presume the peritumoral edema had a marked influence on EEG activities, while affecting the neurologic symptoms only to a mild or subclinical extent. The recovery of EEG slowing and rCBF after removal of the tumor suggests that these functional reductions may be reversible without critical cell damage, such as is seen in the case of cerebral infarction.

Summary

Twelve patients, each with a meningioma or a metastatic brain tumor, were studied with tomographic measurements of rCBF by the xenon-enhanced CT method and EEG tomography. In patients with marked peritumoral edema demonstrated on CT, rCBF in the white matter was found to be uniformly reduced in the regions affected by edema. In contrast, hyperemic areas were observed in the gray matter around the perifocal edema. Hemispheric slowing in the EEG was conspicuous in these patients. The EEG abnormalities, however, were improved and localized after removal of the tumor, in keeping with subsidence of the edema. Such changes in rCBF and EEG were less evident in patients without peritumoral edema.

It is concluded that the evolution of peritumoral edema may result in a significant, but possibly reversible, effect on cerebral blood flow and on EEG activity in the course of brain tumors.

References

1. Karasawa J, Kuriyama Y, Kikuchi H, Sawada T, Kozuka T, Naito H, Sakashita Y, Kuro M (1983) Simultaneous measurement of multi-level 1-CBF by using xenon and a CT scanner – Development of the Shuttle method. Prog CT 5:37–44
2. Nagata K, Mizukami M, Araki G, Kawasa T, Hirano M (1982) Topographic electroencephalographic study of cerebral infarction using computed mapping of the EEG. J Cereb Blood Flow Metab 2:79–88
3. Penn RD (1980) Cerebral edema and neurological function in human beings. Neurosurgery 6:249–254
4. Philippon J, Foncin JF, Grob R, Srour A, Poisson M, Pertuiset BF (1984) Cerebral edema associated with meningiomas: possible role of a secretory-excretory phenomenon. Neurosurgery 14:295–301

Brain Edema and Neurologic Function

T. NAKAMURA [1], K. OHATA, K. KUROSE, Y. INOUE, K. TSUDA, K. TANAKA,
Y. MATSUOKA, M. MAEDA, Y. FU, and S. NISHIMURA

Key words: Cerebral edema, neurological function, water content, specific gravity, ICP

Introduction

Massive brain edema increases intracranial pressure (ICP) and sometimes leads to herniation, which causes severe neurologic deficits. It is still obscure whether increased tissue water content, which is the primary phenomenon of edema, itself leads to neurologic deficits. In this experimental study the assumption that brain edema results in neurologic deficits was investigated in the direct infusion model. The relationship between water content and CT number was also investigated in this model.

Materials and Methods

Adult cats ($n=8$) were anesthetized with pentobarbital (20 mg/kg IP), intubated and ventilated spontaneously. Infusion edema was produced by infusing 0.5 ml serum through a 25-gage needle inserted into the white matter beneath the left sensorimotor area according to stereotaxic coordinates (19AP, 9LAT, 19V) using a motorized syringe pump (Fig. 1). When the animals had completely recovered from the anesthetic (24–48 h after the infusion), their neurologic status was checked with reference to a modification of the five-point ordinal scale [1] originally developed by Tarlov. Then they were anesthetized again with pentobarbital (30 mg/kg IP) and a CT scan (SOMATOM 2) was performed.

After this, ICP and the pressure/volume index (PVI) [2] were measured, and the animals were then sacrificed for measurement of the water content of white matter by the gravimetric method [3].

[1] Dept. of Neurosurgery, Osaka City University, Medical School, 1-5-7 Asahi-machi, Abeno-ku, Osaka 545, Japan

Results

The neurologic status appeared to be unimpaired; all cats had normal motor function (score 5) and could walk and run normally.

The CT scan showed a conspicuous low-density area in the left frontal lobe in all cats, and the average CT number on the edematous side was 24.6 ± 0.6 (mean $\pm$ SE) (control side 35.1 ± 1.0) (Fig. 2).

ICP and PVI were measured in four cats. The opening pressure was 9.1 ± 1.2 mmHg (mean $\pm$ SD) and PVI was 1.26 ± 0.11 ml (mean $\pm$ SE). Both these were within the normal ranges.

When the brain surface was exposed it was observed that the gyrus was flattened at the sensorimotor area. The water content on the edematous side was 79.2 ± 0.7 g H_2O/g tissue (mean $\pm$ SE) (control 67.0 ± 0.4) (Table 1).

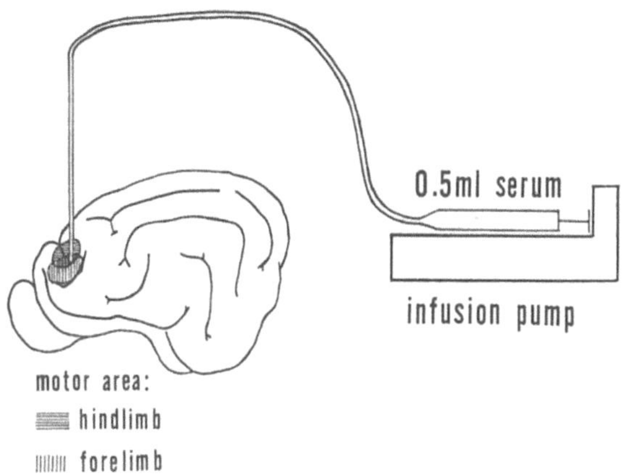

Fig. 1. Experimental model

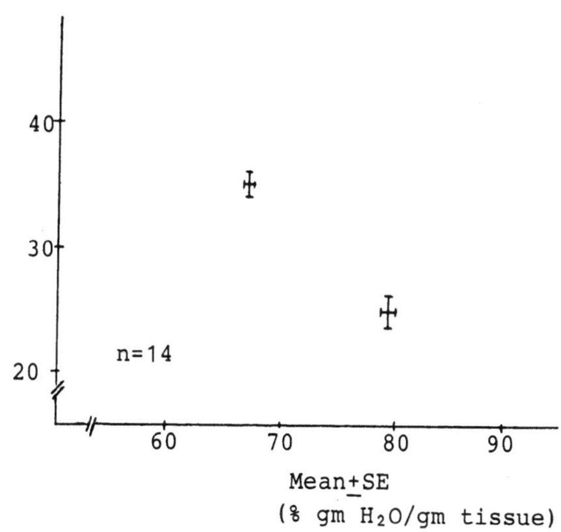

Fig. 2. Water content vs CT number

Table 1. Water content in white matter

No.	E	C
1	79.6	67.0
2	83.5	65.3
3	77.2	67.2
4	78.2	66.2
5	77.9	67.1
6	79.0	69.4
7	79.9	67.1
8	78.6	66.5
$n=8$	79.2±0.7	67.0±0.4

E, edematous side; C, control side (means ±SEM, %g H_2O/g tissue)

Discussion

Edema is often thought to be a reason for neurologic dysfunction. But it was not clear whether the cause of dysfunction is due to increased water content per se or due to the secondary changes produced by edema, such as increased ICP, shifts in neural tissue, and decreased CBF.

Penn reported three patients who had no apparent neurologic dysfunction and concluded that edema did not affect neural activity [5]. The water content in these cases was 72, 74, and 75%g H_2O/g tissue. In a clinical study, it is difficult to find constant edema at the same region as seems to be connected with neurologic function. With the direct infusion model constant edema can be induced in any region. In this experiment all cats had normal motor function, but the water content in the white matter just beneath the sensorimotor area was up to 79.2%g H_2O/g tissue. The values for ICP and PVI were within the normal ranges, and the edema produced in this model seemed to have no remarkable mass effect. With this infusion model, Tanaka et al. [6] observed changes in CBF and somatosensory evoked potential (SEP) after the infusion of 0.5 ml serum and reported a 50% reduction in the white matter blood flow (CBFw) with no latency change in SEP. The water content stays at almost the same level for 3 days after infusion [4]. Therefore, if the decrease in CBF is proportional to the water content there must have been a 50% reduction in CBFw when cat neurologic functions were checked in this experiment. It is concluded that brain edema with about 80%g H_2O/g tissue in the white matter does not directly cause neurologic deficits.

Summary

The assumption that brain edema results in neurologic deficits was investigated. The direct serum infusion model (0.15 ml/h) was used, and edema was produced in the white matter beneath the sensorimotor area in cats. When the cats ($n=8$) recovered from the anesthetic, all of them could walk around and run normally. The water content in the white matter according to the gravimetric method was 79.2 ± 0.7 (mean $\pm$ SE) %g H_2O/g tissue (control side 67.0 ± 0.4). It is concluded that brain edema below the level of 79.2%g H_2O/g tissue does not itself cause any neurologic deficits.

References

1. Faden AI, Jacobs TP, Holaday JW (1981) Thyrotropin-releasing hormone improves neurologic recovery after spinal trauma in cats. N Engl J Med 305:1063–1067
2. Marmarou A, Shulman K, Lamorgese J (1975) Compartmental analysis of compliance and outflow resistance of the cerebrospinal fluid system. J Neurosurg 43:523–534
3. Marmarou A, Poll W, Shulman K, Bhagavan H (1978) A simple gravimetric technique for measurement of cerebral edema. J Neurosurg 49:530–537
4. Marmarou A, Tanaka K, Shulman K (1982) The brain response to infusion edema: dynamics of fluid resolution. In: Hartmann A, Brock M (eds) Treatment of cerebral edema. Springer, Berlin Heidelberg New York, pp 11–18
5. Penn RD (1980) Cerebral edema and neurological function in human beings. Neurosurgery 6(3):249–254
6. Tanaka K, Marmarou A, Shulman K (1981) Regional cerebral blood flow changes associated with direct infusion edema. J Cereb Blood Flow Metab 1 [Suppl 1]:s156–157

Hydro-Hemodynamics in Areas of Periventricular Edema in Normal-Pressure Hydrocephalus

N. TAMAKI[1], N. KOJIMA, T. NAGASHIMA, T. SHIRAKUNI, and S. MATSUMOTO

Key words: Normal-pressure hydrocephalus, periventricular lucency, computed tomography (CT), dynamic CT, hydro-hemodynamics

Introduction

Since the advent of the computed tomography (CT) scanner as a revolutionary diagnostic tool for diseases of the central nervous system, the pathogenesis of many such diseases has been clarified; however, hitherto unknown pathologic conditions have been seen, and it seems this is a problem that should be resolved early. Periventricular lucency in the CT scans of patients with hydrocephalus is one of the pathologic conditions newly recognized since the beginning of the CT era. The pathogenesis of periventricular lucency on CT scans remains obscure.

Clinical Materials and Methods

Twenty-two patients with suspected normal pressure hydrocephalus (NPH) were included in this study. These patients were classified into two groups: (a) Patients with true NPH, who responded to cerebrospinal fluid (CSF) shunting; and (b) patients with false NPH, who did not respond to shunt placement. CT attenuation values were measured in the frontal white matter corresponding to the area of periventricular edema and in the frontal gray matter. The measurements were done three times: preoperatively, and at 1–3 weeks (average: 1.5 weeks) and 4–8 weeks (average: 4.4 weeks) after shunting.

Dynamic CT studies were also performed on three occasions, after measurement of the CT attenuation values. A series of 7 rapid scans and a total of 14 segmented scans were obtained in 40.3 s beginning 0.5 s after injection of 40 ml 65% iodized contrast medium. The contrast material was injected within 4 s by means of an auto-injector, through an 18-gage catheter introduced into a cubital vein. Circulation time, defined as the difference between the arrival time of contrast medium and the center of gravity of the CT density-time curve, was measured in the region of periventricular edema and in the frontal gray matter.

---

[1] Dept. of Neurosurgery, Kobe University School of Medicine, 5-1 Kusunoki-cho 7-chome, Chuo-ku, Kobe 650, Japan

Results

Change in CT Attenuation Values and Circulation Times in Patients with True NPH

CT attenuation values of the periventricular white matter corresponding to the area of periventricular edema in patients with true NPH were significantly low compared with those in normal subjects (Fig. 1, left). However, there was no significant difference in CT attenuation values of the frontal gray matter between the patients with true NPH and normal controls (Fig. 1, right).

CT attenuation values of the periventricular white matter increased significantly 4 weeks after shunt placement (Fig. 2, left), although there was no difference between pre- and postoperative CT attenuation values of the frontal gray matter (Fig. 2, right).

Thus, there was an improvement of hydrodynamics in the periventricular edematous area in patients with true NPH after shunt placement. However, there was no change of hydrodynamics in the frontal gray matter.

Circulation times of the periventricular white matter in patients with true NPH did not differ from those in normal subjects (Fig. 3, left), but circulation times in the frontal gray matter were significantly longer in these patients than in normal subjects (Fig. 3, right).

In patients with true NPH postoperative the circulation times were significantly shorter both in the periventricular white matter and in the frontal gray matter (Fig. 4).

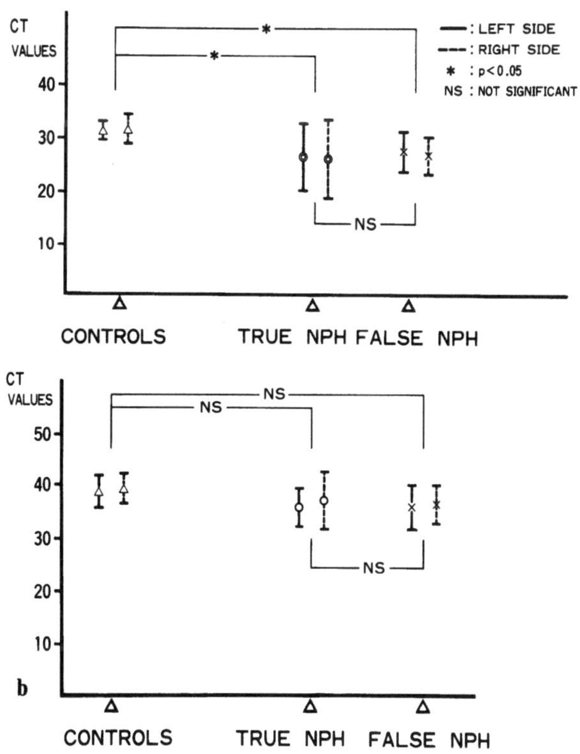

Fig. 1a, b. CT attenuation values of the periventricular white matter (**a**) and the frontal gray matter (**b**) in patients with true and false NPH

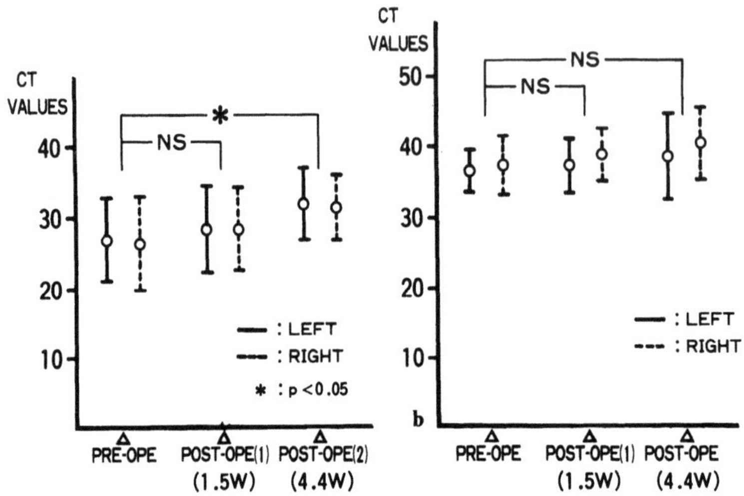

Fig. 2a, b. Postoperative changes in CT attenuation values in periventricular white matter (**a**) and frontal gray matter (**b**) of patients with true NPH

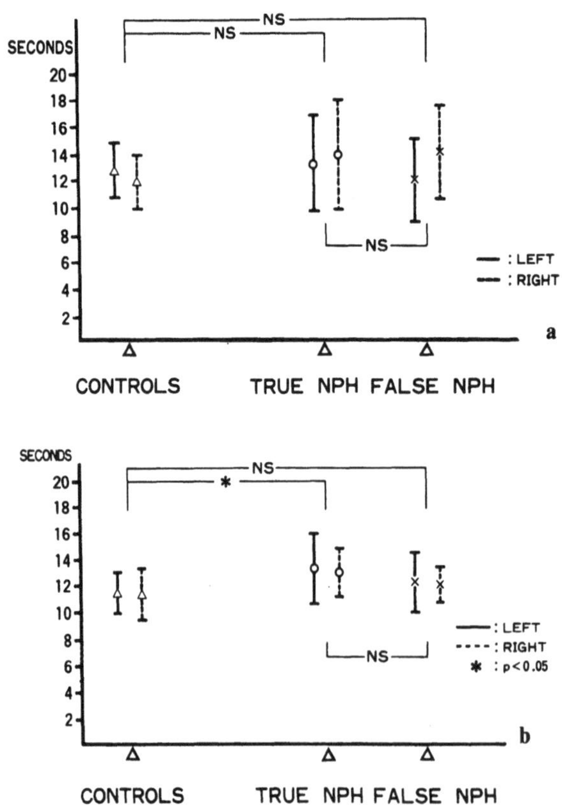

Fig. 3a, b. Circulation times in the periventricular white matter (**a**) and the frontal gray matter (**b**) in patients with true and false NPH

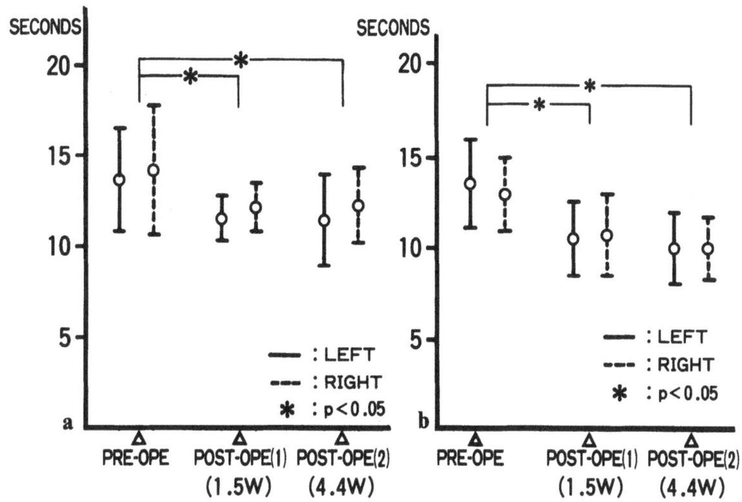

Fig. 4a, b. Postoperative changes in circulation times in periventricular white matter (**a**) and frontal gray matter (**b**) of patients with true NPH

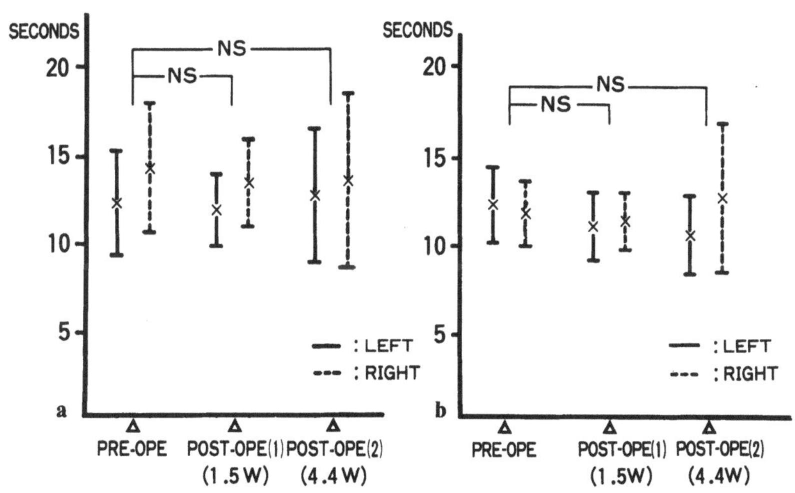

Fig. 5a, b. Postoperative changes of CT attenuation values in periventricular white matter (**a**) and frontal gray matter (**b**) of patients with false NPH

Thus, an improvement of the hemodynamics was achieved both in the periventricular white matter and in the frontal gray matter after CSF shunting.

Changes in CT Attenuation Values and Circulation Times in Patients with False NPH

CT attenuation values of the periventricular white matter in patients with false NPH were also significantly low compared with those in normal controls (Fig. 1, left). In frontal gray matter, however, there was no significant difference between the attenuation values in these patients and those in normal controls (Fig. 1, right).

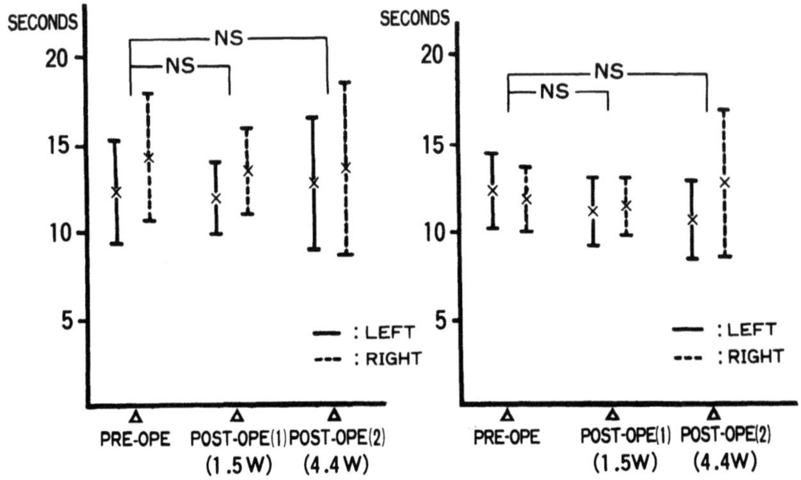

Fig. 6. Postoperative changes of circulation times in periventricular white matter (*left*) and frontal gray matter (*right*) of patients with false NPH

There was no postoperative change in CT attenuation values either in the periventricular white matter or in the frontal gray matter in patients with false NPH (Fig. 5).

Thus, there was no change in hydrodynamics either in the periventricular white matter or in the frontal gray matter in patients with false NPH.

The circulation times in patients with false NPH were not significantly different from those in normal controls either in the periventricular white matter or in the frontal gray matter (Fig. 3); nor was there any significant change between preoperative and postoperative circulation times in either white or gray matter in these patients (Fig. 6).

Thus, there was no change of hemodynamics in either region examined in patients with false NPH.

Discussion

A review of the literature indicates that cerebral blood flow is reduced in patients with hydrocephalus or with dementia of various etiologies, including cerebral degeneration, and that there is no statistical difference in the decrease in cerebral blood flow between patients with NPH and those with dementia resulting from other causes [1–7, 9]. The mechanism of the clinical improvement in patients with NPH after shunt placement is thought to be associated with improvement of the cerebral blood circulation [1, 3, 5, 7, 9, 10].

The results of this investigation are consistent with those previously reported in the literature, although most earlier studies addressed only the question of the regional blood flow in the gray matter [1, 3, 5–7].

Dynamic CT studies enabled us to demonstrate the hemodynamic condition of the deep structures, such as the periventricular white matter, corresponding to the area of the periventricular lucency on plain CT and emission CT or the stable xenon inhalation technique combined with CT [8, 10]. Thus, it became possible to investigate the pathogenesis and pathophysiology of NPH more precisely and in greater detail.

There was no distinguishable difference in cerebral hemodynamics between patients with NPH and patients considered to have false NPH from other causes in the present study. Patients with true NPH had a postoperative improvement in cerebral hemodynamics, while patients with degenerative dementia resulting from hydrocephalus ex vacuo did not. There is presumably some difference in hemodynamics between these two patient groups, which needs further investigation.

Conclusion

The hydrodynamics of the area of periventricular edema in NPH was investigated by analysis of the serial change in CT attenuation values. Patients with NPH had significantly lower attenuation values than normal subjects, which increased after shunt placement. Hemodynamics of the frontal gray and white matter were studied by means of dynamic CT. In patients with NPH the circulation time in the gray matter was longer than normal before shunting, and that in both the gray and the white matter was shorter after CSF shunting.

Our present data suggest that impaired cerebral hemodynamics constitute one of the main pathologic conditions in the periventricular tissue.

Summary

The pathophysiology of the periventricular tissue in normal pressure hydrocephalus (NPH) was investigated by analysis of the changes in attenuation values and a dynamic CT study. Periventricular tissue in patients with true NPH showed significantly lower attenuation values than that in normal controls. The attenuation values increased after shunt operation. Thus, hydrodynamics improved in the periventricular tissue after shunt placement, but there was no change in the hydrodynamics in the frontal gray matter. Hemodynamics were impaired in both areas before surgery, but there was a significant improvement after surgery. There was no significant postoperative change in hydro-hemodynamics in either area in patients with false NPH.

References

1. Greitz TVB, Grepe AOL, Kalmer MSF, Lopez J (1969) Pre- and postoperative evaluation of cerebral blood flow in low pressure hydrocephalus. J Neurosurg 31:644–651
2. Hachinski VC, Iliff LD, Ailhka E, Du Boulay GH, McAllister VL, Mershall J, Russel RWR (1975) Cerebral blood flow in dementia. Arch Neurol 32:632–637
3. Hartman A, Alberti E (1977) Cerebral blood flow and cerebrospinal fluid pressure in patients with communicating hydrocephalus. In: Wüllenweber R, Brock M, Hamer J et al. (eds) Lumbar disc, adult hydrocephalus. Springer, Berlin Heidelberg New York, pp 144–155

4. Ingvar DH, Gustafson L (1970) Regional cerebral blood flow in organic dementia with early onset. Acta Neurol Scand 46 (Suppl 43):42–73
5. Ingvar DH, Gchwarz MS (1975) The cerebral blood flow in low pressure hydrocephalus. In: Lundberg N, Pontein U, Brock M (eds) Intracranial pressure II. Springer, Berlin Heidelberg New York, pp 153–156
6. Mathew NT, Meyer JS, Hartmann A, Otto EO (1975) Abnormal cerebrospinal fluid–blood flow dynamics. Implications in diagnosis, treatment and prognosis in normal pressure hydrocephalus. Arch Neurol 32:557–664
7. Meyer JS, Tachibana H, Hardenberg JP, Dowell RE, Kitagawa Y, Mortel KF (1984) Normal pressure hydrocephalus. Influence on cerebral hemodynamics and cerebrospinal fluid pressure – clinical autoregulation. Surg Neurol 21:195–203
8. Meyer JS, Shaw TG, Okayasu H, Tachibana H (1983) Multi-infarct and Alzheimer dementias differentiated from normal aging by xenon contrast CT CBF measurements. J Cereb Blood Flow Metab (Suppl 1)3:506–507
9. Salmon JH, Timperman AL (1971) Cerebral blood flow in posttraumatic encephalopathy. The effect of ventriculo-atrial shunt. Neurology 21:33–42
10. Tamaki N, Kusunoki T, Wakabayashi T, Matsumoto S (1984) Cerebral hemodynamics in normal pressure hydrocephalus. Evaluation by X-133 inhalation method and dynamic CT study. J Neurosurg 61:510–514

Regional Cerebral Blood Flow in Experimental Hydrocephalus of Dogs, Measured by Xenon-Enhanced CT

H. HIRATSUKA [1], Y. TAKASATO, S. TSURUOKA, T. KUROIWA, K. OKADA, R. SUZUKI, T. FUKUMOTO, M. SEIDA, and Y. INABA

Key words: Cerebral blood flow, hydrocephalus, periventricular edema, periventricular hypodensity, xenon-enhanced CT

Introduction

Hydrocephalic brain edema has become widely recognized since the introduction of computer tomography (CT). On CT scan, edema is seen especially in the periventricular white matter, where it is familiar as periventricular lucency or periventricular hypodensity (PVH) [13, 14, 17]. Our previous study with metrizamide CT scanning showed transependymal migration of metrizamide in the area of PVH. The iodine concentration was highest in the periventricular white matter according to measurement by the cerate-arsenite method. The specific gravity was particularly low in the periventricular white matter of the hydrocephalic brains in which it was measured by means of a gradient column containing kerosene and bromobenzene. On the basis of these facts edema is interpreted as transependymal migration of cerebrospinal fluid (CSF) into the brain [6–8].

Recently, in attempts to characterize the pathophysiologic significance of hydrocephalus, several studies dealing with the change in cerebral blood flow in hydrocephalus have been performed and reported [5, 16, 21]. However, no consistent results have been obtained.

In the work reported in this paper, we studied the changes in regional cerebral blood flow (rCBF) over time and regional differences in rCBF in experimental hydrocephalus. We measured rCBF in kaolin-induced hydrocephalus in dogs by the stable xenon-enhanced CT method, which achieves high anatomic spatial resolution owing to the topographic flow map. Light and electron microscopic observations were also carried out to establish the time course of changes in the ependymal layer and surrounding tissue. Changes in the cerebral microvessel architecture were analyzed by soft X-ray angiogram.

Materials and Methods

Eighteen mongrel adult dogs weighing 8–13 kg were used. The dogs were anesthetized with sodium pentobarbital (13 mg/kg, IV). After tracheal intubation, respi-

---

[1] Department of Neurosurgery, Tokyo Medical and Dental Univsersity School of Medicine, 1-5-45 Yushima, Bunkyo-ku, Tokyo 113, Japan

Table 1. Value recorded on blood gas analysis during CBF measurement

Parameter	Before hydrocephalus (12)	At 1–4 weeks after induction (8)	At 9–13 weeks after induction (4)
Arterial pH	7.41± 0.03	7.43± 0.02	7.38± 0.01
$PaCO_2$ (mmHg)	38.07± 2.15	37.79± 1.71	37.75± 1.53
PaO_2 (mmHg)	203.96±12.52	230.75±12.68	218.10±11.40
Arterial Hb	13.70± 1.00	15.13± 0.80	14.20± 0.76

Each value is the mean ± SE for the number of animals indicated in parentheses at the column head

ration was controlled with pancronium bromide (0.2 mg/kg, IV) to allow adequate blood gas analysis data (Table 1). Experimental hydrocephalus was induced in the dogs by injecting dissolved kaolin in 1 ml saline (30–50 mg/kg) into the cisterna magna. Measurement of rCBF was performed as follows: An IV line was placed in the cubital vein. Then the femoral artery was catheterized for arterial blood sampling. After desaturation of nitrogen from the tissue by pure oxygen inhalation, mixed gas (50% xenon + 50% O_2) was substituted for 25 min. During xenon inhalation ten serial CT scans were performed in the same CT plane with a TOSHIBA TCT-20A CT scanner. Simultaneously, end-tidal concentrations of Xe, O_2, N_2, and CO_2 were continuously analyzed by means of a SHIMAZU Medical Mass Spectrometer model R-MC. Arterial blood samples were taken at the start and end of xenon inhalation to assess the arterial blood gases and the xenon concentration in the blood.

Based on the Fick principle the following equations were used:

$$K = C_i(T) - C_i(O)/\lambda \int_0^T C_a(t)\,dt - \int_0^T C_i(t)\,dt$$

$$f = 100\,\lambda K$$

where Ci and Ca are the tissue and arterial blood xenon concentrations, respectively, K is the tissue buildup flow rate, f is the flow in the chosen compartments (ml/100 g brain tissue/min, and λ is the tissue-blood partition coefficient. λ can be calculated from the formula L = Ci (T)/Ca (T). The above-mentioned process was governed completely by a computer program. Finally, K, λ, and rCBF maps were obtained and displayed on the screen. The rCBF was found by setting the region of interest (ROI) on the screen.

At the end of rCBF measurement the dogs were sacrificed by KCl injection, and microbarium was injected through the common carotid artery (CCA). The ipsilateral external carotid artery and the contralateral CCA were ligated. After 1 week's fixation in 10% formalin solution soft X-ray films were taken with 2-mm slices.

Immediately after sacrifice of each dog, specimens of ventricular wall and the surrounding tissue were taken. Light and electron microscopic examinations were then carried out.

Results

After the kaolin injection, ventricular dilatation became noticeable in 24 h, progressing to reach a peak in about 3–4 weeks. Periventricular hypodensity was extreme at the dorsolateral portions of the anterior horns of the lateral ventricles. On the whole, the appearance of the PVH paralleled the time course of the ventricular dilatation (Fig. 1). After xenon inhalation, a contrast of gray and white matter is

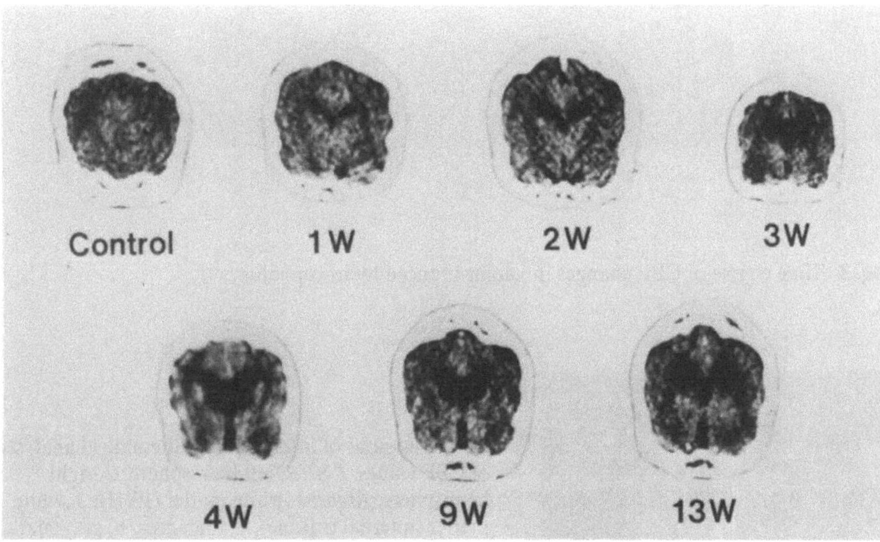

Fig. 1. Time course of changes in ventricular size during kaolin-induced hydrocephalus

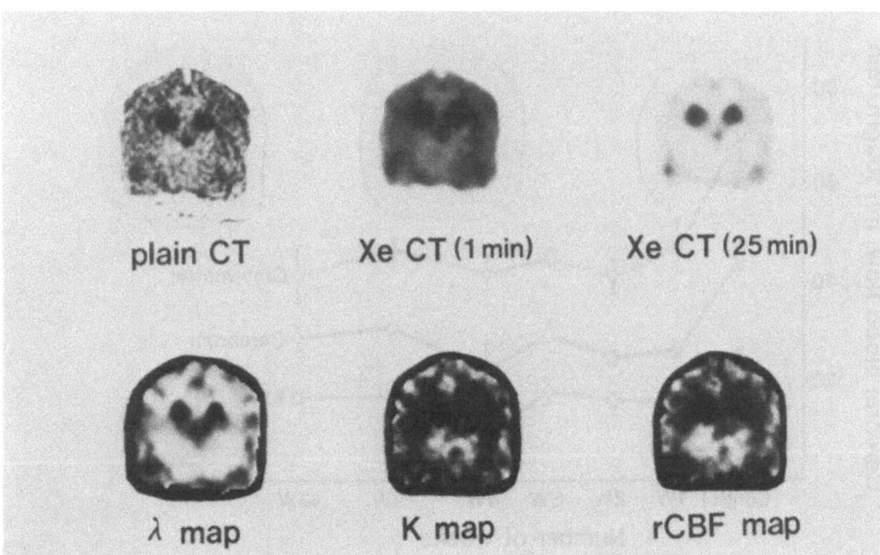

Fig. 2. Plain and xenon-enhanced CT, and λ, K, and rCBF maps in dog 10 at 3 weeks after kaolin injection

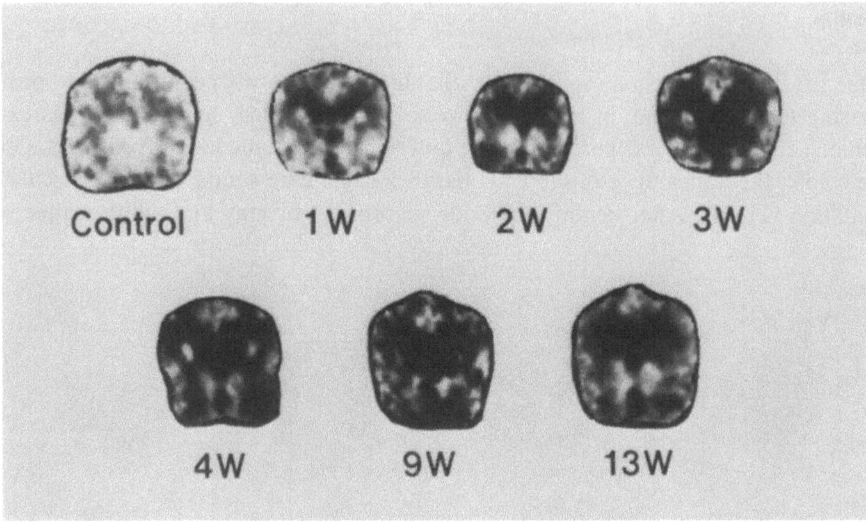

Fig. 3. Time course of CBF changes in kaolin-induced hydrocephalus

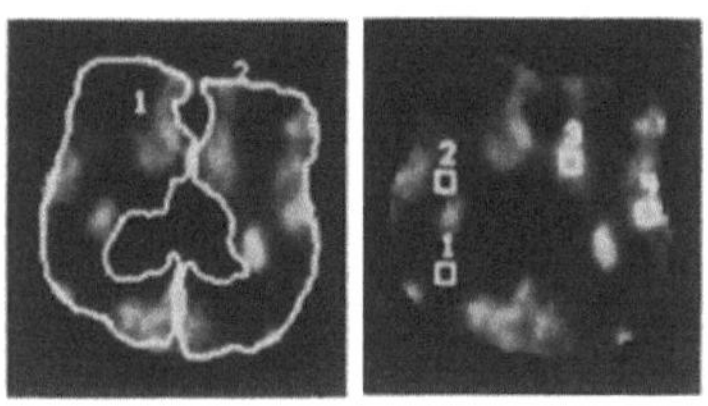

Fig. 4. Regions of interest for mathematical analysis of CBF values. *Left: 1,* left hemisphere; *2,* right hemisphere. *Right: 1,* white matter (PVH); *2,* white matter (internal capsule); *3,* thalamus; *4,* gray matter

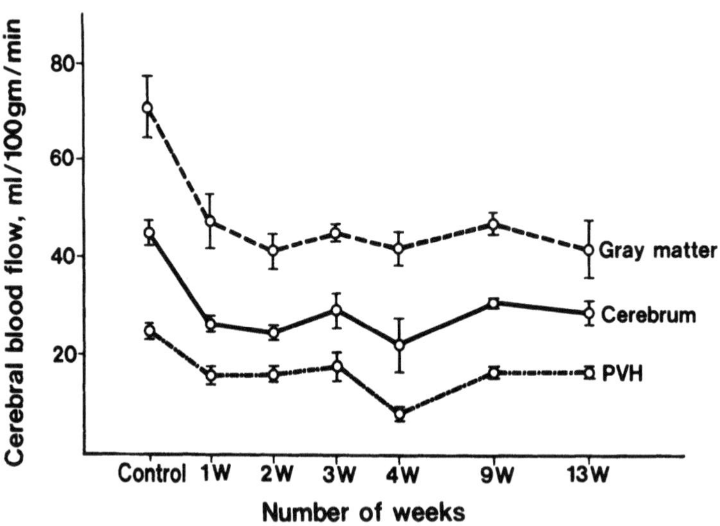

Fig. 5. Time course of CBF changes in kaolin-induced hydrocephalus. *Points,* means; *bars,* SEM

Table 2. Regional cerebral blood flow in control and hydrocephalic dogs

Region	Regional cerebral blood flow (ml/100 g/min)		
	Control (12)	Hydrocephalus for	
		1–4 weeks (8)	9–13 weeks (4)
Hemisphere	44.65±2.69	26.19±1.08[a]	29.59±1.27[a]
Gray matter	70.94±6.54	43.86±2.72[a]	44.81±3.71
White matter (PVH)	24.89±1.29	15.41±1.29[a]	16.68±0.72[a]
White matter (internal capsule)	27.63±1.26	17.59±0.60[a]	21.74±0.83[a]
Thalamus	73.94±6.23	42.00±3.01[a]	46.33±2.63[a]

Each value is the mean ± SE for the number of animals indicated in parentheses.
[a] Differs significantly ($P<0.05$) from control value by Student's *t*-test

well demonstrated with a 1-min xenon inhalation scan, while rather homogeneously enhanced images are obtained with the saturated scan at 25 min. Partition coefficients (λ), transfer constant (K), and rCBF are calculated by using the formulas previously mentioned, and the λ, K, and rCBF maps are obtained as shown in Fig. 2. The time course of CBF changes in kaolin-induced canine hydrocephalus is shown in Fig. 3 in the form of rCBF maps. As shown in Fig. 4, the specific regions of interest are studied for rCBF. Table 2 shows the value of rCBF in each region of interest. After 1 week, the average hemispheric CBF value decreased by approximately 40% compared with the control value. There were no significant regional differences in the decreased rate of rCBF value; that is to say the area of PVH did not specifically have lower CBF values (Fig. 5). The time course of changes revealed by soft X-ray films in kaolin-induced canine hydrocephalus is shown in Fig. 6. The opacification of microvessels became worse with time after kaolin injection. Again there were no significant regional differences in the degree of microvessel opacification between white matter in the area of PVH and in the cerebral cortex.

Light microscopic observation revealed subependymal interstitial edema with relative preservation of ependymal cell linings at 1 week, and progressive damage to ependymal cells and periventricular white matter thereafter (Fig. 7). Electron microscopic examination confirmed the loose organization of parenchymal cellular components in the periventricular white matter (Fig. 8). There is an increase in extracellular fluid space especially in the perivascular area, whereas the endothelial cells seem to be preserved relatively intact.

Discussion

In computed tomography of hydrocephalus, periventricular hypodensity or periventricular lucency has often been recognized, although the pathophysiologic significance has not yet been fully clarified [13, 14, 17].

Our previous reports suggested that the development of PVH is due to increased transit of CSF from the ventricles to the white matter [6–8]. From the pathological

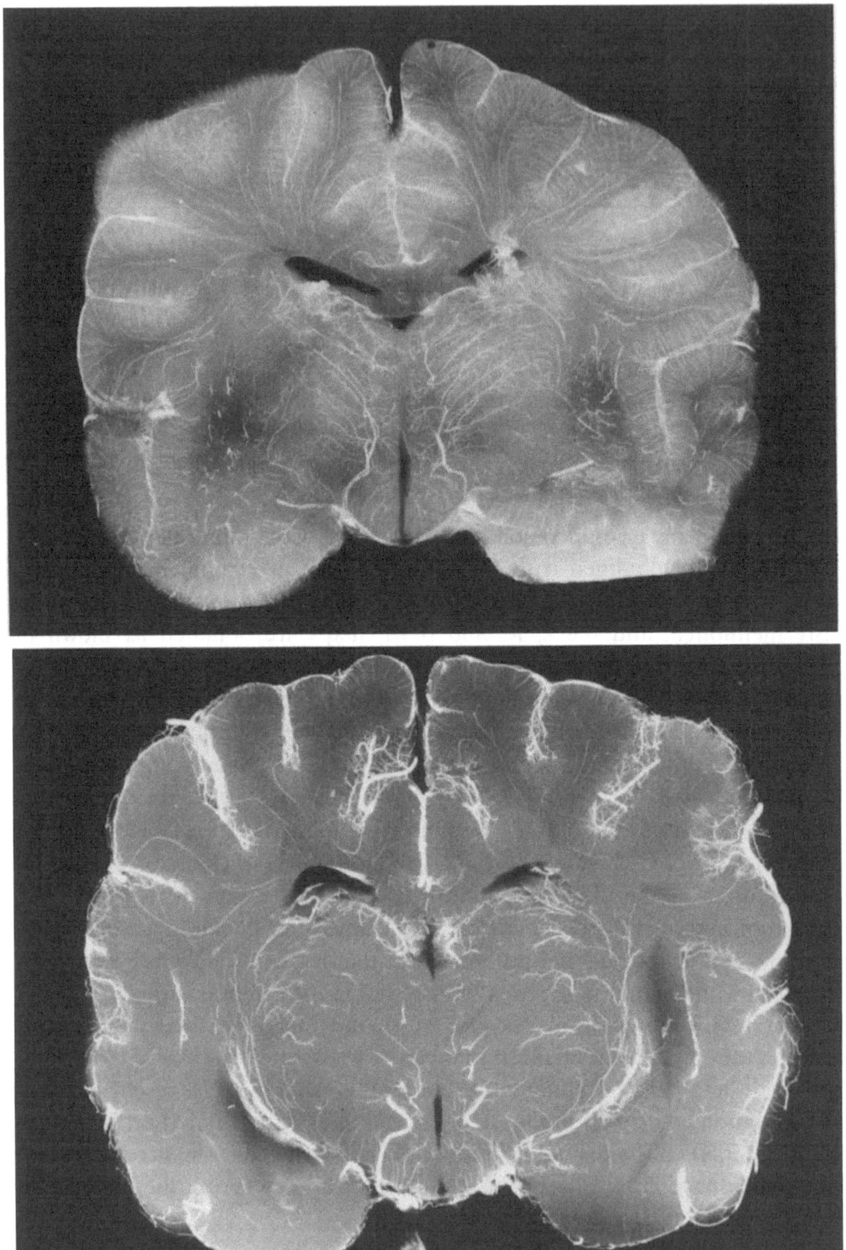

A

B

Fig. 6 A–D. Time course of soft X-ray films in control (**A**) and hydrocephalic (**B–D**) dogs. **B** 1 week; **C** 4 weeks; **D** 13 weeks after kaolin injection

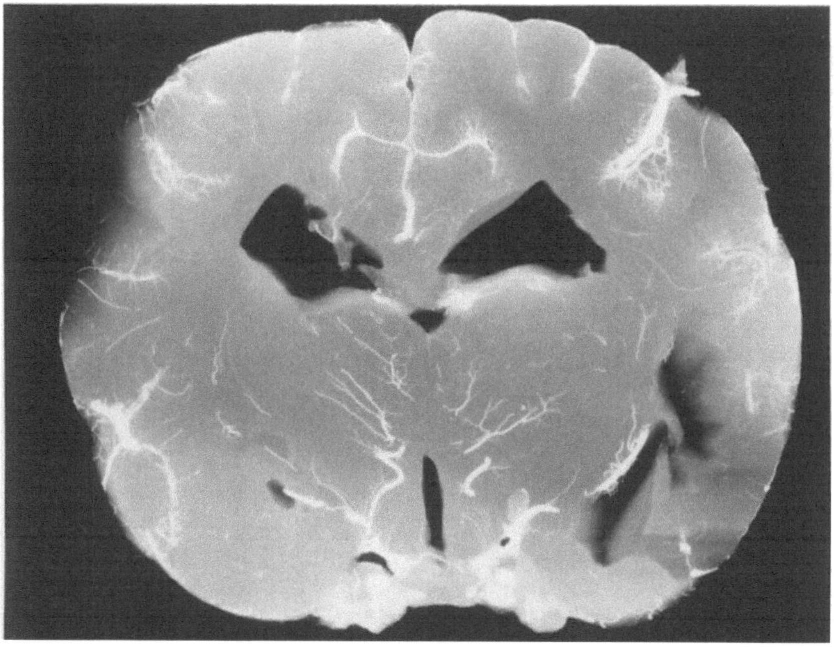

C

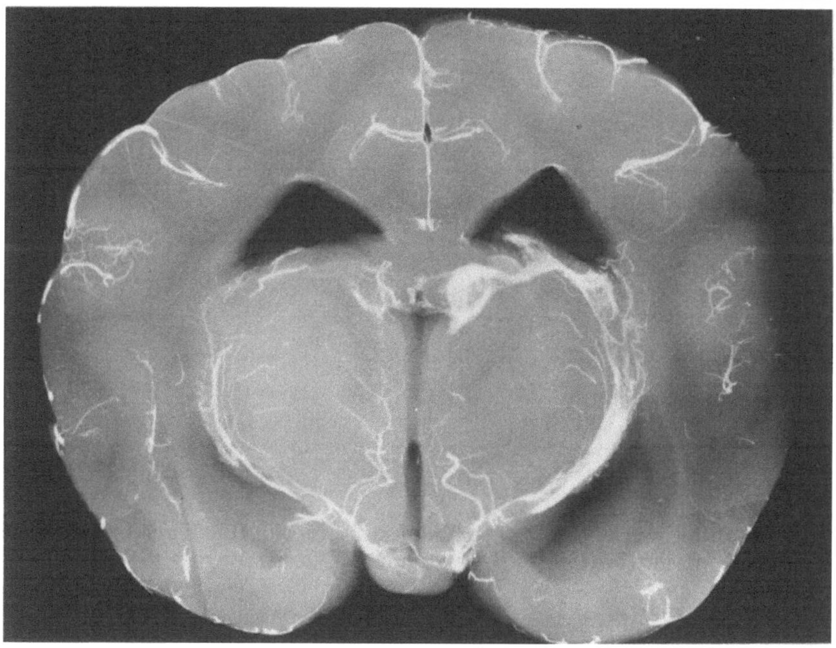

D

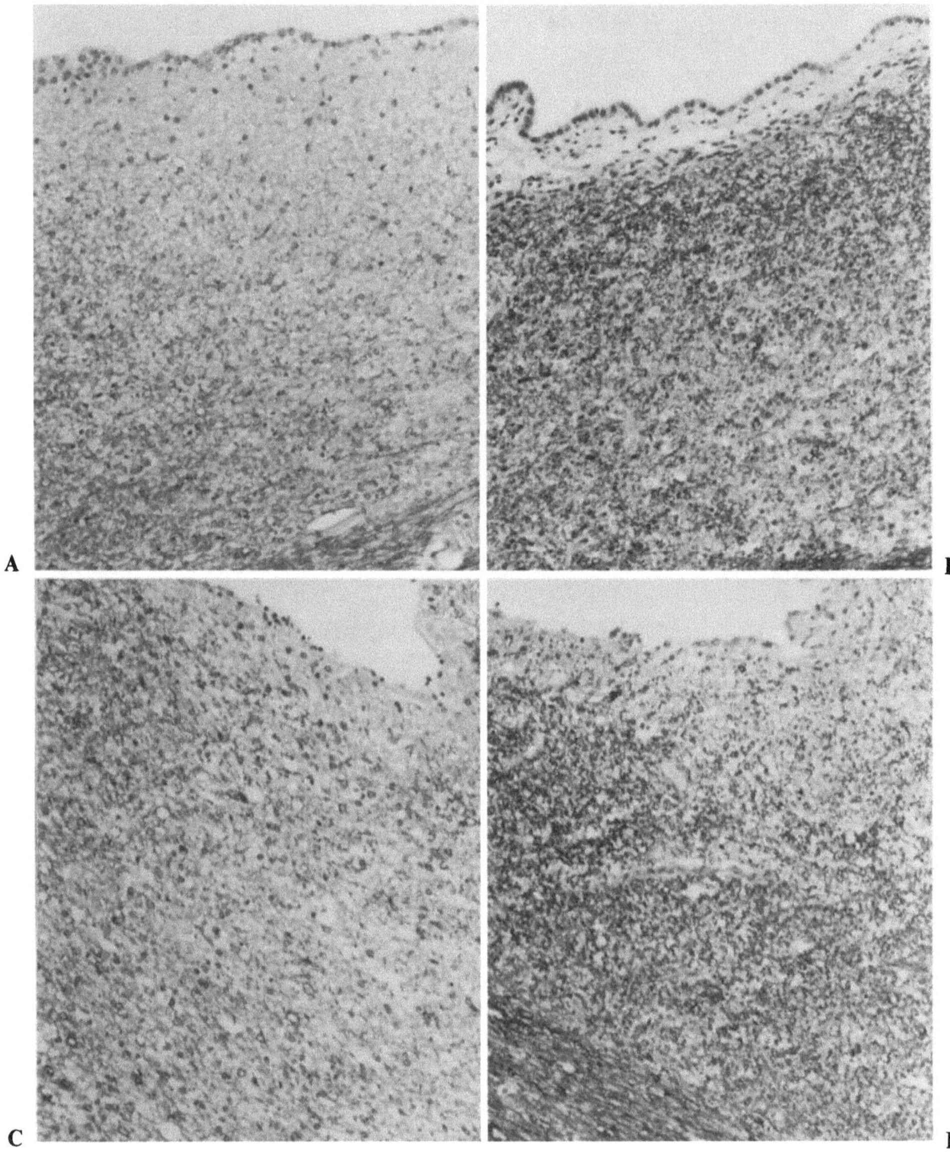

Fig. 7 A–D. Light micrographs of periventricular area with H & E and LFB stain control (**A**) and hydrocephalic (**B–D**) dogs; **B** 1 week after; **C** 3 weeks after; **D** 13 weeks after kaolin injection

standpoint, the histology of the area is compatible with interstitial edema. However, another report has suggested that impaired hemodynamics is involved in the development of PVH [16]. In some reports, in adult patients with chronic hydrocephalus or normal pressure hydrocephalus, the area of PVH is described as revealing demyelination or degeneration, or even infarction, of the white matter [9, 22].

Measurement of rCBF has become an essential tool in the field of neurology and neurosurgery. Until recently, the ^{133}Xe inhalation or IV injection methods, which

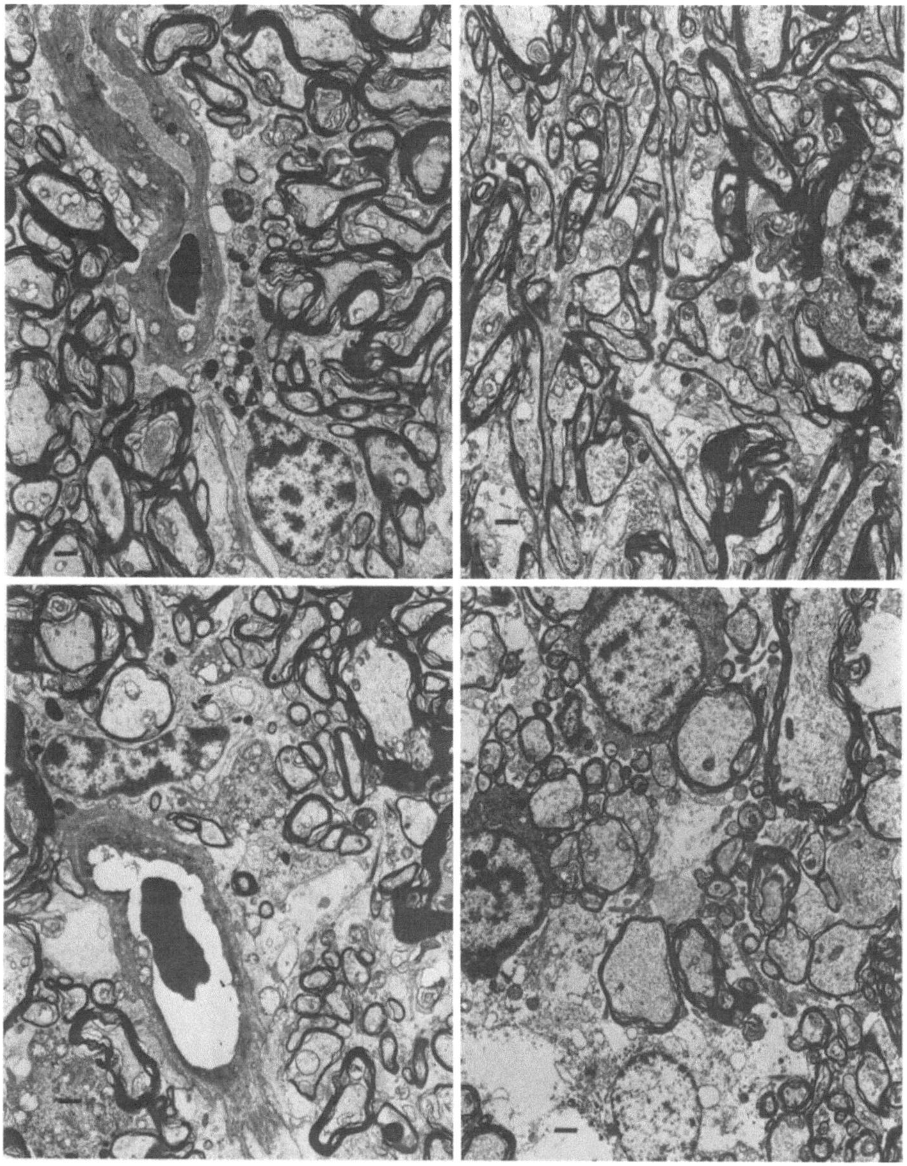

Fig. 8A–D. Electron micrograph of periventricular white matter in control **A,** and hydrocephalic (**B–D**) dogs. **B** 1 week after; **C** 3 weeks after; **D** 13 weeks after kaolin injection. *Scale bar* 1 μm

were first described by Obrist et al. have been widely used [15]. Meanwhile, three-dimensional rCBF mapping techniques have been developed. These are positron emission tomography [5], single photon emission tomography [10], and xenon-enhanced CT [1–4, 11, 12, 19, 20]. Xenon-enhanced CT has many advantages over the others for measurement of rCBF, including high spatial resolution of the tomographic maps facilitating the calculation of actual partition coefficients (λ). This method has been applied both to animal experiments and to clinical use [1–4, 11, 12, 20].

We mapped rCBF, λ, and K in control and hydrocephalic dogs. Decreased CBF values were obtained in hydrocephalic dogs. In the area of PVH, a statistically significant decrease in rCBF compared with the control dogs was noted. Opacification of microvessels also became worse with development of hydrocephalus. However, no significant regional differences were noted in the 13 weeks of this study. Further long-term chronological study may be necessary, because in cases of hydrocephalus in which the circulatory disturbance is initially suggested by PVH the course would be much longer than the duration of this experiment.

Summary

For 3 weeks after kaolin injection into the cisterna magna, ventricular enlargement progressed markedly. After this the ventricle increased in size gradually until the end of 13 weeks.

On the whole, the appearance of PVH paralleled the time course of ventricular dilatation.

After 1 week, the average hemispheric CBF value decreased by approximately 40% compared with the control value.

There were no significant regional differences in the decreased rCBF values.

Opacification of microvessels became worse with time after kaolin injection.

Hydrocephalic brain consistently revealed subependymal interstitial edema with progressive damage to the ependymal cell linings and periventricular white matter.

References

1. Drayer BP, Gur D, Wolfson SK, Cook EE (1980) Experimental xenon enhancement with CT imaging; cerebral applications. Am J Neuroradiol 1:3–8
2. Drayer BP, Wolfson SK, Reinmuth OM, Dujovny M, Boehnke M, Cook EE (1978) Xenon enhanced CT for analysis of cerebral integrity, perfusion, and blood flow. Stroke 9:123–130
3. Gur D, Good WF, Wolfson SK, Yonas H, Shabason L (1982) In vivo mapping of local cerebral blood flow by xenon-enhanced computed tomography. Science 215:1267–1268
4. Gur D, Wolfson SK, Yonas H, Good WF, Shabason L, Latchaw RE, Miller DM, Cook EE (1982) Progress in cerebrovascular disease: local cerebral blood flow by xenon-enhanced CT. Stroke 13:750–758
5. Hassler O (1964) Angioarchitecture in hydrocephalus. An autopsy and experimental study with the aid of microangiography. Acta Neuropathol 4:65–74
6. Hiratsuka H, Fujiwara K, Okada K, Takasato Y, Tsuyumu M, Inaba Y (1980) Modification of periventricular hypodensity in hydrocephalus with ventricular reflux in metrizamide CT cisternography. J Comput Assist Tomogr 2:471–474
7. Hiratsuka H, Tabata H, Tsuruoka S, Aoyagi M, Okada K, Inaba Y (1982) Evaluation of periventricular hypodensity in experimental hydrocephalus by metrizamide CT ventriculograph. J Neurosurg 56:235–240
8. Inaba Y, Hiratsuka H, Tsuyumu M, Tabata H, Tsuruoka S (1984) Evaluation of periventricular hypodensity in clinical and experimental hydrocephalus by metrizamide computed tomography. In: Go G, Baethmann A (eds) Recent progress in the study and therapy of brain edema. Plenum, New York, pp 299–310
9. Ishii N, Momii S, Suzuki T, Ito K (1980) CT findings of multi-infarct dementia with particular reference to periventricular lucency. Neurol Med 12:376–381

10. Lassen NA, Henriksen L, Paulson OB (1981) Regional cerebral blood flow in stroke by xenon-133 inhalation and emission tomography. Stroke 12:284–288
11. Meyer JS, Hayman A, Amano T, Nakajima S, Shaw T, Lauzon P, Derman S, Karacan I, Harati Y (1981) Mapping local blood flow of human brain by CT scanning during stable xenon inhalation. Stroke 12:426–436
12. Meyer JS, Hayman LA, Yamamoto M, Sakai F, Nakajima S (1980) Local cerebral blood flow measured by CT after stable xenon inhalation. Am J Neuroradiol 1:213–225
13. Mosely IF, Radu EW (1979) Factors influencing the development of periventricular lucencies in patients with raised intracranial pressure. Neuroradiology 17:65–69
14. Naidich TP, Epstein F, Lin JP et al. (1976) Evaluation of pediatric hydrocephalus by computed tomography. Radiology 119:337–345
15. Obrist WD, Thompson HK, Wang HS, Wilkinson WE (1975) Regional cerebral blood flow estimated by 133 xenon inhalation. Stroke 6:245–256
16. Ohya M (1984) Changes of cerebral microvasculature in experimental hydrocephalus and its relation to periventricular lucency. Nervous System Children 9:173–181
17. Pasquini U, Bronzini M, Gozzoli E et al. (1977) Periventricular hypodensity in hydrocephalus: a clinicoradiological and mathematical analysis using computed tomography. J Comput Assist Tomogr 1:443–448
18. Phelps ME, Mazziotta JC, Huang SC (1982) Study of cerebral function with positron computed tomography. J Cereb Blood Flow Metab 2:113–163
19. Segawa H, Wakai S, Tamura A, Yoshimasu N, Nakamura O, Ohta M (1983) Computed tomographic measurement of local cerebral blood flow by xenon enhancement. Stroke 14:356–362
20. Suzuki R, Hiratsuka H, Ohno K, Inaba Y, Kimura T, Inoue J (1985) Topographic mapping of regional cerebral blood flow by xenon-enhanced CT – Introducing a simplified method as a routine examination. Brain Nerve 37:73–80
21. Wozniak M, McLone DG, Raimondi AJ (1975) Micro- and macrovascular changes as the direct cause of parenchymal destruction in congenital murine hydrocephalus. J Neurosurg 43:535–545
22. Yamanouchi H, Tohgi H, Tomonaga M, Iio M (1981) Computerized tomographic evaluation of chronic ischemic lesions in cerebral white matter. Jpn J Geriat 18:297–307

Time Course of Tissue Relaxation Time in Cerebral Infarction

M. FURUSE[1], Y. MOTEGI, K. SASO, S. INAO, and N. KAMATA

Key words: Nuclear magnetic resonance, relaxation time, cerebral infarction, brain edema, tissue degeneration

Introduction

The nuclear magnetic resonance (NMR) technique yields various kinds of information depending on proton spin distribution and relaxation times, so that it is presumably possible to obtain any information available on the dynamics of cerebral edema or intracranial degenerative processes.

In the present study, in vivo measurement of spin lattice relaxation times (T_1) were used to assess the pathophysiological status in patients with cerebral infarction. Emphasis was laid upon the time course of the focal tissue T_1 value following cerebral ischemic insults.

Materials and Methods

Thirty patients with cerebral infarction were included in the study, and serial alterations in NMR imagings and in vivo T_1 measurements were examined for each. The age range in this series was 16–86 years (average age 60.2), and the male: female ratio was 1:0.57 (19 m, 11 f).

A whole-body NMR scanner (FONAR QED 80-alpha) was used for the present study. The equipment used has dual functions for sensing information, i.e., anatomy and chemistry modes. A brief description of the method is given below:

a. Anatomy mode (imaging display)
   1. Static magnetic field strength: 433.6 gauss
   2. Scanning method: Projection reconstruction technique
   3. Radiofrequency sequence: Steady state free precession (SSFP) (in general 10 μs pulse width and 5.12 ms repetition cycle)
   4. Slice thickness: 10–20 mm
   5. Spatial resolution: 2 mm

[1] Department of Neurosurgery, Nakatsugawa Municipal General Hospital, Ebisu-Machi, Nakatsugawa 508, Japan

Table 1. Standard T_1 values in healthy brain

Location	Gray matter (frontal lobe)	White matter (frontal lobe)	Cerebellar cortex	Cerebellar white matter	Pons
T_1 value (Mean $\pm$SD, ms)	288 ± 42	227 ± 27	273 ± 29	248 ± 29	250 ± 41

b. Chemistry mode (T_1 measurement)
1. Magnetic field strength of the focused spot: 468.6 gauss
2. Measuring method: Field focusing technique using a pulsed high frequency (around 2 MHz)
3. Pulse sequence: Progressive saturation method ($90°-\tau-90°$)
4. Tau values used: Generally 8–13 points ranging from 25 to 350 ms
5. Spot size: 10–20 mm in diameter

For in vitro calibration of T_1 values, phantoms containing nickel chloride solutions of known concentration were used. The values of T_1 measured in $NiCl_2$ solutions of 5, 7, 10, and 16 mMol/l were 298 ± 10.5, 216 ± 4.8, 155 ± 7.1, and 106 ± 4.6 ms (mean $\pm$ SD), respectively. It was ascertained before and after each clinical measurement that variations in the values in test phantoms remained within 10% of the standardized T_1 values. Table 1 shows the standard T_1 values in the varied sites of normal brain parenchyma. The standardized T_1 in the gray matter was significantly longer than that in the white matter in either the cerebrum or the cerebellum.

Results

NMR Image and T_1 Values Associated with Cerebral Infarction

The infarcted area of the brain was displayed as a high-density zone in SSFP imagings. In general, the shape and size of the area of high signal intensity in the NMR image were in keeping with the distribution of low-density areas found on X-ray CT. On occasion, however, such high-density areas in the NMR image exceeded the extent of low-density areas on X-ray CT. Figure 1 illustrates an example of massive cerebral infarction. Three months before, the patient was suddenly afflicted with right hemiplegia and sensory aphasia caused by occlusion of the left internal carotid artery. NMR-CT revealed an apparently high-density zone in the left parieto-occipital region, in accordance with the area of low density found on X-ray CT. At the core site of infarction T_1 was extremely long, the actual value being in excess of 600 ms. In addition, NMR imaging in this case represented a relatively high density area in the ipsilateral frontal lobe, in which X-ray CT revealed no imaging abnormality. Measurement of relaxation time in the corresponding area indicated a moderate prolongation of T_1. Such increased values for T_1 seemed to reflect the existence of such tissue abnormalities as cerebral edema or circulatory disorder in the area adjacent to the ischemic zone. Figure 2 illustrates another example of cerebral infarction in the chronic stage. This patient had double vascular lesions in the internal carotid system, that is, right-sided complete occlusion of the vessel at the

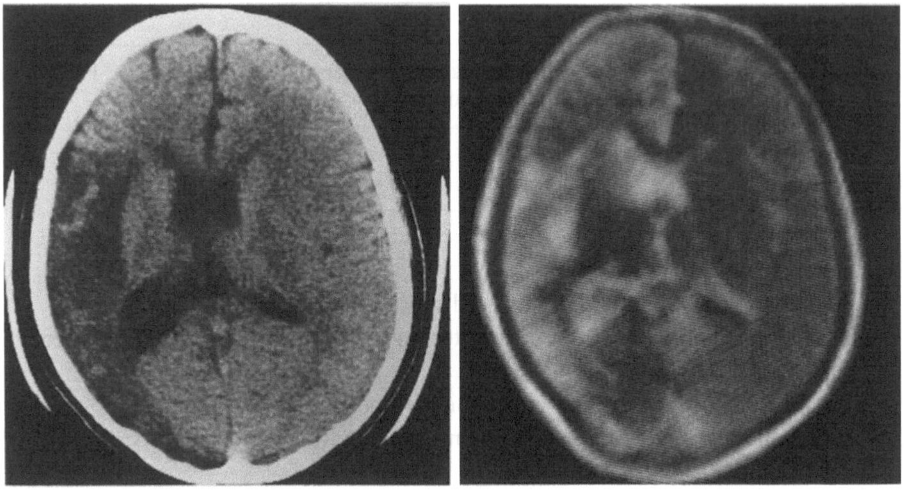

a b

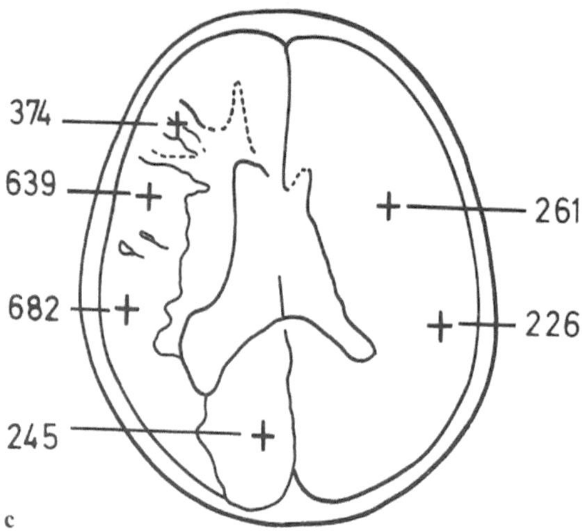

c

Fig. 1a–c. Left cerebral infarction in a 42-year-old woman: **a** X-ray CT; **b** NMR-CT; **c** T_1 values

neck and irregular narrowing at the siphon on left side. X-ray CT showed a unilateral low-density zone in the right frontoparietal region. In contrast, NMR imaging revealed bilateral abnormalities, predominantly in the right cerebral hemisphere. An extremely prolonged T_1 of more than 1000 ms was measured at the core site of the long-standing infarction, where both X-ray CT and NMR revealed prominent abnormalities. Such an extreme value for T_1 suggested drastic changes in the tissue, such as cavitation. In the left frontal white matter, a relatively long T_1 of 376 ms was found despite the absence of any imaging abnormality on X-ray CT. This finding was thought to be a response to intracranial pathology induced by left-sided ICA stenosis.

Time Course of T_1 Values in Cerebral Infarction

T_1 values in the infarcted area changed with time. Usually T_1 measured at the center of an extensive cerebral infarction was consistently prolonged.

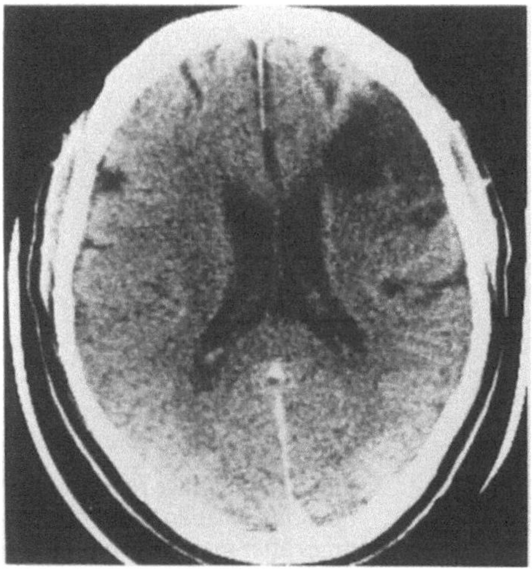

a

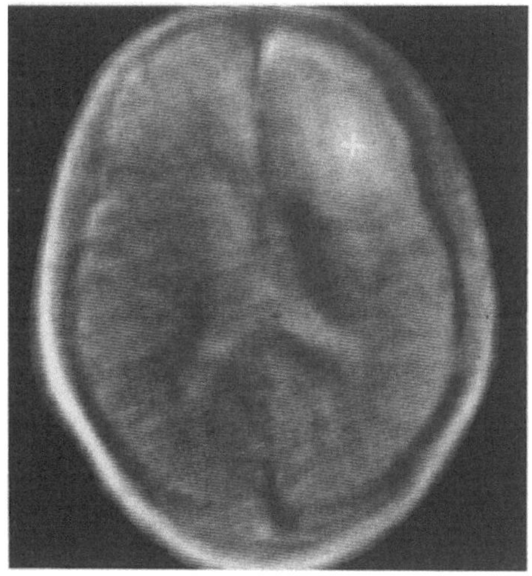

b

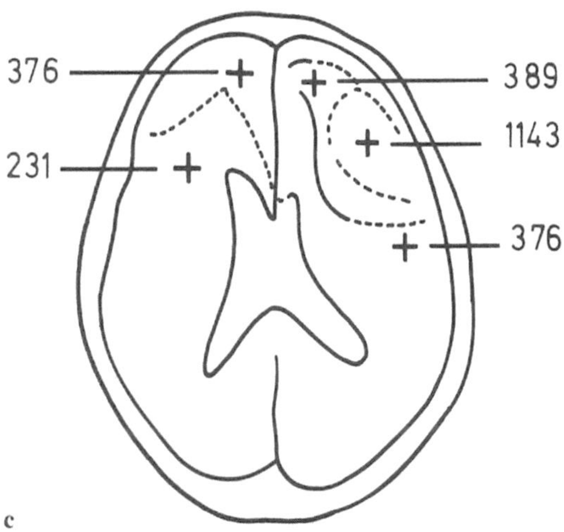

c

Fig. 2a–c. Right cerebral infarction in a 51-year-old man: **a** X-ray CT; **b** NMR-CT; **c** T_1 values

Table 2. Time course of T_1 values in patients with cerebral infarction (means ± SD, ms)

Site \ Period after onset	1–30 days	1–3 months	3– months
Infarcted area	361±81 (*n*=15)	742±389 (*n*=5)	1298±804 (*n*=7)
Border zone	278±40 (*n*=16)	337± 89 (*n*=4)	315± 45 (*n*=8)

Table 2 and Fig. 3 indicate the time courses of T_1 in 20 cases with massive cerebral infarction. As indicated, T_1 values in the central area of cerebral infarction were consistently increased, being on average 361 ms up to 1 month after infarction, 742 ms between 1 and 3 months, and 1298 ms more than 3 months after. In contrast, T_1 values in the border zone of cerebral infarction varied only slightly or moderately, ranging between 278 and 337 ms on average.

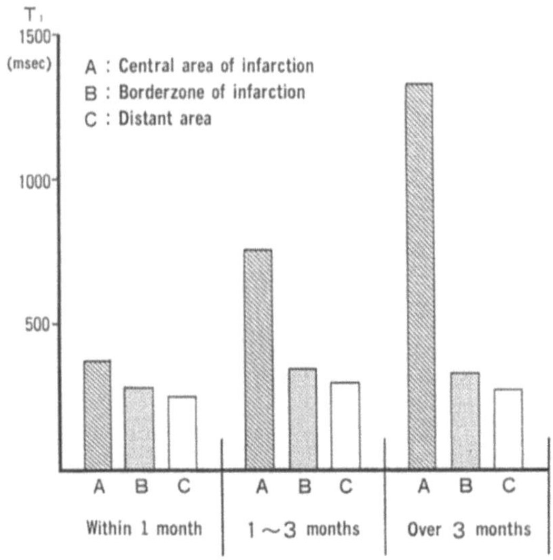

Fig. 3. Spin lattice relaxation times in 20 patients at different times after massive cerebral infarction

Discussion

In vitro proton NMR techniques have been applied to examine the pathophysiology of edema from the viewpoints of biological water dynamics. Bakay [1] and Go et al. [3] studied induced brain edema by means of pulse NMR for chemical use, indicating a proportional relation between tissue water content and in vitro proton relaxation time. Naruse and his coworkers [5] reported, on the basis of studies on various types of experimental brain edema, that prolongation of T_1 was related to the increased volume of water in edematous tissues, and that a biphasic T_2 probably reflected the distribution and content of the edema fluid induced. The results of these investigations strongly support a considerable potential for the exploitation of proton relaxation time measurement in the field of brain edema research. Recent progress in the development of diagnostic NMR equipment is making it possible to extend the applications to the fields of clinical imaging or relaxation time measurement.

As indicated in the present results, T_1 was significantly longer in the core region of cerebral infarction. The values of T_1 were 361 ms on average within 1 month after the stroke. Even within 1 week, T_1 in the central ischemic zone was 384 ms on average. It is reasonable to believe that cerebral infarction causes not only cerebral edema in association with oligemia or complete ischemia, but also the initiation of tissue degeneration, even in its acute phase. Interestingly, such prolonged T_1 times became much longer with time. After 3 months or more, the T_1 values for the central region of cerebral ischemia were far in excess of 1000 ms. These alterations in relaxation are probably different from the T_1 changes observed in acute or subacute phases of cerebral ischemia. Extreme prolongations of T_1 in the chronic stage may be related to denatured processes in the ischemic lesion, probably corresponding to processes of necrotic change and cavity formation as a terminal sequel to tissue degeneration.

It seems that in vivo T_1 measurements in circulatory disorders will make it possible to estimate the severity of the damage in cerebral lesions. The proton relaxation time and its time course may be a suitable means of evaluating the reversibility of the tissue damage. Although further investigations are required for understanding of relaxation phenomena in the biological tissues, in vivo T_1 measurement will yield valuable information that can be used in grading of ischemic brain insults.

Conclusion

Measurement of T_1 in different brain regions reveals various kinds of information on the properties of the lesion site. In an acute or subacute stage, an elevated T_1 within brain parenchyma generally reflects the progression of cerebral edema, whereas marked T_1 prolongation in the chronic stage is likely to have resulted from denaturation in ischemic brain tissue.

Summary

In vivo measurements of spin lattice relaxation time (T_1) were performed to assess the pathophysiologic status in cerebral infarctions. Thirty patients with cerebral infarction were examined by the FONAR QED 80-Alpha system. Infarcted areas showed up as high-density zones in SSFP images. On occasions, high-density areas in the NMR display exceeded the low-density zones found on X-ray CT in extent. This wider extent of density abnormalities probably represents the actual spread of cerebral edema. Infarcted areas were characterized by an apparent prolongation of T_1, which was 361 ms on average within 1 month after the stroke. T_1 values in the infarcted area changed frequently over time. The core region revealed markedly prolonged values of T_1 in chronic edema, with mean values of 742 ms between 1 and 3 months after and 1298 ms more than 3 months after the stroke. This prolongation of T_1 was considered to reflect the processes of tissue degeneration induced by ischemic insults.

References

1. Bakay L, Kurland RL, Parrish RG, Lee JC, Peng RJ, Bartkowshi HM (1975) Nuclear magnetic resonance studies in normal and edematous brain tissue. Exp Brain Res 23:241–248
2. Furuse M, Saso K, Inao S, Motegi Y, Kimura H, Kasai A (1983) NMR images and in vivo T_1 values associated with cerebrovascular diseases. J NMR Med 3:54–60
3. Go KG, Edzes HT (1975) Water in brain edema. Observation by the pulsed nuclear magnetic resonance technique. Arch Neurol 32:462–465
4. Motegi Y, Furuse M, Saso K, Inao S, Izawa A, Kamata N (1984) Estimation on pathophysiology of cerebral infarction by nuclear magnetic resonance. Image Technology Information Display 16:42–48
5. Naruse S, Horikawa Y, Tanaka C, Hirakawa K, Nishikawa H, Yoshizaki K (1982) Proton nuclear magnetic resonance studies on brain edema. J Neurosurg 56:747–752

Clinicopathological Analysis in Severe Head Injury

H. WATANABE, J. OKADA, M. HARA, M. OGASHIWA, M. NUMOTO [1], K. AKAI, and K. TAKEUCHI

Key words: Traffic accident, head injury, diffuse axonal injury, retraction ball

Introduction

In modern societies, the major cause of severe head injuries is probably traffic accidents. We studied CT findings, outcomes [3], and pathologic features of severe head injury cases (Glasgow coma score [4] < 8) and we found that in some cases outcome was poor despite minimal CT abnormalities. These patients became comatose immediately after the insults and never subsequently regained consciousness. The clinical sample was composed of 68 cases among 422 hospitalized patients who had sustained head injuries in traffic accidents between December 1979 and March 1984. Cases with gross intracranial hematomas and primary brain stem damage were excluded. Most of the patients underwent CT scan within 2 h of the accident.

Results

The sex and age distributions (age between 2 and 82 years, mean 30.4 years) are shown in Fig. 1. In this sample, 62% of the patients were under 30 years old, and the male/female ratio was 3:1. The mortality rate of those over 60 years of age was 89%, while that of those under 60 was 54%.

A good correlation between GCS (Glasgow coma score) and outcome was noted, as is apparent from Table 1. The extremely poor outcome in cases with GCS under 5 is stressed. There are four exceptional cases. Two patients with GCS of 3 made a good recovery; both had been under the influence of alcohol at the initial examination. On the other hand, two patients died of complications even though the initial GCS in each was 8.

The outcome in each patient and the various CT findings are shown in Table 2. Diffuse brain swelling [6, 7] was the most frequent feature on CT. Five patients died despite minimal abnormalities on CT, four with small contusions and one with ventricular hemorrhage.

Autopsies were performed in three of the above five cases, and in one case of diffuse brain swelling (Table 3). Extensive diffuse axonal injury [1, 2] with retraction

[1] Department of Neurosurgery, Kyorin University School of Medicine, 6-20-2 Shinkawa, Mitaka-shi, Tokyo 181, Japan

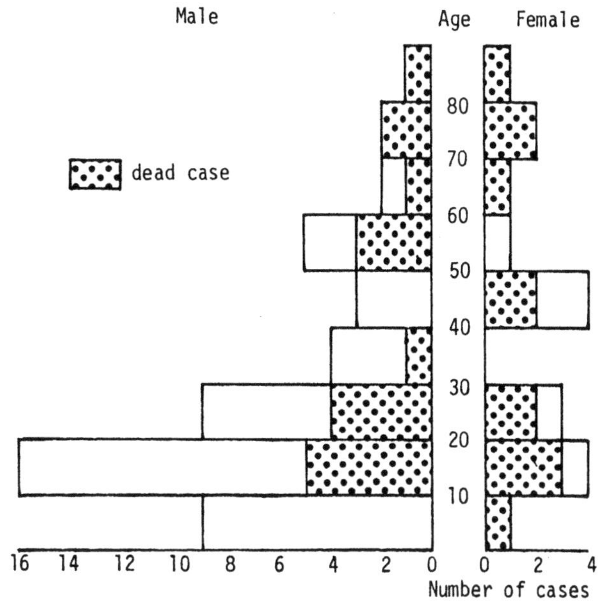

Fig. 1. Sex and age distribution. *Shading* indicates a fatal outcome. GCS≦8 in all cases

Table 1. GCS and outcome of head injury

GCS \ GOS	Good recovery	Moderate disability	Severe disability	Persistent vegetative state	Death	Total
8	9	1	0	0	2	12
7	11	0	0	0	1	12
6	12	1	0	0	1	14
5	1	1	0	0	1	3
4	1	0	1	0	4	6
3	2	0	0	0	19	21
Total	36	3	1	0	28	68

GOS, Glasgow outcome scale

Table 2. CT findings and outcome

	Diffuse brain swelling	Massive contusion	Small contusion	Ventricular hemorrhage	Normal	Not examined
Good recovery	26	0	1	0	8	1
Moderate disablement	2	0	1	0	0	0
Severe disablement	0	0	1	0	0	0
Persistent vegetative state	0	0	0	0	0	0
Death	8 (1)	7	4 (3)	1	0	8
Total	36	7	7	1	8	9

( ), autopsy

Table 3. Findings at autopsy

Pt	Age (years)	Sex	Histopathologic findings
KS	22	F	Diffuse axonal injury, small contusions
NH	16	M	Diffuse axonal injury, small area of necrosis
TK	52	M	Diffuse axonal injury, small contusions
AK	12	F	Diffuse brain swelling, extensive necrosis

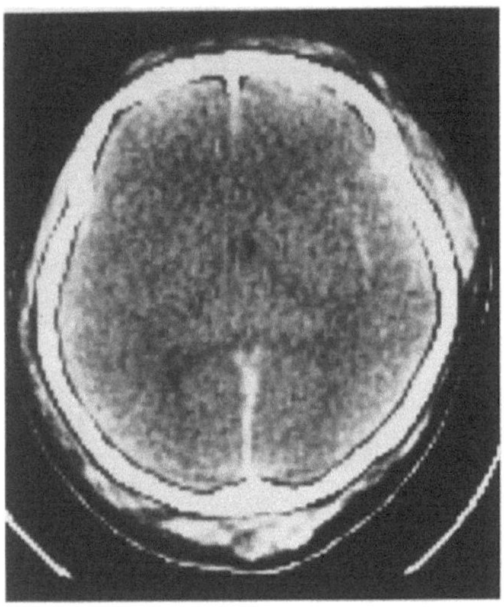

Fig. 2. CT on admission, showing cerebral contusion in right frontotemporal area

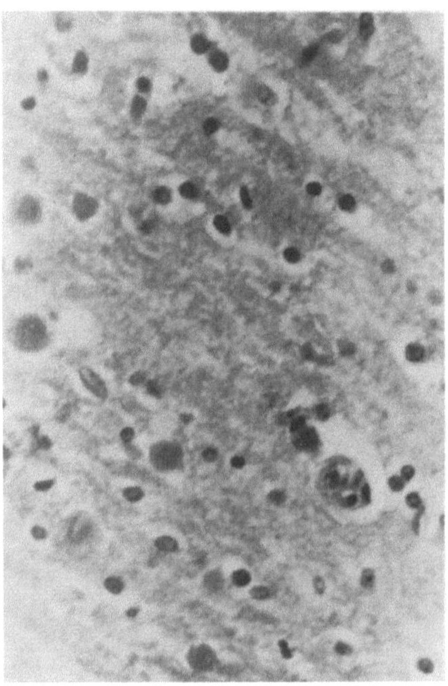

Fig. 3. Photomicrograph of the specimen from the left temporal lobe, showing axonal injury with retraction balls. (H & E; ×270) (Watanabe and Takeuchi [5])

balls was the most striking finding in all three cases with small contusions. The patient with diffuse brain swelling was found to have extensive brain edema and necrosis.

Case Reports

Case 1. A 22-year-old woman driving a motorcycle was thrown onto the road on collision with a truck. She became comatose immediately after the accident. Her GCS, measured in the casualty room, was 4. CT on admission revealed cerebral contusion in the right frontotemporal area (Fig. 2). She died 17 h after the accident. An autopsy was performed. The histopathological findings showed diffuse axonal injuries not only in the contused hemisphere but also in the contralateral hemisphere (Fig. 3).

Case 2. A case with intracranial hematoma is described for reference. A 16-year-old youth driving a motorcycle crashed into a concrete wall. He became comatose im-

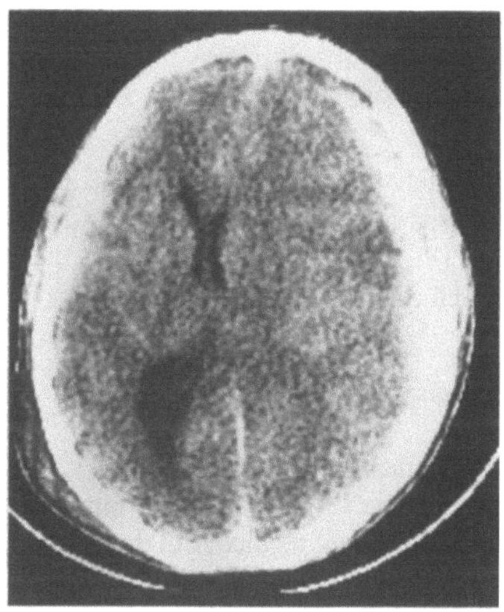

Fig. 4. CT on admission, showing a subdural hematoma on the right and cerebral contusion. Midline shift to the left is evident

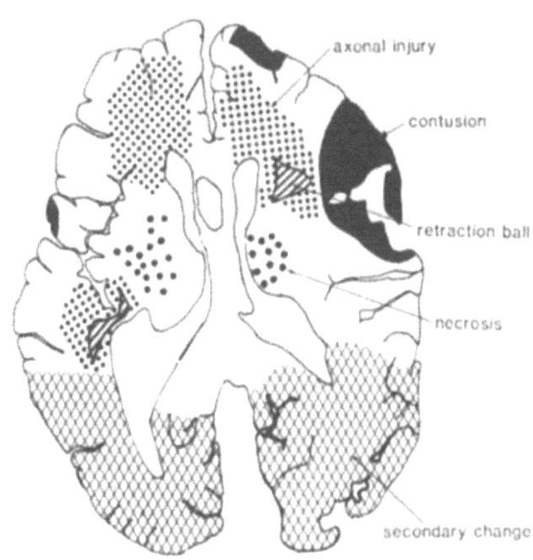

Fig. 5. Schematic mapping of a brain slice. Note bilateral scatter of diffuse axonal injury. (Watanabe and Takeuchi [5])

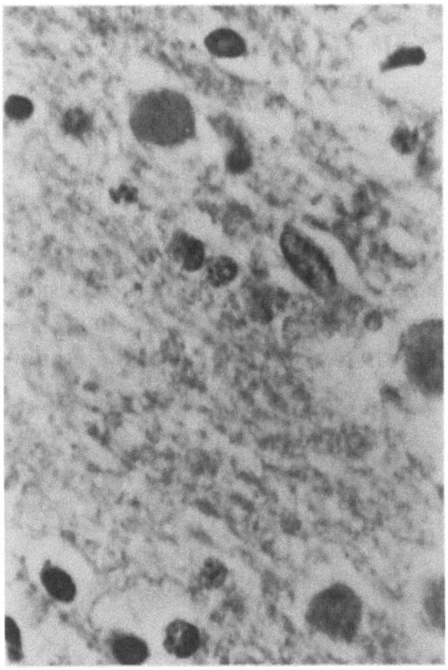

Fig. 6. Photomicrograph of a specimen from the left temporal lobe, showing axonal injury with retraction balls. (H&E; ×270) (Watanabe and Takeuchi [5])

mediately after the insult. His GCS was 3 in the casualty room. CT on admission revealed a subdural hematoma and cerebral contusion in the right frontotemporal area (Fig. 4). He died 57 days after the accident. An autopsy was performed and revealed extensive diffuse axonal injury (Figs. 5 and 6).

Summary

In a clinical study of patients with severe head injuries we noted that in one group of patients the CT findings were minimal compared with the neurological findings, so that CT was not predictive of the outcome in these patients. Autopsy was carried out in three patients in this group, and extensive diffuse axonal injury was the characteristic finding.

Life-threatening phenomena other than gross intracranial hematoma, edema, diffuse brain swelling and ischemia, and diffuse axonal injury may occur in head-injured patients. The primary brain matrix damage in the severely head-injured patient is extensive and varied, which means it cannot be detected by CT. The most prominent histopathological findings are diffuse axonal injury associated with retraction balls, destruction of oligodendroglias, and astrocytosis even far distant from the contused area. Diffuse axonal injury is an irreversible, and perhaps primary, change in axons.

References

1. Adams JH, Graham DI, Murray LS, Scott G (1982) Diffuse axonal injury due to non-missile injury in human. An analysis of 45 cases. Ann Neurol 12:557–563

2. Gennarelli TA, Thibault LE, Adams JH, Graham DI, Thompson CJ, Marcincin RP (1982) Diffuse axonal injury and traumatic coma in primate. Ann Neurol 12:564–574
3. Jennett B, Bond M (1975) Assessment of outcome after severe brain damage. A practical scale. Lancet I:480–484
4. Teasdale G, Jennett B (1976) Assessment and prognosis of coma after head injury. Acta Neurochir (Wien) 34:45–55
5. Watanabe H, Takeuchi K (1984) Head injury caused by traffic accident. Surg Diagn Treat 26:691–692
6. Zimmermann RA, Bilaniuk LT, Bruce D, Dolinskas C, Obrist W, Kuhl D (1978) Computed tomography of pediatric head trauma. Acute general cerebral swelling. Radiology 126:403–408
7. Zimmermann RA, Bilaniuk LT, Gennerlli T (1979) Computed tomography of shearing injuries of the cerebral white matter. Radiology 127:393–396

Relationship Between Size of Hematoma and Blood Flow in Hypertensive Intracerebral Hematoma

T. YAMADA [1], T. SHIMA, S. MATSUMURA, Y. OKADA, H. HATAYAMA, and S. OKITA

Key words: Hypertensive intracerebral hematoma, emission CT, cerebral blood flow

Introduction

CBF studies in cases with hypertensive intracerebral hematoma (HIH) have been performed with a two-dimensional technique [1, 4] involving the disadvantage of an unresolved problem, viz. look-through phenomenon [3]. We used a three-dimensional technique to study the relationship between size of hematoma and serial CBF changes in cases with HIH.

Methods

Eighteen cases (mean age 62 years) were all in mildly disturbed states of consciousness at the beginning of the study. In 10 of the 18 cases the hematoma was located in the putamen; in 5 cases, in the thalamus; and in 3 cases, in the temporal lobe. In 7 cases of hematoma more than 30 ml and 1 of hematoma 17 ml in volume surgery was performed in the acute stage, while in 10 cases of hematoma less than 30 ml in volume no operation was performed.

CBF was measured in a slice 5 cm above the OM line by single photon emission CT (Tomomatic 32) at 1–7 days, 1–2 months, and 2–3 months after the start of the study. We calculated the mean CBF in each cerebral hemisphere with a CBF map. The $PaCO_2$ was maintained between 35 and 43 mmHg during CBF measurement.

Theta and alpha activities in the EEG were also analyzed by computer mapping of the EEG (CME) at 1–7 days, 1–2 months, and 2–3 months. In addition, neurologic deficits were evaluated at 1–7 days and 2–3 months after the start and were compared with CBF and EEG changes.

Results

The size of each hematoma was correlated with the CBF reduction 1–7 days from the start of the study in the affected hemisphere (Fig. 1). However, in the nonaffected hemisphere no such correlation could be found.

[1] Department of Neurosurgery, Chugoku Rousai Hospital, 1477 Hiro-machi, Kure-shi 737-01, Japan

At 1–7 days after the onset, the mean CBF in the effected hemisphere was 40 ml/100 g/min in the cases subjected to surgery, which was markedly lower than the corresponding value (50 ml) in the patients who did not undergo surgery (Fig. 2). In the former group the mean CBF in the affected hemisphere increased markedly to 49 ml at 1–2 months, while in the no surgery group the increase was less pronounced, the value not reaching 55 ml. The mean CBF in the nonaffected hemisphere was slightly lower at first in both groups, but subsequently increased by less than in the affected hemisphere.

CME revealed a tendency to increasing alpha activity with no evident changes in theta activity in the group that underwent surgery. In the other patients CME revealed a tendency to decreasing theta activity with increasing alpha activity.

Improvement of neurologic signs was observed in only 3 of the 8 patients in the surgery group, while 9 of the 10 patients not subjected to surgery experienced improvement. There was some correlation between these neurologic changes and CME findings, but not between neurologic and CBF changes.

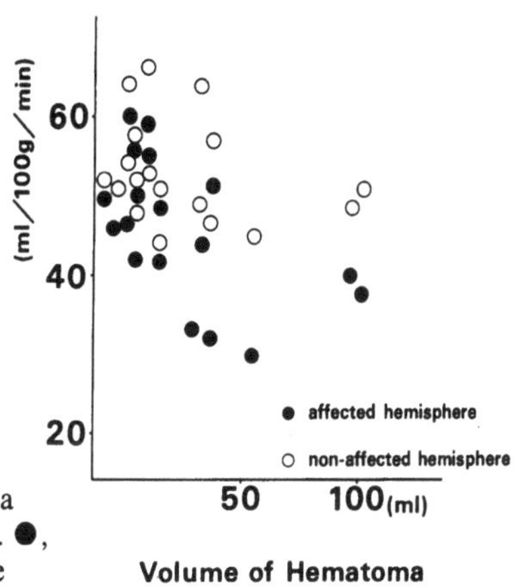

Fig. 1. Correlation between volume of hematoma and mean CBF within 1 week after start of study. ●, affected hemisphere; ○, nonaffected hemisphere

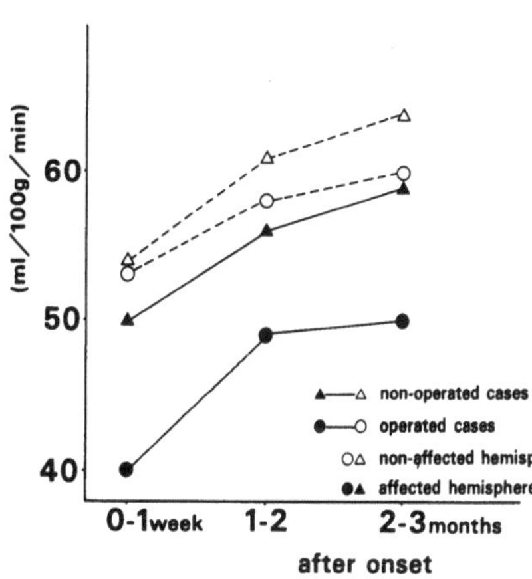

Fig. 2. Comparison of mean CBF changes between cases treated (●–○) and not treated (▲–△) by surgery. ○ △, nonaffected hemisphere; ● ▲, affected hemisphere

Discussion

Our study showed the relationship between the size of hematoma and the degree a CBF reduction in the affected hemisphere in the acute stage of HIH. Some previous reports measuring CBF by a conventional two-dimensional technique had suggested similar results [1, 4]. Two mechanisms of CBF reduction were found [1, 4]. The first was the effect of increased intracranial pressure due to the hematoma and associated brain edema. The second involved transneural depression due to direct destruction of the putamen and/or thalamus by the hematoma itself [4]. Sugiyama [4] showed a nonlinear relationship between the size of hematoma and degree of CBF reduction: CBF was more severely reduced in cases with smaller hematomas. This result could not be explained solely by mass effect, and he suggested that direct destruction of the putamen or thalamus resulted in severe hemispheric CBF reduction. However, in our study, even in a case with massive hematoma in the temporal lobe apart from the thalamus or putamen, a marked reduction of CBF similar in degree to that seen with a putaminal hematoma of the same volume was found. Additionally, in cases with thalamic or putaminal hemorrhage, a marked increase in CBF was found at that time 1–2 months after surgery, whereas the thalamus or putamen appeared to be partly destroyed. Our study suggested that reduction of CBF was caused not only by transneural depression, but by a mass effect. Further investigation with serial ICP and CBF monitoring was thought to be necessary for the explanation of these mechanisms.

Whether surgery is indicated in HIH combined with mildly disturbed consciousness is still a controversial question [2]. In our study, the EEG and neurologic deficits improved to a lesser degree in the patients who underwent surgery than in those who did not. One explanation for this result might be that the hematomas in the patients treated surgically were so large that there was more destruction of the brain at the beginning of the study and this prevented early improvement of the EEG and neurologic findings. Evaluation of the indications for surgery in cases with mildly disturbed consciousness will require a further followup period and investigation of more cases.

Summary

We studied the relationship between size of hematoma and changes in cerebral blood flow (CBF) in an attempt to determine the effects of hematoma on CBF.

Eighteen patients were all in midly disturbed states of consciousness. Seven patients with hematomas more than 30 ml in volume and one with a hematoma 17 ml in volume underwent surgery, while the remaining ten with hematomas less than 30 ml in volume did not. We measured CBF by single photon emission CT at 1–7 days, 1–2 months, and 2–3 months after the start of the stroke.

At the start of the study an inverse relationship between the size of hematoma and the mean CBF in the affected hemisphere was observed. The mean CBF in the nonaffected hemisphere was also reduced. The mean CBF in the affected hemisphere in the patients subjected to surgery was much lower than that in the other patients before surgery, and increased markedly after the operation.

In a case with massive hematoma in the temporal lobe apart from the putamen or thalamus, the mean lowering of CBF at the beginning was similar in degree to that observed with putaminal hematoma of the same size. In this case too, marked improvement of CBF was observed following operation. These two results might suggest that the marked CBF reduction was caused mainly by increased intracranial pressure due to a mass effect, and not by transneural depression.

References

1. Ishii R, Takeuchi S, Oosugi S, Tanaka R, Arai H (1982) Cerebral blood flow in patients with putaminal hemorrhage using Xe-133 inhalation method. Neurol Med Chir (Tokyo) 22:813–821
2. Kanno K, Katada K, Hoshino M, Soda M, Mitsuyama F, Yokoi K, Shinoyama Y, Sano H (1982) Relationship between the mode of hematoma spreading and the prognosis for hypertensive intracerebral hemorrhage. Neurol Med Chir (Tokyo) 22:725–732
3. Olsen TS, Larsen B, Hering M, Skriver EB, Lassen NA (1983) Blood flow and vascular reactivity in collaterally perfused brain tissue. Stroke 14:332–341
4. Sugiyama H (1984) Cerebral blood flow in patients with hypertensive intracerebral hemorrhage. Neurol Med Chir (Tokyo) 24:564–572

Dexamethasone Fails to Prevent the Development of Brain Edema in Temporal Lobe Contusions

E. FACCO[1], M. ZUCCARELLO, G. C. ANDRIOLI, and G. P. GIRON

Key words: Dexamethasone, brain edema, temporal lobe contusion, cimetidine

Introduction

The beneficial effects of steroids in severe head injuries have yet to be unequivocally documented, although they have been used for many years and a vast amount of data is available in the literature.

The clinical syndrome of temporal lobe contusion (TLC), described by McLaurin and Helmer in 1965 [7], allows us to detect and to follow the progression of perilesional hypodensity around the contusion on CT scan in head-injured patients [9].

The aim of our study is to evaluate whether high doses of dexamethasone can prevent the appearance or the progression of perilesional hypodensity and midline shift on CT scan and worsening of the clinical condition in patients with isolated TLC.

Subjects and Methods

A prospective trial was performed in ten patients admitted to the Neurosurgical Department of Padua University with isolated TLC. The age range was 20–58 years, with a mean of 47.4 ± 13.6 (SD); at the time of admission the Glasgow coma score was 10.4 ± 2.8 (mean ± SD); two patients were hemiparetic, three aphasic, and two comatose. All the patients were subjected to a standard management protocol, including mannitol 20% at a dose of 0.25 g/kg body weight [6] every 4 h and prophylactic administration of cimetidine at a dose of 1 g/day IV. Dexamethasone treatment started within 6 h after the trauma: an initial dose of 24 mg IV was followed by 8 mg every 4 h for 7 days. In comatose patients controlled hyperventilation was applied to keep the partial CO_2 pressure in arterial blood between 25 and 30 torr [3].

All the patients were submitted to CT scan examination at the moment of admission; a control CT scan was performed on the 4th day. A further control CT scan was performed 6–9 days after the trauma. CT scan findings were graded according to a four-point scale: (0) absence of perifocal hypodensity; (1) presence of perifocal

[1] Ist. Anestesiologia e Rianimazione, Università degli Studi di Padova, Via C. Battisti 267, 35100 Padova, Italy

hypodensity ("edema"); (2) temporal lobe hypodensity; (3) hemispheric hypodensity. Midline shift was also measured.

Outcome was assessed at 3 and 6 months and classified according to a five-point scale according to Jennett and Bond [5]: Dead (D); Persistent Vegetative State (PVS); Severe Disability (SD); Moderate Disability (MD); Good Recovery (GR).

Results

Table 1 reports the main clinical data, CT scan findings, and outcome recorded in our cases: only two patients did not show any progression of edema on the CT scan during the first week after the trauma; one patient underwent surgical treatment on the 2nd day in hospital and clinical and radiologic improvement was seen on the second CT scan performed on the 4th day. All other patients showed enlargement of the hypodense area around the contusion and the appearance or increase of midline shift on control CT scans (Fig. 1). These radiologic findings correlated with worsening of the clinical condition: three patients became comatose within 4 days of the injury and three more patients, between the 5th and 9th days; three patients were hemiparetic on admission, six at the time of the second CT scan, and seven at the time of the third CT scan; one patient became aphasic on the 3rd day in hospital and another one was aphasic on emergence from coma.

Five of the six comatose patients underwent surgical treatment. Four patients died: two of these developed septic shock and one, severe hemorrhagic shock resulting from massive gastric bleeding. Among the survivors mild gastric bleeding occurred on the 7th day in hospital in one case; dexamethasone was discontinued and the patient recovered.

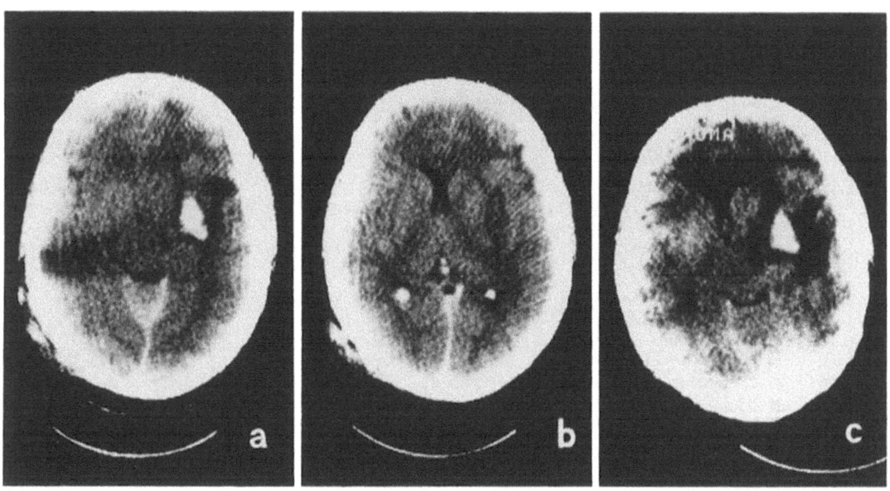

Fig. 1a–c. A typical case of temporal lobe contusion: **a, b** CT scan performed on admission; **c** enlargement of both contusion and perilesional hypodense area with increased midline shift on the 7th hospital day

Table 1. Relationship between clinical course, serial CT scan findings, and outcome in ten patients with temporal lobe contusion

Patient	I CT scan (1st day)					II CT scan (4th day)					III CT scan (6–9th day)					Day of surgery	Extracranial complications	Out-come
	Grade	Shift (mm)	GCS	HP	A	Grade	Shift (mm)	GCS	HP	A	Grade	Shift (mm)	GCS	HP	A			
V. N.	1	0	10	–	–	1	0	15	+	–	1	0	15	+	–	–	–	MD
R. A.	1	0	10	+	+	1	0	10	+	+	1	0	10	+	+	–	Severe gastric bleeding	D
G. G.	0	0	15	–	–	1	0	15	+	–	1	3	15	+	–	–	–	MD
P. G.	1	3	9	–	–	2	6	10	+	+	2	6	10	+	+	–	–	SD
T. U.	1	3	11	–	–	2	6	7	–	?	§	§	10*	–	+	7th	Mild gastric bleeding	MD
N. C.	1	0	13	–	+	2	3	11	–	+	3	6	8	–	?	–	–	SD
S. R.	1	4.5	11	–	+	2	6	10	+	+	3	9	8	+	?	8th	Septic shock	D
Z. F.	1	4.5	7	–	+	3	9	7	–	?	3	12	5	+	–	8th	Septic shock	D
C. V.	2	6	6	+	?	1*	3*	13*	–	–	§	§	14	–	–	2nd	–	MD
T. I.	1	3	12	+	+	3	9	11	+	+	3	9	7	+	?	9th	–	D

HP, hemiparesis; A, aphasia; +, present; –, absent; *, after surgery; ?, not evaluable; §, not performed

Discussion

As is well known, the temporal lobe is the most frequent site of brain contusion. Although TLC may occur with a more diffuse brain injury, McLaurin and Helmer [7] emphasized the importance of recognizing it as a separate entity with a distinct clinical presentation, course, and treatment. Recently the CT features of temporal lobe contusion and the correlation between clinical course and serial CT examinations have been described [9]: worsening of patients' conditions seems to be associated with the progressive appearance of a hypodense area (edema) surrounding the contusion. Therefore, the clinical syndrome of TLC allows us both to detect the onset and to follow the progression of brain edema on CT scan.

There are conflicting opinions about the usefulness of steroids in head-injured patients: Gobiet et al. [4] detected significant beneficial effects following the administration of high doses of dexamethasone, but other trials [2, 11, 1] have shown no significant effects of steroids on morbidity or mortality; nevertheless steroids seem to exert many beneficial metabolic effects on traumatized brain, such as inhibition of arachidonic acid release and improvement of regional glucose utilization [10].

A recent paper has reported on the effectiveness of cimetidine in the prevention of gastrointestinal hemorrhage in severely head-injured patients [8].

In our series only two patients out of ten showed no neurologic deterioration during the clinical course; the only patient who had improved by the time of the second CT scan had been operated on the day after the injury: therefore we cannot rule out the possibility that this improvement was due to the surgical treatment. In all other patients there was a deterioration in the clinical condition, accompanied by progression of the hypodense area around the contusion on CT scan in the first week after the injury. Four patients died and five required surgical treatment; moreover, two patients had gastric bleeding, which was fatal in one case, and two developed late septic shock.

Our results suggest that steroids may have no beneficial effects in reducing perifocal hypodensity in patients with parenchymal contusions, and may even be harmful, causing severe extracranial complications: definitive confirmation of this idea requires further study.

The value of our conclusions is limited owing to the restricted number of patients, but our study suggests that: (a) dexamethasone failed to prevent the occurrence and/or the development of brain edema in post-traumatic TLC; (b) dexamethasone seemed to enhance the risk of extracranial complications, e.g., gastrointestinal bleeding; (c) cimetidine at a dosage of 1 g daily did not prevent upper gastrointestinal tract bleeding; and (d) neurologic status, clinical course, and CT scan were closely related, as reported by Nelson et al. [9].

Summary

The clinical syndrome of temporal lobe contusion (TLC) provides a good opportunity to detect and to follow the progression of brain edema around the contusion on CT scan in head-injured patients.

A prospective study was performed in ten patients; dexamethasone treatment at a dose of 48 mg/day and prophylactic administration of cimetidine at a dose of 1 g/day started within 6 h of the trauma. CT scans were performed at the time of admission, on day 4, and on days 6–9.

Seven patients showed neurologic deterioration in the first week after the trauma, associated with appearance or progression of the hypodense area around the contusion and midline shift on CT scan.

Six patients became comatose; five underwent surgical treatment; and four died: two of these had developed septic shock and one, a severe hemorrhagic shock due to massive gastric bleeding.

One surviving patient had mild gastric bleeding on the 7th day.

Our results, although based on a limited sample, suggest that dexamethasone at a dose of 48 mg/day fails to prevent the development of brain edema in TLC, and may even enhance the risk of severe extracranial complications; cimetidine lacks effectiveness in the prevention of gastric hemorrhage in steroid-treated head-injured patients.

References

1. Braakman R, Schouten HJA, Blaaw-van Dishoek M, Minderhoud J (1983) Megadose steroids in severe head injury. Result of a prospective double-blind clinical trial. J Neurosurg 58:326–330
2. Cooper PR, Moody S, Clark WK, Kirkpatrick J, Maravilla K, Gould AL, Drane W (1979) Dexamethasone and severe head injury. A prospective double-blind study. J Neurosurg 51:307–316
3. Crockard HA, Coppel DL, Morrow WFK (1973) Evaluation of hyperventilation in treatment of head injuries. Br Med J 4:634–640
4. Gobiet W, Bock WJ, Liesegang J, Grote W (1976) Treatment of acute cerebral edema with high dose of dexamethasone. In: Becks JWF, Bosch DA, Brock M (eds) Intracranial pressure III. Springer, Berlin Heidelberg New York, pp 231–235
5. Jennett B, Bond M (1975) Assessment of outcome after severe brain damage. A practical scale. Lancet 1:480–484
6. Marshall LF, Smith RW, Rausher LA, Shapiro HM (1978) Mannitol dose requirement in brain-injured patients. J Neurosurg 48:169–172
7. McLaurin RL, Helmer F (1965) The syndrome of temporal-lobe contusion. J Neurosurg 23:296–304
8. Mouawad E, Deloof T, Genette F, Vandesteene A (1983) Open trial of cimetidine in the prevention of upper gastrointestinal haemorrhage in patients with severe intracranial injury. Acta Neurochir 67:239–244
9. Nelson PB, Rosembaum AE, Moossy J, Maraon JC (1982) Delayed deterioration in the syndrome of temporal lobe contusion: evaluation by computed tomography (CT). J Trauma 22/1:39–42
10. Pappius HM, Wolfe LS (1984) Effects of drugs on local cerebral glucose utilization in traumatized brain: mechanisms of action of steroids revisited. In: Go KG, Baethmann A (eds) Recent progress in the study and therapy of brain edema. Plenum, New York, pp 11–26
11. Saul TG, Ducker TB, Saleman M, Carro E (1981) Steroids in severe head injury: A prospective randomized clinical trial. J Neurosurg 54:596–600

Amelioration of Ischemic Brain Edema by a Free Radical Scavenger, AVS: Experimental Analysis of Its Action in the Cat MCA Occlusion Model

T. ASANO [1], H. JOHSHITA, T. KOIDE, and K. TAKAKURA

Key words: Cerebral ischemia, cerebral edema, free radicals, brain energy metabolism, radical scavengers

Introduction

Cerebral edema resulting from an ischemic insult is of great clinical importance, because it aggravates brain damage by way of an elevation of intracranial pressure, frequently leading to brain herniation.

The currently available therapy against ischemic brain edema consists of administration of hyperosmolar agents, steroids, and other drugs, combined with hyperventilation or CSF drainage. The effects are mostly transient, however, and have not been found to be sufficiently powerful as to have a favorable influence on the final outcome. Therefore, there is a need to develop an effective therapeutic agent against ischemic cerebral edema, whose action presumably will address a novel pathomechanism.

Based on the free radical hypothesis suggested by Demopoulos et al. [4], we have been investigating the effects of a novel radical scavenger, AVS (1,2-bis(nicotine-amide)-propane, Chugai Pharmaceutical Co., Ltd) on ischemic cerebral edema and cerebral vasospasm following subarachnoid hemorrhage (SAH). Our previous data indicate that AVS significantly inhibits the occurrence of chronic vasospasm in the canine SAH model [2] and that the drug attenuates hemispheric edema developing in the rat MCA occlusion model [5]. A study of the in vitro action of AVS showed that AVS scavenges the hydroxyl radical in the Udenfriend's system [7] and suppresses the lipoxygenase activity, that is decreases the production of hydroxyacids, of the rat brain microvessel [8] or the canine basilar artery [6].

For further examination of the antiedema effect of AVS on ischemic brain edema, the present study was carried out in the cat MCA occlusion model.

Materials and Methods

The effects of AVS on the cerebral cortical blood flow (lCBF) and specific gravity (coSG) 4 h after middle cerebral artery occlusion in cats were studied in experiment

---

[1] Department of Neurosurgery, University of Tokyo Hospital, 7-3-1, Hongo, Bunkyo-ku, Tokyo 113, Japan

I, and its effect on the energy metabolites in the cerebral cortex was studied in experiment II. The same experimental model and conditions were used in both experiments.

Experiment I

Adult cats of both sexes weighing 3–4 kg were divided into the control group receiving saline (10 cats) and the AVS group treated with AVS (10 cats). AVS was dissolved in saline and administered IV at the rate of 1 mg/kg/min. The same amount of saline (50 ml) was infused in the same way to the control animals.

Cats were anesthetized by inhalation of halothane and intubated. The femoral artery and vein were catheterized and the skull was fixed in a stereotaxic holder. Six hydrogen-sensitive platinum electrodes were then implanted at the predetermined positions of the MCA territory of the left hemisphere (Fig. 1). The bared tip of each electrode was inserted into the cerebral cortex for a depth of 1 mm through a small burr hole in the cranium. The left internal carotid artery and the middle cerebral artery (MCA) were exposed by the transorbital approach and freed from the surrounding structures so that clips could easily be applied later. After the above operative procedures, halothane was turned off. Each cat was immobilized by IV administration of gallamine and ventilated with 70% N_2O/30% O_2. The end-expiratory CO_2 and O_2 tensions were continuously monitored with a gas analyzer (San-ei, Expired gas monitor 2H21A). The arterial gases were analyzed every hour with ABL-1. The base deficits and alteration of pCO_2 were corrected each time. The rectal temperature was monitored with a thermistor and was kept within the range of 37.5 ± 0.5 °C with the aid of a warming blanket and an infrared electric lamp.

After the systemic arterial pressure (SAP), rectal temperature, and blood gases had stabilized within the physiological ranges following immobilization, the first measurement of lCBF was carried out by the hydrogen clearance method. Then, the previously exposed left MCA and internal carotid artery were individually occluded with clips (Zen clip, Ohwa Tsusho). In

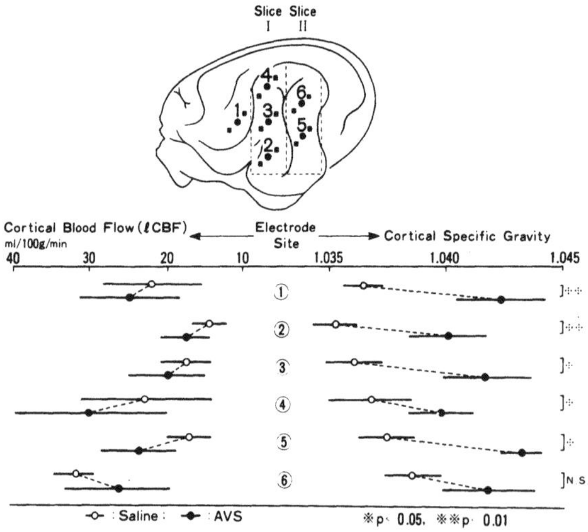

Fig. 1. The sites of hydrogen-sensitive electrodes (*above,* ●) and of sampling for the measurement of specific gravity in tissue topographically corresponding to each electrode (○). The *hatched area* represents the cortical area excised for the measurements of water and electrolyte contents and of the energy metabolites. Values (means ± SEM) recorded at each electrode site in control and experimental groups after MCA occlusion for lCBF (*below, left*) and for coSG (*below, right*)

the present study, the internal cerebral artery at the lateral margin of the optic nerve was also clipped in addition to the MCA, because this was believed to cause a more severe and more reliably reproducible ischemic lesion than NCA occlusion alone.

The lCBF was measured at 10, 30, 60, 90, 120, 150, 180, and 210 min after arterial occlusion. Immediately after the lCBF measurement at 10 min the IV infusion of saline with or without AVS was started, which continued until the end of the experiment. At 4 h after the arterial occlusion the cat was sacrificed by IV injection of KCl. The skull was removed and samples of the cerebral cortex were excised around each electrode. These samples were excised in duplicate, within several millimeters from each electrode, so that the coSG values were thought to correspond topographically to the lCBF values of each electrode. The coSG was measured by the gravimetric technique described by Marmarou et al. [9]. After the measurement of coSG, which took about 10 min, the remaining areas of cerebral cortex in the left and right MCA territory were excised as shown in Fig. 1. The water content and the sodium and potassium contents of these specimens were measured by the comparison of dry and wet weight and by flame photometry, respectively.

Experiment II

In experiment II, cats were divided into three groups, these being the control group and two ischemia groups (with and without AVS administration). In the control group (8 cats) cats were anesthetized with halothane inhalation, intubated, and artificially ventilated with 70% N_2O/30% O_2, as in experiment I. The artificial ventilation was maintained for 4 h and then the cats were sacrificed. In the remaining two groups, arterial occlusion by the transorbital approach was carried out as in experiment I. Saline (MCA-saline group: 6 cats) or AVS (MCA-AVS group: 7 cats) was then administered as in experiment I. At 4 h after the initiation of artificial ventilation in the normal control group and 4 h after arterial occlusion in the remaining groups, the skull was widely opened on both sides. As described by Welsh [11], the brain was frozen in situ with liquid nitrogen. Then the cat was sacrificed and decapitated. The head was immersed in liquid nitrogen and stored in a deep freezer (–80 °C).

The frozen head was cut in the coronal plane as shown in Fig. 1, in a cold room using a precooled electric saw. The cortical area corresponding to that for the measurement of water and electrolyte contents was chiseled out and homogenized by mincing in liquid nitrogen. Aliquots of the specimen were used for the analysis of energy metabolites. ATP, ADP, AMP, phosphocreatine, lactate, and pyruvate were measured by specific enzymatic techniques. All determinations were carried out with kits provided by Boehringer-Mannheim.

In the text, values are expressed as means ± SE. For statistical analysis, Student's two-tailed *t*-test was used.

Results

Experiment I

Between the control and AVS groups there was no significant difference in the values for blood gases. The SAP was stable around 140 mmHg in both groups for the first 2 h. Thereafter, the SAP dropped significantly ($P < 0.05$) by 10–20 mmHg in the AVS group.

The mean lCBF value at each electrode site ranged from 69 to 110 ml/100 g/min before arterial occlusion. After arterial occlusion it ranged from 13 to 30 ml/100 g/min (Fig. 1). The topographically corresponding mean value for coSG at each electrode is also shown in Fig. 1. At all the electrode sites the mean coSG was greater in the AVS group than in the control group, and the difference was significant at electrode sites 1, 2, 3, 4, and 5 (Fig. 1).

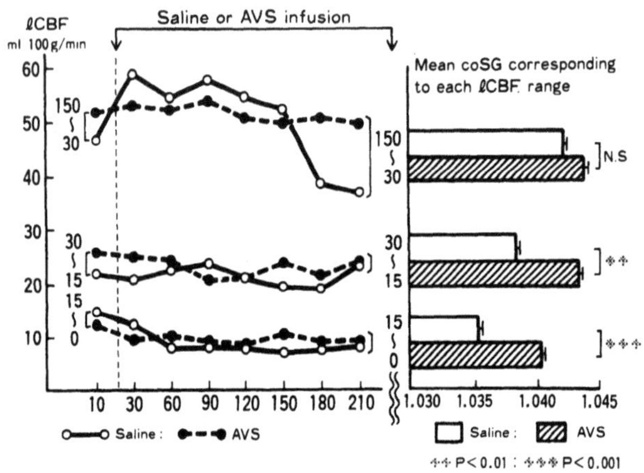

Fig. 2. Time course of lCBF in each lCBF range (*left*) and corresponding mean coSG values (*right*)

Table 1. Cortical contents of water, sodium, and potassium

		Water	Na	K
L-I	Control	83.52±0.76*	647.9±67.6*	489.1±26.8
	AVS	80.77±0.68*	458.7±35.7*	436.3±23.0
L-II	Control	82.46±0.66*	567.9±50.0*	431.3±24.4
	AVS	80.04±0.78*	416.0±25.7*	403.5±34.9
R-I	Control	79.91±0.73	386.2±24.7	509.1±31.1
	AVS	79.18±0.42	358.8±11.1	508.6±21.7
R-II	Control	79.94±0.66	368.7±18.1	526.2±19.7
	AVS	79.18±0.42	342.4±13.7	468.7±22.0

* $P<0.05$

Table 2. Values for energy metabolites

	MCA-Saline $n=6$	Normal control $n=8$	MCA-AVS $n=7$
ATP	1.557± 0.172	1.806±0.058	1.541±0.061
ADP	0.597± 0.054	0.498±0.018	0.506±0.034
AMP	0.177± 0.035	0.088±0.016*	0.105±0.027
Adenine nucleotide pool	2.331± 0.239	2.392±0.076	2.153±0.062
Energy charge	0.792± 0.018	0.860±0.008**	0.834±0.018
Lactate	17.183± 4.757	2.205±0.206*	8.316±1.564
Pyruvate	0.208± 0.032	0.273±0.021	0.314±0.057
L/P ratio	79.412±27.050	8.958±0.922*	31.186±3.815
Phosphocreatine	2.078± 0.315	2.733±0.212	3.141±0.573

MCA-saline vs. Normal control or MCA-AVS
* $P<0.05$; ** $P<0.01$ (Student's *t*-test)

To analyze the effect of AVS on lCBF and coSG, all the electrode sites were considered together in each experimental group, and they were grouped according to the lCBF values measured 10 min after arterial occlusion. The lCBF ranges were set as 0–15, 15–30, and 30–150 ml/100 g/min. The result of this stratified analysis is shown in Fig. 2. In no lCBF range was any significant difference in the time course of lCBF found (Fig. 2, left), but the fall in coSG was significantly less pronounced in the AVS group (Fig. 2, right). The values for water, sodium, and potassium contents of the cortical samples are shown in Table 1. There were significant differences in the water and sodium contents between the control and AVS groups on the affected side (L-I, and L-II).

Experiment II

The mean values for ATP, ADP, AMP, calculated adenine nucleotide pool, energy charge, lactate, pyruvate, lactate: pyruvate ratio (L/P ratio), and phosphocreatine are shown in Table 2. The ATP levels in the normal control and the MCA-occluded groups compare well with the value given in the preceding report [10]. Compared with the normal control group, the increase in the AMP, lactate, and L/P ratio and the decrease in E.C. were significant in the MCA-saline group. These changes were less pronounced in the MCA-AVS group, although the difference from the MCA-saline group did not reach a significant level in the present study.

Discussion

The topographical distribution of cortical ischemia induced by the occlusion of the internal carotid artery and MCA was found to be similar in the control and AVS groups. At no electrode site was there any significant difference between the two groups in mean lCBF values. When the electrode sites were grouped according to the lCBF value measured 10 min after the arterial occlusion, which is considered to represent the severity of ischemia in the region, no difference in the time course of lCBF was found between the control and AVS groups. These results indicate that AVS exerts no particular influence on lCBF in the present model.

On the other hand, both the depression of coSG and the increase in the cortical contents of water and sodium following ischemia were significantly attenuated by the administration of AVS. Since the lCBF was not affected, this antiedema effect of AVS may be ascribed to its actions affecting the cerebral metabolism or the dysfunction of the blood-brain barrier (BBB) following ischemia. The result concerning the cortical content of energy metabolites showed that AVS ameliorated the derangement of energy metabolism induced by ischemia to some extent. Although it is assumed on the basis of the free radical theory that AVS prevents ischemic damage to the energy-producing system, it is difficult to decide from the present data whether this improvement in the energy metabolism, albeit small, was the cause or the result of edema suppression.

Concerning the mechanism of action of AVS, we have obtained some data indicating that AVS suppressed the influx of water and sodium across the BBB by modulating the arachidonate metabolism in the cerebral microvessel (MV). In a study using the rat MCA occlusion model it was shown that the eicosanoid synthetic activity of the MV was significantly increased 24–72 h after the induction of ischemia [3]. In that model, AVS significantly suppressed the increases in the hemispheric contents of water and sodium in the corresponding period [5]. Also, AVS suppressed the enhanced eicosanoid synthetic activity of the MV prepared from the ischemic hemisphere [8]. To find which agents caused the enhancement of the eicosanoid synthetic activity of the MV, the effects of norepinephrine, dopamine, dibutyryl cyclic AMP, and 15-hydroperoxy arachidonic acid (15-HPAA) were examined in vitro [8]. The biogenic amines showed no effect, whereas 15-HPAA induced a remarkable enhancement of the eicosanoid synthetic activity of the MV. This effect of 15-HPAA was significantly inhibited by radical scavengers such as vitamin E, hydroquinone, and AVS [8]. The above results indicate the possibility that the eicosanoid synthetic activity of the MV is enhanced by generation of free radicals and/or lipid hydroperoxides following ischemia, which subsequently leads to dysfunction of the BBB and development of brain edema. It is also tempting to assume that the antiedema effect of AVS is based on the suppression of the above mechanism. In this connection, it may be worthy of mention that AVS suppressed only the lipoxygenase activity of the rat MV [8], while indomethacin, which did not prevent edema in the rat MCA occlusion model [1], suppressed only the cyclooxygenase activity of the rat MV. This may suggest that the lipoxygenase activity rather than the cyclooxygenase activity of the MV is relevant to the mechanism underlying ischemic brain edema. The recent finding that the rat MV predominantly produced 11-HETE [Usui et al. 1984, this volume] would lend support to such a view. At present the mechanism of action of AVS remains speculative, but the antiedema effect of AVS, as shown in the present and preceding studies, would merit further investigation.

Summary

The cat MCA occlusion model was used to study the effect of a free radical scavenger, AVS (1,2-bis(nicotineamide)-propane), on cortical blood flow, edema, and energy metabolites. The severity of cortical edema 4 h after MCA occlusion was assessed by the measurement of specific gravity and of the water and electrolyte content. Compared with the control group receiving saline, the AVS group showed a significant amelioration of the cortical edema, while the cortical blood flow was not influenced. The changes induced in the energy metabolites by ischemia were also improved by AVS. The results indicate that AVS mitigates the development of cortical edema following the MCA occlusion. The possible mechanism of action of AVS is discussed with reference to the arachidonate metabolism of the brain microvessel.

References

1. Asano T (1983) Metabolic changes of membrane lipids following cerebral ischemia with special reference to the possible pathways of arachidonate metabolism. Brain Nerve 35:41–50

2. Asano T, Sasaki T, Koide T, Takakura K, Sano K (1984) Experimental evaluation of the beneficial effect of an antioxidant on cerebral vasospasm. Neurol Res 6:49–53
3. Asano T, Gotoh O, Koide T, Takakura K (1985) Ischemic brain edema following occlusion of the middle cerebral artery in the rat: II. Alteration of the eicosanoid synthesis profile of brain microvessels. Stroke 16:110–113
4. Demopoulos HB, Flamm ES, Seligman M, Poser R, Pietronigro D, Ransohoff J (1976) Molecular pathology of lipids in CNS membranes. In: Jöbris FF (ed) Oxygen and physiological function. Professional Information Library, Dallas, p 491
5. Gotoh O, Koide T, Asano T, Takakura K, Tamura A, Sano K (1984) A model to study ischemic brain edema in rats and the influence of drugs. In: Go KG, Baethmann A (eds) Recent progress in the study and therapy of brain edema. Plenum, New York, p 499
6. Koide T, Neichi T, Takato M, Matsushita H, Sugioka K, Nakano M, Hata S (1982) Possible mechanisms of 15-hydroperoxyarachidonic acid-induced contraction of the canine basilar artery in vitro. J Pharmacol Exp Ther 221:481–488
7. Koide T, Noda Y, Asano T, Matsushita H (1983) Lipid peroxidation and cerebral vasospasm: a beneficial pharmacological approach by AVS (a radical scavenger). Proceedings of the 11th Symposium on drugs and actions, Sendai, Japan, pp 121–125
8. Koide T, Gotoh O, Asano T, Takakura K (1985) Alterations of the eicosanoid synthetic capacity of the rat brain microvessel following ischemia: relevance to ischemic brain edema. J Neurochem (in press)
9. Marmarou A, Poll W, Shulman K, Bhagavan H (1978) A simple technique for the measurement of cerebral edema. J Neurosurg 49:254–260
10. Schuier F, Hossmann KA (1980) Experimental brain infarcts in cats: II. Ischemic brain edema. Stroke 11:593–601
11. Welsh F, Rieder W (1978) Evaluation of in situ freezing of cat brain by NADH fluorescence. J Neurochem 31:299–309

Experimental DMSO and Glycerol Treatment for Postischemic Focal Brain Edema with Special Reference to the Topographic Differences

T. OKAMURA [1] and H. AOKI

Key words: Ischemic brain edema, vasogenic brain edema, dimethyl sulfoxide, glycerol, cat MCA occlusion

Introduction

Both the dynamics and the extent of the blood-brain barrier opening after the occurrence of transient focal ischemia are highly controversial topics [2, 3, 8–11, 14, 16, 18].

Our investigation was designed to determine how the extension pattern of vasogenic brain edema in the MCA territory [6] is modified after treatment with dimethyl sulfoxide (DMSO) [1, 4, 5, 7, 12, 15, 17] or glycerol [13, 15].

Materials and Methods

Thirty-six cats were used for the experiments. All animals were anesthetized with Nembutal (30 mg/kg IP) and then received succinylcholine for muscle relaxation and were ventilated by means of a respirator via an endotracheal tube. The femoral artery and vein were cannulated, and cats were covered with warm mats. Blood gases were constantly recorded. In 12 cats (group I) the proximal MCA was clipped by the transorbital approach and the clips left in place for 3 h, hypotension with mean arterial pressure (MAP) 50–80 mmHg was achieved and maintained for 1 h by removal of 15 ml blood/kg. After rCBF measurement at the bilateral middle ectosylvian gyrus and the caudate nucleus by the hydrogen clearance method over time, reperfusion and Evans blue infusion were performed. The animals were sacrificed 24 h later and each 5-mm coronal brain slice (slice A-O on biauricular line; slice A-5, 5-mm anterior to slice A-0; slice A-10, 5-mm anterior to slice A-55, etc.) was studied. In eight cats (group IIa), DMSO (2.5 g/kg in 15% solution) was infused before MCA clipping and 4 h later. In eight cats (group IIb) the same dosage of DMSO was infused shortly after MCA clipping and again 4 h later. In six cats (group III) glycerol (20 ml/kg) was infused shortly after MCA clipping and 3 h later. In two cats an rCBF study without MCA clipping was conducted as a sham operation.

---

[1] Department of Neurosurgery, Yamaguchi University, 1144 Kogushi, Nishi-ku, Ube, Yamaguchi 755, Japan

Results

During the 24-h followup, 6 of 12 cats (group I) died owing to extended vasogenic edema, with a marked midline shift and tentorial pressure cone. In contrast, mortality was low in groups IIa (1/8), IIb (1/8) and III (1/6). Water content was measured by means of wet and dry weight in gray matter, white matter, and basal ganglia from slice A-0-5. On the experimental side the increase in the water content was confirmed; it was most pronounced in the white matter.

Topographical Analysis

Regional CBF

In group I and the sham operation cases, rCBF in the left middle ectosylvian gyrus was 48.6 ± 6.6ml/100 g/min (mean ± SD, $n = 14$), and that in the left caudate nucleus was 42.3 ± 4.7 ml/100 g/min ($n = 7$). In group I, the rCBF of the left middle ectosylvian gyrus fell to 17.4 ± 8.1 shortly after clipping, then to 13.1 ± 8.5 during hypotension; it reversed to 43.7 ± 16.9 shortly after reperfusion and to 40.0 ± 18.3

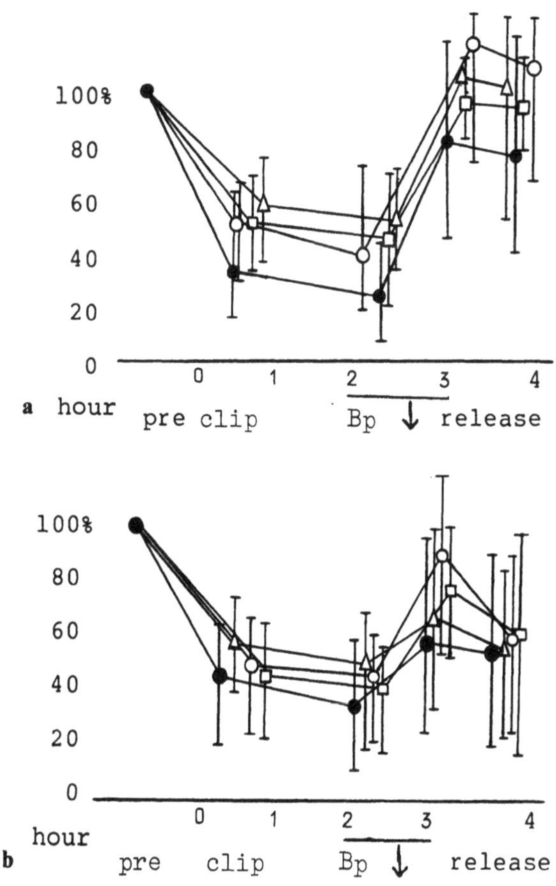

Fig. 1 a, b. Regional CBF in left middle ectosylvian gyrus (**a**) and in left caudate nucleus (**b**), presented as percentages of corresponding control values. ●, group I; ○, group IIa; △, group IIb; □, group III

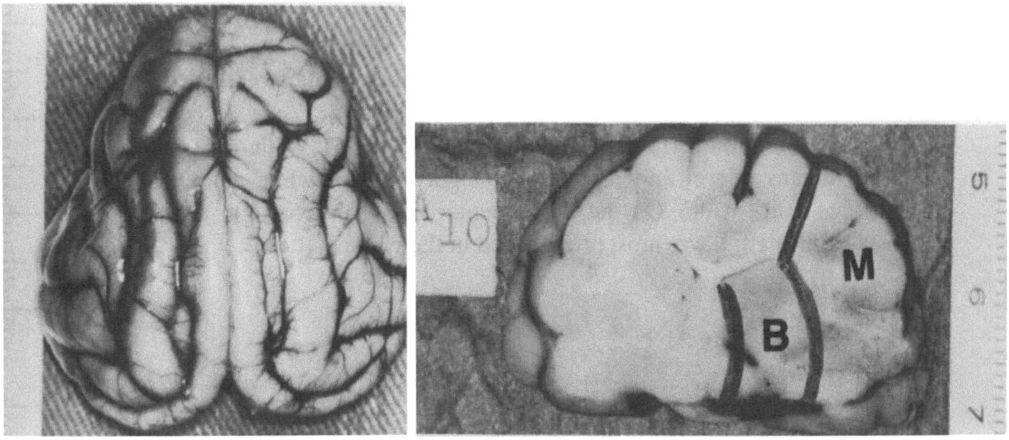

a

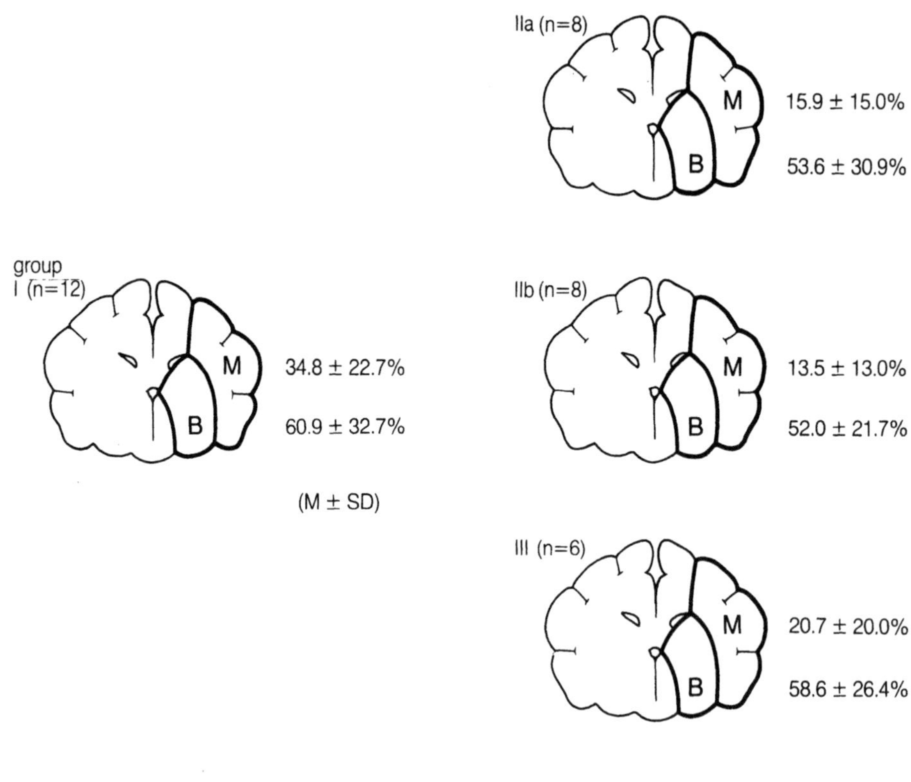

b M: IIa, IIb <III <I (P(to) >0.05)

Fig. 2. **a** Evans blue extravasation in the cerebral mantle and basal ganglia of a case in group I. *Left,* extensive extravasation throughout MCA territory; *right,* heterogeneous extravasation in slice A-10, in which MCA territory is schematically divided into mantle (*M*) and basal ganglia (*B*) according to a modification of Kamijo's method [6]. **b** Sizes of areas of extravasation in M and B in different groups, presented as percentages of corresponding control values

1 h later. The rCBF in the left caudate nucleus fell to 17.1 ± 7.3 shortly after clipping, then to 11.8 ± 6.0 during hypotension, reversing to 24.7 ± 17.7 shortly after institution of reperfusion. In contrast, rCBF in the left middle ectosylvian gyrus on clipping and hypotension was 19.1 ± 10.1 in group IIa, 20.0 ± 8.8 in group IIb, and 18.0 ± 5.8 in group III. The rCBF change in each part is shown as a percentage of the appropriate control value (Fig. 1a, b). In treated groups, the rCBF reduction during ischemia tended to be less extensive in the left middle ectosylvian gyrus, while treatment was less effective in the caudate nucleus. After the restoration of blood flow, low perfusion in the caudate nucleus was significant.

Evans Blue Leakage

The MCA territory of an A-10 slice was divided into mantle (M) and basal ganglia (B). The B part contained mainly deep perforating arteries, and the M part, cortical branches, as Kamijos reported [6].

Patterns of Evans blue leakage were quite variable and heterogeneous. The size of the area of extravasation in each part was measured by perimetry mater and is shown as a percentage for each part (Fig. 2b). In group I the size of the area of leakage was 34.8% ± 22.7% (mean ± SD) in the mantle and 60.9% ± 32.7% in the basal ganglia. In the mantle, the mean sizes were 15.9% ± 15.0% (IIa), 13.5% ± 13.0% (IIb), and 20.7% ± 20.0% (III).

On the other hand, in the basal ganglia the size was 53.6% ± 30.9% (IIa), 52.0% ± 21.7% (IIb), and 58.6% ± 26.4% (III), respectively. This indicates that a narrowing tendency resulting from treatment was profound in the mantle, but only a very slight tendency in the basal ganglia.

Micromorphological Change (A-10∼15 slice)

Pathological findings in the area of leakage were not homogeneous. The necrotic and slight histological changes were coincident, as revealed by HE and KB stains. Fluorescein microscopy without additional staining revealed Evans blue diffusely, while around the capillaries brilliant staining appeared. In the basal ganglia brilliant Evans blue leakage was found surrounding both the arterioles and the capillaries.

Discussion

In this study an attempt was made to elucidate the topographical differences responsible for the spreading of postischemic focal brain edema, with special reference to the therapeutic aspects. Both DMSO and glycerol had beneficial effects, but DMSO seemed to be more beneficial than glycerol in this experiment. It is still the subject of discussion whether DMSO is effective against ischemic insult or not [5, 7, 12, 15, 17]. It seems that the differences in the reported effect are mainly due to the use of different models. In brain edema caused by transient focal ischemia, as in the present study, DMSO seemed to improve low perfusion by redistributing blood flow from the perifocal area [7]. This action is marked in the cerebral mantle, where rCBF is easy to relate to collateral circulation, but it is weak in the basal ganglia. Another cause of this poor result in the basal ganglia is thought to be long-standing postischemic low perfusion.

Summary

The extension pattern of vasogenic edema after focal cerebral ischemia was investigated. In the cat, transorbital proximal clipping of the MCA was performed and left in place for 3 h with hemorrhagic hypotension to 50–80 mmHg (MAP). After rCBF measurements were taken on several points, and restoration and Evans blue infusion were performed. The animal was sacrificed 24 h later and each coronal brain slice was investigated.

The animals were divided into four groups: I, no treatment ($n=12$); IIa, preischemic treatment with DMSO before MCA clipping ($n=8$); IIb, postischemic treatment with DMSO ($n=8$); and III, postischemic treatment with glycerol ($n=6$).

During followup, the high mortality in group I (6/12) was found to be due to extensive vasogenic brain edema. Low mortality was found in groups IIa (1/8), IIb (1/8), and III (1/6). The extension pattern of vasogenic edema showed heterogenicity. A significant topographical difference in the effects of DMSO and glycerol was confirmed.

The extension pattern was ameliorated more easily in the cerebral mantle than in the basal ganglia. The cause of the difference was discussed.

References

1. Brown FD, Johns LM, Mullan S (1980) Dimethyl sulfoxide in experimental brain injury, with comparison to mannitol. J Neurosurg 53:58–62
2. Furuse M, Brock M, Hasuo M, Dietz H (1981) Relationship between brain tissue pressure gradients and cerebral blood flow distribution studied circumscribed vasogenic cerebral edema. Neurochirurgia (Stuttg) 24:10–14
3. Hossmann KA (1976) Development and resolution of ischemic brain swelling. Springer, Berlin Heidelberg New York, pp 219–227
4. James HE, Camp PE, Harbaugh RD, Marshall LF, Werner L (1982) Comparison of the effects of DMSO and pentobartone on experimental brain edema. Acta Neurochirurgica (Wien) 60:245–255
5. Dela Torre UR, Surgeon JW (1976) Dexamethasone and DMSO in experimental transorbital cerebral infarction. Stroke 7(6):577–583
6. Kamijo Y, Garccia J (1975) Carotid arterial supply of the feline brain application to the study of regional cerebral ischemia. Stroke 6:361–369
7. Kassell NF, Sprowell JAS, Boarini DJ, Olin JJ (1983) Effect of Dimethyl Sulfoxide on the cerebral and systemic circulations of the dog. Neurosurgery 12:24–28
8. Klatzo I (1967) Neuropathological aspects of brain edema. J Neuropathol Exp Neurol 26:1–14
9. Kogure K, Busto R, Scheinberg P (1981) The role of hydrostatic pressure in ischemic brain edema. Ann Neurol 9:273–282
10. Little JR (1976) Microvascular alterations and edema in focal cerebral ischemia. Springer, Berlin Heidelberg New York, pp 236–243

11. Marmarou A, Pöll W, Shapiro K, Shulman K (1976) The influence of brain tissue pressure upon local cerebral blood flow in vasogenic edema. In: Becks JWF, Bosch DA, Brock M (eds) Intracranial pressure III. Springer, Berlin Heidelberg New York, pp 10–13
12. Marshall LF, Camp PE, Bowers SA (1984) Dimethyl sulfoxide for the treatment of intracranial hypertension: a preliminary trial. Neurosurgery 14:659–663
13. Meyer JS, Fukuuchi Y, Shimazu K, Ohuchi T, Ericsson AD (1972) Effect of intravenous infusion of glycerol on hemispheric blood flow and metabolism in patients with acute cerebral infarction. Stroke 3:168–180
14. Reulen HJ, Graham R, Spatz M, Klatzo I (1977) Role of pressure gradients and bulk flow dynamics of vasogenic brain edema. J Neurosurg 46:24–35
15. Rosenblum WI, El-Sabban F (1982) Dimethyl sulfoxide (DMSO) and glycerol, hydroxyl radical scavengers, impair platelet aggregation within and eliminate the accompanying vasodilatation of, injured mouse pial arterioles. Stroke 13:35–39
16. Tamura A, Sano K (1979) The temporary occlusion of middle cerebral artery in cats – The correlation between the rCBF and the histological changes. Brain Nerve 31:1005–1015
17. Tung H, James HE, Laurin R, Marshall LF (1983) Modification of the effect of dimethyl sulfoxide on intracranial pressure, brain water, and electrolyte content by indomethacin. Acta Neurochirurgica 68:101–110
18. Waltz AG, O'Brien MD, Hayakawa T, Heiss WD (1976) Ischemic cerebral edema and hypermia in the process of cerebral infarction. Springer, Berlin Heidelberg New York, pp 262–267

Effectiveness and Mode of Action of Glycerol in Brain Edema Therapy

Clinical, Biochemical, and Neurophysiological Investigations

E. Csanda[1], Z. Bácsy, I. Tulok, A. Balogh, Ágnes Köves, and S. Komoly

Introduction

In 1963, at the Second European Congress of Neurosurgery, we learned from Cantore et al. [1] of the usefulness of oral glycerol therapy for space-occupying lesions. We have been using glycerol ever since, and have extended its indications to include brain edema (BE) of ischemic, toxic, metabolic, and inflammatory origin. Our experience is based on more than 2000 patients. From the beginning the CSF pressure was continuously measured by the manometric method in 75 patients. EEGS were initially evaluated visually, but since 1975 offline and online computerized methods of analysis have been used. The glycerol content of the plasma and CSF was measured 5, 10, 30, 60 and 120 min after oral administration. The 24-h glycerol excretion in the urine was determined. In addition, K^+, Na^+, Ca^{2+}, phosphate, ketonic bodies, and dextrose level in the plasma were monitored.

To clarify some aspects of the mode of action of glycerol animal experiments were performed. We used the hexachlorophene BE model, with and without glycerol treatment.

Clinical Examinations

The most constant finding following oral glycerol administration was the very rapid absorption from the gastrointestinal tract even in profoundly comatose patients, to whom glycerol was administered through a nasogastric tube. In 5 min the serum glycerol level was increased to over 5 mg%, which establishes the osmotic difference needed for the lowering of intracranial pressure (ICP). The higher the initial increase in ICP, the more pronounced was the percentage reduction, whose peak fell between 30 and 60 min. The speed and duration of this lowering effect are dose dependent. Following 0.5 g/kg body weight the ICP rose again slowly after 120 min, reaching the initial level and never producing a rebound effect. When 2 g/kg was given the lowest ICP was maintained at a constant level with repeated administration every 4 h. The time needed for an effective decrease in ICP to start varied, but was never longer than 15–20 min. The slow increase in CSF glycerol content must be mentioned, it sometimes slightly exceeded that in blood with no rebound in CSF pressure.

[1] Institute of Neurology, Semmelweis Medical University, Budapest, Hungary

In general, no significant plasma electrolyte changes are provoked by glycerol, but in a study of 17 patients who received therapy lasting more than 1 week a slight decrease in K^+ and organic phosphate was observed.

Blood sugar was slightly increased at the beginning of administration, but soon returned to the initial level. Ketonic body content was decreased and the blood urea level, unchanged. We administered glycerol to diabetic patients and observed a favorable effect, which can be related to the fact that glycerol enhances aerobic glycolysis, influencing the Krebs cycle. Glucose is metabolized in the presence of glycerol without needing insulin, taking part in the energy supply of cerebral tissue.

Visual analysis of EEG recordings revealed changes within as little as 5–6 min: the background activity became faster, and diffuse slow waves were reduced, except in the damaged area. This phenomenon makes it possible to determine the site of the lesion more precisely, which is especially helpful if the whole EEG recording is extremely disturbed and the comatose state makes it difficult to evaluate the clinical signs. In 30–60 min after glycerol a dramatic arousal effect was seen both in the clinical condition and in electrical activity.

By means of longer recordings (3–5 h) with online analysis by the BERG-Fourier method in 32 patients, we observed an energy power decrease in the slow bands and increased energy of the alpha band. The peak frequency of the alpha band became faster. In 30 min we observed an increase of 0.5–1.0 Hz, which remained constant throughout the recording (Fig. 1). Glycerol was observed to regularize the rhythm, especially in the alpha band.

Animal Experiments

Experimental brain edema was induced by hexachlorophene administered to rats at a dose of 10 mg/kg body weight per day IP. The development of brain edema was followed by an increase in the water content of the brain tissue (5.2% on the 4th day), which was accompanied by a decrease in the $K^+:Na^+$ ratio and the brain energy potential counted in the brain tissue homogenate $\left(\frac{\text{ATP} + 1/2\,\text{ADP}}{\text{ATP} + \text{ADP} + \text{AMP}}\right)$; the latter decreased by nearly 50%. Administration of 3 g/kg glycerol prevented the development of brain edema and the above-mentioned accompanying phenomena.

New Solvent for Dilution of Glycerol

Both clinical and experimental observations demonstrate the active participation of glycerol in the ion transport processes. In consequence of this, a moderate decrease in serum K^+ and phosphate concentration may occur. To prevent these undesirable changes we propose a new solvent for dilution for both oral (50%) and IV (10%) administration, in preference to the widely accepted NaCl (0.9%) solvent. The new solvent contains (mmol/liter) Na^+ (77), K^+ (50), Cl^- (102), P_a (25). In a comparative study in 17 patients, the absorption of glycerol given in the new solvent proved to be as rapid as with NaCl solvent, and in some patients even faster.

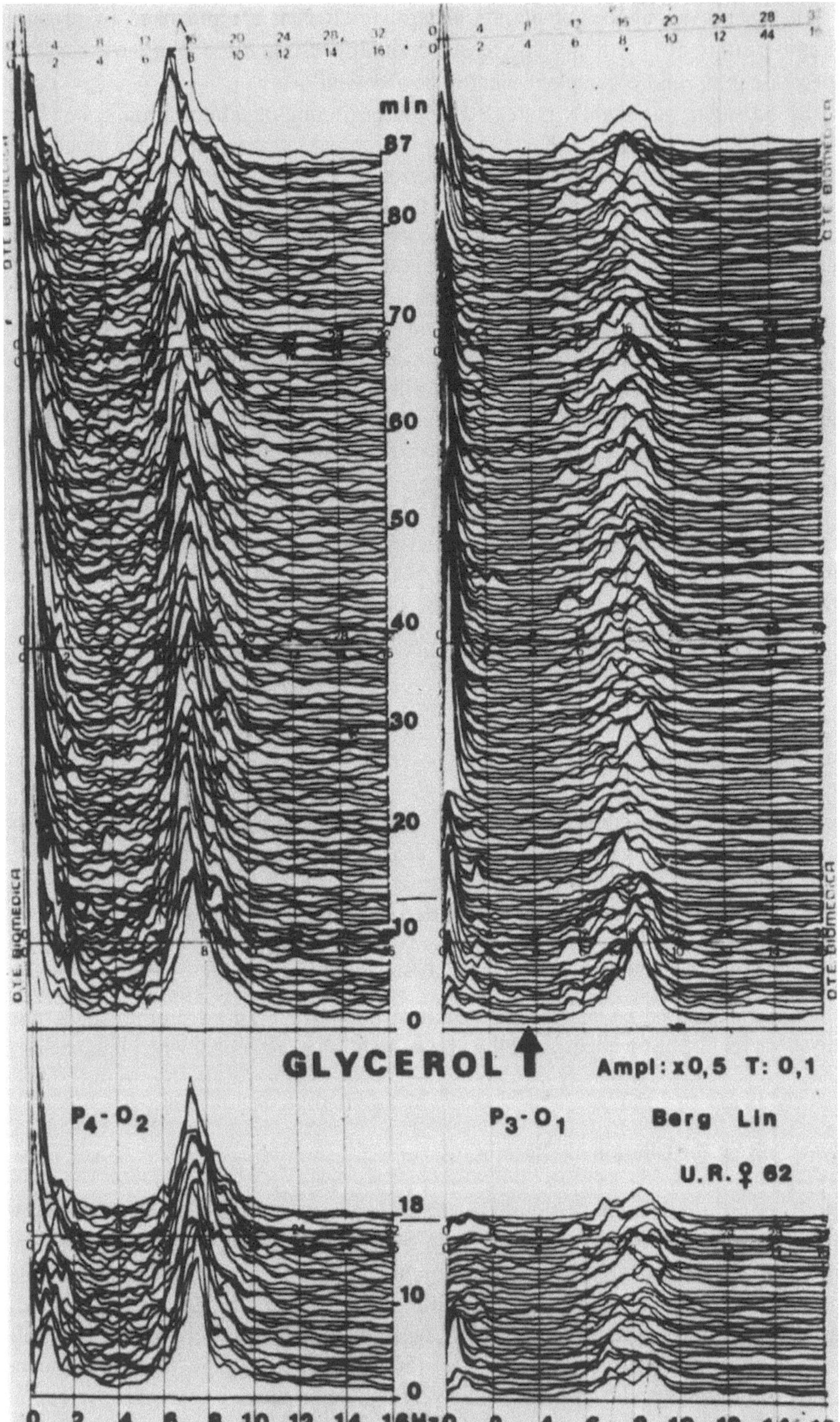
min
87
80
70
60
50
40
30
20
10
0
GLYCEROL
Ampl: x0,5 T: 0,1
P_4-O_2
P_3-O_1
Berg Lin
U.R. ♀ 62
18
10
0
0 2 4 6 8 10 12 14 16Hz
0 2 4 6 8 10 12 14 16
OTE BIOMEDICA

◀ **Fig. 1.** Patient aged 62 years, with occlusion of the left internal carotid artery. After glycerol dominant alpha frequency increases (0.5 Hz), as does its amplitude

Summary

Glycerol has been used in the therapy of brain edema in space-occupying lesions, acute cerebrovascular disorders, inflammatory diseases, subarachnoid hemorrhage, and various anoxic states (status epilepticus, toxifications, diabetic and other metabolic encephalopathies) since 1963. It has proved to be very effective in decreasing high intracranial pressure, can be administered both PO and in the form of IV perfusions, causes no rebound effect, and has no toxic effects.

In the present study the effect of glycerol on CSF pressure, serum electrolyte concentrations, acid/base balance, and glucose metabolism was investigated in human subjects, and its effect on cerebral energy supply in animals. EEG was examined by visual evaluation and online BERG-Fourier analysis. The effect of glycerol was also investigated in experimental brain edema induced by hexachlorophene in rats.

According to the results, glycerol is highly effective in reducing brain edema of all types, whether given PO or IV. Its effect is based on osmotic and metabolic actions. The osmotic effect can be sustained for long periods, and is dose dependent. Metabolic influences are also supported by biochemical and neurophysiological findings. With both oral and IV administration a new solvent containing K^+ and phosphate has proved to be a better dilutent for glycerol than the classic NaCl solvent.

References

1. Cantore G, Guidetti B, Virno M (1964) Oral glycerol for the reduction of intracranial pressure. J Neurosurg 21:278
2. Csanda E (1978) Actual problems in brain edema treatment (in Hungarian). Orvosi Hetilap 119:2982

Effects of Indomethacin on the Pathophysiology of Temporary Focal Ischemia

K. ARITAKE[1] and M. BROCK

Key words: Brain edema, temporary ischemia, cerebral blood flow, indomethacin, arachidonic acid

Introduction

Interest has increased in the role of arachidonic acid metabolism in cerebral ischemia and associated brain edema. In the gerbil, reperfusion of the brain after brief ischemic episodes is followed by the occurrence of large amounts of arachidonic acid metabolites [3, 7]. It therefore appears likely that reestablishment of blood flow, that is, the sudden supply of oxygen to ischemic brain tissue rich in arachidonic acid, results in an explosive enhancement of arachidonic acid conversion via cyclooxygenase.

At the same time, keen attention has been given to factors such as hyperperfusion, immediate or delayed hypoperfusion, and associated brain edema following ischemia, all of which can limit recovery from the ischemic insult. Disproportionate production of prostanoids, including thromboxane A_2 and prostacyclin, has been shown to be responsible for such postischemic flow alterations [6]. Moreover, arachidonic acid metabolism, particularly by way of cyclooxygenase, has been reported to contribute to the development of ischemic edema, although this is still a matter of controversy [1, 2, 5]. Thus, it is highly probable that cyclooxygenase is involved in the outcome of an ischemic event.

In the present study we investigated the effects of indomethacin (Ind.), a potent cyclooxygenase inhibitor, on both the temporal pattern of reperfusion flow changes and edema formation in temporary focal ischemia.

Materials and Methods

A total of 23 cats (11 controls, 12 pretreated with Ind.) were subjected to middle cerebral artery (MCA) occlusion for 1 h, followed by subsequent reperfusion. Sequential measurement of blood flow values was achieved by the hydrogen clearance method (cf. Aritake and Brock, this volume). Five hydrogen clearance electrodes were implanted in three different cortical regions: the core of the MCA territory

[1] Department of Neurosurgery, Universitätsklinikum Steglitz, Free University of Berlin, Hindenburgdamm 30, D-1000 Berlin 45

(sylvian and ectosylvian gyri), its margin (the suprasylvian gyrus), and its periphery surrounding the MCA territory (the marginal gyrus). One electrode was used for monitoring in the nonischemic hemisphere to provide control values. The water content of cortical tissue surrounding the hydrogen electrode was measured by the vacuum freeze-drying method. The pretreated animals received continuous administration of Ind. (total dose 5 mg/kg) before MCA occlusion.

Results

In untreated animals the mean preocclusion flow was 61 ± 14 ml/100 g/min (62 examined sites, mean ± SD). The consequences of MCA occlusion were not restricted to its territory proper, but were also observed in more collaterally perfused regions (periphery) (Table 1). Immediate flow measurement after reperfusion revealed hyperperfusion in the MCA field (core and margin) and depressed perfusion (hypoperfusion) in the remaining region (periphery). Sustained hyperperfusion was observed in the severely ischemic core, whereas the final flow measurement revealed a reduction in the periphery (Tables 1 and 2).

The mean preocclusion flow was significantly reduced, from 67 ± 22 to 49 ± 15 ml/100 g/min, following the administration of Ind. (67 sites, $P < 0.05$). In pretreated animals the distribution of blood flow in the ischemic brain was altered, particularly in the region surrounding the MCA territory (Table 1). Following restoration of the blood supply hyperperfusion was not curtailed in the densely ischemic core, but in the moderately ischemic margin. Moreover, depressed flow in the periphery was improved by Ind. in the immediate reperfusion period (Tables 1 and 2).

Table 1. Mean blood flow values before, during, and after MCA occlusion, based on regional differences (mean ± SD, ml/100 g/min)

Treatment	Region	Pre-occlusion values	Occlusion values	Initial post-occlusion values	Maximal post-occlusion values	Final post-occlusion values
Untreated	C (27)	62 ± 14	11 ± 11[b]	107 ± 42[b]	120 ± 50[b]	88 ± 49[a]
	M (11)	56 ± 14	17 ± 14[b]	96 ± 42[b]	105 ± 44[b]	78 ± 46
	P (13)	59 ± 10	42 ± 17[b]	33 ± 11[b]	50 ± 15	40 ± 11[b]
	Contr. (11)	67 ± 18	66 ± 20	67 ± 18	77 ± 25	59 ± 21
Pretreated	C (31)	53 ± 16	15 ± 14[b]	72 ± 35[b]	89 ± 43[b]	55 ± 34
	M (12)	44 ± 13	17 ± 14[b]	56 ± 27	69 ± 28[a]	48 ± 29
	P (12)	49 ± 12	47 ± 12	51 ± 27	66 ± 29	44 ± 14
	Contr. (12)	47 ± 13	56 ± 19	55 ± 22	62 ± 25	50 ± 30

C, M, P: core, margin, periphery of MCA territory (see text)
Contr.: nonischemic hemisphere; ( ) number of cases
[a] $P<0.05$; [b] $P<0.01$: significant differences from corresponding mean preocclusion flow values

Table 2. Mean blood flow values before, during and after MCA occlusion, based on the degree of flow reduction during the ischemic period (ischemic levels) (mean ± SD, ml/100 g/min)

Treatment	Ischemic level	Pre-occlusion values	Occlusion values	Initial post-occlusion values	Maximal post-occlusion values	Final post-occlusion values
Untreated	0–10 (21)	62±14	5±3[b]	119±46[b]	129±43[b]	98±49[b]
	11–20 (14)	56±13	15±3[b]	75±32	84±35[a]	61±37
	21–40 (8)	63±18	33±7[b]	64±44	88±78	62±50
	41– (8)	58±10	54±8	45±25	63±21	42±11[b]
Pretreated	0–10 (20)	48±17	4±4[b]	71±42[b]	97±44[b]	53±33
	11–20 (9)	54±15	15±3[b]	67±27	79±41	46±38
	21–40 (16)	50±13	32±5[b]	58±22	62±21	53±15
	41– (10)	50±14	51±8	56±27	70±32	47±25

( ) Number of data cases
[a] $P<0.05$; [b] $P<0.01$: significant differences from corresponding mean preocclusion flow values

The mean tissue water content in the nonischemic hemisphere of pretreated animals (78.80% ± 1.90%, mean ± SD) did not differ from that in untreated animals (78.91% ± 1.41%) (Fig. 1). Edema developed when the ischemic blood flow was reduced to less than 15 ml/100 g/min in untreated animals. Indomethacin increased the critical threshold for edema formation from 15 to 20 ml/100 g/min. In contrast, the degree of edema formation was significantly decreased only in the occlusion flow range between 0 and 5 ml/100 g/min.

Discussion

Indomethacin appears to be suitable for testing the hypothesis that enhancement of the cyclooxygenase route of arachidonic acid metabolism in temporary ischemia is involved in postischemic events. With regard to hemodynamic changes in pretreated animals, however, the interpretation of the data we obtained is complicated by the very fact that Ind. reduced the preocclusion (basal) flow values.

Our regional analysis of blood flow indicates that the sudden occlusion or reopening of the occluded MCA results in interregional redistribution of blood supply between regions of less and more intensive involvement, altering over time. Indomethacin did not reduce the degree of hyperperfusion in the densely ischemic core, but in the moderately ischemic regions. This may indicate that the drug modifies the distribution of blood supply in less ischemic areas through its vasoconstrictive effect [4]. It also seems unlikely that postischemic production of prostacyclin plays a major role in vascular dilatation in the immediate reperfusion period.

With regard to modification of the development of edema, Ind. seems to make the ischemic brain more susceptible to edema formation. Harris et al. reported that Ind. worsened edema formation in permanent ischemia [4]. However, no aggravation of

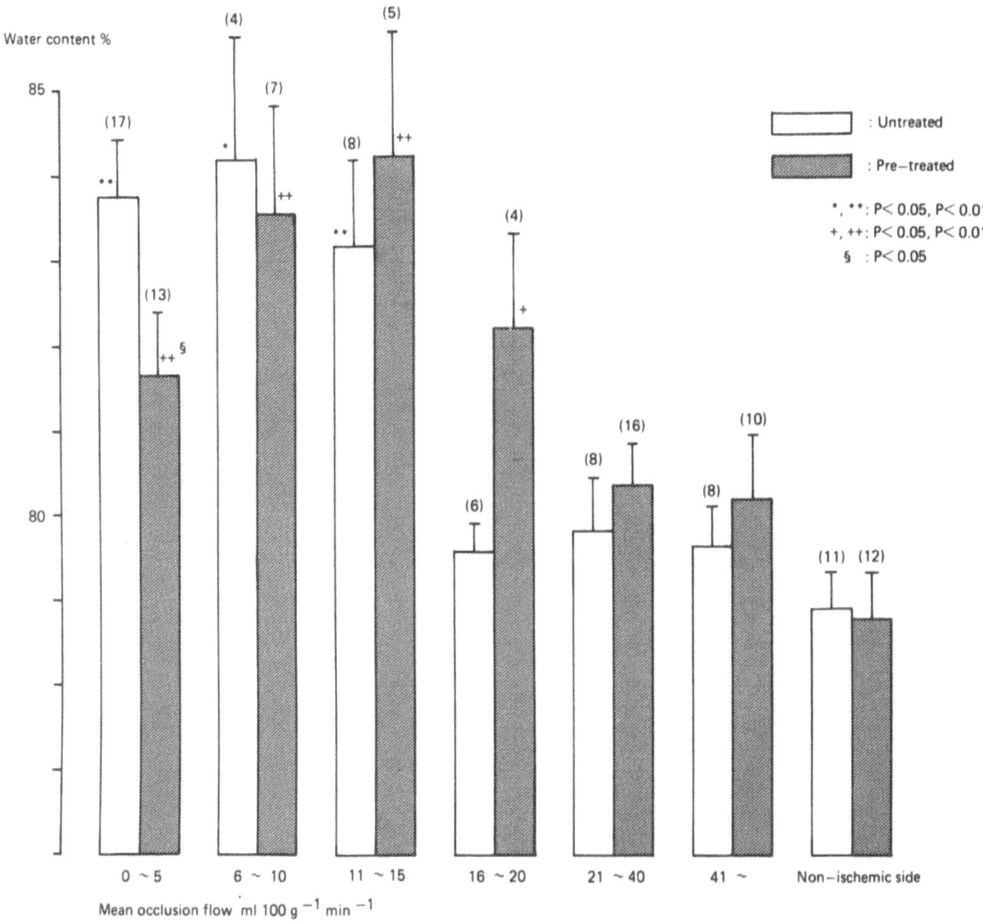

Fig. 1. Correlation of water content and occlusion flow. Mean values (± SEM) of water content are shown for 5 ml/100 g/min blood flow increments. ( ), number of cases; *, **, significantly different from mean water content on the nonischemic side in untreated animals; +, + +, significantly different from mean water content on the nonischemic side in pretreated animals; §, significantly different from mean water content for the corresponding 5 ml/100 g/min blood flow interval in untreated animals

edema formation was observed at ischemic flow rates of less than 15 ml/100 g/min in temporary ischemia. Incomplete suppression of the development of edema by Ind. in temporary ischemia may reflect the fact that the drug not only inhibits the cyclooxygenase route but also secondarily stimulated the lipoxygenase route, since the latter has been known to contribute to changes in vascular permeability [4]. It is, therefore, possible that the effects of Ind. on edema formation in temporary ischemia might be curtailed by secondary augmentation of the lipoxygenase route, which conversely results in aggravation of edema formation. Moreover, it seems likely that the lipoxygenase route is preponderant in permanent ischemia without reperfusion/reoxygenation, while the cyclooxygenase route is of more importance in temporary ischemia with recirculation.

Summary

The effect of indomethacin (5 mg/kg, IV) on either ischemic brain edema or hemodynamic changes was examined in a model of acute temporary focal ischemia. A total of 23 cats (11 controls, 12 pretreated with indomethacin) were subjected to middle cerebral artery (MCA) occlusion for 1 h with the corresponding regional blood flow determined by the hydrogen clearance method. Edema formation was correlated with occlusion flow values. Brain edema developed at ischemic levels of less than 15 ml/100 g/min. Following recirculation, hyperperfusion developed in the formerly ischemic MCA territory. Indomethacin considerably diminished the degree of edema formation in the occlusion flow range below 5 ml/100 g/min. However, it also increased the critical threshold for edema formation from 15 to 20 ml/100 g/min. Indomethacin significantly reduced the basal blood flow values. The drug curtailed hyperperfusion only in moderately ischemic regions following reperfusion, which possibly led to alterations in the distribution of blood flow. Possible pathomechanisms of temporary focal ischemia are discussed.

References

1. Aritake K, Wakai S, Asano T, Takakura K (1983) Peroxidation of arachidonic acid and brain edema. Brain Nerve 35:965–973
2. Chan PH, Fischman RA (1978) Brain edema: induction in cortical slices by polyunsaturated fatty acids. Science 201:358–360
3. Gaudet RJ, Alam J, Levine L (1980) Accumulation of cyclooxygenase products of arachidonic acid metabolism in gerbil brain during reperfusion after bilateral common carotid artery occlusion. J Neurochem 35:653–658
4. Harris RJ, Bayhan M, Branston NM, Watson A, Symon L (1982) Modulation of the pathophysiology of primate focal cerebral ischemia by indomethacin. Stroke 13:17–24
5. Iannotti F, Crockard A, Ladds G, Symon L (1981) Are prostaglandins involved in experimental ischemic edema in gerbils? Stroke 12:301–306
6. Shohami E, Rosenthal J, Lavy S (1982) The effects of incomplete cerebral ischemia on prostaglandin levels in rat brain. Stroke 13:494–499
7. Yoshida S, Inoh S, Asano T, Sano K, Kubota M, Shimazaki H, Ueda N (1980) Effect of transient ischemia on free fatty acids and phospholipids in the gerbil brain. Lipid peroxidation as a possible cause of post-ischemic injury. J Neurosurg 53:323–331

Effect of a Calcium Antagonist, Nicardipine, on Ischemic Brain Edema Formation

H. JOHSHITA [1], T. ASANO, and K. TAKAKURA

Key words: Calcium antagonist, nicardipine, cerebral blood flow, hydrogen clearance, specific gravity

Introduction

The effects of calcium antagonists on cerebral ischemia or anoxia have been widely discussed [1, 2]. But there is some controversy about their beneficial effects. We studied the influence of a calcium antagonist [3], nicardipine, on the cortical blood flow (lCBF) and specific gravity (SG) following focal cerebral ischemia.

Materials and Methods

The experiment was carried out in 31 cats (11 saline controls, 11 post-treated and 9 pretreated with nicardipine), which were subjected to focal ischemia by left MCA occlusion. Conditions of the experiment are shown in Fig. 1. Cortical lCBF was measured by the hydrogen clearance method at six fixed positions within the ipsilateral MCA territory before and during the 4 h of ischemia. At the end of the experiment cats were sacrificed by KCl injection, samples of the cortical tissue around each electrode were quickly excised, and the specific gravity (CoSG) of each was measured with the aid of a bromobenzene-kerosene column [4]. Data were evaluated by analysis of variance and Duncan's multiple range test.

Results

Nicardipine significantly lowered the mean arterial blood pressure in both the pre- and the post-treated groups. In all the experimental groups the electrode sites were grouped according to the lCBF values measured 10 min after MCA occlusion which reflected the severity of ischemia at each location (site A: 0–20; site B: 20–40; site C: > 40 ml/100 g/min) (Fig. 2). In the severely ischemic cortical area (site A), in both pre- and post-treated groups nicardipine caused significant decreases in the SG values (Fig. 3), whereas the time courses of lCBF were not affected (Fig. 2). In a moderately ischemic area (site B) in the pretreated group the time course of lCBF

[1] Department of Neurosurgery, University of Tokyo Hospital, 7-3-1 Hongo, Bunkyo-ku, Tokyo 113, Japan

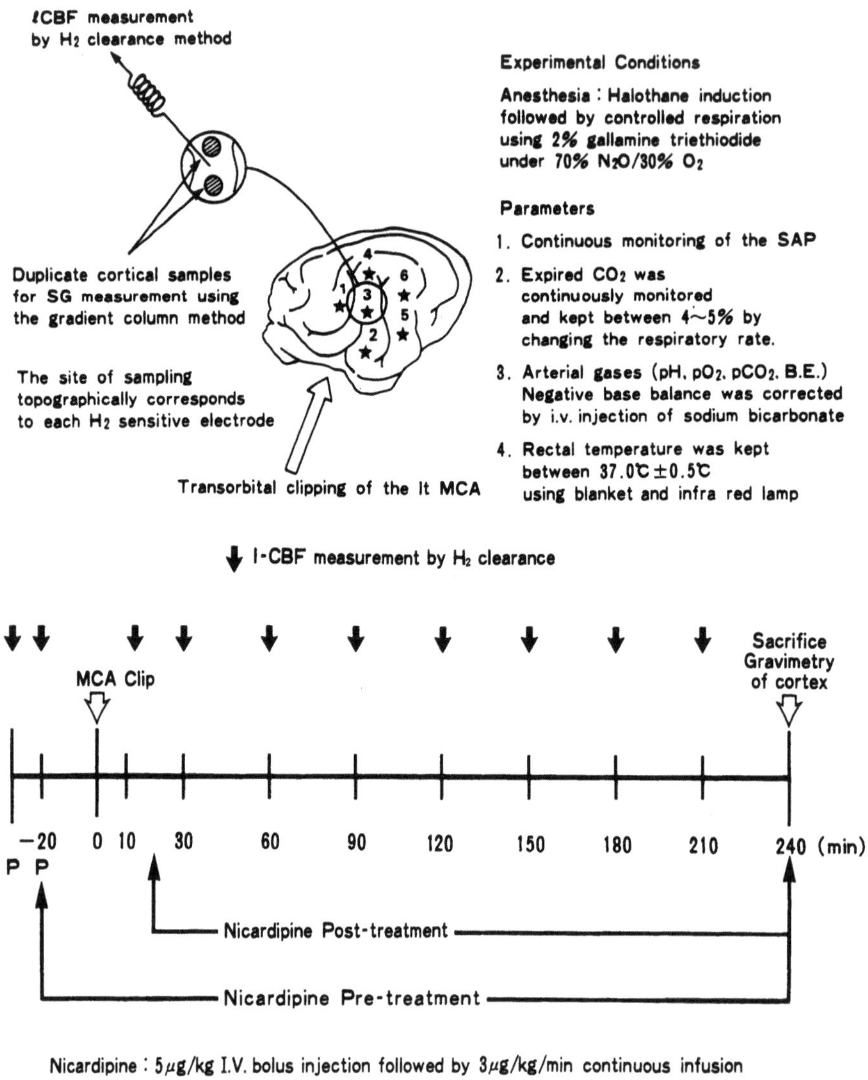

Fig. 1. Experimental design

was not different from that of the control group (Fig. 2), whereas the mean SG was lower than that of the control group (Fig. 3). In site B in the post-treated group, nicardipine administration caused an immediate increase in lCBF, which continued throughout the experiment (Fig. 2). But the mean SG at this site was no better than in the control group (Fig. 3). The relative frequency distribution histogram of SG values (Fig. 4) reveals a decrease in both drug-treated groups, in which the SG values were significantly lower than in the control group ($P < 0.05$).

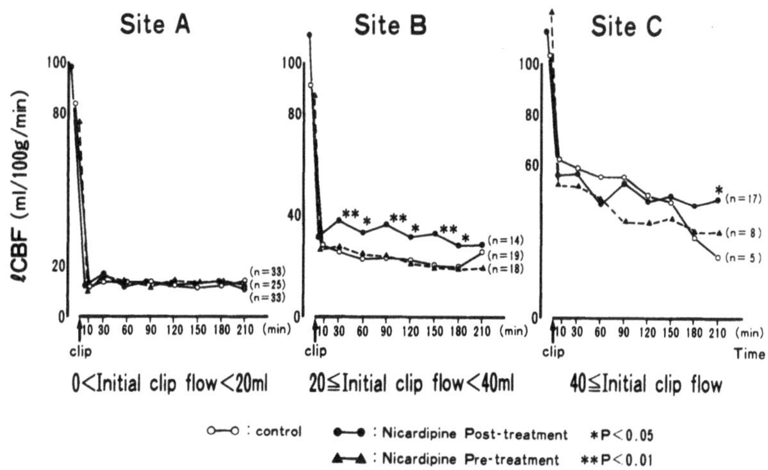

Fig. 2. Changes in lCBF over time, grouped by initial value of flow measured 10 min after MCA occlusion

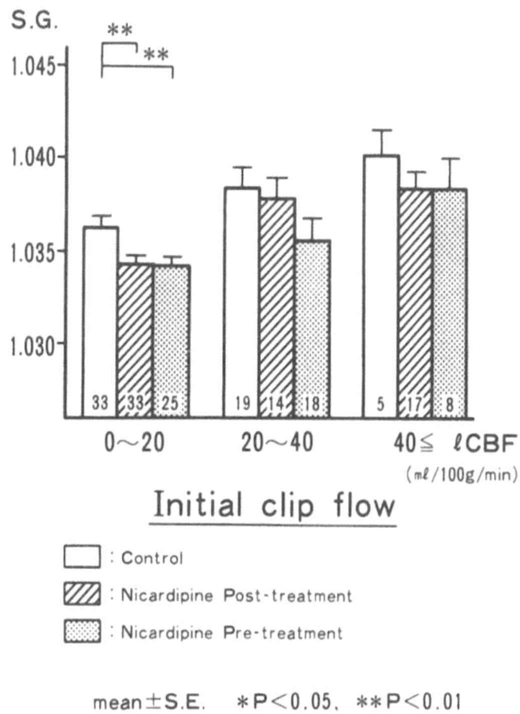

Fig. 3. Effect of nicardipine on brain edema, grouped by initial value of flow measured after MCA occlusion

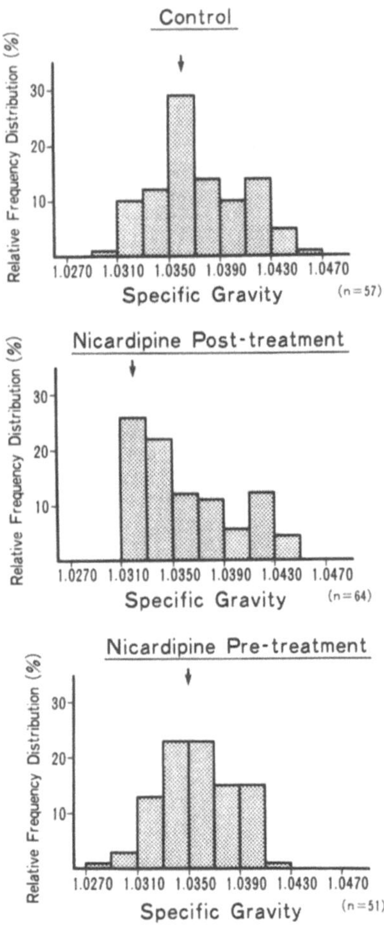

Fig. 4. Relative frequency distribution histograms of Co-SG values

Conclusion

In the present study, nicardipine caused a significant increase in lCBF of the normal cerebral cortex in spite of a decrease in the systemic arterial pressure (SAP). After MCA occlusion nicardipine, like nimodipine [3], significantly enhanced edema formation in the severely ischemic areas in both the pre- and the post-treated groups, without any significant changes of the lCBF. In the pretreated group it is not clear whether or not the preceding general increase in lCBF exerted any influence on edema formation in this experiment. In the post-treated group, however, a significant increase in lCBF was observed in the moderately ischemic area. The fact that the lCBF in the severely ischemic area did not change negates the occurrence of a steal phenomenon. This hemodynamic change induced by the drug did not have a beneficial influence on the development of edema, but neither did it exert a detrimental effect on brain edema formation in this moderately ischemic area. The above results indicate that nicardipine induces a significant alteration in cortical blood flow, but exacerbates the development of early cortical edema through some mechanism not related to its hemodynamic effect.

Summary

Using the cat middle cerebral artery (MCA) occlusion model, the effect of a calcium antagonist, nicardipine, on cortical blood flow (lCBF) and specific gravity (SG) was studied. Before MCA occlusion, nicardipine induced a significant increase in lCBF in spite of a significant drop in the systemic arterial pressure. When the drug was administered after MCA occlusion, CBF in the moderately ischemic cortical area (20 < lCBF < 40 ml/100 g/min) significantly increased, whereas lCBF in the severely ischemic area (lCBF < 20 ml/100 g/min) did not change. When the SG values in the cortical areas exposed to similar ischemic flow ranges in the control, pre-, and posttreatment groups were compared it was shown that nicardipine significantly decreased SG values regardless of its hemodynamic effect. Although nicardipine is water soluble, results of the present study indicate that the drug, like nimodipine, exacerbates early ischemic edema through a mechanism not directly related to its hemodynamic effect.

References

1. Kazda S, Garthoff B, Krause HP, Schlossmann K (1982) Cerebrovascular effect of the calcium antagonistic dihydropyridine derivative nimodipine in animal experiments. Drug Res 32:331–338
2. Harris RJ, Branston NM, Symon L, Bayhan M, Watson A (1982) The effect of a calcium antagonist, nimodipine, upon physiological responses of the cerebral vasculature and its possible influence upon focal cerebral ischaemia. Stroke 13:759–764
3. Takenaka T, Handa J (1979) Cerebrovascular effects of YC-93, a new vasodilator, in dogs, monkeys and human patients. Int J Clin Pharmacol Biopharm 17:1–11
4. Marmarou A, Poll W, Shulman K, Bhagavan H (1978) A simple gravimetric technique for measurement of cerebral edema. J Neurosurg 49:530–537

Effects of Direct Administration of Pentobarbital into Subcortical Structures on Increased Intracranial Pressure

M. Hayashi[1], Y. Handa, H. Kobayashi, H. Ishii, and H. Kawano

Introduction

Barbiturates are effective in lowering raised intracranial pressure. When administered IV they produce depression of the central nervous system, and because of the low selectivity of their action, it is impossible to achieve the desired effect without evidence of general depression of the central nervous system. In this study we administered pentobarbital directly into some subcortical sites of the brain, with the intention of analyzing the effects of barbiturate so administered on increased intracranial pressure in a state of acute experimental intracranial hypertension.

Materials and Methods

Animal Preparation and Intracranial Pressure Recording

Twenty-five adult mongrel dogs were used for this study. The animals were anesthetized with IV thiopental sodium and paralyzed with gallamine triethiodide. The initial doses were 15 and 1.5 mg/kg, and the maintenance dosages were 3 and 1 mg/kg/h, respectively. The animals were tracheotomized and ventilated with room air from a respirator. With the animal prone and the head elevated and fixed in a stereotaxic frame, the calvaria was adequately exposed. The intracranial pressure was recorded through a needle inserted stereotaxically in the lateral ventricle or the cisterna magna and connected with a pressure transducer.

Stereotaxic Insertion of Tubing into Subcortical Sites

Appropriate small holes were made for placement of cannulae for the administration of pentobarbital into the posterior hypothalamus, the pontine reticular formation, and the medullary reticular formation. Placement of the cannulae in the desired subcortical sites was achieved by a stereotaxic method. The locations of the cannula tip in the posterior hypothalamus corresponded anatomically to the nucleus hypothalamicus dorsomedialis; that in the pontine reticular formation, to the nucleus reticularis tegmenti pontis; and that in the medullary reticular formation, to the nucleus reticularis paramedialis.

---

[1] Department of Neurosurgery, Fukui Medical School, Matsuoka-cho, Yoshida-gun, Fukui 910-11, Japan

Induction of Intracranial Hypertension

The subarachnoid injection of autogenous incubated blood was utilized to increase the intracranial pressure; the blood was injected through a needle into the chiasmatic cistern.

Protocol

The animals were randomly divided into four groups. Group I consisted of seven dogs that received subarachnoid injections of the incubated blood into the chiasmatic cistern. The animals in this group received no pentobarbital, but were treated for control studies by injection of 0.3–0.5 ml physiological saline into the subcortical sites. Group II consisted of six dogs that received subarachnoid injections of blood followed by the introduction of pentobarbital into the posterior hypothalamus. Group III consisted of six dogs that received subarachnoid injections of blood and then pentobarbital injected into the pontine reticular formation. Group IV consisted of six dogs that received subarachnoid injections of blood followed by the administration of pentobarbital into the medullary reticular formation. A pentobarbital sodium concentration of 1 mg/ml was injected into the desired subcortical sites with a microinjection apparatus. Pentobarbital was administered when the intracranial pressure rose to 20 mmHg or more after the intracisternal blood injection. In group II and III animals pentobarbital was introduced bilaterally, and in group IV animals, unilaterally. Usually, 0.3 mg pentobarbital was introduced through each cannula.

Results and Conclusions

Controls

Group I animals all had intracranial hypertension after the intracisternal blood injection. Figure 1 illustrates an example of the intracranial hypertension that followed a 10-ml intracisternal blood injection. The intracranial pressure rose to about 45 mmHg during the blood infusion, subsequently falling to the original level within a few minutes. Thereafter, the trace showed slowly increasing pressure over the course of the next few hours, with frequent intracranial pressure irregularities. The pressure reached levels of about 55 mmHg 17 h after the intracisternal injection. In control experiments physiological saline was injected into the subcortical sites when the intracranial pressure rose to 20 mmHg or more after the intracisternal blood injection. The intracranial pressure after the injection of physiological saline into the subcortical sites was quite similar to that of the animals that did not receive any saline.

Pentobarbital Application to Posterior Hypothalamus and Pontine Reticular Formation

In group II animals, four out of six had a transient decrease followed by a steep rise in intracranial pressure. This steep increase in intracranial pressure was always ac-

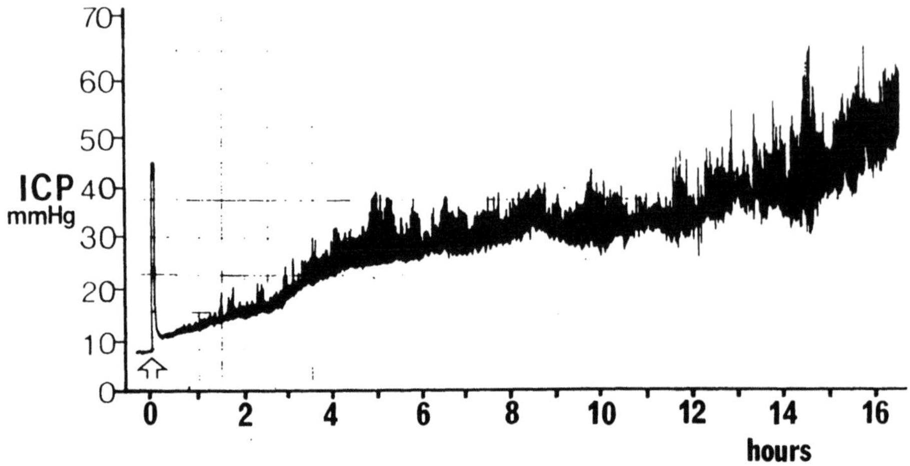

Fig. 1. Intracranial hypertension following a 10-ml intracisternal injection of incubated blood. Paper chart speed is 2 cm/h. *Open arrow,* time of intracisternal injection of blood; *ICP,* intracranial pressure

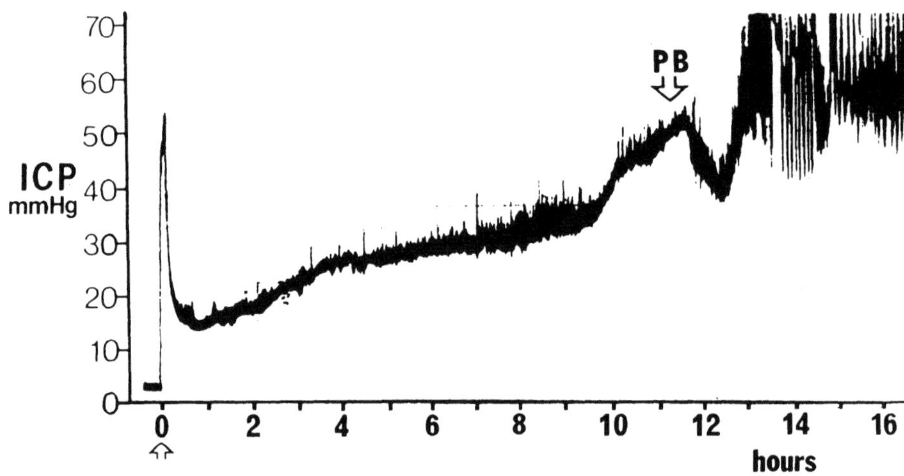

Fig. 2. Intracranial pressure (*ICP*) curve before and after pentobarbital application into the bilateral posterior hypothalamus (*PB* with *large open arrow*) during intracranial hypertension. Paper chart speed is 2 cm/h. *Small open arrow,* time of intracisternal blood injection

companied by more frequent and larger amplitude intracranial pressure irregularities than in the controls. In two animals, however, only a decrease and no subsequent rise in intracranial pressure was observed after pentobarbital administration. Figure 2 shows an intracranial pressure curve, in which a transient depression followed by a steep rise after the administration of pentobarbital into the bilateral posterior hypothalamus can be seen.

In group III animals, three out of six dogs had an intense rise in intracranial pressure, accompanied by intracranial pressure irregularities, and the other three animals initially manifested only a marked increase in intracranial pressure irregularities followed within 6–8 h by a steep rise in intracranial pressure.

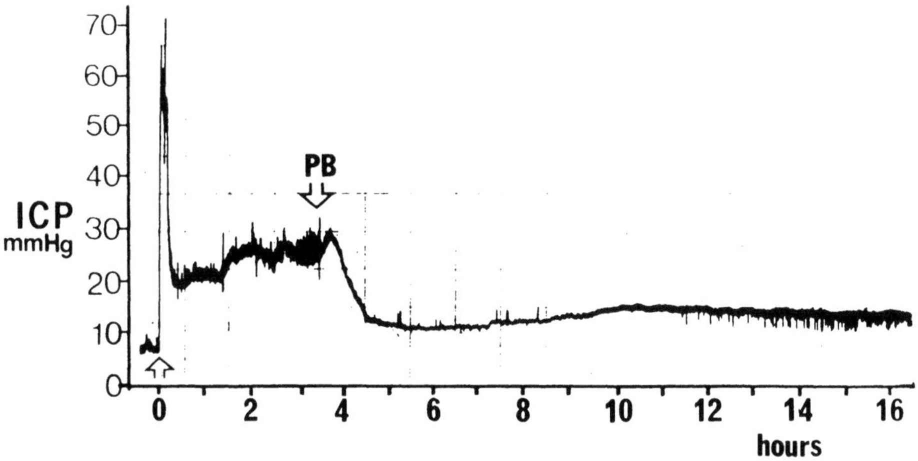

Fig. 3. Intracranial pressure (*ICP*) curve before and after injection of pentobarbital into the medullary reticular formation (*PB* with *large arrow*) during intracranial hypertension. Paper chart speed is 2 cm/h. *Small open arrow*, time of intracisternal injection of blood

Pentobarbital Administration into Medullary Reticular Formation

Group IV animals all showed either stabilization of intracranial pressure irregularities or a significant drop in intracranial pressure after pentobarbital administration into the medullary reticular formation. Figure 3 illustrates an example of the intracranial pressure curve in an animal in this group.

In the present study, the administration of pentobarbital into the posterior hypothalamus and the pontine reticular formation produced a marked increase in intracranial pressure accompanied by frequent intracranial pressure irregularities, suggesting the development of cerebrovascular excitatory responses. On the other hand, administration of pentobarbital into the medulla oblongata depressed both the increased level and the irregularities of intracranial pressure, suggesting a depression of cerebrovascular responses. The results suggest that the effectiveness of barbiturates in reducing raised intracranial pressure may be due to sedation of the vasomotor center of the medullary reticular formation.

Summary

Intracranial hypertension was induced in dogs by intracisternal injection of autogenous incubated blood. Changes in intracranial pressure were studied in animals that had received pentobarbital administered directly into the posterior hypothalamus, the pontine reticular formation, and the medullary reticular formation during the course of intracranial hypertension. Arterial oxygen and carbon dioxide pressure were maintained in the normal ranges. In animals in which pentobarbital had been given into the posterior hypothalamus and the pontine reticular formation, both a more marked elevation in intracranial pressure and more frequent intracranial pressure irregularities were observed than in the control animals. Following administration into the medullary reticular formation, either a stabilization of intracranial pressure irregularities or a significant decrease in intracranial pressure was noted. The results suggest that the effectiveness of barbiturates in reducing increased intracranial pressure may result from sedation of the vasomotor center of the medullary reticular formation.

New Therapies for Brain Edema

D. M. LONG [1]

Introduction

Brain edema is still an extremely important complication of brain tumors and strokes; it is the principle factor responsible for the secondary effects which complicate these brain diseases [15]. There has been no major advance in therapy since glucosteroids were introduced by Galicich and French in 1959 [17]. At the same time there has been a dramatic improvement in our understanding of the pathologic process since the first Brain Edema Symposium in 1965 [23]. If the therapy of edema is to progress it is likely that this will occur through an increased understanding of the pathophysiology of the process and assessment of the secondary effects of edema upon the brain. An immediate need is to understand these secondary effects [29]. It is also necessary to have some technique for evaluating and monitoring the degree of edema in patients.

Computerized axial tomography has revolutionized our ability to diagnose and quantify edema in the human [8, 39]. Magnetic resonance imaging may prove even more satisfactory in quantification and localization of the edema mass [19]. Furthermore, the ability to study energy metabolism with these techniques will undoubtedly be useful in defining the secondary effects of edema. Positron emission tomography gives us the capability of studying blood flow, oxygen metabolism, blood volume, cerebral metabolic rate, and protein metabolism [37]. However, none of these techniques will allow the immediate assessment or the regular monitoring of the edema process [34].

The therapy of brain edema began in the early part of this century. Weed described the effects of hyperosmolar solutions upon the brain, and clinical applications began in the 1930s [31]. The principle agents in use at that time were sugar solutions. Javid introduced urea and really provided the basis for our ubiquitous use of the osmotic diuretics in clinical practice. In the 1960s both glycerol and mannitol were introduced. Mannitol has now become the standard [5]. In the 1970s Diamox and furosemide were introduced based upon data reported by Long et al. [27, 29]. These have now become important adjuncts to the management of brain edema and have found real use in the treatment of another disorder of brain water, hydrocephalus. The inference that steroids would be of value in the treatment of brain edema was made well before their introduction for that purpose. Prados first described steroid protection of the exposed cortex in the course of studies designed to

[1] Department of Neurosurgery, Johns Hopkins University School of Medicine, Baltimore, MD 21205, USA

reduce morbidity from extensive operations for epilepsy [40]. Galicich and French described dramatic improvement in patients with glioblastoma and correctly deduced that this was achieved through an effect on edema, and not on the tumor itself [17]. Long, Galicich, and French then undertook a series of studies which demonstrated improvement in patients with brain injuries of non-neoplastic origin [33]. Rasmussen described the dramatic effects of steroids upon the morbidity of craniotomy for temporal lobectomy [44]. Since then, a wide variety of studies have validated the use of steroids in edema-producing disease states [2, 6, 9, 33].

A laboratory investigation on the value of steroids in brain edema began shortly after the clinical observations were made. In 1960, Long, Hartman, and French began a series of studies designed to delineate the effect of steroids upon edema [25, 26, 32]. It was first necessary to prove that steroids had an effect upon the water content of the brain (Fig. 1). This was done in investigations utilizing the cold injury model originally described by Klatzo [22]. A number of studies have confirmed these original measurements. However, Pappius has emphasized that the changes in volume abnormality may not be the only or even the most important effect of steroids [36, 38]. She has demonstrated improved glucose metabolism when steroids are used in the same model. Subsequent studies have shown that glocusteroids are equipotential in their effect (Fig. 2). In 1972, Choi and Long demonstrated that furosemide and acetazolamide had a strong influence upon brain edema [29]. The combination of these drugs with glucosteroids was more effective than the glucosteroids alone (Fig. 3). However, the electrolyte abnormalities which attend the use of these nonosmotic diuretics are of such a kind that it has been extremely difficult to use them widely [5]. The current therapy of brain edema requires the use of osmotic diuretics for short-term reduction of intracranial pressure. Glucosteroids are the only effective therapy for the long-term reduction of edema and improvement in func-

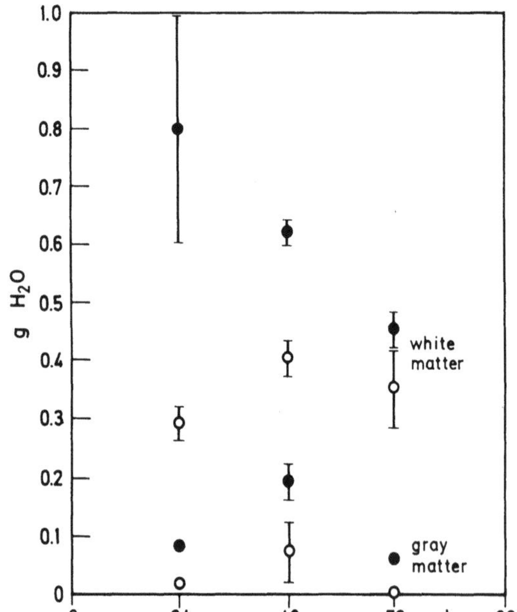

Fig. 1. Comparison of steroid-treated (*open circles*) and non-steroid-treated (*closed circles*) cold injury edema

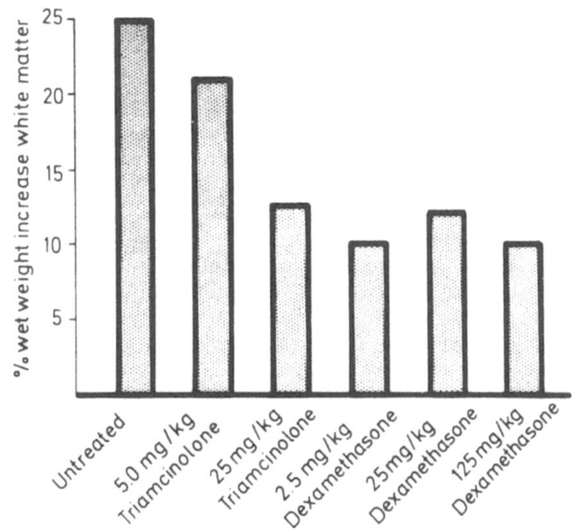

Fig. 2. Comparison of differing steroids and doses

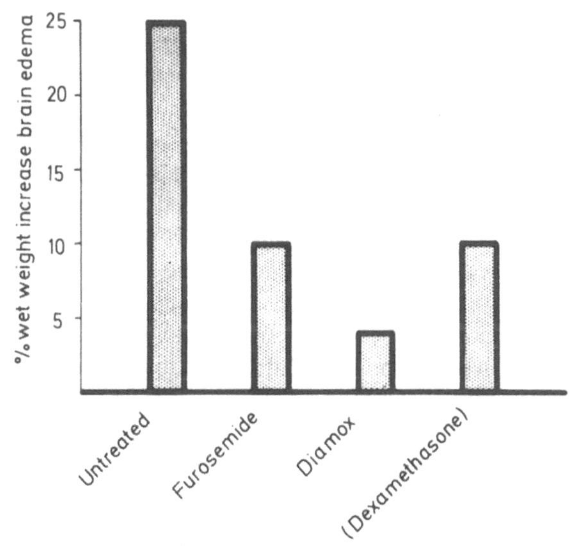

Fig. 3. Effect of nonosmotic diuretics and steroids on edema

tion. Furosemide is useful in prolonging and intensifying the effects of the osmotic diuretics. Acetazolamide has not been used in any significant way [35]. While these therapies are partially effective, they have not been improved upon in the past 25 years and it is time for a major new effort in brain edema therapy.

Evolution and Resolution of Vasogenic Brain Edema

It is now well accepted that vasogenic brain edema occurs because of a focal breakdown or absence of the blood-brain barrier (Table 1). Klatzo has previously demonstrated this effectively by the use of multiple-tracer dye techniques [21–23]. Follow-

Table 1. Evolution and resolution of vasogenic edema

1) Focal Insult: Breakdown or absence of blood brain barrier
2) Extravasation of a protein-rich fluid into extracellular space
3) Cellular swelling
4) Increased tissue pressure and migration of edema fluid
5) Functional changes in the lesion or in the surrounding area
a) Metabolism
b) Mediators
c) Blood flow – the spreading fire effect
6) Phagocytosis by astrocytes and histiocytes
7) Discharge into vascular system
8) Discharge into the ventricular system
9) Gliosis

We have no way of monitoring either the development or the resolution of brain edema

ing the injury there is extravasation of a protein-rich fluid into the extracellular space [4, 11]. This is promptly followed by a dramatic expansion of the extracellular space, particularly in the white matter. There is a concomitant cellular swelling, which appears to develop quickly in the cortex and much more slowly in the white matter. The cortical swelling is mostly astrocytic, but dendritic enlargement does occur [26, 32]. Go and Reulen have independently demonstrated the importance of local increases in tissue pressure [45–47]. Fenstermacher has shown that the edema fluid migrates by bulk flow [14]. The functional changes which occur during this time are not nearly as well understood as the anatomical abnormalities. There are clearly changes in metabolism [20, 37, 38]. Potential mediators of edema have been studied extensively by Baethmann and others [10, 12, 13, 30, 41, 50]. There is a progressive abnormality within the edematous process which relates to blood flow. Klatzo has described this as the "forest fire" or the "spreading fire" effect. Increased tissue pressure apparently decreases blood flow, leading to progressive ischemia, breakdown of the barrier, cellular swelling, and a steady expansion of the edema process. It is well accepted that this is important in ischemic edema. Its role in vasogenic edema is not so certain. There is a great need for expansion of our knowledge of the secondary effects upon brain function which come from the edematous process.

There is relatively rapid dissociation of protein and water following the extravasation [3, 7]. Phagocytosis of astrocytes and histocytes is common, particularly in the pericellular region. Astrocytic swelling occurs, and it appears that long chains of astrocytes, which are potentially in functional continuity, can be demonstrated spreading across the edematous cortex in particular [26]. Klatzo has suggested that there is a discharge of the phagocytosed protein into the vascular system and Reulen has clearly shown the discharge of this material into the ventricular system [48].

Development of Ischemic Edema

Ischemic edema follows a similar but somewhat different course (Table 2). The ischemic insult occurs first, and cellular swelling and cell death are prominent early features (Fig. 4). Breakdown of the blood-brain barrier occurs, but is much less important and occurs later in the course of the edema. There is extravasation of fluid into the extracellular space, resulting both from cellular lysis and from breakdown of the barrier (Fig. 5). The continuation of the process in the periphery through the spreading fire effect is most important in ischemic edema. Long has studied the microvascular changes which occur in this situation [24]. It appears that there is an early enlargement of the basement membrane and a progressive collection of fluid, first within the basement membrane and then in the disrupted perivascular space (Fig. 6). This culminates in collapse or disruption of small blood vessels, with extravasation of intravascular contents and surrounding cellular injury which is apparently ischemic. These descriptive studies do not allow a functional analysis of the changes, and this is an area of great importance for subsequent study. Klatzo and his colleagues have demonstrated changes in blood flow which are progressive in areas of cold-induced edema and an apparent functional concomitant of the abnormalities described by Long [16, 24, 51].

The therapeutic options may be reviewed with reference to what is known about the evolution and resolution of brain edema (Table 3). One possibility is to seal the blood-brain barrier. In the presence of tumors this may be difficult, because the defects are anatomical and not functional [28, 43]. However, there may be a functional component at the tumor margin, and it is extremely important to determine whether this is the case. In ischemia, sealing the barrier has the potential of reducing the ongoing involvement of the microvasculature, and it may be possible to stop the spreading fire effect in this way [49]. It is also possible that mediators may spread the derangement of permeability. A number of these have been studied, but no effective antagonists have yet been found.

Table 2. Development of ischemic edema

1) Ischemic insult
2) Cell swelling and death
3) Breakdown of blood-brain barrier
4) Extravasation into extracellular space
5) Continuation of the process at the periphery

Table 3. Therapeutic options

1) and 2) Seal the blood-brain barrier
a) Tumors: Defects are anatomical, not functional; margins may have functional component
b) Ischemia: Compromise of microvasculature is ongoing and may be reversible
c) Mediators or ischemia may spread derangement of permeability: may be reversible
1) Remove the lesion
2) Improve the microcirculation
3) Control mediators
4) Cellular swelling

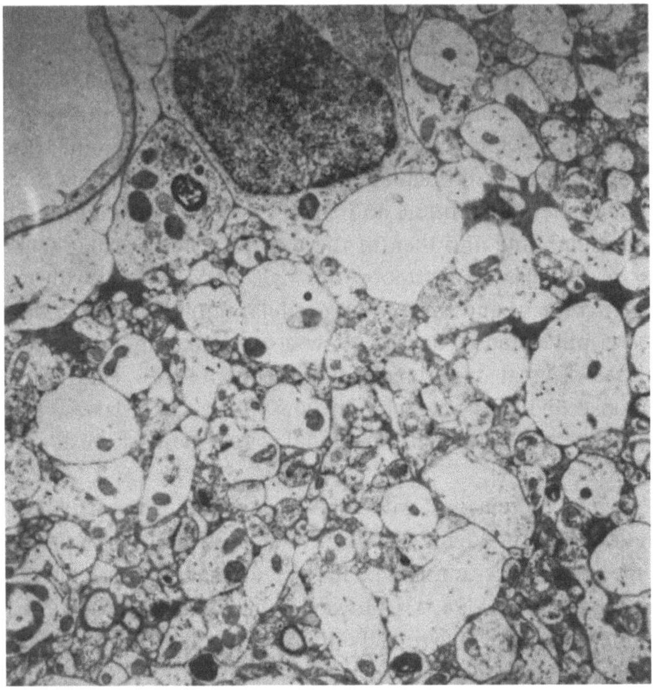

Fig. 4. Swollen astrocytes and dendrites near an area of ischemia; model, carotid occlusion in the gerbil

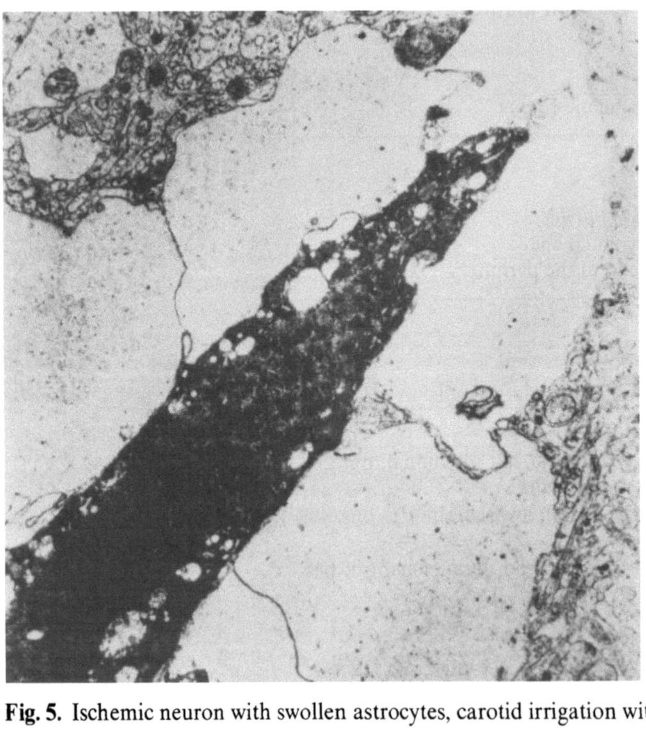

Fig. 5. Ischemic neuron with swollen astrocytes, carotid irrigation with saline, for 6 min

One way to seal the barrier is to remove the lesion (Fig. 7). Arabi and Long have demonstrated that excision of the cortical cold lesion virtually eliminates edema. Replacement of the injured brain does not reinstitute the edematous process [1]. It appears that microvasculature is mandatory for the development of the edema process. Blood pressure is another factor which can be manipulated. Klatzo et al. demonstrated long ago that hypotension retarded the edematous process and hypertension greatly accelerated it [23]. The manipulation of blood pressure must be balanced with the degree of tissue ischemia, which might be influenced adversely by reductions in blood pressure. At least hypertension should be avoided. As we learn more about the microvasculature and the role of ischemia in the edematous process, it may be possible to manipulate the blood pressure to control the extravasation of fluid. With regard to mediators, it will be necessary to identify those that are most important in the development of edema before antagonists can be found. Serotonin and the biogenic amines have been studied [41]. The prostaglandins have been implicated. Various members of the arachidonic cascade have been studied [15] and the renins are currently under investigation [50]. Free radicals remain a strong possibility [12], and satisfactory free radical scavengers are now being investigated. Long and associates have studied a broad spectrum of vasoactive drugs without finding any which had a potentially beneficial effect upon cold injury edema [27].

It may be possible to treat edema effectively by improving the ventricular drainage of the extravasated protein-rich fluid (Table 4). Since phagocytosis of proteins is an important part of the resolution process, it is possible that manipulations which would improve phagocytosis might be useful. Before this can become practical we will need to learn much more about the role of protein metabolism in the edematous process. Ventricular drainage and reduction of cerebrospinal fluid production both appear to be feasible ways of speeding the edematous process, but clinical trials will be required to prove this. The late gliosis which develops in untreated edema can be improved by steroids.

The role of intraneural mechanisms remains undefined. Raichle has shown that locus ceruleus stimulation increases vascular permeability [42], and Gann has shown the importance of intraneural mechanisms in homeostasis following trauma [18]. This is another fruitful area for potential therapeutics.

Table 4. Possible ways of reducing spread of edema

Increased tissue pressure
Colloidal influence of extravasated protein
Remove focus
Decrease hydrostatic force
Increase elimination of protein
Increase fractionation and phagocytosis
Increase protein metabolism
Reverse flow of protein/water
Increase effluent CSF
Lower CSF pressure
Diamox-furosemide
Drainage

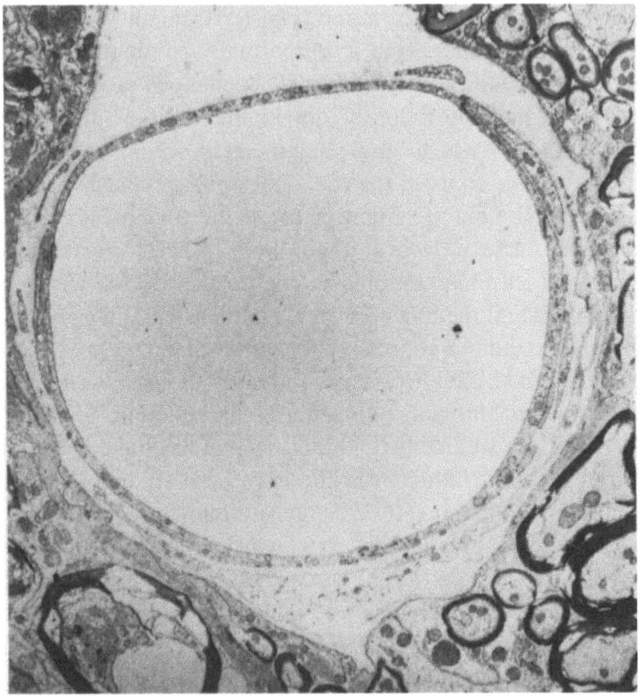

a

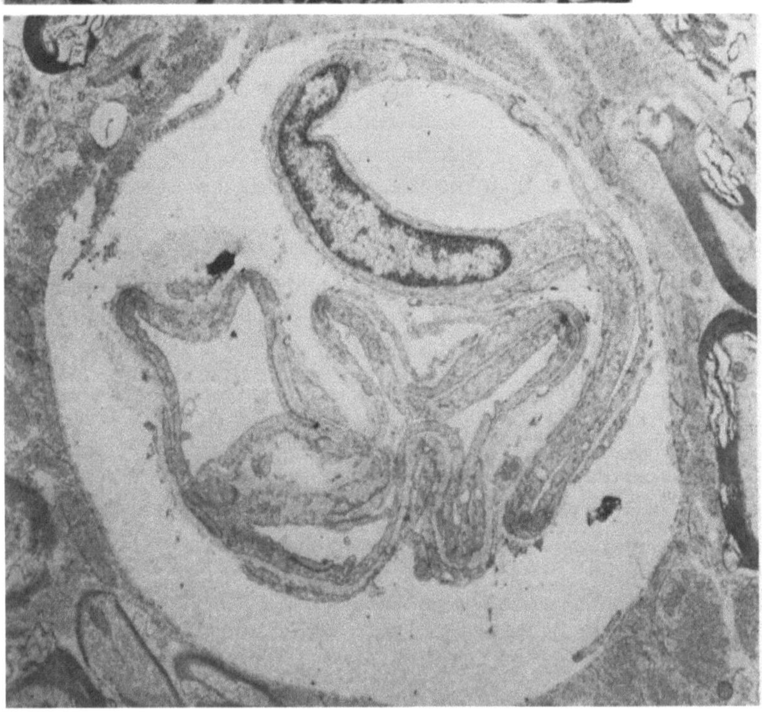

b

Fig. 6a–c. Ischemic capillary with widened basement membrane (**a**), collapse, (**b**), and dissolution of wall (**c**)

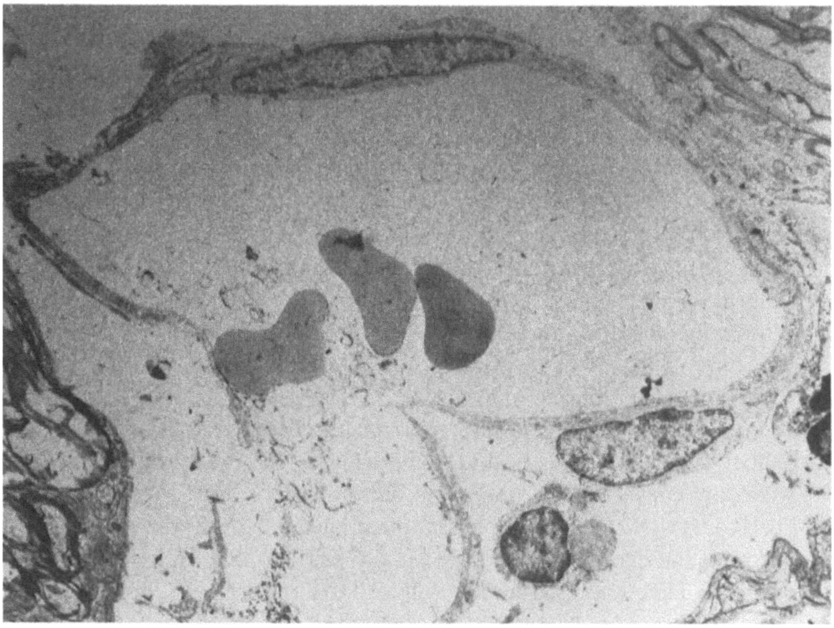

6c

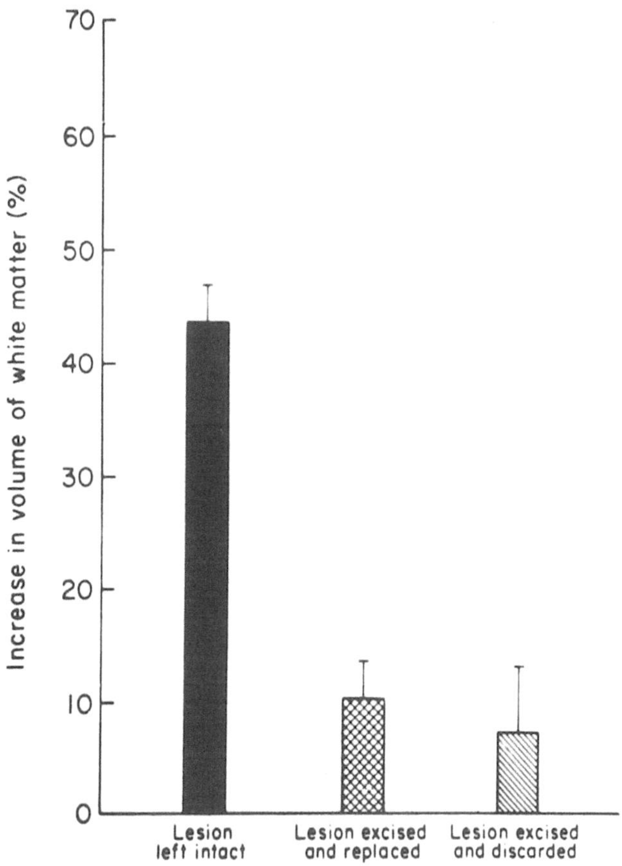

Fig. 7. Histogram showing increase in volume of white matter as a function of procedure followed with regard to the edematous focus

Since it is not possible to control the focus of edema production, it is probable that our activities must be concentrated on the spread of edema and the secondary effects of the edematous process. Areas for therapeutic investigation will include ways of decreasing tissue pressure and eliminating the colloidal influence of the extravasated protein. It is now possible to remove the focus in some situations, but not in all. When it is not possible to remove the focus a decrease in the hydrostatic force can be useful, but the value of blood pressure reduction must be weighed against the effects upon cerebral blood flow. It should be possible to increase the elimination of protein by increasing fractionation and phagocytosis, by increasing protein metabolism, or by reversal of the flow of protein water. This is probably best accomplished by increasing the amount of effluent CSF through lower cerebrospinal fluid pressure. This may be possible through combinations of acetazolamide and furosemide or by ventricular drainage [48].

The therapy of brain edema remains a major challenge. We have seen little improvement in the past 25 years, and brain edema is still the most important cause of the secondary effects of both stroke and brain tumors. Future therapeutic effort can take two courses. We must have a continued elucidation of basic mechanisms with correction of the derangements. It is equally possible that an indirect attack upon the secondary effects of brain tumors will lead to improvements in treatment.

Summary

Brain edema is still a major factor in the outcome following stroke or the development of a brain tumor. There has been no major advance in therapy since 1959. Current treatment utilizes hyperosmolar solutions and glucosteroids. New therapies are needed. A review of the current understanding of the evolution and resolution of brain edema may lead to the development of new treatments.

One direction for therapy is suggested by the well-known abnormalities of the blood-brain barrier. Attention should be directed to the possibility of sealing the abnormal barrier. The spread of edema by bulk flow may be modifiable by techniques which retard or accelerate that flow. Functional changes which occur in the brain surrounding areas of edema, particularly compromise of the microcirculation, are not well understood and offer a potential for treatment if they can be defined. Potential mediators of edema have been explored. The possibility of antagonists to those mediators is important. Techniques for improving the resolution of edema include acceleration of the elimination of protein, particularly through its discharge into the ventricular system. The development of new therapies depends upon continued elucidation of basic mechanisms of edema formation and on better understanding of the secondary effects of brain edema.

References

1. Arabi B, Long DM (1979) The role of an intact vascular bed in the production and propagation of vasogenic brain edema. J Neurosurg 51:779–784
2. Beks JWF, Doorenbos H, Walstra GJM (1972) Clinical experiences with steroids in neurosurgical patients. In Reulen H, Schurmann K (eds) Steroids and brain edema. Springer, Berlin Heidelberg New York, pp 233–238

3. Blasberg RG (1976) Clearance of serum albumin from brain extracellular fluid: a possible role in cerebral edema. In: Pappius HM, Feindel W (eds) Dynamics of brain edema. Springer, Berlin Heidelberg New York, pp 38–102
4. Bodsch W, Mies G, Paschen W, Hossmann KA (1984) Regional quantitative biochemistry and autoradiography of protein synthesis and serum extravasation in brain edema. In: Go KG, Baethmann A (eds) Recent progress in the study and therapy of brain edema. Plenum, New York, pp 27–35
5. Bourke RS, Kimelberg HK, Daze MA, Popp AJ (1979) Studies on the formation of astroglial swelling and its inhibition by clinically useful agents. In: Popp AS et al. (eds) Neural trauma. Raven, New York
6. Brock M, Wiegand H, Zillig C, Zywietz C, Mock P, Dietz H (1976) The effect of dexamethasone on intracranial pressure in patients with supratentorial tumors. In: Pappius HM, Feindel W (eds) Dynamics of brain edema. Springer, Berlin Heidelberg New York, pp 330–336
7. Bruce DA, Ter Weeme C, Kaiser G, Ghostine S (1979) Mechanisms and time course for clearance of vasogenic cerebral edema. In: Popp et al. (eds) Neural trauma. Raven, New York
8. Clasen RA, Huchman MS, Pandolfi S, Laing I, Jacobs J (1976) Computed tomography of vasogenic cerebral edema. In: Pappius HM, Feindel W (eds) Dynamics of brain edema. Springer, Berlin Heidelberg New York, pp 278–282
9. Cooper PR, Moody S, Clark WK, Kirkpatrick J, Marovilla K, Gould AL, Drane W (1979) Dexamethasone and severe head injury. A prospective double blind study. J Neurosurg 51:307–316
10. Costa JL, Ito U, Spatz M, Klatzo I, Demirjian C (1974) 5-Hydroxytryptamine accumulation in cerebrovascular injury. Nature 248:135–136
11. Cserr HF, Cooper DN, Milhorat TH (1976) Production, circulation and absorption of brain interstitial fluid. In: Pappius HM, Feindel W (eds) Dynamics of brain edema. Springer, Berlin Heidelberg New York, pp 95–97
12. Demopoulos HB, Flamm ES, Seligman ML, Mitamura JA, Ransohoff J (1979) Membrane perturbations in central nervous system injury: theoretical basis for free radical damage and a review of the experimental data. In: Popp et al. (eds) Neural trauma. Raven, New York
13. Fenske A, Sinterhauf K, Reulen HJ (1976) The role of monoamines in the development of cold-induced edema. In: Pappius HM, Feindel W (eds) Dynamics of brain edema. Springer, Berlin Heidelberg New York, pp 150–154
14. Fenstermacher JD, Patlak CS (1976) The movements of water and solutes in the brains of mammals. In: Pappius HM, Feindel W (eds) Dynamics of brain edema. Springer, Berlin Heidelberg New York, pp 87–94
15. Fishman RA (1975) Brain edema. N Engl J Med 293:706–711
16. Frei HJ, Wallenfang TH, Poll W, Reulen HJ, Schubert R, Brock M (1973) Regional cerebral blood flow and regional metabolism in cold induced oedema. Acta Neurochir (Wien) 29:15–28
17. Galicich JH, French LA (1961) Use of dexamethasone in the treatment of cerebral edema resulting from brain tumors and brain surgery. Am Pract 12:169–174
18. Gann D, Ward D, Baertschi A, Carlson D, Maran J (1977) Neural control of ACTH release in response to hemorrhage. Ann NY Acad Sci 297:477–497
19. Go KG, Van Dijk P, Luiten AL, Teelken AW (1984) Proton spin tomography in brain edema. In: Go K, Baethmann A (eds) Recent progress in the study and therapy of brain edema. Plenum, New York, pp 283–291
20. Heller V, Poch B, Gaab M, Sold M, Heissler HE (1984) O_2 availability and O_2 metabolism in cold induced brain edema. In: Go KG, Baethmann A (eds) Recent progress in the study and therapy of brain edema. Plenum, New York, pp 397–405
21. Herrmann HD, Neuenfeldt D (1972) Development and regression of a disturbance of the blood-brain barrier and of edema in tissue surrounding a circumscribed cold lesion. Exp Neurol 34:115–120
22. Klatzo I, Piraux A, Laskowski E (1958) The relationship between edema, blood brain barrier, and tissue elements in local brain injury. J Neuropathol 17:548–563

23. Klatzo T (1967) Presidential address: neuropathological aspects of brain edema. J Neuropathol Exp Neurol 26:1–14
24. Long DM: Microvascular changes in cold injury edema. In: Go KG, Baethmann A (eds) Recent progress in the study and therapy of brain edema. Plenum, New York, pp 45–54
25. Long DM, Hartmann JF, French LA (1966) The response of human cerebral edema to glucosteroid administration. An electron microscopic study. Neurology 16:521–528
26. Long DM, Maxwell RE, French LA (1971) The effects of glucosteroids upon cold induced brain edema. II. Ultrastructural evaluation. J Neuropathol Exp Neurol 30(4):680–697
27. Long DM, Maxwell RE, Choi KS, Cole HO, French LA (1972) Multiple therapeutic approaches in the treatment of brain edema induced by a standard cold lesion. In: Reulen HJ, Schurmann K (eds) Steroids and brain edema. Springer, Berlin Heidelberg New York, pp 87–94
28. Long DM (1970) Capillary ultrastructure in human malignant brain tumors. J Neurosurg 32:127–144
29. Long DM, Maxwell R, Choi KS (1976) A new therapy regimen for brain edema. In: Pappius HM, Feindel W (eds) Dynamics of brain edema. Springer, Berlin Heidelberg New York
30. Maier-Hauff K, Lange M, Schurer L, Guggenbichler Ch, Vogt W, Jacob K, Baethmann A (1984) Glutamate and free fatty acid concentrations in extracellular vasogenic edema fluid. In: Go KG, Baethmann A (eds) Recent progress in the study and therapy of brain edema. Plenum, New York, pp 183–192
31. Masserman JW (1935) Effects of intravenous administration of hypertonic solutions of sucrose. Johns Hopkins Hosp Bull 57:12–21
32. Maxwell RE, Long DM, French LA (1971) The effects of glucosteroids on experimental cold-induced brain edema: gross morphological alterations and vascular permeability changes. J Neurosurg 34:477–487
33. Maxwell RE, Long DM, French LA (1972) The clinical effects of a synthetic glucocorticoid used for brain edema in the practice of neurosurgery. In: Reulen HJ, Schurmann K (eds) Steriods and brain edema. Springer, Berlin Heidelberg New York, pp 219–232
34. Meinig G, Aulich A, Wende S, Reulen HJ (1976) The effect of dexamethasone and diuretics on peritumor brain edema: comparative study of tissue water content and CT. In: Pappius HM, Feindel W (eds) Dynamics of brain edema. Springer, Berlin Heidelberg New York, pp 301–305
35. Meinig G, Reulen HJ, Simon RS, Schurmann K (1980) Clinical, chemical and CT evaluation of short-term and long-term antiedema therapy with dexamethasone and diuretics. Adv Neurol 28:271–291
36. Pappius HM (1972) Effects of steroids on cold injury edema. In: Reulen HJ, Schurmann K (eds) Steroids and brain edema. Springer, Berlin Heidelberg New York, pp 57–63
37. Pappius HM (1980) Mapping of cerebral functional activity with radioactive desoxyglucose application in studies of traumatized brain. Adv Neurol
38. Pappius HM, Wolfe LS (1984) Effect of drugs on local cerebral glucose utilization in traumatized brain: mechanisms of action of steroids revisited. In: Go KG, Baethmann A (eds) Recent progress in the study and therapy of brain edema. Plenum, New York, pp 11–26
39. Penn RD (1976) Cerebral edema and blood volume in man measured by CT scan. In: Pappius HM, Feindel W (eds) Dynamics of brain edema. Springer, Berlin Heidelberg New York, pp 288–292
40. Prados M, Strowger B, Feindel W (1945) Studies on cerebral edema. II. Reaction of the brain to exposure to air; physiological changes. Arch Neurol Psychiatry 54:290–300
41. Osterholm JL, Bell J, Meyer R et al. (1969) Experimental effects of free serotonin on the brain and its relation to brain injury, Part 1. The neurological consequences of intracerebral serotonin injections. J Neurosurg 31:408–412
42. Raichle ME, Eichling JO, Grubb RL, Hartman BK (1976) Central noradrenergic regulation of brain microcirculation. In: Pappius HM, Feindel W (eds) Dynamics of brain edema. Springer, Berlin Heidelberg New York, pp 11–17
43. Rapoport SI, Matthews K, Thompson HK (1976) Absence of brain edema after reversible osmotic opening of the blood-brain barrier. In: Pappius HM, Feindel W (eds) Dynamics of brain edema. Springer, Berlin Heidelberg New York, pp 18–22

44. Rasmussen T, Gulati DR (1962) Cortisone in the treatment of postoperative cerebral edema. J Neurosurg 19:535–544
45. Reulen JH, Kreysch HG (1973) Measurement of brain tissue pressure in cold induced cerebral oedema. Acta Neurochir (Wien) 29:29–40
46. Reulen HJ, Graham R, Fenske A, Tsuyumu M, Klatzo I (1976) The role of tissue pressure and bulk flow in the formation and resolution of cold-induced edema. In: Pappius HM, Feindel W (eds) Dynamics of brain edema. Springer, Berlin Heidelberg New York, pp 103–112
47. Reulen HJ, Graham R, Spatz M, et al. (1977) Role of pressure gradients and bulk flow in dynamics of vasogenic brain edema. J Neurosurg 46:24–35
48. Reulen HJ, Tsuyumu M, Tack A, Fenske AR, Prioleau GR (1978) Clearance of edema fluid into cerebrospinal fluid. J Neurosurg 48:754–764
49. Spatz M, Rap ZM, Rapoport SI, Klatzo I (1972) The effects of hypertonic urea on the blood-brain barrier and on the glucose transport in the brain. In: Reulen HJ, Schurmann K (eds) Steroids and brain edema. Springer, Berlin Heidelberg New York, pp 19–27
50. Unterberg A, Maier-Hauff K, Wahl M, Lange M, Baethmann A (1984) Cerebral uptake and consumption of plasma-kininogens in vasogenic brain edema: Recent findings of kinin-mechanisms. In: Go KG, Baethmann A (eds) Recent progress in the study and therapy of brain edema. Plenum, New York, pp 175–182
51. Wallenfang T, Schubert R, Grote J, Schaaf W, Reulen HJ (1973) Regional cerebral blood flow and regional cerebrovascular reactivity following local brain injury. Adv Neurosurg 1:176–183

Comparative Nuclear Magnetic Resonance Study of Brain Edema in Immature and Adult Rats

M. MASUMURA[1], M. YAMAGUCHI, T. SHIRAKUNI, T. NAGASHIMA, N. TAMAKI, S. MATSUMOTO, and M. SUGIURA

Key words: Experimental brain edema, immature rat brain, proton relaxation time, water content

Introduction

In recent years, brain water content has been studied in various types of neurologic conditions by using proton nuclear magnetic resonance (proton NMR). Thus, it is possible to illustrate the brain water status on the basis of such parameters as proton density, longitudinal relaxation time (T_1), and transverse relaxation time (T_2). However, the literature dealing with basic studies of various types of information obtained with NMR is very small [1, 3, 6, 7]. Since little is known about the immature brain [2, 4, 5], we have measured the water content and the relaxation times (T_1 and T_2) in cerebral gray and white matters over time. The age range of the animals used extended from the 20th day of gestation to 8 weeks after birth.

Further, we have induced cold injury to produce brain edema in these young animals to obtain more detailed data on the relaxation times during this pathologic condition. The information obtained would contribute much to the reading and interpretation of clinical NMR images recorded in human infants in the future.

Materials and Methods

Physiologic Changes in the Brain Water Content, T_1, and T_2 with Aging

Measurement of Water Content

Animals used in this experiment were Wistar strain male rats except for the fetuses, which were difficult to sex with certainty. The water content was determined by the dry weight method. In all, 95 animals were used in this work (8 rats of 20 days' gestation; 15 rats aged 1 week, 13 aged 2 weeks, 10 aged 3 weeks, 20 aged 4 weeks, 18 aged 5 weeks, and 11 rats aged 8 weeks).

[1] Department of Neurological Surgery, Kobe University School of Medicine, 7-5-1 Kusunoki-cho, Chuo-ku, Kobe 650, Japan

Measurement of Relaxation Times

As for the measurement of water content, 32 rats (4 fetuses of 20 days' gestation, and 6 subgroups of 4–6 each of rats aged 1–8 weeks) were decapitated, and specimens (15–30 mg each of the gray and the white matter) were prepared for the determination of relaxation times. The NMR spectrometer used was the Varian XL 200 (200 MHz). T_1 was measured by the inversion recovery method, while T_2 was measured by the Carr-Purcell-Meiboon-Gill method. These measurements were completed within 6 h after sacrifice.

Cold Injury Brain Edema

Cold injury brain edema was produced as follows: in rats aged 7 days (group A) a metal rod cooled to –70 °C with acetone dry ice was pushed through the skin and into the right parietal area without anesthesia. In rats aged 5 weeks (group B), a burr hole was made over the parietal area under light anesthesia with ether, and a metal rod at –70 °C was advanced to the dura to produce experimental brain edema. On the 1st or 7th experimental day the water content and relaxation times were determined on gray and white matter specimens from groups A and B.

Results

Changes in the Brain Water Content, T_1, and T_2 with Aging

It was almost impossible to separate the white matter from the gray matter of 20-day fetuses. The cerebral water content was estimated for the whole brain specimen. The water content of the fetal brain was found to be 87.40% ± 3.08%. Immediately after birth, the water content was highest in the cerebellum, followed by brain stem, cerebral white matter, and cerebral gray matter in declining order. Thereafter, the water content decreased with age. In rats aged 2 weeks or more the water content was highest in the gray matter, followed by the white matter, cerebellum, and brain stem in declining order.

Water Content, T_1, and T_2 in Gray Matter

The water content and T_1 decreased almost in parallel. In rats aged 4 weeks the water content was 81.73% ± 1.31% and T_1 was 1.370 ± 0.026 s. Thereafter, few changes in these parameters were noted until the age of 8 weeks. On the other hand, T_2 decreased at a relatively rapid rate. In rats aged 4 weeks, T_2 was 59.00 ± 2.09 ms. Thereafter, no significant difference was noted between the 4-week-old group and the mature group.

Water Content, T_1, and T_2 in White Matter

In rats aged 5 weeks the water content reached 79.45% ± 2.39% and no significant decrease was noted thereafter. In rats aged 2 weeks, T_1 was 1.400 ± 0.169 s. This value is close to T_1 in the mature animals. The value for T_2 in the 5-week-old group was 56.70 ± 1.46 ms and no significant decrease was observed after this age.

Water Content and Relaxation Times in Edematous Brains in Groups A and B

The water content of edematous brains is shown in the Tables 1 and 2 and Fig. 1. When the water content of the brain had decreased to 83% T_1 was at almost normal values without exception; T_1 was always significantly prolonged if the water content was over 83%.

Table 1. Water content and T_1 and T_2 in gray (G) and white (W) matter of specimens prepared from group A animals on days 1 and 7 after cold injury compared with normal control values

	24 h after cold injury (normal control)	1 week after cold injury (normal control)
Water content (%)	G: 90.30 ± 1.00[d]	G: 83.56 ± 1.08
	(84.26 ± 2.72)	(82.94 ± 1.60)
	W: 89.34 ± 0.05[d]	W: 83.71 ± 1.03[d]
	(82.48 ± 2.21)	(81.30 ± 0.34)
T_1 (s)	G: 1.770 ± 0.131[a]	G: 1.625 ± 0.075[d]
	(1.565 ± 0.151)	(1.416 ± 0.015)
	W: 1.752 ± 0.199[d]	W: 1.604 ± 0.114[d]
	(1.400 ± 0.169)	(1.346 ± 0.035)
T_2 (ms)	G: 97.0 ± 12.0[c]	G: 83.0 ± 6.1[d]
	(73.1 ± 6.5)	(61.3 ± 1.8)
	W: 92.8 ± 8.8[b]	W: 83.4 ± 2.7[d]
	(69.8 ± 12.8)	(60.7 ± 2.8)

[a] $P<0.05$; [b] $P<0.025$; [c] $P<0.01$; [d] $P<0.005$

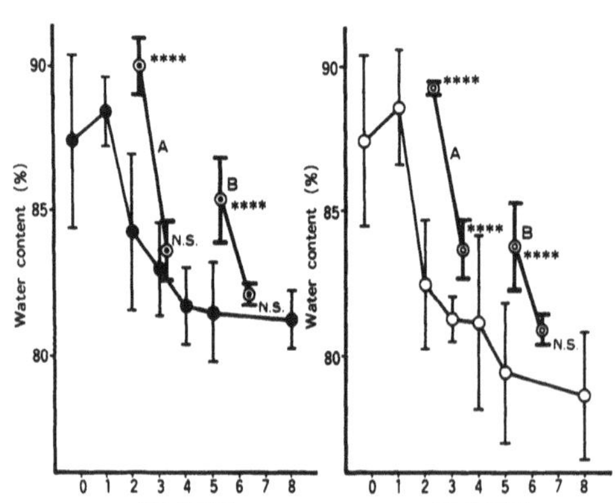

Fig. 1. Changes in water content of gray (◉, ●) and white (◎, ○) matter after cold injury in 7-day-old rats (*A*) and 5-week-old rats (*B*). *N.S.*, not significant; *$P < 0.05$; **$P < 0.025$; ***$P < 0.01$; ****$P < 0.005$

Table 2. Water content and T_1 and T_2 in gray (G) and white (W) matter of specimens prepared from group B animals on days 1 and 7 after cold injury, compared with normal control values

	24 h after cold injury		1 week after cold injury, edema side
	Edema side (normal control)	Opposite side	
Water content %	G: 85.37 ±1.52^{d} (81.47 ±1.67)	G: 84.21 ±0.24^{c}	G: 82.08 ±0.69
	W: 83.83 ±1.50^{d} (79.45 ±2.39)	W: 81.60 ±0.63	W: 80.98 ±0.53
T_1 (s)	G: 1.451±0.003^{c} (1.387±0.041)	G: 1.394±0.014	G: 1.428±0.044^{c}
	W: 1.353±0.011^{b} (1.278±0.036)	W: 1.366±0.011^{c}	W: 1.392±0.018^{c}
T_2 (ms)	G: 57.9 ±1.3 (58.7 ±2.7)	G: 54.7 ±2.0	G: 58.9 ±0.2
	W: 58.5 ±1.0 (56.7 ±1.5)	W: 57.4 ±1.6	W: 58.5 ±0.1

^{a} $P<0.05$; ^{b} $P<0.025$; ^{c} $P<0.01$; ^{d} $P<0.005$

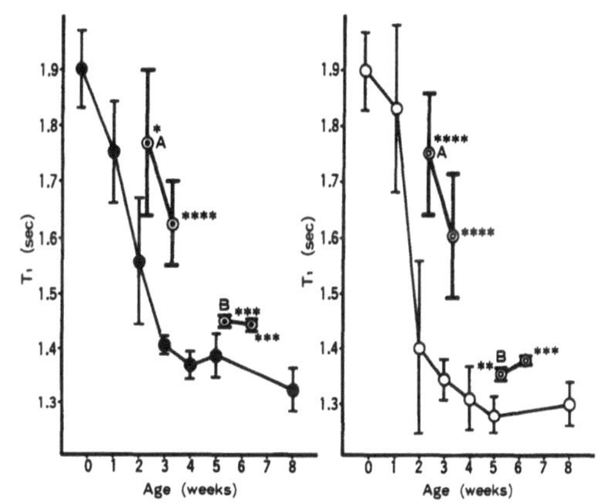

Fig. 2. Changes in T_1 in gray (◉, ●) and white (◎, ○) matter after cold injury in 7-day-old rats (*A*) and 5-week-old rats (*B*). $*P < 0.05$; $**P < 0.025$; $***P < 0.01$; $****P < 0.005$

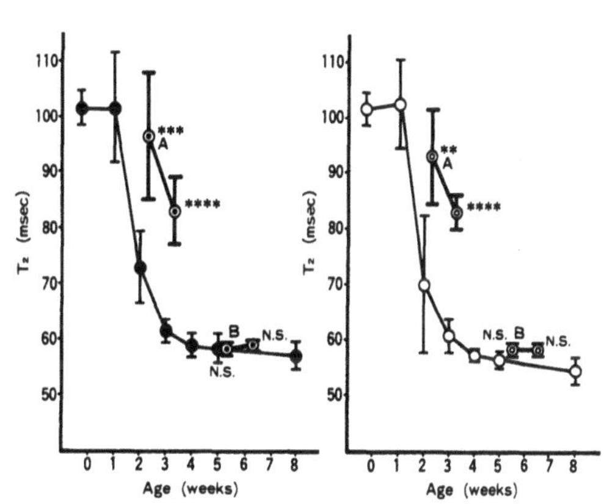

Fig. 3. Changes in T_2 of gray (◉, ●) and white (◎, ○) matter after cold injury in 7-day-old rats (*A*) and 5-week-old rats (*B*) *N.S.*, not significant; $*P < 0.05$; $**P < 0.025$; $***P < 0.01$; $****P < 0.005$

T_2 was always significantly prolonged in group A, while no significant deviation from the control value was determined in group B when it was estimated 24 h and 7 days after the insult. There was thus a major difference in the behavior of T_1 and T_2 in the experimental conditions (Figs. 2 and 3).

Discussion

Changes in Water Content and Relaxation Times with Normal Aging

At first, the authors were not confident about the development of edema in hyperhydrated brains of fetal or neonatal rats. We ascertained that water content, T_1, and T_2 decreased with age from gestation to 8 weeks after birth. We believe, therefore, that the water content, T_1, and T_2 of any pathologic brain tissue should be always evaluated in comparison with physiological changes on aging. Examination of the trends in detail revealed that T_1 was strikingly prolonged in the brain tissue when the water content was over 83% in either gray or white matter. The result also revealed that the T_2 was consistently shortened with age even if the water content reached almost to the range normal in mature animals.

Water Content and Relaxation Times During Brain Edema

There was a delicate difference between T_1 and T_2 during brain edema, as already mentioned. It was noted that in the mature group T_2 remained constantly normal. This may be because the relaxation time we measured was not separated into the "two components" shown by Go [3] and Naruse [6] in the edematous state. The T_2 we measured may be either the rapid moiety of the so-called two components or a value affected strongly by the "fast component" itself. It is also suggested that the fast component of T_2 may not be prolonged in the edematous brain of mature animals (S. Naruse, personal communication). In group A, T_2 was strikingly prolonged and did not recover the normal range even 7 days after the edema-producing insult. To the best of our knowledge, no publication has appeared about the T_2 change following edema development in such young experimental animals.

In conclusion, it is considered that the measurement of proton relaxation times is quite valuable in the investigation of such pathologic brain conditions as edema.

Summary

On the basis of in vitro measurement of NMR signals, it is generally accepted that the water content in the brain tissue of immature animals is the main causative factor in prolongation of proton relaxation times [longitudinal (spin-lattice) and transverse (spin-spin) relaxation times, T_1 and T_2, respectively]. Water content, T_1, and T_2 were estimated in specimens taken from rats with a wide age distribution ranging from fetal age (20 days of gestation) to 8 weeks after birth, and the values obtained tended to decrease gradually with advancing age in both gray and white matter. Except for T_1 in the white matter, parameters measured in the gray and white matter of animals aged 4 weeks or less were significantly higher than those in rats aged 8 weeks.

In assessing edema in the 7-day-old rat brain over time, the water content and T_1 and T_2 were estimated and compared with the corresponding values for 5-week-old rats. When the brain edema was produced by cold injury in immature rats, prolonged T_1 and T_2 were observed in preparations taken from animals at 1 and 7 days after the insult. In the group of 5-week-old rats T_2 was not prolonged on days 1 and 7 after the insult. In the edematous brain, T_1 differed from T_2 in that it did become longer in the course of aging. This is ascribable to the involvement of the minute cell structure or the degree of myelination process.

References

1. Bakay L, Kurland RJ, Parrish RG, Lee CC, Peng RJ, Bartkowski HK (1975) Nuclear magnetic resonance studies in normal and edematous brain tissue. Exp Brain Res 23:241–24B
2. Buonanno FS, Pykett IL, Brady TJ, Vielma J, Burt CT, Goldman MR, Hinshaw WS, Pohost GM, Kistler JP (1983) Proton NMR imaging in experimental ischemic infarction. Stroke 14:178–184
3. Go KG, Edzes HT (1975) Water in brain edema. Observations by the pulsed nuclear magnetic resonance technique. Arch Neurol 32:462–465
4. Johnson MA, Pennock JM, Bydder GM, Steiner RE, Thomas DJ, Hayward R, Byrant DRT, Payne JA, Levene MI, Whitelaw A, Dubowitz LMS, Dubowitz V (1983) Clinical NMR imaging of the brain in children. Am J Radiol 141:1005–1018
5. Levene MI, Whitelaw A, Dubowitz V, Bydder GM, Steiner RE, Randell CP, Young IR (1982) Nuclear magnetic resonance imaging of the brain in children. Br Med J 285:774–776
6. Naruse S, Horikawa Y, Tanaka C, Hirakawa K, Nishikawa H, Yoshizaki K (1982) Proton nuclear magnetic resonance studies on brain edema. J Neurosurg 56:747–752
7. Zawadzki MB, Bartkowski HM, Ortendahl DA, Pitts LH, Hylton NM, Nishimura MC, Crooks LE (1984) NMR in experimental cerebral edema: Value of T1 and T2 calculation. AJNR 5:125–129

Nuclear Magnetic Resonance Study of Periventricular Edema in Hydrocephalus

N. Tamaki[1], T. Shirakuni, N. Kojima, M. Masumura, and S. Matsumoto

Key words: Hydrocephalus, nuclear magnetic resonance (NMR), periventricular high intensity (PVHI), computed tomography (CT), periventricular lucency (PVL)

Introduction

Nuclear magnetic resonance (NMR) studies display not only a satisfactory amount of morphological detail of the normal and pathologic anatomy of the brain, but also dynamic conditions in various diseases of the central nervous system.

Experience with NMR imaging of patients with hydrocephalus of various causes suggests that this is a very promising approach for investigation of the pathogenesis and pathophysiology of the periventricular tissue in hydrocephalus.

Materials and Methods

Thirty patients with hydrocephalus were included in this study. The types of hydrocephalus represented were: normal pressure hydrocephalus (NPH) (17 cases), hydrocephalus resulting from aqueduct obstruction (5 cases), hydrocephalus due to posterior fossa tumor (6 cases), and hydrocephalus associated with primary degenerative dementia (2 cases). The age of the patients ranged from 7 to 87 years, with a mean age of 55.

The patients were examined with a 0.15 T resistive NMR imaging unit. The NMR imager used (Picker International Co., Inc., Ohio) incorporated a 1.5-kG resistive magnet with a 30-cm aperture head coil. The slice thickness was 10 mm and a multislice technique was used to allow examination of eight slices simultaneously.

Both the spin echo (SE) and inversion recovery (IR) techniques were used. For the SE technique the repetition time was set at 2100 ms and the echo times were 40 ms and 80 ms. For the IR technique, the repetition time was set at 2100 ms and the time of inversion was 500 ms. Slices were transverse in addition to coronal. All the patients were examined by X-ray computed tomography (CT), which was used as a standard against which the NMR findings were compared.

Of the 30 patients, 18 had continuous monitoring of the intracranial pressure (ICP) for 24 h; in 18 of the patients the regional cerebral blood flow was measured

[1] Department of Neurosurgery, Kobe University School of Medicine, 5-1 Kusunoki-cho, 7-chome, Chuo-ku, Kobe 650, Japan

by the xenon-133 inhalation method; and in 22 of the patients CT cisternography with metrizamide was performed. The results of these examinations were compared with the NMR findings.

Results

The pathologic condition of the periventricular tissue in hydrocephalus was most prominently delineated as a periventricular high signal intensity (PVHI) by the SE technique with a repetition time of 2100 ms and echo time of 80 ms (SE 2100/80). In normal subjects the signal intensity of the periventricular tissue is lower than or equal to that of the gray matter with the spin echo technique at a pulse sequence of 2100/80 ms. It is therefore considered pathologic when the periventricular tissue has a higher intensity than that of the gray matter (Fig. 1). The PVHI was characterized by a change in its intensity and extent after cerebrospinal fluid (CSF) shunting (Fig. 2), and by its absence in patients with marked hydrocephalus caused by aqueduct obstruction. All four of the patients with marked hydrocephalus associated with aqueduct obstruction since early in life had no PVHI on NMR images (Fig. 3 and Table 1).

Classification of PVHI on NMR

The PVHI was classified into four types on the basis of the grade of its extension (Table 2 and Fig. 4). Type 0 is seen in normal or negative subjects, in whom the periventricular linear shadow has the same signal intensity as that of the gray mat-

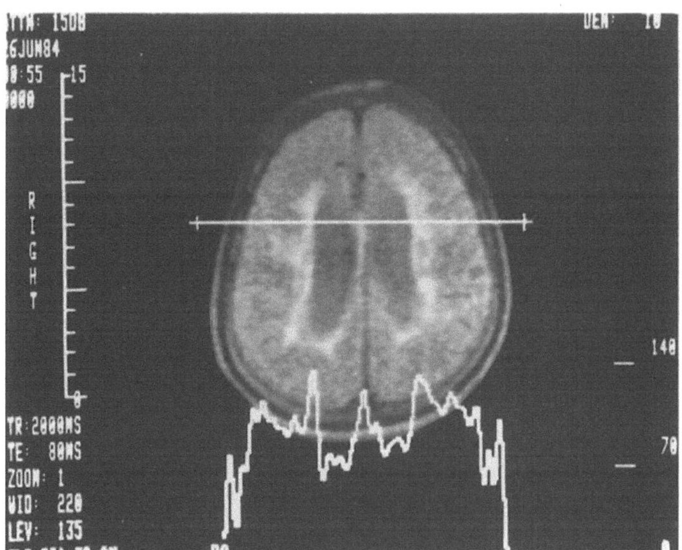

Fig. 1. Periventricular high intensity (PVHI) demonstrated on NMR images by spin echo technique at repetition time of 2100 ms and echo time of 80 ms (SE 80/2100)

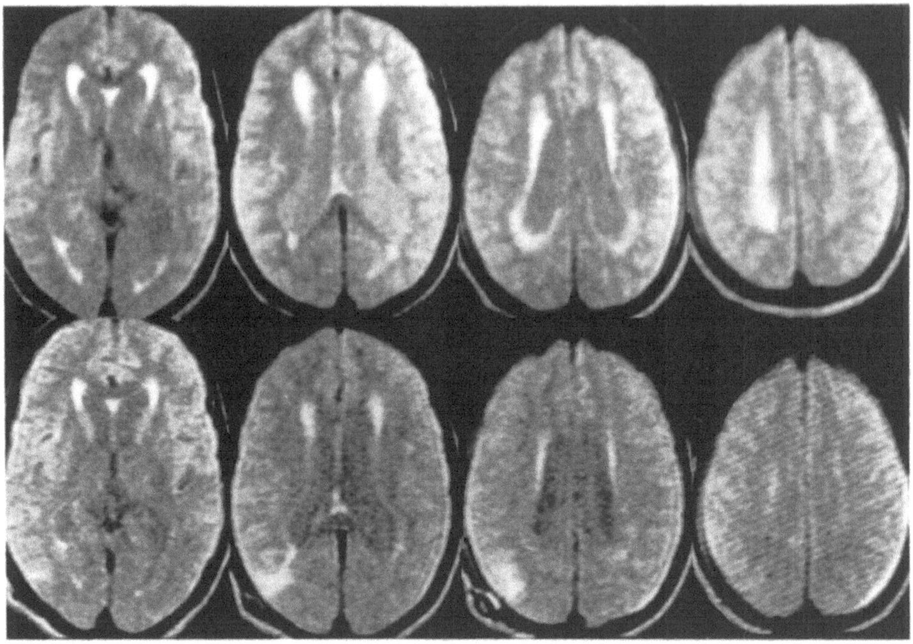

Fig. 2. Periventricular high intensity before (*above*) and after (*below*) shunt

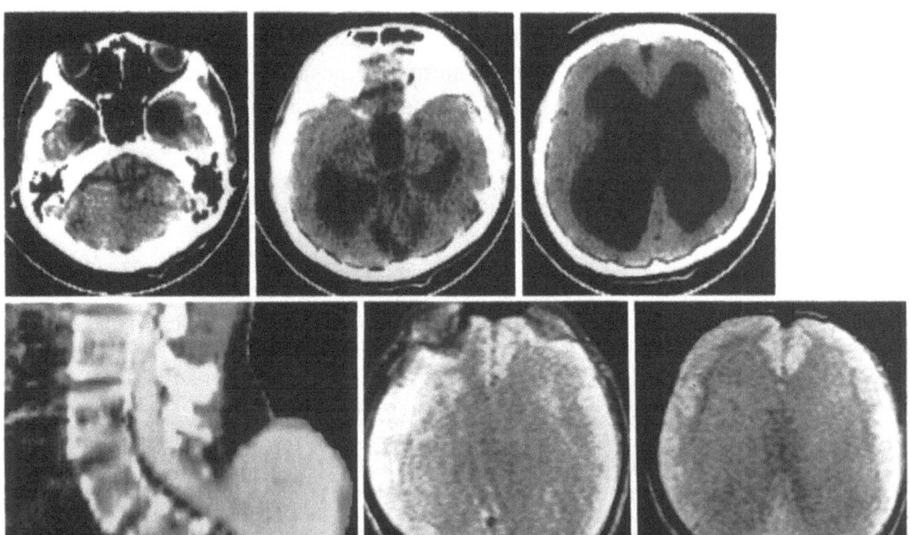

Fig. 3. NMR images of the patient with marked hydrocephalus associated with aqueduct obstruction and myelomeningocele who had no periventricular high intensity

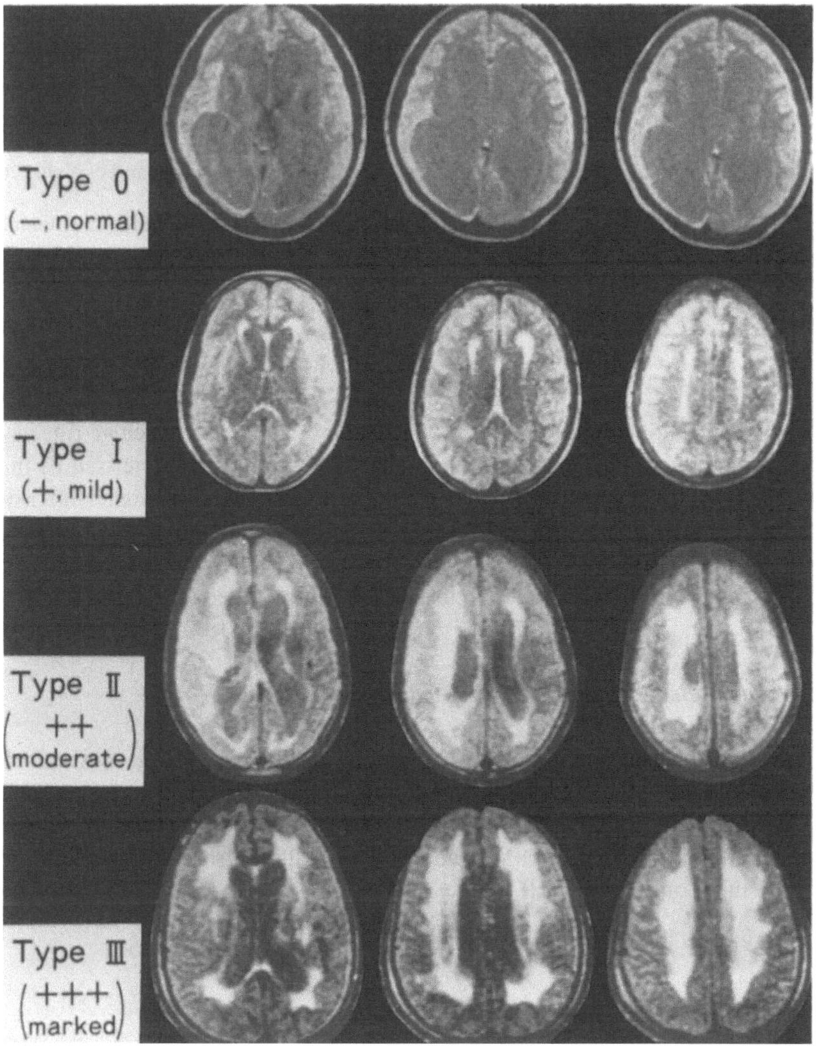

Fig. 4. NMR images demonstrating the classification of periventricular high intensity

Table 1. Clinical summary of patients with aqueduct obstruction

Patient	Age	Sex	Dementia score	Etiology	Hydro-cephalus	PVHI on NMR
I. M.	20	M	32.5	Myelomeningocele Arnold-Chiari malformation	Marked	–
W. M.	26	F	32.5	Meningitis (at 2 years)	Marked	–
T. M.	33	M	24	Congenital (at 6 months)	Marked	–
A. K.	39	M	32.5	Arteriovenous malformation	Moderate	–

Table 2. Classification of periventricular high intensity on NMR images

Type 0 (–, normal)	Periventricular linear shadow with same intensity as gray matter
Type I (+, mild PVHI)	Periventricular rim in narrow bands of higher intensity than gray matter
Type II (+ +, moderate PVHI)	Periventricular rim in wider band of higher intensity than gray matter; PVHI extends to half of the width of white matter, the margin of which is sometimes irregular
Type III (+ + +, marked PVHI)	Periventricular high intensity occupies almost all of white matter

ter. Type I involves mild PVHI, in which there is a periventricular rim in narrow bands of higher intensity than the gray matter. Type II is characterized by moderate PVHI, in which the periventricular rim is in a wider band of higher intensity than the gray matter and which extends across half the width of the white matter. The margin of the PVHI is sometimes irregular. Type III is characterized by marked PVHI, in which PVHI occupies almost all the white matter.

Correlation Between Type of Hydrocephalus and PVHI on NMR

Patients with suspected NPH showed various grades of PVHI on NMR; 2 of 16 patients had no PVHI, 3 had mild, 7 moderate, and 4 had marked PVHI on NMR.

It is of interest that patients with marked hydrocephalus due to aqueduct obstruction had no PVHI on NMR, and patients with hydrocephalus due to posterior fossa tumor, only mild PVHI (Table 3).

Table 3. Relationship between kinds of hydrocephalus and PVHI on NMR

PVHI on NMR \ Kinds of hydrocephalus	NPH	AO	PFT	DD
–	2	4	1	1
+	3	1	5	1
+ +	7			
+ + +	4			1

NPH, normal-pressure hydrocephalus; AO, aqueduct obstruction, PFT, posterior fossa tumor; DD, degenerative dementia; PVHI, periventricular high signal intensity; NMR, nuclear magnetic resonance

Correlation Between Clinical Symptoms and PVHI on NMR

All patients with suspected NPH were scored by Hasegawa's dementia test. Patients showing marked PVHI (type III) on NMR had an average score of 10.5 in Hasegawa's test; patients showing moderate PVHI (type II), an average score of 19.3; and patients with mild PVHI (type I), an average score of 26.1. Patients with no PVHI on NMR (type 0) had a score of 29.5, which is considered subnormal in Hasegawa's dementia test. Thus, there was a close correlation between dementia score and grade of PVHI on NMR images. In these patients with suspected NPH, the more severe the clinical symptoms of dementia were the more prominent was the PVHI on their NMR image (Fig. 5). There was no dementia in the patient with marked hydrocephalus due to aqueduct obstruction with no PVHI on NMR images.

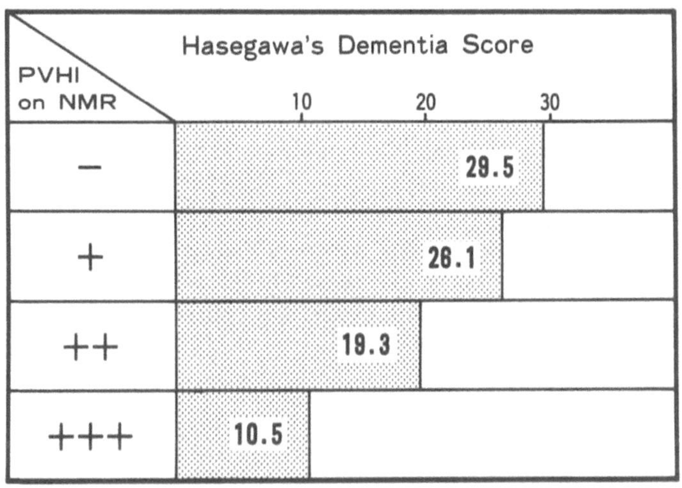

Fig. 5. Correlation between dementia in NPH and grade of periventricular high intensity

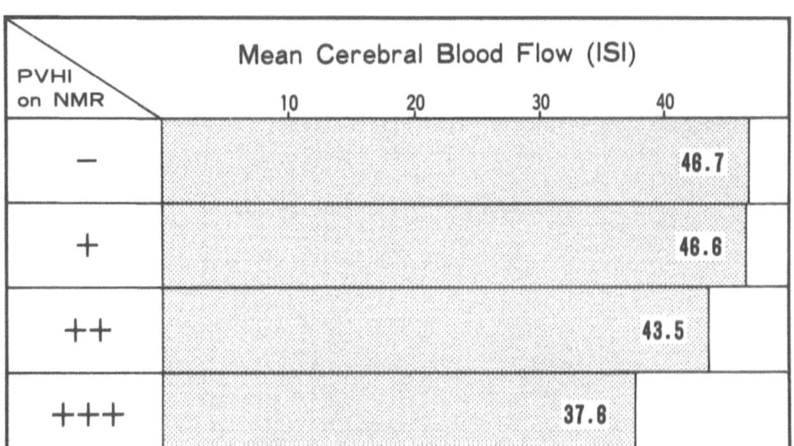

Fig. 6. Correlation between CBF and grade of periventricular high intensity

Influence of Cerebral Blood Flow on PVHI on NMR

The initial slope index (ISI) was used as a parameter of cerebral hemodynamics according to Risberg [12]. Patients with marked PVHI on NMR images (type III) had an average ISI of 37.6; those who had moderate PVHI (type II) had an average ISI of 43.5; and patients who had mild PVHI or none at all had an average of 46.6 or 46.7 respectively. It is, therefore, reasonable to argue that there is a tendency for CBF to decrease in accordance with the grade of PVHI (Fig. 6).

Correlation Between NMR and CT Findings

Periventricular lucency (PVL) on CT scans was also graded into type 0, in which there was no PVL, and types I, II, and III according as whether mild, moderate, or marked PVL was observed. Comparison of PVHI on NMR with grade of PVL on CT revealed that patients with mild PVL had either mild or moderate PVHI on NMR, while patients with moderate PVL had either moderate or marked PVHI on NMR (Table 4). Thus, NMR imaging is a more sensitive reflection of the periventricular pathology than CT scans. NMR imaging, therefore, appears to be very useful for investigating the pathophysiology and pathogenesis of periventricular pathology in hydrocephalus.

The relationship between degree of ventriculomegaly and grade of PVHI was examined. There was no correlation between the degree of ventriculomegaly and the grade of PVHI in NMR, except that patients with marked ventriculomegaly on CT scans had no PVHI in NMR.

Influence of Intracranial Pressure on PVHI

The relationship between the incidence of β-waves within a 24-h recording of the CSF pressure and the grade of PVHI was examined. Patients with marked PVHI on NMR images had β-waves in 33.9% of the recording time; patients with moderate

Table 4. Correlation between periventricular high intensity on NMR images and periventricular lucency on CT scans

PVL on CT \ PVHI on NMR	–	+ (Mild)	+ + (Moderate)	+ + + (Marked)
–	8	7		
+ (Mild)		4	5	
+ + (Moderate)			1	3
+ + + (Marked)				2

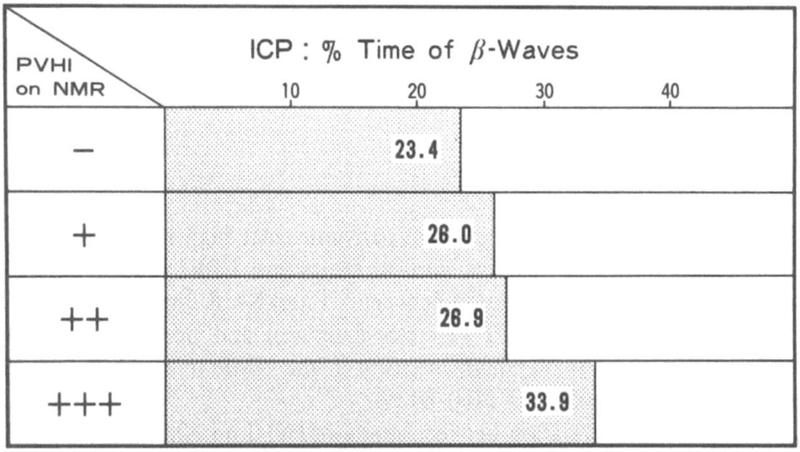

Fig. 7. Influence of ICP on periventricular high intensity on NMR images

PVHI had β-waves in 26.9%; and patients showing mild PVHI had β-waves in 26.0%. The patient with no PVHI had β-waves in only 23.4% of the recording time. Rising frequency of β-waves was accompanied by increasing severity of the grade of PVHI in NMR images (Fig. 7).

Discussion

Since the initial description of normal pressure hydrocephalus (NPH) by Hakim and Adams [4], questions regarding reliable diagnostic criteria and patient selection for the CSF shunting have been presented and discussed, so far without any solution. The mechanism of the syndrome of NPH has been gradually clarified by using various new techniques, such as CT scanning, CT cisternography, continuous ICP monitoring, measurement of CBF, emission tomography, and NMR imaging.

For several years, since the advent of X-ray CT, periventricular lucency seen on CT scans has continued to attract the attention of neurosurgeons, neurologists, psychiatrists, and neuroradiologists [1, 7–11, 13–15]. It is generally assumed that the periventricular lucency seen on CT scans represents the migration of the CSF from ventricles into the intercellular spaces in the periventricular white matter [2, 6, 16].

On the basis of studies by CT scanning, the periventricular lucency appears more frequently in high pressure hydrocephalus, especially that of the noncommunicating type [1, 7–10, 13–15]. It can also be seen in normal or low pressure hydrocephalus. In this study we attempted to investigate the periventricular pathology in hydrocephalus by NMR imaging. The NMR findings correlate well with the CT findings. But there were characteristic findings of the NMR study. NMR imaging visualizes periventricular pathology more extensively and precisely. Differentiation of periventricular CSF edema seen in hydrocephalus from subcortical degenerative encephalopathy seen in hypertensive arteriosclerosis or Binswanger's disease is imperative for differential diagnosis of dementia patients [3, 5, 15]. It is expected that the pathophysiology and mechanism of periventricular pathology in hydrocephalus will be clarified by further study with NMR imagers, positron emission tomography, and other new methods.

Conclusion

The correlations among the grade of periventricular high intensity (PVHI) seen on NMR images and CT findings, clinical symptoms, CBF, and ICP dynamics were analyzed. The overall correlation between CT and NMR findings was good. Areas of periventricular lucency on CT were especially well, and more extensively, visualized as areas of periventricular high intensity in the NMR images with the echo technique at a pulse sequence of 2100/80 ms.

There was no correlation between grade of PVHI on NMR images and extent of ventriculomegaly, except for the absence of PVHI in the patients with marked hydrocephalus due to aqueduct obstruction. Areas of PVHI improved and decreased in size after CSF shunting in patients who responded to shunt placement.

The more extensive the PVHI is, the more severe the clinical symptoms, the lower the CBF, and the higher the incidence of β-waves. It is suggested, therefore, that symptoms of NPH may be related to PVHI, occurrence of which is correlated with cerebral hemodynamics and ICP dynamics.

Summary

The correlation between nuclear magnetic resonance (NMR) and computed tomography (CT) findings was attempted with special reference to the periventricular pathology in hydrocephalus. We classified the periventricular high signal intensity (PVHI) on NMR images into four types according to the extension and grade of the PVHI. Factors influencing the development and extension of the PVHI in patients with hydrocephalus were assessed. The overall correlation between CT and NMR findings was good, except that there was more prominent visualization on NMR images. The clinical picture correlated well with the extent of PVHI in NMR images, which was also linked with cerebral hemodynamics and intracranial pressure dynamics.

References

1. Asada M, Tamaki N, Kanazawa Y, Matsumoto S, Matsuo M, Kimura S, Fujii S (1978) Computer analysis of periventricular lucency on the CT scan. Neuroradiology 16:207–211
2. Fisherman RA (1975) Brain edema. N Engl J Med 293:706–711
3. Goto K, Ishii N, Fukasaw H (1981) Diffuse white-matter disease in the geriatric population. A clinical, neuroradiologic, and CT study. Radiology 141:687–695
4. Hakim S, Adams RD (1965) The special clinical problem of symptomatic hydrocephalus with normal cerebrospinal fluid pressure. Observation on cerebrospinal fluid hydrodynamics. J Neurol Sci 2:307–327
5. Loizow LA, Kendall BE, Marshall J (1981) Subcortical arteriosclerotic encephalopathy: a clinical and radiological investigation. J Neurol Neurosurg Psychiatry 44:294–304

6. Manz HJ (1974) The pathology of cerebral edema. Hum Pathol 5:291–313
7. Mori K, Handa H, Murata T, Nakano Y (1980) Periventricular lucency in computed tomography of hydrocephalus and cerebral atrophy. J Comput Assist Tomogr 4:204–209
8. Mori K, Murata T, Nakano Y, Handa H (1977) Periventricular lucency in hydrocephalus on computerized tomography. Surg Neurol 8:337–340
9. Moseley IF, Radu EW (1979) Factors influencing the development of periventricular lucencies in patients with raised intracranial pressure. Neuroradiology 17:65–69
10. Murata T, Handa H, Mori K, Nakano Y (1981) The significance of periventricular lucency on computed tomography; experimental study with canine hydrocephalus. Neuroradiology 20:221–227
11. Naidich TP, Epstein F, Lin JP, Kiricheff II, Hochwald GM (1976) Evaluation of pediatric hydrocephalus by computed tomography. Radiology 119:337–345
12. Risberg J, Ali Z, Wilson EM, Wills EL, Halsey JH (1975) Regional cerebral blood flow by Xenon-144 inhalation. Preliminary evaluation of an initial slope index in patients with unstable flow compartments. Stroke 6:142–148
13. Pasquini U, Bronzini M, Gozzali P, Mancini F, Menichelli F, Salvolini U (1977) Periventricular hypodensity in hydrocephalus; a clinico-radiological and mathematical analysis using computed tomography. J Comput Assist Tomogr 1:443–448
14. Rosenberg GA, Baland L, Kyner WT (1983) Pathophysiology of periventricular tissue changes with raised CSF pressure in cats. J Neurosurg 59:606–611
15. Sprung CH, Grumme TH (1983) Differentiation of periventricular lucency and other type of hypodensity in various forms of hydrocephalus. Intracranial pressure 15:660–668
16. Weller RD, Mitchel J (1980) Cerebrospinal fluid edema and its sequelae in hydrocephalus. Adv Neurol 28:111–123

Effect of CSF Albumin Concentration on NMR Relaxation Parameters*

M. E. Castro[1], D. P. Boisvert, E. O. Treiber, J. A. Lunt, and P. S. Allen

Key words: Nuclear magnetic resonance, brain edema, proton-relaxation, cerebrospinal fluid, albumin

Introduction

Imaging with nuclear magnetic resonance (NMR) is a sensitive indicator of the location and extent of brain edema [1, 2]. Indeed, preliminary studies indicate that NMR imaging gives better definition of the extent and mass effects of edema than is achievable at present with X-ray computed tomography (CT) [1, 3]. CT gives information only on tissue density (i.e., the coefficient of linear X-ray absorption), whereas proton NMR provides information related to the density of mobile hydrogen and to its relaxation behavior; i.e., the longitudinal (T_1) and transverse (T_2) relaxation times. The corresponding relaxation rates are given as $1/T_1$ and $1/T_2$.

The increased water content of edematous brain prolongs both T_1 and T_2 relaxation of the protons [4–7], in a relationship that is usually linear [6, 7]. However, variable T_1 and T_2 values may be obtained for different types of brain edema with similar water content [5], and the induction of "vasogenic edema" [8] in rats is not accompanied by a linear decrease in the transverse relaxation rate over the entire range of increase in water content [6]. It was suggested on the grounds of the studies cited that changes in the serum protein content of the edema fluid might be responsible for this effect. It is well known that the introduction of macromolecules such as proteins produce marked changes in the relaxation behavior of water protons [9, 10].

We used cerebrospinal fluid (CSF) containing various concentrations of albumin and electrolytes as a simple model of edema fluid. Proton relaxation times were measured to determine the quantitative basis for the effect of these variations in edema fluid in vivo.

---

* The study described in this paper was supported by grants from the Alberta Heritage Foundation for Medical Research (major equipment) and the Alberta Heritage Savings Trust Fund for Applied Research – Cancer (H-184: H-340). MEC is an Alberta Heritage Foundation for Medical Research Fellow.

[1] Departments of Surgery, University of Alberta, Edmonton, Alberta, Canada

Materials and Methods

Samples (2–3 ml) of CSF from the fluid withdrawn during routine lumbar myelography in adults ($n=24$) were centrifuged immediately. The supernatant fluid was tested at once or was stored for up to 7 weeks at –20 °C. Frozen samples were thawed at room temperature before testing. Each sample was divided into aliquots for biochemical and NMR determinations.

Concentrations of CSF total protein and glucose were determined by spectrophotometry (ACA III; DuPont Instruments, Wilmington, Del), and albumin and IgG were measured with a laser nephelometer (Behring model; Hoechst Pharmaceuticals, Frankfurt, W. Germany). Sodium and potassium were measured with ion-specific electrodes, and chloride with a coulometric generator (Astra 8; Beckman Instruments, Brea, Calif); pH was determined with a Fisher Accumet meter, model 610 A.

The NMR determination of relaxation times of protons was carried with a wide-bore spectrometer (CXP model; Bruker Instruments, Karlsruhe, W. Germany) operating at 100 MHz. T_1 was determined by the inversion recovery sequence ($180° - \tau - 90°$); an interval at least 10 times as long as T_1 was allowed between readings, to ensure reestablishment of thermal equilibrium. T_2 was determined by the Carr-Purcell technique as modified by Meiboom and Gill [11], using only the even points of the decay curve ($n=8$ points). The temperature inside the radiofrequency coil enclosure, monitored with probes, was kept constant at (37 ± 0.2) °C by a flow of warm air. Samples were placed inside the coil enclosure and were tested when they reached 37 °C. The probes had no apparent effect on homogeneity of either the static or the radiofrequency magnetic field across the sample. Several of the individual CSF samples were tested at 25 °C and 29 °C and then at 37 °C to assess the effect of temperature changes on the relaxation times.

The remainder of each CSF sample was pooled. The pooled sample was divided into three lots: one was diluted twofold with distilled deionized water; one had NaCl added to give approximately twice the sodium concentration of normal CSF; and the third was not altered. All three lots were subjected to the same biochemical and NMR measurements. Human albumin (crystallized and lyophilized; Sigma Chemical Co., St. Louis, Mo) was added in steps to give concentrations ranging from 0.27 g/liter to 50.27 g/liter, and NMR determinations were made at each concentration.

The magnetization, M, was plotted semilogarithmically against *tau* for both T_1 and T_2 data, and the least-squares analysis was applied to plots from pooled samples containing high albumin concentrations. Values are reported as means $\pm$ SD.

Results

In the individual samples of CSF, concentrations of electrolytes were within the normal range for adults and concentrations of albumin and total protein were normal or only slightly elevated (Table 1). The mean pH was 9.00 ± 0.25. No relationship was found between the range of these values and the relaxation times.

In the pooled CSF batches (Table 1), increasing the albumin concentration reduced both T_1 and T_2 of the protons (Table 2). Plotting the relaxation rates ($1/T_1$

Table 1. Biochemical composition and proton relaxation times of human cerebrospinal fluid (CSF)

	Individual CSF samples		Pooled CSF		
	n	Mean ± SD	Na 50%	Na normal	Na 200%
Albumin (g/liter)	24	0.27 ± 0.12	0.13 [a]	0.27	0.27
Total protein (g/liter)	24	0.49 ± 0.18	0.22 [a]	0.43	0.44
Sodium (mmol/liter)	23	145.0 ± 2.5	80.0	146.0	286.0
Potassium (mmol/liter)	23	2.87 ± 0.17	1.6	2.8	3.0
Chloride (mmol/liter)	23	128.0 ± 3.2	62.0	125.0	268.0
T_1 (s)	24	3.8 ± 0.1	3.9	3.9	3.9
T_2 (s)	23	2.6 ± 0.2	2.6	2.5	2.6

[a] Not measured; calculated (for 50% dilution) from normal value

Table 2. Relationship between albumin concentrations and proton relaxation times in pooled CSF with various sodium levels

Albumin [a] (g/liter)	Na 200%		Na normal		Na 50%	
	T_1 [b]	T_2	T_1	T_2	T_1	T_2
Control	3.9	2.6	3.9	2.5	3.9	2.6
10	3.7	1.7	3.7	1.8	3.7	1.7
20	3.5	1.4	3.4	1.4	3.6	1.4
30	3.3	1.1	3.3	1.1	3.3	1.1
40	3.1	0.9	3.2	0.9	3.2	0.9
50	3.0	0.8	3.0	0.8	3.1	0.7

[a] Values for other than control samples are rounded to the nearest whole numbers; they represent the amount of albumin added to the CSF aliquots
[b] Values are given in seconds

Table 3. Relationship between albumin concentration and rates of proton relaxation in pooled CSF with various sodium levels

Pooled CSF	$1/T_1$			$1/T_2$		
	Slope [a]	Intercept [b]	*r*	Slope	Intercept	*r*
Na Normal	0.0015	0.256	0.9940	0.018	0.391	0.9933
Na 50%	0.0013	0.258	0.9938	0.020	0.358	0.9935
Na 200%	0.0015	0.258	0.9805	0.018	0.392	0.9939

[a] Values are given in $s^{-1}\ g^{-1}\ l^{-1}$
[b] Values are given in s

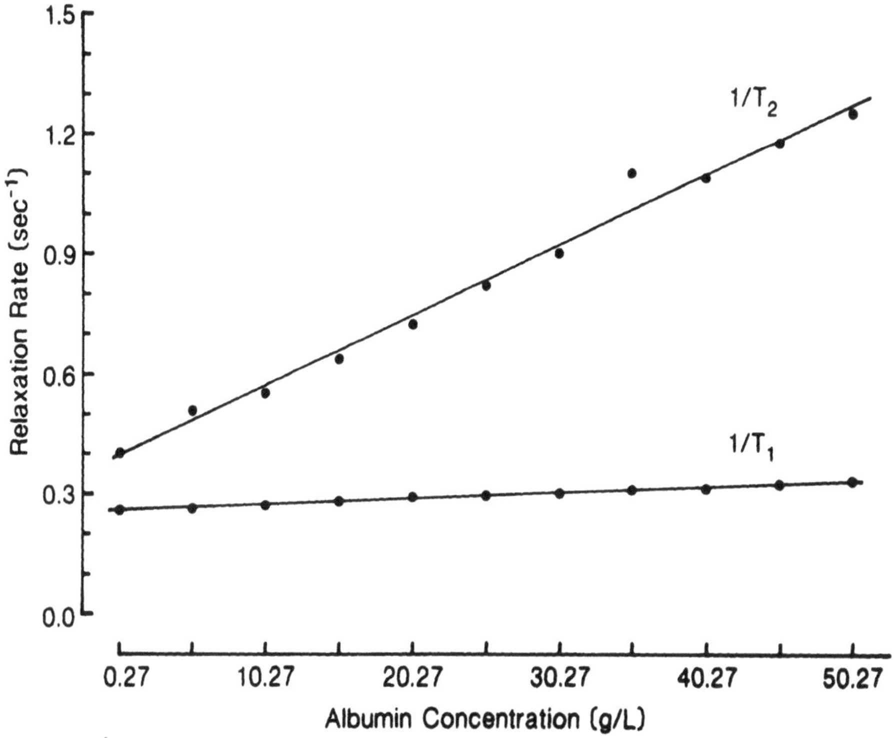

Fig. 1. Effect of increasing albumin concentration on the proton relaxation rates of untreated (pooled) CSF

and $1/T_2$) against albumin concentration ([Alb]) showed a linear relationship, with a gradient of increase approximately 10 times greater for T_2 than for T_1. This linear relationship, which is shown for untreated CSF (Fig. 1), was almost identical for the samples with varied electrolyte concentrations (Table 3).

Semilogarithmic plots showed a linear relationship between the magnetization and *tau* for T_1. However, least-squares analysis of the T_2 data of pooled samples with higher albumin content, showed evidence of a weak second component of $< 1\%$ weighting and with a much longer characteristic time constant. This weak component had negligible effect on the values shown in Table 2.

Discussion

The use of CSF with altered concentrations of albumin and electrolytes as a model for cerebral edema fluid is based on several observations. The ventricles communicate with the extracellular space of the brain via the ependyma that line them and allow the passage of fluid from the brain tissue to the CSF [12]. As this cerebral extracellular fluid accounts for a considerable proportion of total CSF production [13], its chemical composition is similar to that of CSF. Thus, the addition of albumin to CSF simulates the protein-rich extracellular fluid that constitutes the edema fluid in vasogenic edema.

Several indices provided by proton NMR give information on the freedom of movement of hydrogen nuclei (protons). T_1 and T_2 relaxation times are among the more commonly used measures, especially in the investigation of biological systems. In this study, the use of the NMR technique clearly showed that increased albumin content in the CSF is associated with markedly decreased relaxation times (i.e., increased $1/T_1$ and $1/T_2$). Extensive studies of this effect with protein solutions [9] have led to the hypothesis that it results from interactions between water molecules and compounds such as proteins. By adsorbing to the surface of large macromolecules, water molecules restrict their ability to move freely relative to their surroundings [10]; conversely, water molecules not thus associated have unrestricted mobility. The type of macromolecule, its concentration, and its structure determine how much water it binds and to what extent [10]. As the bound and free fractions of water possess individual relaxation times, and because water molecules are free to exchange between fractions, it is thought that NMR provides information on the average relaxation efficiency of the water protons [9].

Changes in temperature affect the mobility of water molecules and thus affect the proton relaxation times in biological specimens [14]. Our measurements in the individual CSF samples showed increases in both T_1 (124%) and T_2 (116%) when the temperature was raised from 25 °C to 37 °C, reflecting increased mobility of protons. This effect must be taken into account when comparing studies done in vitro at room temperature and those performed in vivo.

Changes in the ionic composition also alter the relaxation process [15]; for example, electrolytes could increase the relaxation times by displacing protons from proteins. However, although brain edema is characterized by changes in electrolyte concentrations, mainly increased sodium and decreased potassium [16], we found no correlation with the relaxation times in the range of electrolyte concentrations studied (Table 1). Changes in pH occur in certain types of brain edema, and it has been reported that pH is decreased (< 1 unit) in brain tumors [17], reflecting increased lactate production by neoplastic cells. Although changes in pH may affect the relaxation of protons [18], we found no evidence of this in our CSF samples with pH ranging between 8.40 and 9.45; however, the reported change was in the alkaline range and cannot be directly extrapolated to variations toward acidic.

The chief determinants of the change in relaxation efficiency appear to be the interactions between water and macromolecules [9, 10]. NMR studies of brain edema in vitro have shown good correlation of increasing water content of the tissues with increasing proton relaxation times, both T_1 and T_2 [4–7]; this accords with experimental data from several types of tissue [19–21]. However, T_1 and T_2 values were found to differ between various types of brain edema in which the water content was similar [5], and in vasogenic edema the correlation of increased water content with decreased T_2 relaxation rate was not linear after 4 h [6]. In both these studies the authors attributed these effects to changes in concentrations of serum proteins in the edema fluid. The albumin concentrations we tested reflect the potential range of changes in the fluid of vasogenic edema; they strongly affected the relaxation behavior, particularly T_2 (Fig. 1), by modifying the water–macromolecule interactions.

Although NMR is a sensitive technique for the detection of brain edema in vivo, its specificity remains unproven. Reports on NMR imaging of edematous brain in vivo have commented on the difficulty of distinguishing lesions, especially brain tumors, from surrounding edema [1–3]. Such lesions usually have increased water content and relaxation times compared with normal brain [3]. In most cases, however, the imaging parameters designed to highlight T_2 differentiate tumor from edema [22] by showing differences in the degree of change in T_2. These findings and those of the present study indicate that, when alterations in biochemical composition predominate over changes in water content within brain lesions, T_2-dependent images will provide better delineations; on the other hand, the effect of regional variations in brain water content per se on T_2 may not be observed, due to differences in biochemical composition. On the other hand, images which highlight T_1, which is affected to a lesser degree by changes in biochemical composition, should provide a better assessment of serial changes in the water content of brain tissue.

Summary

Individual and pooled samples of cerebrospinal fluid containing various concentrations of albumin and electrolytes were used as a model for cerebral edema fluid in studies to determine the effects of these variations on proton relaxation times measured with nuclear magnetic resonance (NMR). The pH and concentrations of total protein, albumin, IgG, glucose, Na^+, K^+, and Cl^- were established, and longitudinal (T_1) and transverse (T_2) relaxation times were measured at 100 MHz and 37 °C. In untreated samples, the mean T_1 was (3.8 ± 0.1) s and the mean T_2 was (2.6 ± 0.2) s. Increasing the albumin concentration produced a linear increase in both rates of relaxation, which was 10 times greater in the transverse than in the longitudinal rate, whereas changes in electrolyte concentration had no noticeable effect. We conclude that the albumin content influences the rate of relaxation of protons in edema fluid, and thus is a major determinant of contrast in NMR images of edematous brain tissue.

Acknowledgement. The assistance of Mrs. U. Matthews and Mrs. A. El Zanaty in preparing this manuscript is gratefully acknowledged.

References

1. Bydder GM, Steiner RE, Young IR, Hall AS, Thomas DJ, Marshall J, Pallis CA, Legg NJ (1982) Clinical NMR imaging of the brain: 140 cases. Am J Roentgenol 139:215–236
2. Brant-Zawadzki M, Davis PL, Crooks LE, Mills CM, Norman D, Newton TH, Sheldon P, Kaufman L (1983) NMR demonstration of cerebral abnormalities: comparison with CT. Am J Roentgenol 140:847–854
3. Randell CP, Collins AG, Young IR, Haywood R, Thomas DJ, McDonell MJ, Orr JS, Bydder GM, Steiner RE (1983) Nuclear magnetic resonance imaging of posterior fossa tumors. Am J Roentgenol 141:489–496
4. Bakay L, Kurland RJ, Parrish RG, Lee JC, Peng RJ, Bartkowski HM (1975) Nuclear magnetic resonance studies in normal and edematous brain tissue. Exp Brain Res 23:241–248
5. Bartkowski HM, Bederson J, Nishimura M, Moon K, Pitts LH (1983) Nuclear magnetic resonance imaging and spectroscopy in experimental cerebral edema: proceedings of a symposium. Society of Magnetic Resonance in Medicine, second annual meeting, San Francisco

6. Naruse S, Horikawa Y, Tanaka C, Hirakawa K, Nishikawa H, Yoshizaki K (1982) Proton nuclear magnetic resonance studies on brain edema. J Neurosurg 56:747–752
7. Go KG, Edzes HT (1975) Water in brain edema. Observations by the pulsed nuclear magnetic resonance technique. Arch Neurol 32:462–465
8. Klatzo I (1967) Neuropathological aspects of brain edema. J Neuropathol Exp Neurol 26:1–14
9. Hazlewood CF (1979) A review of the significance and understanding of the physical properties of cell-associated water. In: Drost-Hansen W, Clegg J (eds) Cell-associated water. Academic, New York, pp 165–259
10. De Vré RM (1979) The NMR studies of water in biological systems. Prog Biophys Mol Biol 35:103–134
11. Meiboom S, Gill D (1958) Modified spin-echo method for measuring nuclear relaxation times. Rev Sci Inst 29:688–691
12. Milhorat TH (1975) The third circulation revisited. J Neurosurg 42:628–645
13. Pollay M, Curl F (1967) Secretion of cerebrospinal fluid by the ventricular ependyma of the rabbit. Am J Physiol 213:1031–1038
14. Fung BM, McGaughy TW (1974) The state of water in muscle as studied by pulsed NMR. Biochim Biophys Acta 343:663–673
15. Hazlewood CF, Nichols BL, Chang DC, Brown B (1971) On the state of water in developing muscle: a study of the major phase of ordered water in skeletal muscle and its relationship to sodium concentration. Johns Hopkins Med J 129:117–131
16. Pappius HM, McCann WP (1969) Effects of steroids on cerebral edema in cats. Arch Neurol 20:207–216
17. Jähde E, Rajewsky MF, Baumgärtl H (1982) pH distribution in transplanted neural tumors and normal tissues of BDIX rats as measured with pH microelectrodes. Cancer Res 43:1498–1504
18. Fung BM, Puon PS (1981) Nuclear magnetic resonance transverse relaxation in muscle water. Biophys J 33:27–37
19. Saryan LA, Hollis DP, Economov JS, Eggleston JC (1974) Nuclear magnetic resonance studies of cancer IV. Correlation of water with tissue relaxation times. J Natl Cancer Inst 52:599–602
20. Fung BM (1977) Correlation of relaxation time with water content in muscle and brain tissues. Biochim Biophys Acta 497:317–322
21. Kirikuta IC, Simplăcneau V (1975) Tissue water content and nuclear magnetic resonance in normal and tumor tissues. Cancer Res 35:1164–1167
22. Weinstein MA, Modic MT, Pavlicek W, Keyser CK (1984) Nuclear magnetic resonance for the examination of brain tumors. Sem Roentgenol 19:139–147

In Vitro Proton NMR Spectroscopy and In Vivo Imaging in Traumatic Brain Edema

T. Hashimoto [1], H. Pitts, M. E. Moseley, and H. M. Bartkowski

Key words: Brain edema, head injury, nuclear magnetic resonance (NMR), proton relaxation time (T_1, T_2)

Introduction

Edematous tissues associated with various kinds of brain pathology prolong proton longitudinal and transverse relaxation times (T_1, T_2). Proton magnetic resonance imaging (MRI) readily depicts brain edema experimentally and clinically [1–3]: mechanically induced traumatic brain edema, however, has not been characterized by means of nuclear magnetic resonance (NMR) techniques, and this is the subject of this study.

Methods

Male Sprague-Dawley rats (350–400 g) were anesthetized by IP injection of chloral hydrate solution and allowed to breathe spontaneously. A circular craniectomy approximately 4 mm in diameter was made over the right temporal bone. A polyethylene impact tube (PE-350, Clay Adams) was placed against the dura, cemented to the skull, and connected to a fluid percussion device [6]. A transient fluid impact pressure of 4 atm was delivered by releasing a pendulum from a predetermined angle. The animals were divided into six groups: Group 1, normal anesthetized controls; group 2, sham-operated controls; and groups 3, 4, 5, 6, in which the animals were sacrificed 2, 6, 12, 24 h after impact, respectively. The brains were removed rapidly and sliced coronally through the impact lesion. Tissue from the injured cortex beneath the impact tube, the contralateral cortex, and both basal ganglia was subjected to NMR spectroscopy for measurement of T_1 and T_2, and to a gradient column method for determination of brain specific gravity. In vitro T_1 and T_2 were measured at a resonant frequency of 100 MHz using inversion recovery and Carr-Purcell-Meiboom-Gill pulse sequences at 23 °C. Brain water content was determined in terms of brain specific gravity by means of a microgravimetric gradient column composed of bromobenzene and kerosine [4]. In vivo MRI was performed 2 and 6 h after impact with a 0.35 Tesla magnet and a resonance frequency of 15 MHz

[1] Department of Neurosurgery, University of California, San Francisco, California, USA

for protons. A spin echo pulse sequence with a repetition interval (TR) of 2 s and an echo delay time (TE) of 28 ms and a two-dimensional Fourier transform reconstruction technique were used.

Results

Cortex T_1 in normal and sham controls was about 1 s. The length of T_1 in injured cortex increased progressively with time after impact up to 12 h after impact ($P < 0.001$) and then began to decrease. In the contralateral cortex T_1 did not change (Fig. 1). Cortex T_2 in normal and sham controls was about 66 ms; in injured cortex T_2 increased with time after impact up to 12 h ($P < 0.002$) and then began to diminish (Fig. 2). Water content in injured cortex increased up to 12 h ($P < 0.001$) (Fig. 3). Basal ganglia T_1 in controls was about 0.9 s, i.e., shorter than the T_1 of cortex. Basal ganglia ipsilateral to the impact first showed T_1 prolongation 24 h after impact ($P < 0.05$) (Fig. 4). The basal ganglia T_2 in controls was about 66 ms, the same as that of cortex. There were no changes in basal ganglia T_2 throughout the experiment (Fig. 5). Brain water increased in the basal ganglia ipsilateral to the im-

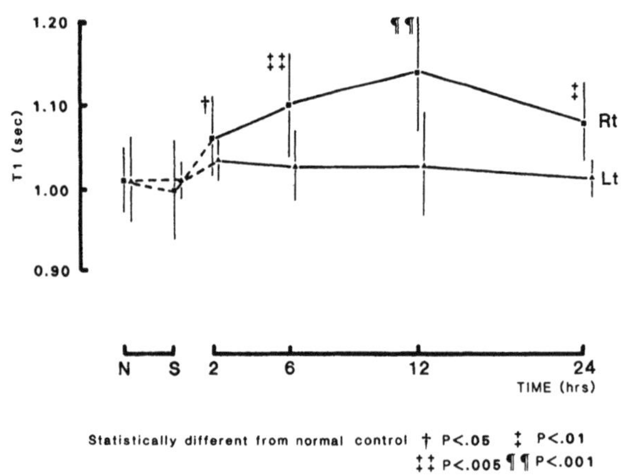

Fig. 1. Longitudinal relaxation times (T_1) in the cortex after impact injury. Values given are means ± SD

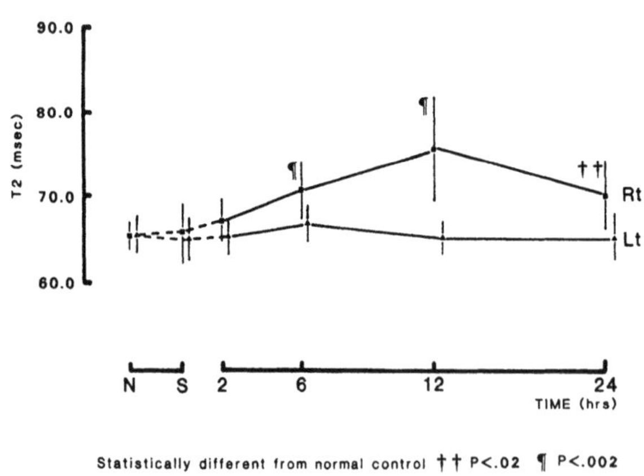

Fig. 2. Transverse relaxation times (T_2) in the cortex after impact injury. Values given are means ± SD

Fig. 3. Water content of cortex after impact injury (means ± SD)

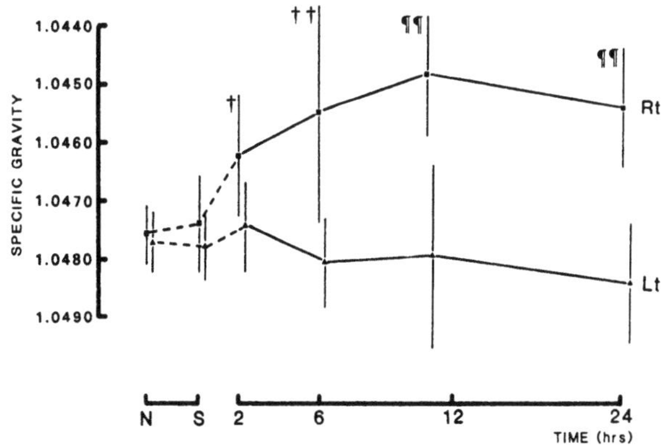

Statistically different from normal control † P<.05 †† P<.02 ¶¶ P<.001

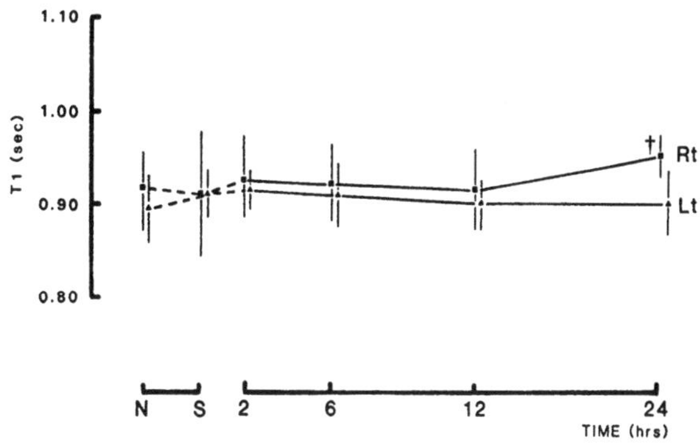

Fig. 4. Longitudinal relaxation times (T_1) in basal ganglia after impact injury (means ± SD)

Statistically different from normal control † P<.05

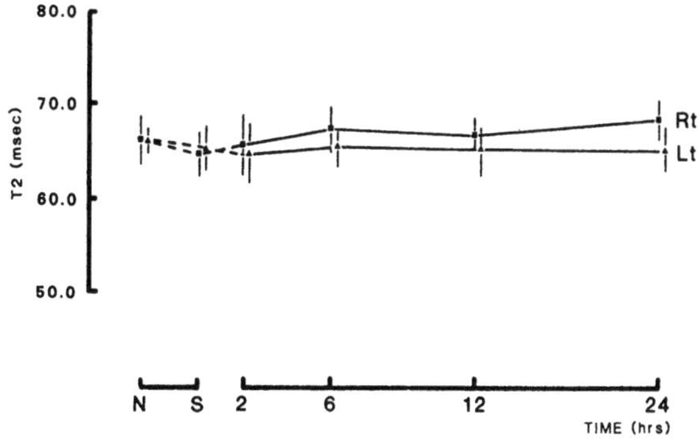

Fig. 5. Transverse relaxation times (T_2) in basal ganglia after impact injury (means ± SD)

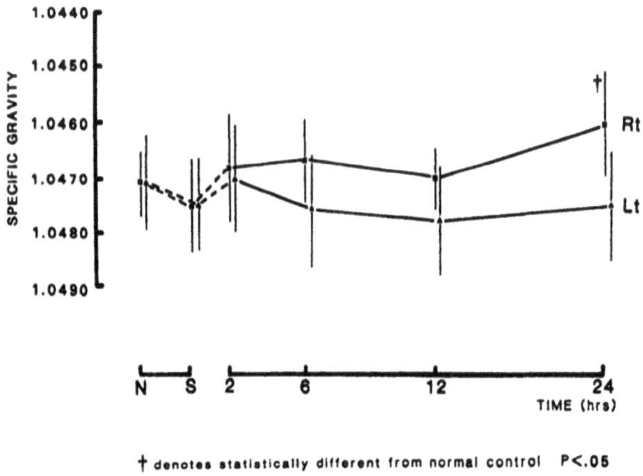

Fig. 6. Water content of basal ganglia after impact injury (means ± SD)

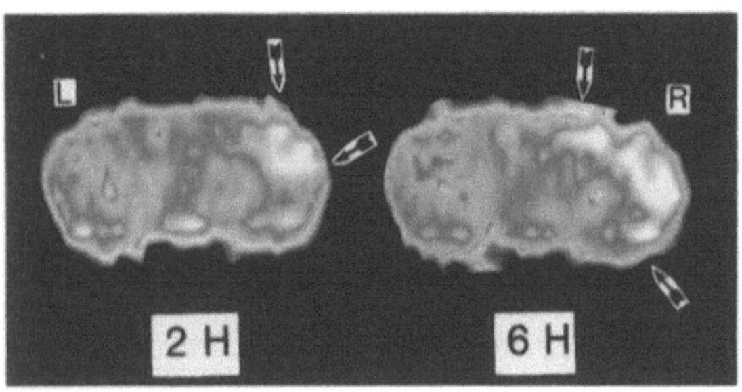

Fig. 7. MRI image of basal ganglia 6 h after impact injury; no abnormalities are seen

pact, but not until 24 h after impact ($P < 0.05$) (Fig. 6). When MRI was performed 2 h after impact this demonstrated relatively localized brain edema as a region of high signal intensity at the impact site. This region of high signal intensity was spreading away from the injured cortex 6 h after impact. No basal ganglia abnormalities had developed by 6 h after the impact (Fig. 7).

Comments

T_1 and T_2 in the injured cortex became progressively longer up to 12 h after impact and then began to decrease, correlating well with the brain water increases. These results are similar to earlier observations after cold injury [5], except that maximal edema was seen 24 h after cold injury, i.e., later than in our experiment. The basal ganglia in the injured hemisphere did not show prolongation of T_1 until 24 h after injury (with no significant change in T_2), by which time the brain water content had also increased, possibly due to the spread of edema from the injured cortex and accounting for the decreases in T_1, T_2, and brain water content of the injured cortex after 12 h. MRI readily showed the extent and progression of traumatic brain edema over the injured cortex. The high signal intensity region correlated with the increases in T_1, T_2, and brain water content. MRI clearly documented the spread of traumatic brain edema in single animals in vivo. Improved MRI resolution will also allow better qualification of some of these changes by accurate T_1 and T_2 determination.

Summary

In vitro proton relaxation times, in vivo magnetic resonance imaging, and brain microgravimetry were examined to document the evolution of traumatic brain edema in rats. In injured cortex proton relaxation times became progressively longer and the brain water content increased progressively up to 12 h after fluid percussion impact and then began to decrease. Basal ganglia ipsilateral to the impact also showed increases in T_1 and water content but not until 24 h after impact. Magnetic resonance imaging readily showed the evolution of traumatic brain edema.

References

1. Asato R, Handa H, Hashi T et al. (1983) Chronological sequences and blood-brain barrier permeability change in local injury as assessed by nuclear magnetic resonance (NMR) images from sliced rat brain. Stroke 14:191–197
2. Buonanno FS, Pykett IL, Brady TJ et al. (1982) Proton NMR imaging in experimental ischemic infarction. Stroke 14:178–184
3. Bydder GM, Steiner RE, Young IR et al. (1982) Clinical NMR imaging of the brain: 140 cases. AJNR 3:459–480
4. Nelson SR, Mantz ML, Maxwell JA (1971) Use of specific gravity in the measurement of cerebral edema. J Appl Physiol 30:268–271
5. Naruse S, Horikawa Y, Tanaka C, et al. (1982) Proton nuclear magnetic resonance studies on brain edema. J Neurosurg 56:747–752
6. Sullivan HG, Martinez J, Becker DP, et al. (1976) Fluid percussion model of mechanical brain injury in the cat. J Neurosurg 45:520–534

Assessment of Brain Edema Associated with Cerebral Hemorrhage by Nuclear Magnetic Resonance

M. Furuse [1], S. Inao, K. Saso, Y. Motegi, and N. Kamata

Key words: Cerebral hemorrhage, perifocal edema, nuclear magnetic resonance, relaxation time, surgical indication

Introduction

Brain edema of varying degrees arises in association with cerebrovascular accidents, and it undoubtedly affects the prognosis. Proton NMR studies on cerebrovascular diseases are an attractive field of clinical application and are seen as an approach to the dynamics of cerebral edema [2; Furuse et al., this volume].

This paper describes the findings recorded by means of NMR imaging and in vivo measurement of spin lattice relaxation time (T_1) in cases of cerebral hemorrhage, with special reference to the time courses of focal T_1 values measured in patients without and with intracranial surgery.

Materials and Methods

Twenty-five patients with intracranial hematoma and ranging in age from 25 to 74 years (mean 55.6) were examined with the aid of a whole-body NMR scanner based on the FONAR QED-80-Alpha system. The equipment possesses dual function modes of imaging display and focal T_1 measurement with a static magnetic field strength of 433 gauss. The details of the method used are described by Furuse et al. elsewhere in this volume. In the actual procedure of NMR examination transverse SSFP (steady state of free precession) images were displayed as the first step, and then absolute values of T_1 in the regions of interest were measured. The T_1 values used in this study were obtained from the direct spin-lattice relaxation curve based upon a Tau sequence of multiple measuring points. Standard T_1 values for healthy brain in this series were 288 ± 42 and 227 ± 27 ms (mean $\pm$ SD) in cerebral gray and white matter, respectively.

[1] Department of Neurosurgery, Nakatsugawa Municipal General Hospital, 1-33 Ebisu-Machi, Nakatsugawa, 508 Japan

Results

Changes in NMR Images and T_1 Values Associated with Intracerebral Hematoma

In all instances of cerebral hemorrhage the site of hematoma was revealed as a high-density area in the SSFP image. Usually the extent of hematoma observed in NMR images corresponded closely to the spread of high-density regions seen on X-ray CT. On occasion however, the NMR image showed a much larger lesion than was apparent from the X-ray CT findings. This large zone of high NMR signal intensity was thought to reflect the spread of edema around the intracerebral hematoma. In T_1 measurements prolonged relaxation times were commonly observed in such perifocal high intensity zones.

Figure 1 shows images recorded with X-ray CT and NMR-CT in a patient suffering from hypertensive cerebral hemorrhage for comparison.

In the examination data recorded on the first day NMR-CT already showed apparently larger high-density areas than those revealed by X-ray CT. Measurement of T_1 revealed rather longer periods here than in the hematoma itself. No surgical intervention was performed in these circumstances. After 14 days of conservative treatment high-intensity zones in the NMR image were seen to be rather enlarged and much brightened, despite evidence that the high-density area was consistently reduced on X-ray CT. The T_1 values measured in perifocal brain tissue remained high, and some were substantially prolonged.

Figure 2 is another example of NMR images and T_1 values observed in a patient subjected to surgery. In this case both X-ray CT and NMR were examined within 6 h of the onset of drowsiness and left hemiparesis. The SSFP image revealed a double-layered shadow of high signal intensity in the right ganglionic region, corresponding to the site of intracerebral hematoma. According to the corresponding X-ray CT findings, the inner area of relatively high tone must be the clot itself. The annular outer layer with strong signal intensity seemingly reveals a liquefied component of the hematoma and also perifocal edema. The existence of a liquefied part around the intracerebral clot was actually confirmed by craniotomy performed on the same day. Such findings of extensive high-density areas around intracerebral masses have been observed in acute phases and also in serious conditions after stroke.

On the 10th postoperative day the high-intensity area still corresponded to the site of the hematoma evacuated. The T_1 value corresponding to the perifocal brain tissue was found to be substantially decreased. These findings observed in the surgical series illustrate a considerable capacity of NMR studies for estimating the effects of medical treatment and deciding whether surgical treatment is indicated.

Time Courses of T_1 in Intracerebral Hematoma and Surrounding Brain

The T_1 value of the intracerebral hematoma itself remained within a rather limited range during its initial phase, followed by prolongation with increasing lapse of time. This seemed to reflect alterations in the properties of hematoma, such as clot formation in the earlier phase and resolution in the later phase. Table 1 summarizes the time course of T_1 values obtained from the hematoma site and from the sur-

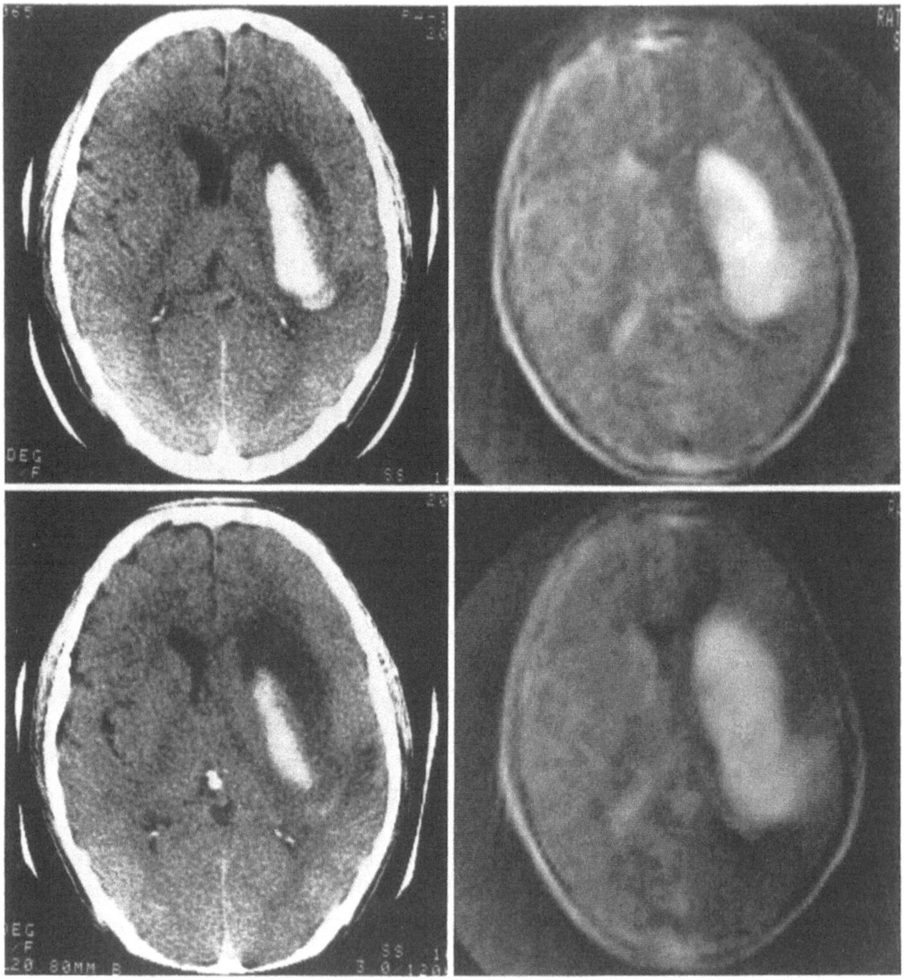

a b c d

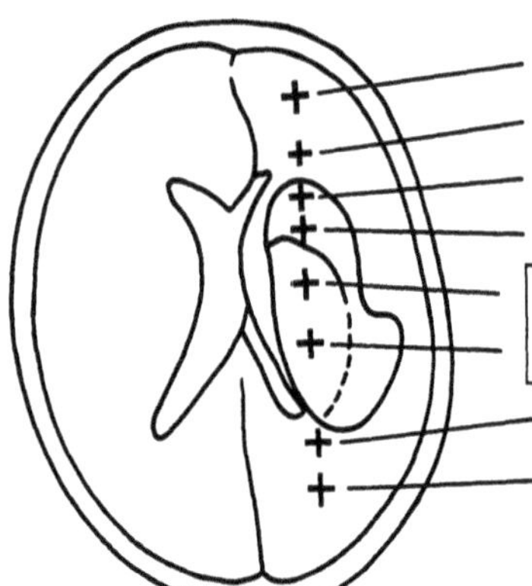

e

	1st day		14th day
D_1	267	→	208
N_1	365	→	380
P_1	377	→	414
P_2	432	→	396
H_1	306	→	281
H_2	295	→	278
N_2	295	→	252
D_2	265	→	259

Fig. 1a–e. Changes in X-ray CT (**a**, **c**) and NMR-CT (**b**, **d**) on days 1 (**a**, **b**) and 14 (**c**, **d**) after surgery and T_1 distribution (**e**) on days 1 and 14. *D*, distant; *N*, neighboring; *P*, perifocal; *H*, site of hematoma

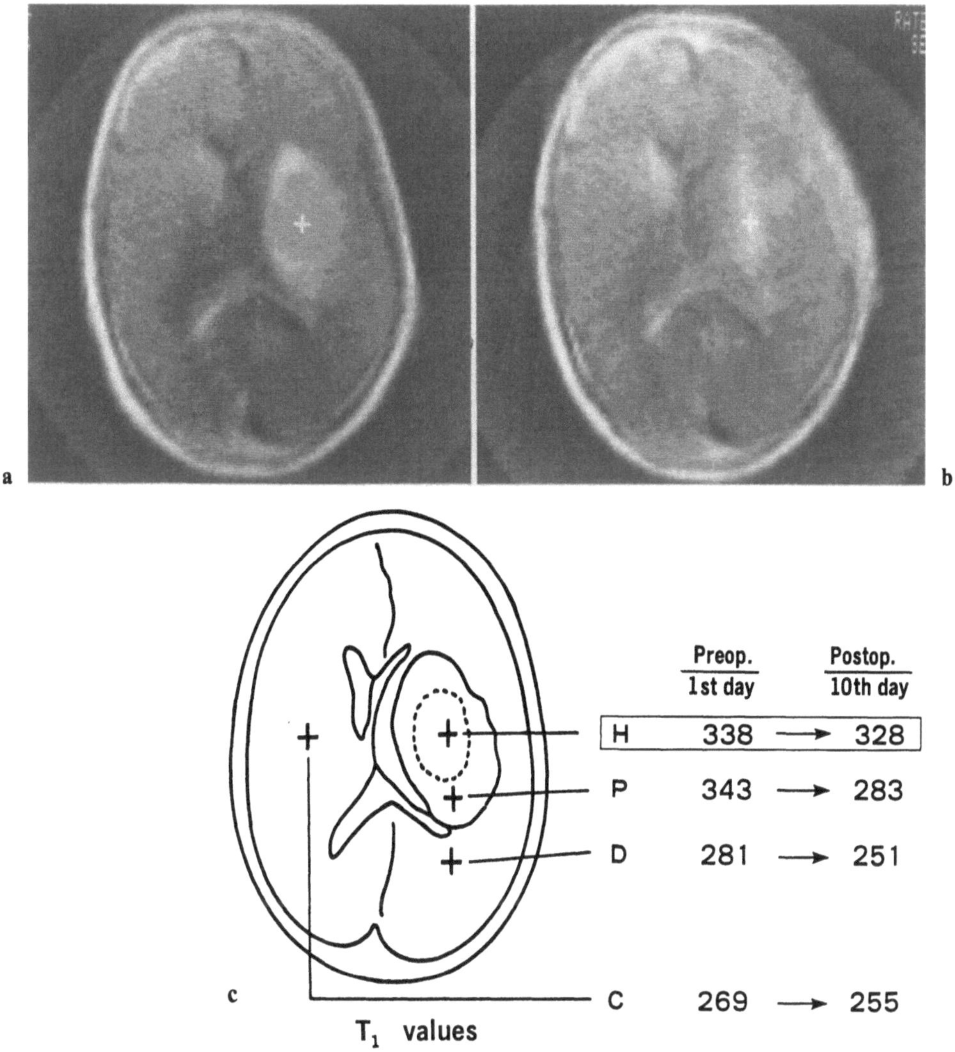

Fig. 2.a Pre- and **b** postoperative SSFP images and **c** T_1 changes in a case with intracerebral hematoma

Table 1. Time course of T_1 values in intracerebral hematoma (ms; mean ± SD)

	1–3 days	4–15 days	16–30 days	30 + days
Hematoma	286 ± 32 (*n* = 8)	263 ± 24 (*n* = 9)	305 ± 32 (*n* = 12)	313 ± 40 (*n* = 5)
Perifocal brain [surgery (–)]	285 ± 29 (*n* = 8)	313 ± 21 (*n* = 8)	315 ± 23 (*n* = 11)	304 ± 36 (*n* = 5)
Perifocal brain [surgery (+)]	–	285 ± 18 (*n* = 7)	298 ± 23 (*n* = 4)	285 ± 18 (*n* = 6)

rounding brain tissue in patient series with and without surgical intervention. The T_1 values in hematomas were 286 ms on average in the acute stage. This became longer with the passage of time, averaging 313 ms by 1 month after stroke.

In contrast, prolongation of T_1 in the brain tissue surrounding the hematoma was observed in the earlier phase, with a maximum duration of 315 ms around 2–4 weeks after the onset, after which the T_1 value tended to normalize. This time course probably reflects the natural processes of formation and regression of perifocal brain edema.

In the patient series in which surgical procedures were carried out the T_1 values measured in the surrounding tissue were found to be consistently lowered in both the subacute and the chronic stages.

Discussion

It was of great interest that different values for T_1 were demonstrated in accordance with changes in intracranial pathology not only in hematoma but also in the surrounding brain tissue. The intracerebral hematoma revealed rather shorter T_1 values than initially expected, being 286 ms on average within 3 days after stroke. This T1 value in the hematoma was substantially shorter than that for whole blood, which was 439 ± 29 (SD) ms. When blood is extravasated from the vessels T_1 values are necessarily shortened by the coagulation process. In other cases with massive cerebral hemorrhage T_1 values for hematoma tended to be prolonged during the chronic stage. Such T_1 prolongation in hematoma is probably due to the natural changes in the clot, such as resolution or liquefaction.

Brain edema is a pathologic process characterized by an abnormal accumulation of water. The increase in total tissue water is closely related to the increase in free water.

As seen in studies of the time course of vasogenic brain edema [1] and cerebral ischema (Inao et al., this volume), the free water fraction constitutes by far the larger part of brain water increase. Prolongation of proton T_1 is also closely related to the increases in free water fraction and in total water content [3]. Changes in T_1 values in normal biological tissues must be available as these constitute a valuable indicator allowing estimation of the degree of brain edema.

Measurements of T_1 in the region adjacent to hematomas may be considered useful in evaluation of the status of the brain. Prolongation of T_1 values in the tissues adjacent to an intracerebral hematoma can reasonably be supposed to reveal progression of brain edema, particularly in the acute or subacute stages after a stroke. As noted in the illustrated cases with cerebral hemorrhage, the prolonged T_1 periods in the perifocal area can be accepted as an indicator that is useful not only in estimation of the prognosis of the illness but also in decisions regarding treatment.

It has also been strongly emphasized that substantial differences in T_1 time course were noted between patient groups with and without surgery. An adequate procedure for the removal of hematomas can be expected to improve the edematous state caused by compression resulting from the intracerebral hematoma. In vivo T_1 measurement offers a convincing and clinically effective means not only of establishing operative indications but also of estimating degrees of tissue damage.

Conclusions

In vivo T_1 measurement and proton NMR imaging have a high clinical potential for assessment of the status of cerebral edema. The values of T_1 measured in the perifocal region of intracerebral hematoma may be useful not only in evaluation of the edematous state but also in decisions as to what kind of surgical intervention is indicated, if any.

Summary

The present study describes time courses for tissue T_1 values and the NMR images associated with intracerebral hematoma. The extent of an intracerebral hematoma was revealed as a high-intensity area. In some cases NMR-CT showed much larger high-signal areas than were found on X-ray CT. Prolonged T_1 times were recorded in such high-intensity zones. These large high-density areas were regarded as reflecting the spread of perifocal brain edema. The T_1 values in the brain tissue surrounding the hematoma was prolonged in the earlier stage up to 1 month, with a tendency to gradual normalization after this. This alteration in T_1 probably reflects the processes of edema formation and regression in the perifocal region. Otherwise, in surgical series there was rapid normalization of perifocal T_1 following hematoma evacuation. The T_1 values measured in the perifocal region might be useful for evaluation of edematous states.

References

1. Furuse M, Gonda T, Kuchiwaki H, Hirai N, Inao S, Kageyama N (1984) Thermal analysis on the state of free and bound water in normal and edematous brains. In: Go KG, Baethmann A (eds) Recent progress in the study and therapy of brain edema. Plenum, New York, pp 293–298
2. Furuse M, Saso K, Motegi Y, Izawa A (1984) Studies on cerebrovascular diseases by means of nuclear magnetic resonance. Magnetic Resonance in Medicine 1 (2):153–154
3. Mizuno M, Izawa A, Inao S, Furuse M (1984) Observations on correlation between water structure (free and bound water) and T1 value – Comparative study in gelatin solutions by means of thermal analysis and proton NMR. J NMR Med 4 [Suppl]:116–117

Chronological Changes in Brain Edema in Hypertensive Intracerebral Hemorrhage Observed by CT and Xenon-Enhanced CT

R. SUZUKI[1], K. OHNO, H. HIRATSUKA, and Y. INABA

Key words: Hypertensive intracerebral hemorrhage, brain edema, regional cerebral blood flow, CT scan, xenon-enhanced CT

Introduction

Patients with hypertensive intracerebral hemorrhage (HIH) are thought to deteriorate neurologically during the 2nd week after onset, even after the initial treatment has been successful and neurologic recovery has been noted earlier. Correspondingly, several authors have revealed that the mass effect shown on the CT scan is most prominent at 10–15 days after the onset of HIH [9, 13, 19]. The low-density area encircling the hematoma, which appears late and causes augmentation of the mass effect, has been thought to be the vasogenic type of brain edema [1, 8].

However, many of the reported animal experiments concerning the vasogenic brain edema caused by cold lesion [5], brain abscess [20], and infusion [11] have revealed that the resolution of vasogenic edema starts within 4–7 days of the lesion. No reasonable explanation has been found for discrepancies between the clinical aspects of vasogenic brain edema in patients with HIH and experimental vasogenic brain edema.

In the present study we examined patients with HIH by CT scan and also performed xenon-enhanced CT for assessment of changes in regional cerebral blood flow (rCBF) over time. Although several authors have reported rCBF measurements in patients with HIH [3, 7, 15], three-dimensional rCBF measurements have not been studied intensively, and the data may reveal some of the pathophysiology of the brain edema occurring in patients with HIH.

Clinical Materials and Methods

Chronologic Changes Observed by CT Scan

Twenty-one patients with HIH whose clinical course had been examined by CT scan were selected for the present study. All the patients survived, though half (cases 1–10 in Fig. 2) received conservative and the other half, surgical treatment. Because

[1] Department of Neurosurgery, Tokyo Medical and Dental University, 1-5-45 Yushima, Bunkyo-ku, Tokyo 113, Japan

of the requirements for the operation all the patients who underwent surgery had larger hematomas than those treated conservatively. Various sites and sizes of the hematomas were also noted in the group of patients treated conservatively. To assess the progression of the edema, changes in mass effect caused by perifocal low-density area (PFLD) and Hounsfield units (HU) were plotted from the CT images for each patient.

Chronologic Changes in rCBF Measured by Xenon-Enhanced CT

The simplified method of Suzuki et al. [16] was used to perform xenon-enhanced CT in 6 patients at various periods, giving a total of 17 examinations. Each patient was positioned on the CT table and had an arterial line, a venous line, and monitoring electrodes for ECG, blood pressure, and respiration attached. First of all, pure oxygen was inhaled to denitrogenate, and then 40%–50% xenon in an oxygen mixture was inhaled for 4 min, after which xenon inhalation was discontinued. During the xenon inhalation serial CT scans were performed in the same CT plane every 60 s and the expired xenon concentration was also continuously recorded by a mass spectrometer. Arterial blood samples were taken at the start and end of xenon inhalation to assess the arterial blood gas and the xenon concentration in the blood.

The formula used for the calculation of rCBF is as follows:

$$K = [C_i(T) - C_i(O)] / \left[\lambda \int_0^T C_a(t)\,dt - \int_0^T C_i(t)\,dt \right],$$
$$f = 100\,\lambda K,$$

where C_i and C_a are the tissue and arterial blood xenon concentrations, respectively, K is the tissue buildup flow rate, f is the flow in the chosen compartments, and λ is the tissue blood partition coefficient, which was fixed as 1.0 for the simplified xenon-enhanced CT method. The values obtained for rCBF in the chosen cerebral regions were converted with a gray scale, giving a topographic flow map with a resolution of 3×3 mm.

rCBF Changes Before and After Glycerol Infusion

To evaluate the effectiveness of the treatment, xenon-enhanced CT was also performed in four patients before and 30 min after infusion of 200 ml 10% glycerol. All these patients had a significant mass effect due to brain edema during the administration of glycerol.

Results

Chronological Changes Observed by CT Scan

In the group of patients treated conservatively, growth of the hematoma was complete within the 1st day of onset; on the next CT scan, which was usually performed on the 2nd or 3rd day from the onset, a perifocal low-density area (PFLD) was noted. This PFLD spread into the white matter afterwards, extending to produce a mass effect in the ipsilateral hemisphere. It is evident that PFLD is most prominent in size on the 11–20th day from the onset, and correspondingly that any existing mass effect seen on CT images is also at its maximum on the same day. Thereafter the PFLD decreases gradually in size.

In the group of patients treated surgically, enlargement of PFLD was also noted until the 2nd week from the onset. Figure 1 shows a CT observation of case 18 over time. The first postoperative scan shows diminution of the midline shift due to removal of the hematoma. However, afterward PFLD spread and produced a mass effect lasting until the 13th day from the onset.

CT scans were performed on 84 occasions in 21 patients in the acute phase of the disease. All the CT findings were plotted by days (Fig. 2). In most cases the mass effect lasted longer than 10 days from the onset, and its peak was around 10–20 days after the onset in both conservative and surgical treatment groups. Though one plot (case 9) shows a decrease in mass effect after the early scan, the patient suffered a relatively small thalamic hemorrhage. PFLD noted on the CT plane spread mainly in the neighboring white matter of the hematoma. The HU in PFLD gradually decreased in number from the onset, reaching the lowest level at 11–20 days after the onset.

Chronologic Changes in rCBF

Xenon-enhanced CT were performed on 12 occasions in 6 patients, which made chronologic analysis of rCBF measurements possible. The hemispheric rCBF values were plotted in Fig. 3 and indicate that ipsilateral flow reached the lowest level during 11–20 days after the onset. Figure 4 shows the chronologic changes in CT images and rCBF maps in case 18, revealing that hypoperfusion involved the whole hemisphere as well as the PFLD area at 20 days after the onset. On the 80th day, though the ipsilateral flow was still low the flow in the cortex apparently recovered and then the area with low flow was clearly visible owing to the surrounding areas in which normal flow was maintained. In contrast, in case 2, whose hematoma was

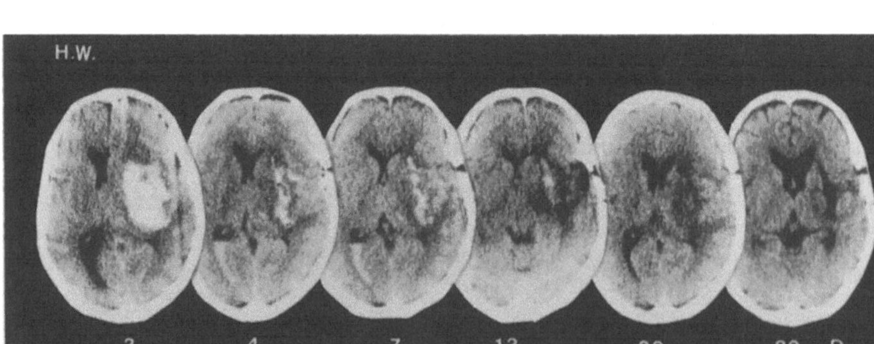

Fig. 1. Serial CT scan images performed in case 18, showing that mass effect reaches its maximum on the 13th day from the onset

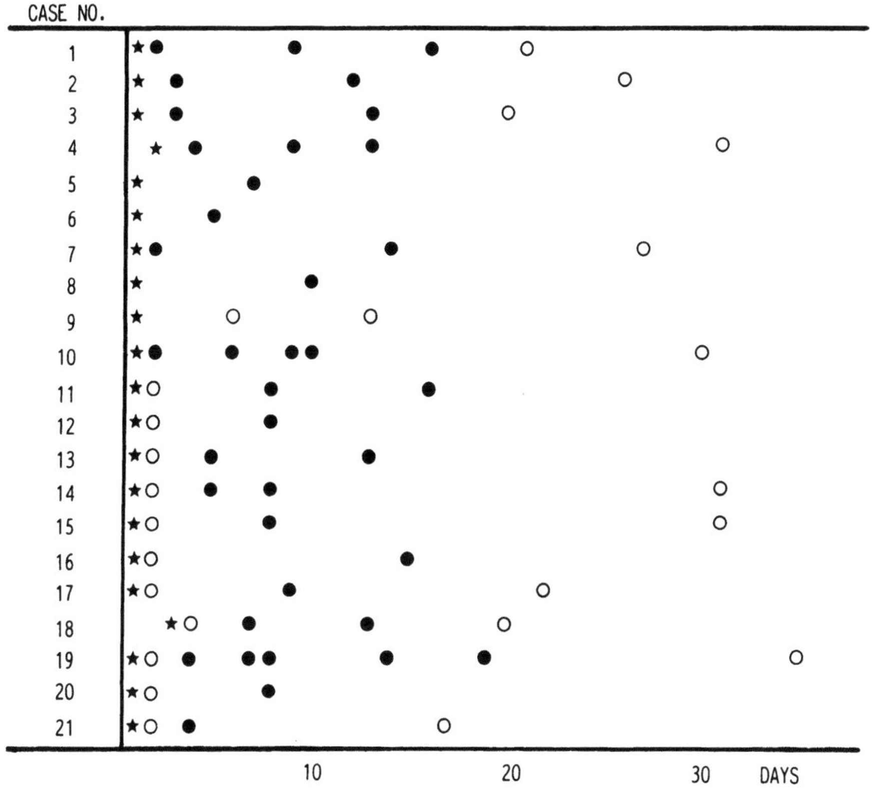

Fig. 2. Plotted CT scans of the patients by days. Scans that showed an increased mass effect compared with the previous one were marked with *black circles,* and those that showed a decreased mass effect compared with the previous one, with *empty circles.* Increasing mass effects were noted until the 15th day from the onset in all patients except case 9

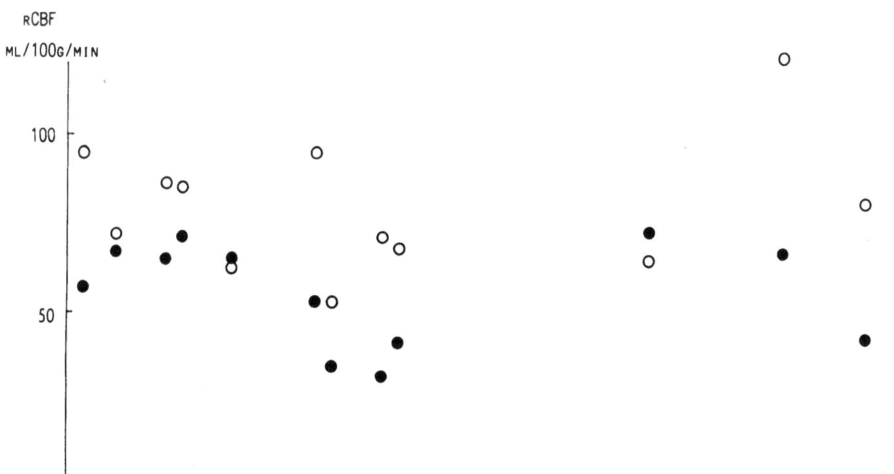

Fig. 3. rCBF values in ipsilateral hemisphere (*black circle*) and contralateral hemisphere (*empty circle*) plotted by days. Flows in the ipsilateral hemisphere reach their lowest value during 10–20 days after the onset. Flows in the ipsilateral hemisphere then start to improve gradually, though still significantly lower than in the contralateral hemisphere even at 2–3 months after the onset

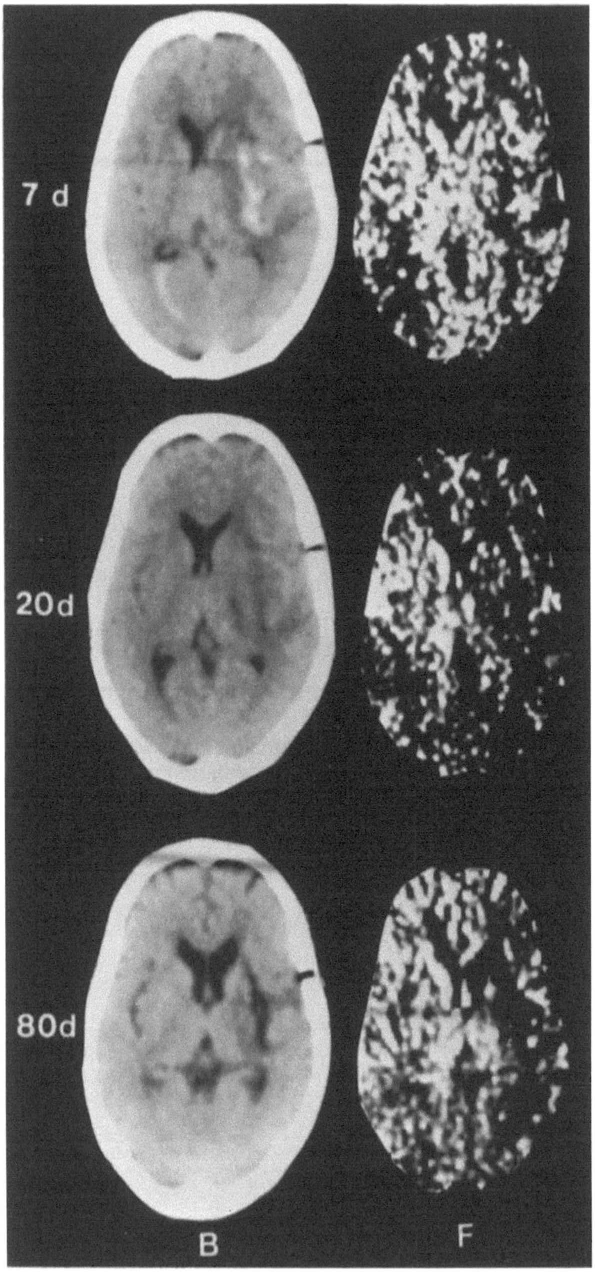

Fig. 4. CT images and rCBF maps for three different periods in case 18. Note diffuse decrease in flow in the ipsilateral hemisphere on the rCBF map for day 20

small, there were no differences in rCBF in the two hemispheres during the observation periods.

The flow in PFLD was parallel to the hemispheric flow. The flow in PFLD reached the lowest values around 11–20 days after the onset, then recovered gradually; however, full receovery was not achieved during the examination period. The flow in PFLD during the first week was rather well maintained.

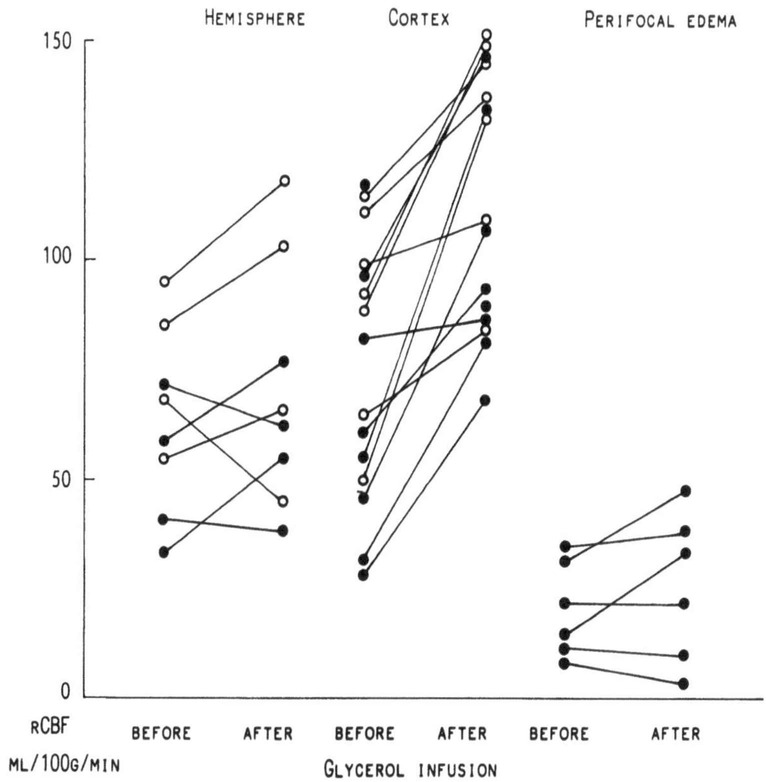

Fig. 5. rCBF changes in different regions before and after glycerol infusion. *Black circles,* rCBF in ipsilateral hemisphere; *empty circles,* rCBF in contralateral hemisphere. Most prominent increase in rCBF was seen in the gray matter

The data on the effect of glycerol on rCBF are summarized in Fig. 5. Glycerol had a positive effect on rCBF in patients with HIH, which was most potent on cortical gray matter thought to be intact primarily and smallest on the perifocal edema. It was well demonstrated that rCBF in the contralateral hemisphere also increased, with nearly the same rate of increase as in the ipsilateral hemisphere.

Discussion

The data presented confirm that brain edema in patients with HIH reached its maximum at 11–20 days after the onset. The PFLD seen on the CT scan in patients with HIH is not due solely to the resolving fluid from the hematoma, since the data (Figs. 1, 2) show that the mass effect increases similarly until 11–20 days in patients treated surgically as well as those treated conservatively. And the PFLD can be identified as mostly vasogenic brain edema, owing to its white matter predominancy. In confirmation, Ishii et al. [4] showed experimentally that the late developing brain edema was conspicuous even after complete removal of the hematoma was achieved. In addition, Mizukami et al. [13] reported that intracranial pressure reached its maximum during the 2nd week after the onset of HIH. Those results support the data presented here concerning the maximum mass effect showing on CT.

Concerning the rCBF changes in patients with HIH, the data indicated a close correlation between extension of the edema and decrease in rCBF. The earlier reports indicated that a decrease in rCBF was noted during the first week, and low perfusion continued constant over a long duration [7, 15]. However, our data suggest that rCBF gradually decreased during the first 10 days, reaching the lowest values during the second 10 days and then starting to recover. The sequential changes described here are more likely than the reported data mentioned above, since edema has been believed to decrease the blood flow by its volume-expansive nature [2]. The three-dimensional flow maps obtained by xenon-enhanced CT revealed that when rCBF reached its lowest values pathologically intact gray matter also showed low rCBF values, though it is a transient phenomenon, as proved by later assessment. It may be due to the volume expansion of brain edema, since after resolution of the brain edema low perfusion in the gray matter improved. However, hemispheric flow on the same side as the hematoma did not show full recovery even 80 days after the onset which may have been due to diaschisis (transneural depression) [12] within the ipsilateral hemisphere.

We have revealed that the deterioration of vasogenic brain edema causes a decrease in rCBF. However, the etiology of longer lasting edema in patients with HIH is still unclear. Experimentally, the vasogenic brain edema resolved within 7–10 days. In contrast, Takasugi et al. [18] reported that growth of the edema was initially rapid until the 4th day, then continued slowly up to 15 days in patients with HIH. These data suggest that initially vasogenic brain edema develops as a result of mechanical destruction of the blood-brain barrier by the hematoma. It may possibly be resolved within 7–10 days, while edema fluid of unknown origin was produced with some delay, and it exaggerates the initially recognized brain edema. Mizukami (1983) hypothesized that the secondary ischemia was due to deformation of the brain by the mass effect of the hematoma, which triggered further aggravation of cerebral edema in the area surrounding the hematoma. This is unlikely, since our data indicated that the brain edema continued to extend even after removal of the hematoma was achieved, which was confirmed by Ishii et al. [4] experimentally. And Hossmann [2] suggested that the edema fluid did not cause microcirculatory compression.

Zimmerman et al. [21] reported the appearance of ring enhancement in the area surrounding the hematoma with contrast-agent-enhanced CT scan from 6 days to 6 weeks after the onset of HIH, and Takasugi [17] demonstrated in experimental animals in which hematoma was produced artificially that newly developed capillaries with prominent activity of pinocytotic actions were found in the areas surrounding the hematoma at the earliest 9 days after the insult. He and also Liliequist [9] suggested that these newly developed capillaries may be responsible for the ring enhancement seen on CT scan. On the other hand, Maeda [10] recently studied the dynamics of cerebrospinal fluid (CSF) by performing radioisotope cisternography on patients with HIH, and proved that a subarachnoid block over the ipsilateral convexity was noted during the first month after the onset. He suggested that this subarachnoid block was caused by the mass effect of the hematoma and the brain edema. According to these observations it may be possible to say that the secondary edema fluid is produced from the newly developed capillaries and the resolution of edema fluid is delayed by an existing subarachnoid block, since CSF clearance has been demonstrated as one of the major mechanisms responsible for the resolution of the edema fluid [11, 14]. Hypertension may also play an important role in the production of edema fluid.

Concerning the effect of the glycerol on rCBF, we confirmed the other reports which show improvement of rCBF after glycerol infusion [13]. Our data show that glycerol mainly improved rCBF in the pathologically intact regions, such as gray matter and the contralateral hemisphere. But the results showed that glycerol seemed to have little effect on the edematous area. It may be logical, since hyperosmolar solutions reduce intracranial pressure by reducing the intracranial volume mainly of normal brain tissue and not the edematous tissue volume [6].

In conclusion, we have demonstrated that the clinical course in patients with HIH corresponds to the exacerbation of brain edema and secondary hypoperfusion in the affected hemisphere. Brain edema occurring in patients with HIH has been shown to prolong the clinical deterioration, which may have affected the patients' outcome. Further research is necessary to find an ideal approach to the treatment of patients with HIH from the viewpoint of brain edema.

Summary

There is an impression that patients with hypertensive intracerebral hemorrhage (HIH) deteriorate neurologically during the 2nd week after the onset. Gradual recovery then occurs during the next month. To find what factors might be responsible for the delayed deterioration, changes in CT findings and regional cerebral blood flow (rCBF) distribution measured by xenon-enhanced CT were observed over time in a total of 21 patients with HIH. Also, to evaluate the effectiveness of the treatment, xenon-enhanced CT was performed before and after glycerol infusion in 4 patients.

CT findings correlated well with the clinical course. The CT scan revealed that brain edema reached its peak within 10–20 days in most patients and the mass effect gradually disappeared in the next month. Xenon-enhanced CT showed a gradual decrease in rCBF in the ipsilateral hemisphere during the first 10 days after the onset, and rCBF reached its lowest values during the second 10 days, subsequently improving. However, even at day 80 after onset, rCBF in the ipsilateral hemisphere had not recovered fully. Correspondingly, Hounsfield units and rCBF in perifocal low density areas reached their lowest values within 10–20 days after the onset. Glycerol revealed its effectiveness on rCBF. Regional CBF increased after glycerol infusion in both hemispheres. The regional increase in CBF was slight in the edematous tissue, though it was most obvious in the morphologically intact gray matter.

References

1. Clasen RA, Huckman MS, Pandolfi S, Laing I, Jacobs J (1976) Computed tomography of vasogenic cerebral edema. In: Pappius HM, Feindel W (eds) Dynamics of brain edema. Springer, Berlin Heidelberg New York, pp 278–282

2. Hossmann K-A (1982) Pathophysiology of vasogenic and cytotoxic brain edema. In: Hartmann A, Brock M (eds) Treatment of cerebral edema. Springer, Berlin Heidelberg, pp 1–10
3. Ishii R, Takeuchi S, Ohsugi S, Tanaka R, Arai H (1982) Cerebral blood flow in patients with putaminal hemorrhage. Using ^{133}Xe inhalation method. Neurol Med Chir (Tokyo) 22:813–821
4. Ishii S, Koike J, Hatashita S (1983) Brain edema in hypertensive intracerebral hemorrhage. In: Mizukami M, Kanaya H, Kogure K, Yamori Y (eds) Hypertensive intracerebral hemorrhage. Raven, New York, pp 11–17
5. Klatzo I, Chui E, Fujiwara K, Spatz M (1980) Resolution of vasogenic brain edema. Adv Neurol 28:359–373
6. Klein HJ, Schmidt K (1982) Hyperosmolar solutions and diuretics in the treatment of brain edema. In: Hartmann A, Brock M (eds) Treatment of cerebral edema. Springer, Berlin Heidelberg New York, pp 81–93
7. Kuroda K (1982) Regional cerebral blood flow in patients with hypertensive intracerebral hemorrhage – patients with putaminal hemorrhage treated surgically. Brain Nerve 34:561–569
8. Lanksch WR (1982) The diagnosis of brain edema by computed tomography. In: Hartmann A, Brock M (eds) Treatment of cerebral edema. Springer, Berlin Heidelberg New York, pp 43–80
9. Liliequist B (1983) Computerized axial tomography in cerebrovascular disease. In: Mizukami M, Kanaya H, Kogure K, Yamori Y (eds) Hypertensive intracerebral hemorrhage. Raven, New York, pp 19–26
10. Maeda Y, Taneda M (1984) Time course of the dynamics of cerebrospinal fluid (Tokyo) Circulation in hypertensive intracerebral hemorrhage. Neurol Med Chir (Tokyo) 24:240–244
11. Marmarou A, Tanaka K, Shulman K (1982) The brain response to infusion edema: Dynamics of fluid resolution. In: Hartmann A, Brock M (eds) Treatment of cerebral edema. Springer, Berlin Heidelberg New York, pp 11–18
12. Meyer JS, Naritomi H, Sakai F, Ishihara N, Grant P (1979) Regional cerebral blood flow, diaschisis, and steal after stroke. Neurol Res 1:101–119
13. Mizukami M, Tazawa T (1983) Theoretical background for surgical treatment in hypertensive intracerebral hemorrhage. In: Mizukami M, Kanaya H, Kogure K, Yamori Y (eds) Hypertensive intracerebral hemorrhage. Raven, New York, pp 239–247
14. Reulen HJ, Tsuyumu M, Tack A, Fenske A, Prioleau G (1978) Clearance of edema fluid into CSF: a mechanism for resolution of vasogenic brain edema. J Neurosurg 48:754–764
15. Sugiyama H (1984) Cerebral blood flow in patients with hypertensive intracerebral hemorrhage. With regard to differences in the mechanism of flow reduction between putaminal and thalamic hemorrhage. Neurol Med Chir (Tokyo) 24:564–572
16. Suzuki R, Hiratsuka H, Ohno K, Inaba Y, Kimura T, Inoue J (1985) Topographic mapping of regional cerebral blood flow by xenon-enhanced CT – Introducing a simplified method as a routine examination. Brain Nerve 37:73–80
17. Takasugi S (1980) Cause of ring enhancement in computed tomographic image of intracerebral hematomas – An experimental histological study. Neurol Med Chir (Tokyo) 20:689–700
18. Takasugi S, Soga T, Masuda T, Yamashita S, Matsumoto K (1979) Management of hypertensive intracerebral hemorrhage – based on the natural course of the hematoma observed by repeated CT scan. Neurol Med Chir (Tokyo) 19:261–269
19. Tomita Y (1980) The perifocal low density around hematoma on computed tomography in hypertensive intracerebral hemorrhage. Brain Nerve 32:545–553
20. Wallenfang T, Bohl J, Kretzschmar K (1980) Evolution of brain abscess in cats – formation of capsule and resolution of brain edema. Neurosurg Rev 3:101–111
21. Zimmerman RD, Leeds NE, Naidich TP (1977) Ring Blush associated with intracerebral hematoma. Radiology 122:707–711

Acute Brain Swelling, Contusional Brain Edema, and Ischemic Brain Damage in Acute Head Injury

U. ITO[1], M. SEIDA, S. TOMIDA, S. YAMAZAKI, and Y. INABA

Key words: Brain contusion, brain edema, acute brain swelling, ischemic brain damage, intracranial pressure

Introduction

Recent evidence provided by CT scans has shown that the secondary clinical deterioration after acute head injury (HI) is not always associated with decreased density reflecting increased tissue water content [7, 15]. The aim of the present study was to elucidate the deterioration process occurring secondary to HI.

Chronological Changes of Acute Brain Swelling and Brain Edema due to Brain Contusion

Changes in acute brain swelling (ABS) and in brain edema due to brain contusion (BEBC) were studied over time in the acute stage of head injury (HI), mainly by repeated serial CT images and intracranial pressure (ICP) monitoring. Serial CT scans were performed in 125 patients who had Glasgow Coma Scale (GCS) scores of less than 14 on admission. Among them, 48 patients who underwent emergency craniectomy were eliminated from this study to avoid secondary modification due to intracranial surgery.

The remaining 77 patients were made up of 51 adults (17–81 years; average 31.8 years) and 26 children (1–16 years; average 10.2 years). Each group was further divided into subgroups with higher (8–14) and lower (3–7) GCS scores on admission. Continuous hyperventilation and hyperosmolal therapy were performed in all patients who had lower admission GCS scores and/or severe acute brain swelling as revealed by CT on admission.

ABS was seen on the CT image as a diffuse homogeneous swelling of the cerebral hemisphere, with iso- or slight hyperdensity. Grades of ABS were classified into three categories according to the CT image: (1) Mild; ventricles and cisterns were narrower on the CT image in the acute stage than those on the CT image more than 3 weeks after the HI. (2) Moderate; in addition, the sylvian fissure and cortical gyri were not visualized. (3) Marked; in addition, the perimesencephalic cisterns were not visualized.

---

[1] Department of Neurosurgery, Musasino Red-Cross Hospital, 1-26-1, Kyonan-cho, Musasino-city, Tokyo 180, Japan

BEBC appeared on the CT image as a low-density area (LDA) spreading into the white matter from the cortical contusion. Intracerebral hematomas more than 3 cm in diameter were operatively removed when local mass signs were recognized on the CT image. On the serial CT image planimetry of the BEBC was carried out. The planimetric size of the LDA resulting from BEBC at the same CT slice level was studied over time.

The catheter-tip pressure gauge transducer (Goelteck) was sub- or epidurally placed in the temporal lobe of the injured hemisphere. The ICP was monitored continuously in eight patients with both ABS and BEBC.

Results

Case History 1. A 29-year-old man was admitted to our hospital with HI sustained in a traffic accident. On admission, GCS score was 7 and signs of neither oculomotor palsy nor motor and/or sensory deficit were found. He underwent hyperventilation and hyperosmolar therapy. An ICP sensor was placed in the left subtemporal space. From 3 to 18 h after HI the ABS was severe, becoming mild 4 days later. The ICP was moderately high from 3 h to 2 days after HI and fell to a mildly elevated level by 3 days after HI. On the other hand, BEBC appeared at 18 h after HI in the bilateral frontal lobe, and increased in size from 3 to 19 days thereafter (Fig. 1).

ABS occurred in 48 (62%) of all 77 patients and was almost equally distributed between higher (58% of 57 patients) and lower (75% of 20 patients) admission GCS groups, and between adults (71% of 51) and children (46% of 26). The degree of ABS on the CT image was plotted against time for each case. The ABS appeared immediately after HI and became less severe 1–2 days after HI (Fig. 2).

Brain contusion occurred in 30 (39%) of the 77 patients, and more frequently in patients with moderate to marked brain swelling than in those patients without or with only mild acute swelling (Table 1). The planimetric size of the LDA resulting from BEBC at the same CT slice level was plotted against time for each case (Fig. 3).

Table 1. Frequency of brain contusion among all patients with acute brain swelling by clinical grade

Group	Clinical grades on admission (GCS)[a]	Grades of ABS[b] None	Mild	Moderate	Marked	Total
Adult	8–14	2/12 (17%)	2/6 (33%)	8/11 (73%)	3/6 (50%)	14/35 (43%)
	3–7	1/3 (33%)	0/1 (0%)	5/7 (71%)	5/5 (100%)	11/16 (69%)
Child	8–14	0/12 (0%)	0/6 (0%)	1/2 (50%)	1/2 (50%)	2/22 (9%)
	3–7	1/2 (50%)	0/0 (0%)	1/1 (100%)	0/1 (0%)	2/4 (50%)
Total		4/29 (14%)	2/13 (15%)	15/21 (71%)	9/14 (64%)	30/77 (39%)

[a] Glasgow Coma Scale
[b] Acute brain swelling (diffuse)

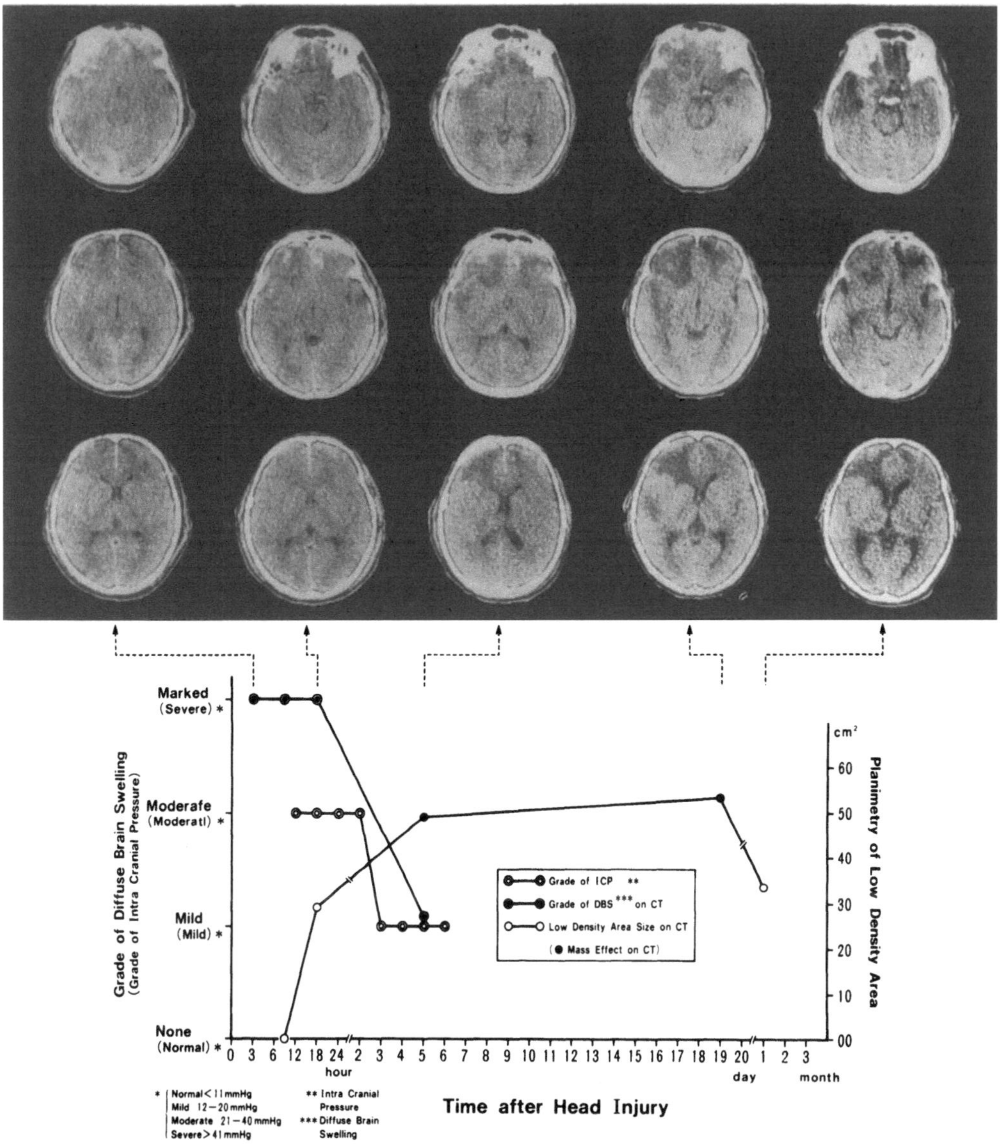

Fig. 1. CT scan and changes over time in severity of diffuse brain swelling and intracranial pressure and in size of low-density area seen on CT in a 29-year-old man after a head injury sustained in a traffic accident

The BEBC usually appeared from 24 h after HI, intensified during days 3–10 after HI, and then decreased. The local mass signs on the CT image were recognized in 11 (37%) of all 30 patients with brain contusion.

Changes in the degree of raised ICP were plotted over time for each of the 8 patients who had both ABS and BEBC (Fig. 4). The ICP was usually markedly elevated in the acute stage of HI and decreased from 4 to 5 days after HI.

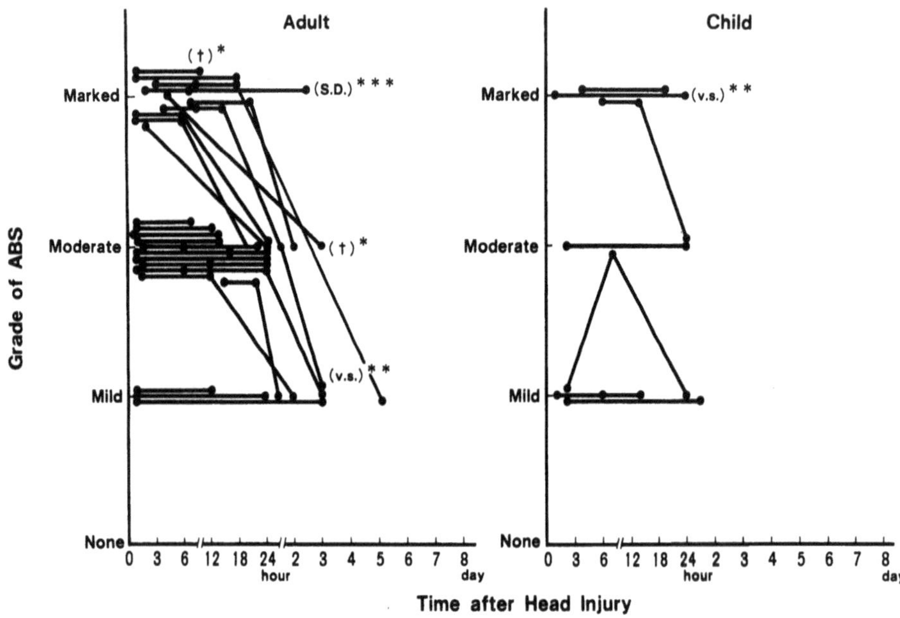

Fig. 2. Time course of severity of acute brain swelling (ABS) after head injury, as seen on CT image. * death, ** vegitative state, *** severe disability

Table 2. Outcome in all 77 patients by GCS score, grade of acute brain swelling (ABS), and brain contusion (BC) on admission

GCS	ABS	BC	Glasgow Outcome Scale				
			Good recovery	Moderate disability	Severe disability	Vegetative state	Death
8–14	None	+	○				
		−	○○○○○○○○○○○○ ●●●●●●●●●●●●●	○			
	Mild	+	○○				
		−	○○○ ●●●●●●				
	Moderate	+	○○○○○○ ●	○			
		−	○○○				
	Marked	+	○ ●		○		
		−	○○○ ●				
3–7	None	+	●				○
		−	○ ●				○
	Mild	+					
		−	○○				
	Moderate	+	○○○				
		−	○○				
	Marked	+	○○			○	○○○ ●
		−				●	○

○ Adult, ● Child

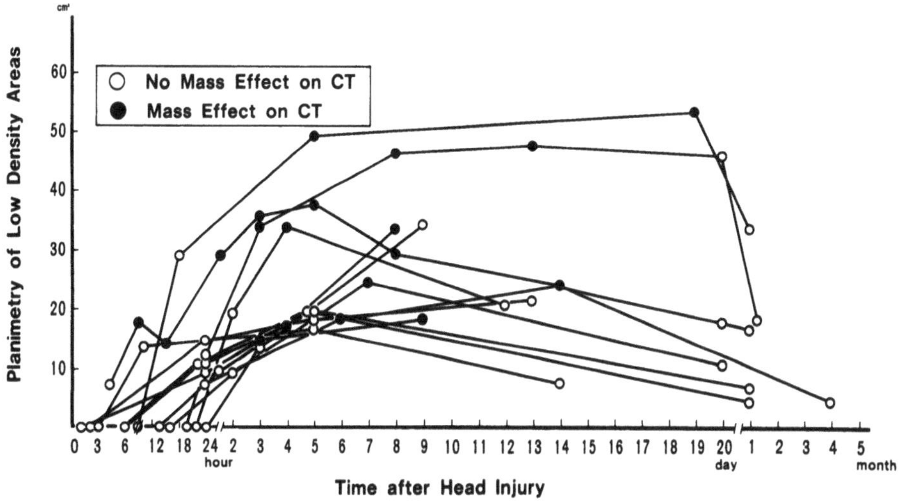

Fig. 3. Time course of size of low-density areas at same CT slice level after head injury

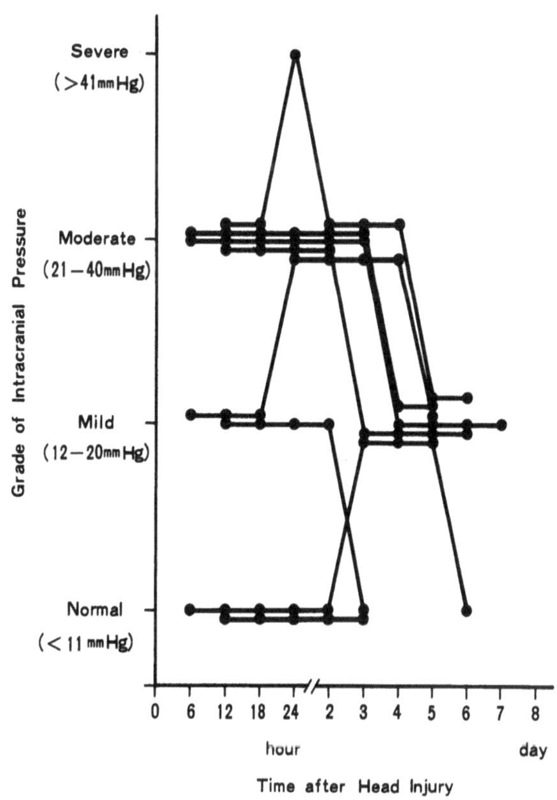

Fig. 4. Time course of grade of intracranial pressure after head injury

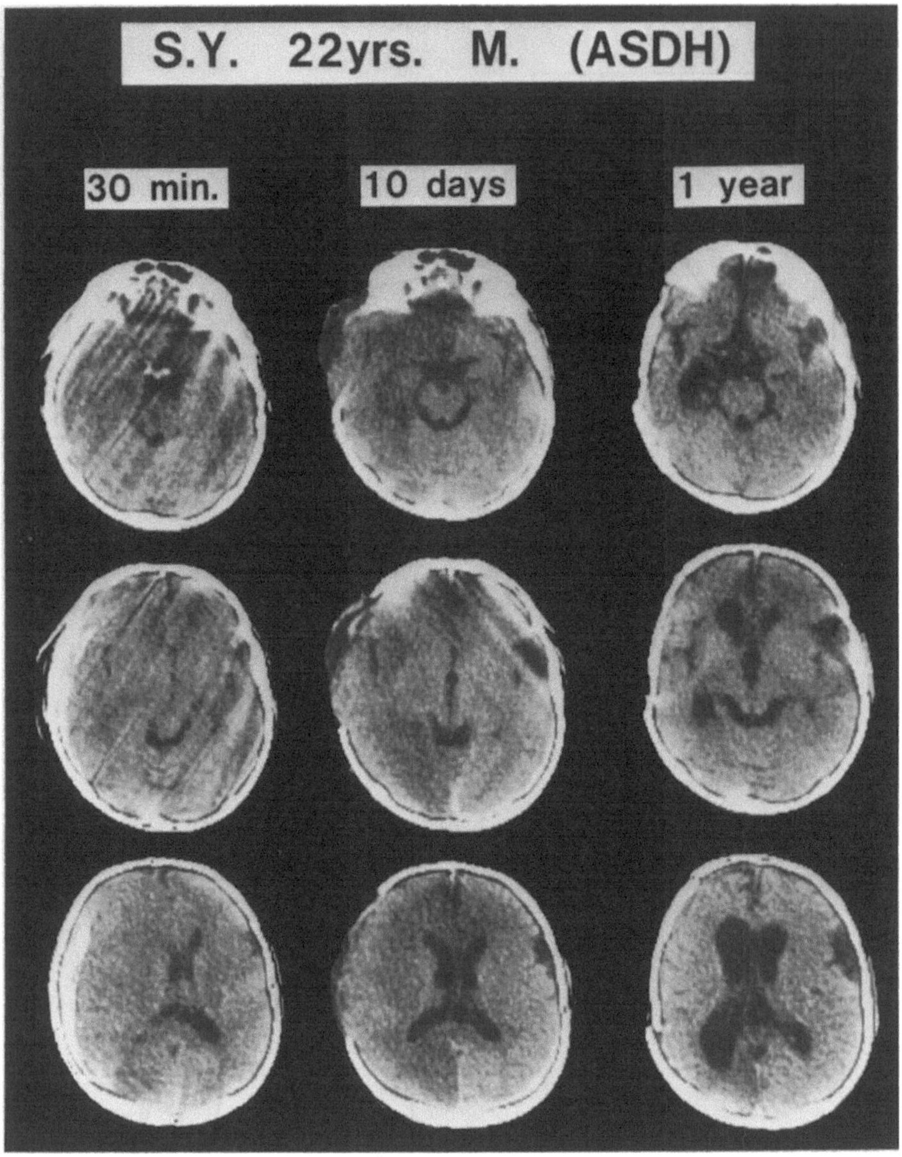

Fig. 5. CT images recorded in a 22-year-old man at different times after head injury; acute brain swelling with acute subdural hematoma and ischemic brain damage

Table 2 shows the outcome in all 77 patients with reference to admission GCS, grade of ABS, and existence of brain contusion. Although the outcome was poor in 10 patients, this was due to death or severe disability resulting from extracranial lesions in 8 cases. In most patients with brain contusion the outcome was good (Table 2).

Factors Involved in Deterioration Following Acute Head Injury – Ischemic Brain Damage

Factors involved in the deterioration following acute HI were analyzed in 42 patients with poor outcomes, including surgically and nonsurgically treated patients (10 severely disabled and in vegetative states and 32 deaths) among 505 patients admitted with acute HI. Among the 42 patients with a poor outcome, in 11 (26%) this was caused by other factors than head injury, and 16 patients (38%) died within a few days of HI owing to extremely severe primary brain damage sustained with the first impact to the brain. Therefore, we analyzed the secondary deterioration factors after acute HI in the remaining 15 patients (36%) with reference to the repeated serial CT image, ICP monitoring, CBF measurement by Kety's method, and clinical course.

Results

Case History 2. A 22-year-old man was able to give his name and address to a policeman soon after the traffic accident. His admission GCS score was 5. Acute subdural hematoma (ASDH) and marked ABS were noted in the left cerebral hemisphere on the admission CT. Two days after the emergency operation diffuse global low density appeared in the left cerebral hemisphere. Later, marked brain atrophy persisted in the same hemisphere (Fig. 5).

Table 3. Intracranial factors in outcome in 15 patients who survived more than 3 days after head injury

	DAI or PBI with			Ischemic brain damage with					
	ABS	ABS + BEBC	ABS + IH	ABS	ABS + IH				
					AEDH	ASDH	ICH	ASDH + ICH	Total
Not Operated on									
SD + vegetative state	0	1	0	1	0	0	0	0	0
Death	1	0	0	0	0	0	0	1	1
Operated on									
SD + vegetative state	0	0	1	0	2	2	2	0	6
Death	0	0	0	0	0	4	0	0	4
Total	1	1	1	1	2	6	2	1	11

ABS, acute brain swelling; AEDH, acute epidural hematoma; ASDH, acute subdural hematoma; BEBC, brain edema due to brain contusion; DAI, diffuse axonal injury; ICH, intracerebral hematoma; IH, intracranial hematoma; PBI, primary brainstem injury; SD, severe disability

Table 4. Frequency of ischemic brain damage among patients with various intracranial mass lesions by clinical grade

Clinical Grades on: Discharge (GOS)	Admission (GCS)	AEDH	AEDH + ABS	ASDH	ASDH + ABS	ICH	ICH + ABS	ASDH + ICH + ABS	BEBC	BEBC + ABS	ABS	Total
Good recovery, and moderate disability	8–14	0/13	0/20	0/3	2/12	0/5	1/6	1/6	0/1	0/17	0/20	4/93
	3–7	0/0	1/4	0/1	0/3	0/0	0/1	0/0	0/0	0/0	0/0	1/9
	Total	0/13	1/24	0/4	2/15	0/5	1/7	1/6	0/1	0/17	0/20	5/102 (4.9%)
Severe disability, vegetative state, and death	8–14	0/0	0/0	0/0	0/0	0/0	1/1	0/0	0/0	0/0	0/0	1/1
	3–7	0/0	2/2	0/0	6/7	0/0	1/1	1/1	0/0	0/1	1/2	11/14
	Total	0/0	2/2	0/0	6/7	0/0	2/2	1/1	0/0	0/1	1/2	12/15 (80.0%)

GOS, Glasgow Outcome Scale; GCS, Glasgow Coma Scale; AEDH, acute epidural hematoma; ABS, acute brain swelling; ASDH, acute subdural hematoma; ICH, intra-cerebral hematoma; BECB, brain edema due to brain contusion

Of the 15 patients who survived more than 3 days after HI, 12 (80%) had ipsilateral or bilateral hemispheric swelling and LDAs with uncontrollable increase in ICP and decreased CBF by Kety's method. These indications of ischemic brain damage (IBD) were seen on the CT 3.1 ± 1.2 days after HI (mean $\pm$ SD). In 11 of the 12 patients with IBD there was ABS combined with intracranial hematoma (Table 3), and in 10 of these IBD was seen on the CT image after removal of the intracranial hematoma. The 11 intracranial hematomas were made up of 6 ASDHs, 2 acute epidural hematomas (AEDHs), 2 intracerebral hematomas (ICHs), and 1 ASDH with ICH (Table 3).

IBD was found in only 4.9% of the patients with intracranial mass lesions in whom the outcome was good, and in 80% of the patients with poor outcome. Distribution of the intracranial lesions was the same in both groups (Table 4).

Discussion

It has been reported that ABS was found more in children (29%) than in adults, and about 2.7 times more frequently in the group with low GCS scores (less than 7) than in the group with higher scores [1]. In the present study, ABS occurred in 62% of patients with admission GCSs of less than 14 and in 75% of the adult group. There was no difference in the percentage frequency between lower and higher admission GCS groups [5]. As ABS appeared on the CT image as a diffuse homogeneous hemispheric swelling with a Hounsfield's number of 37.5 ± 6.2 (control 33.6 ± 6.1), vascular engorgement due to acute vasoparalysis has been considered to be a factor [7, 14]. However, recent experimental studies have revealed a hemispheric increase in tissue water content after water percussion head injury to cats [Marmarou et al., this volume; 16].

Brain contusion was found more in patients with moderate to marked ABS than in patients with mild ABS or none at all (Table 1) [5]. The BEBC spreads to the adjacent white matter from the cortical contusion as in the vasogenic brain edema model based on cortical cold injury [8]. ABS occurred immediately after HI and subsided within several days (Fig. 2) [5]; however, BEBC appeared from 24 h after HI and intensified during the 3–10 days after HI, decreasing thereafter (Fig. 3) [5]. Therefore, BEBC was not found on the CT image in the acute stage of HI [2, 3]. Local mass signs on the CT image were recognized in only 37% of our patients with BC [5]. The ICP was moderately high in the acute stage of HI and decreased 4–5 days after HI, while the BEBC intensified on the CT image over 3–10 days after HI (Fig. 4) [5]. Many of the patients with good outcome were found in the groups with BC (Table 2) [2, 5, 14].

Thus, ABS and/or BEBC per se did not always seem to be the secondary deteriorating factors causing deterioration in the acute HI [5, 7, 14]. On analysis of the 42 patients with poor outcome, the most important secondary factors in deterioration seemed to be simultaneous ABS and intracranial hematoma, especially acute subdural hematoma (Tables 3 and 4) [3, 4, 6, 9–12]. Acute diffuse cortical compression seemed to produce the secondary global ischemic damage via acute venous congestion [4, 6, 10–12].

Summary

Chronological changes and prognosis in acute brain swelling (ABS), brain edema due to brain contusion (BEBC), and ischemic brain damage (IBD) were studied in the acute stage of head injury (HI) by serial CT and ICP monitoring of 168 of 505 patients admitted with HI. ABS was seen on the CT image as a diffuse homogeneous swelling of the cerebral hemisphere with iso- or slight hyperdensity. Grades of ABS were classified as mild, moderate, and marked on the CT image. ABS appeared immediately after HI and decreased in severity 1–2 days later. The BEBC appeared on the CT image as a low density area (LDA) spreading into the white matter from the cortical contusion. Planimetry of the LDA was carried out. BEBC was apparent from 24 h after HI and intensified over 3–10 days after HI, subsequently decreasing. The ICP was monitored by an ipsilateral subdurally placed catheter tip pressure gauge transducer. IBD appeared in the ipsilateral or bilateral cerebral hemisphere of patients with ABS combined with intracranial hematoma, on average around 3.1 ± 1.2 days after HI, as a diffuse global LDA and swelling of the hemisphere with uncontrollably increased ICP, followed by marked hemispheric atrophy. The IBD was found in 80% of patients in whom the outcome after acute HI was poor. In the patients with both ABS and BEBC the ICP was high in the acute stage of HI and decreased 4–5 days after HI. However, in the patients with IBD, the ICP remained high for more than a week. As the BEBC occurred and intensified gradually after the ABS subsided, it did not always produce intracranial hypertension. However, IBD that occurred immediately after the head injury and was combined with the ABS and intracranial hematoma produced a severe increase in ICP. Therefore, BEBC seems to be a less and the IBD a more harmful factor occurring secondary to acute HI.

References

1. Bruce DA, Alavi A, Bilaniuk L, Dolinskas C, Obrist W, Uzzel B (1981) Diffuse cerebral swelling following head injuries in children: the syndrome of "malignant brain edema". J Neurosurg 54:170–178
2. Clifton GL, Grossman RG, Makela ME, Handel S, Sadhu V (1980) Neurological course and correlated computerized tomography findings after severe closed head injury. J Neurosurg 52:611–624
3. Cooper PR, Moody S (1978) Neurodiagnostic studies and management of head injury. Computertomographie 2:197–206
4. Graham DI, Adams JH, Doyle D (1978) Ischemic brain damage in fetal non-missile head injuries. J Neurol Sci 39:213–234
5. Ito U, Kito K, Okada K, Tomita H, Inaba Y (1983) Chronological changes of diffuse brain swelling and contusional edema in acute head injury. Neurotraumatology 6:39–48
6. Ito U, Tomida S, Seida M, Tomita H, Inaba Y (1984) Ischemic brain damage in acute head injury. Study on deteriorating factors. Neurotraumatology 7:143–152 (in Japanese)
7. Jennett G (1981) Clinical brain swelling: edema or engorgement. In: de Vlieger M, de Lange SA, Beks JWF (eds) Brain edema. Wiley, New York, pp 61–65
8. Klatzo I, Wisniewski H, Steinwall O, Stricher E (1967) Dynamics of cold injury edema. In: Klatzo I, Seitelberger F (eds) Brain edema. Springer, Vienna New York, pp 554–563
9. Koo AH, LaRoque RL (1977) Evaluation of head trauma by computed tomography. Radiology 123:345–350

10. Langfitt TW, Gennarelli TA (1982) Can the outcome from head injury be improved? J Neurosurg 56:19–25
11. Lanksch W, Baethman A, Kazner E (1981) Computed tomography of brain edema. In: de Vlieger M, de Lange SA, Beks JWF (eds) Brain edema. Wiley, New York, pp 67–98
12. McPherson P, Graham DI (1978) Correlation between angiographic findings and the ischemia of head injury. J Neurol Neurosurg Psychiatry 41:122–127
13. Merindo-de Villasante J, Taveras JM (1976) Computed tomography (CT) in acute head trauma. Am J Roentgenol 126:765–778
14. Miller JD, Corales RL (1981) Brain edema as a result of head injury: fact or fallacy. In: de Vlieger M, de Lange SA, Beks JWF (eds) Brain edema. Wiley, New York, pp 99–115
15. Tornheim PA, McLaurin RL (1981) Acute changes in regional brain water content following experimental closed head injury. J Neurosurg 55:407–413

Quantification of Brain Edema by Measurement of Brain Conductivity

D. M. LONG [1] and H. W. KO

Introduction

Measurement of brain edema in the laboratory has so far been a cumbersome procedure requiring sacrifice of the animal and dry weight determinations or measurement of specific gravity. There is a need for a simple and rapid way of achieving accurate measurements of the water content of tissue in the study of brain edema.

There are no techniques which allow accurate ongoing measurement of edema in the human. The CAT, MRI, and PET techniques allow one-time estimation of edema, but it is extremely difficult to utilize them for determination of changes, because of the logistics of moving the patient to the scanner and doing the scan. There is a real need for a measurement technique which will allow the progression or regression of brain edema to be estimated at the bedside.

To solve these two problems, we have begun an investigation of the feasibility of measuring brain conductivity by invasive probes and by noninvasive coil techniques. This presentation is a preliminary note demonstrating the feasibility of this approach for quantification of brain edema.

Rationale

It has been known for some time that impedance or conductance can be measured to provide an assessment of the fluid content of the brain. The techniques involved have not been practical for rapid use. It is well known that the conductivity of white matter is approximately 0.10 S/m and that of gray matter significantly greater, with 0.23 S/m, while the conductivity of CSF and extracellular fluid varies between 1.5 and 1.75 S/m. Theoretically, it should be possible to detect the increased conductivity in brain tissue produced by the intrusion of the higher conductivity edema fluid. A number of previous investigations prove the theoretical feasibility of this approach. Some have used inductive measures, but most have utilized contacting electrodes or wheatstone bridge techniques. None of the methods involved have attempted a spatial or temporal assessment.

[1] Department of Neurosurgery, The Johns Hopkins Hospital, Baltimore, Maryland 21205, USA

An Invasive Test Probe For Measurement of Brain Edema

We have created a prototype probe which is bipolar in configuration and utilizes 0.10-in. discs as the electrode. This original probe is designed for test purposes only. Final electrode spacing is projected to be 0.010 in. Brain conductivity or impedance is read directly from a commercially available impedance meter.

Preliminary Results

Original instrumentation and calibration indicated properformance accurate at better than 1% with calibrated ionic solutions of 5, 2.2, and 0.27 S/m. Measurement with 1 MHz in 0.9% saline indicated our probe measurement as 0.152 S/m, as against the generally accepted figure of 1.50 obtained by all other current means. Furthermore, our probe results indicated that we could sample 88%–92% of an edge-limited area. These results were encouraging enough to warrant utilizing the probe in a normal brain sample. For this purpose, a normal rabbit was sacrificed in accordance with accepted laboratory techniques, after which the brain was immediately removed and tested with the probe. The results are shown in Fig. 1. Conductivity varies as a function of temperature, but the figures are within those expected for gray and white matter based upon estimates from other techniques. These studies were repeated using 1, 2, and 4 MHz. The results are seen in Table 1. There is enough difference between gray and white matter to predict that the technique would allow accurate measurement of changes in conductivity.

The project was then expanded to include the study of gray and white matter conductivity in tumor-bearing animals. The VX2 carcinoma has been carried in rabbits in our laboratory for several years. Brain edema develops with this tumor. Its time course has been well studied, and the animals consistently die of edema. The results are seen in Table 2. There is a significant increase in the impedance of the edematous gray matter around the tumor and a definable difference in the white matter. Normal white matter had conductance readings of 0.12, while comparable samples on the tumor-bearing side had 0.15. White matter in the tumor-bearing hemisphere well away from the tumor measured 0.14. All samples were obtained by removing the brain in its entirety, slicing it, and then sampling similar spots on the tumor-bearing and non-tumor-bearing sides (Fig. 2). The figures represent the averages of multiple samples in each hemisphere.

Table 1. Preliminary results and observations in normal brain (M78)

APL, 1984 2 MHz, 12 °C to 22 °C	Gray 0.19±0.01 S/m	White 0.01±0.03 S/m
1 KHz, body temp. and 39 °C [ ]	0.23 S/m	0.10 S/m

Normal gray and white values consistent with literature; normal gray values distinctly higher than normal white values at 1, 2, 4 MHz. Average conductivity difference between normal gray and normal white matter 0.14 S/m at 21–22 °C, 2 MHz

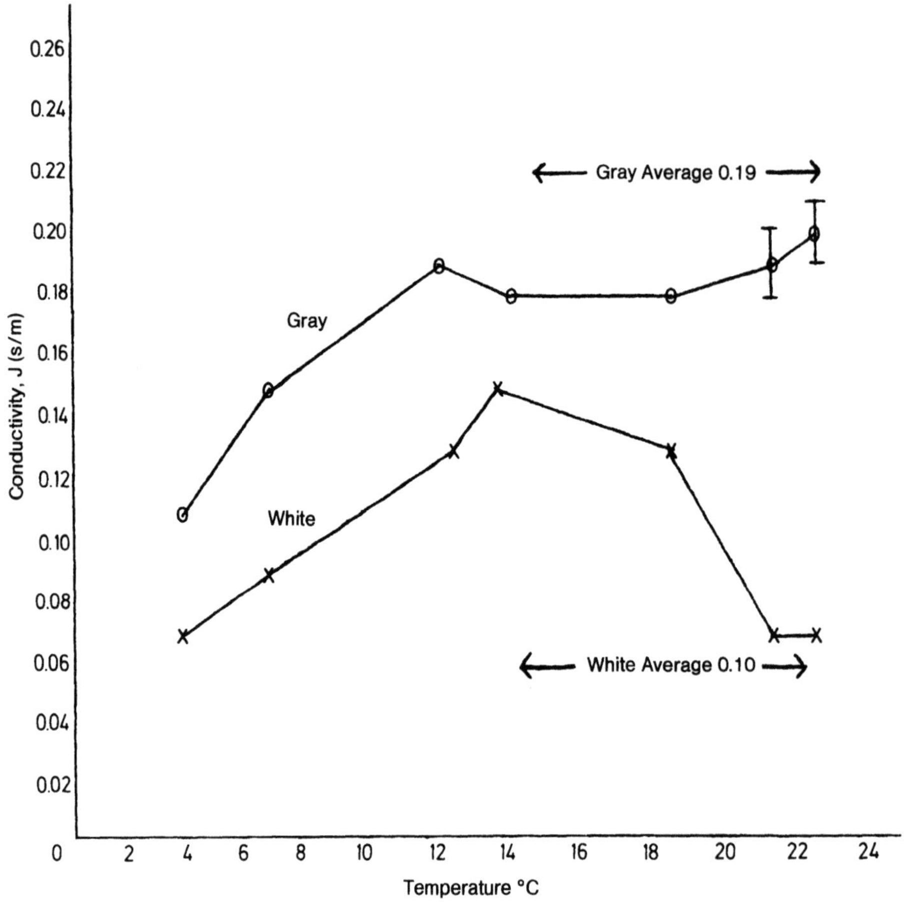

Fig. 1. Conductivity measured in normal brain with the prototype probe at different temperatures

Table 2. Preliminary results and observations in brain with tumor (R65) at 1 MHz

	18 °C	20 °C
Gray, edematous	0.30, 0.34	0.24, 0.29
Tumor	0.28	0.26
Gray, normal	0.17, 0.19	0.18, 0.20
White, edematous	0.15	0.15
White, normal	0.12, *0.14*	0.12, *0.14*

Normal hemisphere: gray and white matter values consistent with M78 normal brain; tumor hemisphere

Fig. 2. Detection of different biological impedance values

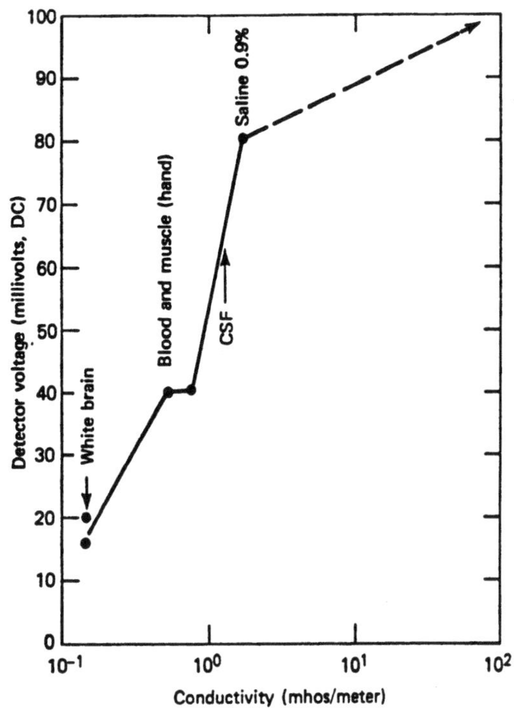

It appears from these studies that there will be a measurable and significant difference in the edematous tissue. Furthermore, it appears that the measurements conform to the assessment of edema visually and by traditional techniques. Development of a small probe for rapid, accurate, and ongoing measurement of brain edema in the laboratory animal appears to be feasible.

Measurement of Brain Edema by an External Coil

The technique utilizes a planar coil placed around the head of the animal, which is sensitive to conductivity changes in the plane of the loop. The basic principle requires a stable oscillation source to energize the coil. The conductor (the brain) is placed in the field and the conductance of the tissue in the field causes eddy currents in the plane. These eddy currents produce a secondary magnetic field which can be detected. In the megahertz range conductance dictates the changes in the secondary magnetic field. Changes outside the coil produce no effect.

Preliminary Results

Our original studies have demonstrated that accurate measurement of differences in conductivity in biological materials is possible with this technique. Figure 3 demonstrates the conductivity changes obtained by moving a metal washer through a column of mock cerebrospinal fluid. This study was undertaken to determine the

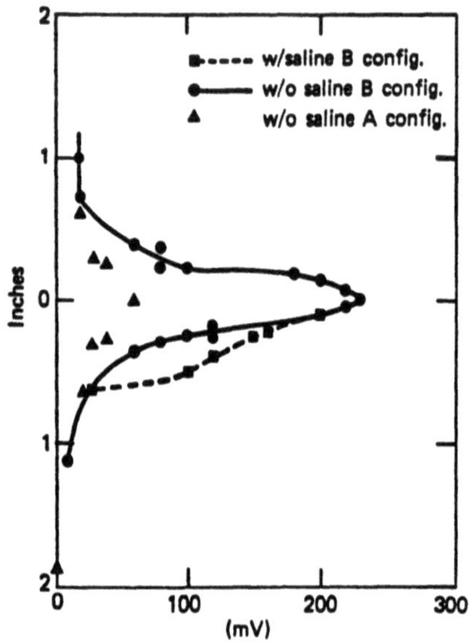

Fig. Changes in conductivity obtained by moving washer up and down through coil

feasibility of spatial localization using the coil technique. Our current project is to refine the coil and the sensors to carry out parallel studies between the invasive probes and the coil technique.

Our preliminary data indicate that it should be possible to define a system for successful measurement of brain edema in the laboratory through the use of conductance measurements. The technique appears to be as accurate as any currently in use and has the great advantage of being rapid and adaptable to continuous monitoring. Ongoing measurement of brain edema in the human using the coil technique appears to be feasible. Much improvement in design will be necessary before the technique can come into general use, but it appears to hold real promise for providing an accurate way of monitoring brain edema in the human.

Summary

Currently there is no method for ongoing measurement of developing or resolving brain edema either in the laboratory or in humans. Measurement of impedance or conductance is a known method of estimating brain water, but techniques currently available are not applicable to the usual laboratory or clinical situation. Measurement of changes in conductance offers the possibility of a longitudinal estimation of brain edema. Preliminary studies using an imposed magnetic field indicate that indwelling probes or external coils may be a feasible way of measuring brain edema. This preliminary work describes the use of these techniques to quantify changes in brain water. The results obtained with these techniques appear to warrant further exploration of the topic.

References

1. Carson BS et al. (1982) An improved rabbit brain tumor model amenable to diagnostic radiographic procedures. Neurosurgery 11:603–608
2. Geddes LA, Baker LE (1967) The specific resistance of biological material. Med Biol Eng 5:271–293
3. Lin JC, Clarke MJ (1982) 4. Imaging of cerebral edema. Proc. IEEE 70:523–524
4. Rannck JB (1963) Specific impedance of rabbit cerebral cortex. Exp Neurol 7:144–152
5. Schwan HP (1957) Electrical properties of tissue and cell suspensions. In: Advances in biology and medical physics, vol. 5. Academic, New York
6. Schwan HP (1961) Determination of biological impedances. In: Physical techniques in biological research, vol 5. Academic, New York
7. Tarjan PP, McFee R (1968) Electrodeless measurements of the effective resistivity of the human torso and head by magnetic induction. IEEE Trans Biomed Eng 15:266–278
8. Van Harreveld A (1972) The extracellular space in the vertebrate central nervous system. In: Bourne GH (ed) The structure and function of nervous tissue, vol 4. Academic, New York, pp 447–511
9. Yedlin M et al. (1974) Electrical conductivity in cat cerebellar cortex. Exp Neurol 43:555–569

Effects of Dexamethasone on the Blood-Brain Distribution of [^{125}I] Albumin and [^{14}C] Alpha-Aminoisobutyric Acid in Vasogenic Cerebral Edema

M.-H. YEN [1], D. WRIGHT, H. NAKAGAWA, R. BLASBERG, C. PATLAK, and J. FENSTERMACHER

Key words: Cerebral edema, dexamethasone, radiolabeled albumin, alpha-aminoisobutyric acid, interstitial bulk flow

Introduction

For a number of years, dexamethasone (Dex) has been used effectively to treat various kinds of cerebral edema, yet the mechanism of this drug's action remains unknown. Among the suggested mechanisms are the stabilization of membranes (e.g., capillaries) and the reduction of plasma protein and ion leakage into the brain [5]. In the present study, cerebral edema was induced in untreated and Dex-treated rats by cortical freezing, and the local distribution of two labeled markers, [^{125}I]serum albumin (RISA) and [^{14}C]alpha aminoisobutyric acid (AIB), in and around the lesion was examined by quantitative autoradiography. The findings indicate that Dex does not appreciably alter the transfer of RISA and AIB across damaged brain microvessels but does diminish the flow of RISA – and probably edema fluid – from the damaged vessels within the primary lesion into the adjacent or perilesional tissue.

Theory

The principal feature of cerebral edema is the accumulation of tissue water; accordingly, investigation of the uptake and flow of water or fluid within the blood brain CSF system is paramount for the understanding of this condition. For various physiological and technical reasons, bulk or convective flow in this system is most often studied by following the distribution of a tracer solute which is thought to be carried or entrained in the flowing "stream" of edema fluid, and not by following the distribution of tracer water. The usage of solute tracers as markers of water flow is fraught with problems, however.

The distribution of a marker in this, or any other system, depends on the rates of its diffusional and convective transfer (a) within the microvessels, (b) across the capillaries, (c) through the interstitium and CSF, and (d) across neuronal, glial, ependymal, and pia-glial membranes, and also on (e) the sizes of the various blood

[1] National Defense Medical Center, Taipei, Taiwan, Republic of China

and tissue compartments which the marker enters. In addition, the distribution pattern which is found for any marker reflects the times when blood and tissue are sampled; accordingly the sampling times are important variables in the experimental design and the interpretation of the data.

In the normal animal the cerebral plasma flow delivers RISA to CNS microvessels, where RISA very slowly penetrates into the neural parenchyma. Accordingly, RISA is often used in short-term studies (< 10 min) of normal animals as a marker of the tissue's plasma volume. In studies where the permeability of the microvessels to RISA is markedly increased, or in long-term experiments, appreciable amounts of RISA will pass across the microvessels into the surrounding interstitium. Subsequently, this RISA will move through the interstitium by diffusion and, in the presence of bulk interstitial fluid flow, by convection. In view of all this, relatively short-term RISA studies provide fairly specific information about plasma flow and the volume of the plasma compartment plus the "tightness" of the capillaries, whereas long-term ones reflect not only these processes and the plasma volume but also the rates and mechanisms of RISA distribution within the interstitium. Finally, RISA distribution depends heavily on the shape of the plasma-time curves in both short- and long-term experiments. Judicious selection of the experimental periods and the time course of plasma RISA concentration makes it possible to examine the permeability of the microvessels and the mechanisms of interstitial distribution in both control and drug-treated animals.

Tracer AIB is distributed between plasma and CNS tissue in a different manner than RISA. Both substances are carried to the tissue by the plasma; however, AIB crosses intact CNS microvessels somewhat more rapidly than RISA and is taken up by brain cells much more rapidly than RISA. Consequently, AIB tends to be trapped locally (i.e., immediately around the microvessels it passes through), and its distribution within the tissue is relatively unaffected by the bulk flow of interstitial fluid, providing that the local cellular uptake systems for AIB are not greatly compromised. Furthermore, when experimental periods (e.g., 10 min) are selected any interstitial movement of AIB will be minimized, regardless of the condition of the cellular uptake systems, and AIB distribution will primarily indicate local plasma volume and local capillary permeability.

Having applied the preceding reasoning to our study of Dex's effect on freeze-lesion-induced cerebral edema, we have chosen to investigate microvascular permeability with 30-min RISA and 10-min AIB experiments, and interstitial diffusional and convective flow with 4-h RISA experiments. All these three types of experiments were performed in both untreated and Dex-treated rats immediately after and approximately 1 day after freezing of a small portion of the right frontal cortex.

Methods

Male Sprague-Dawley rats weighing 350–400 g were divided into two groups: (a) an untreated control group, and (b) a treatment group, which was given Dex, 1.5 mg/kg IM twice daily starting 48 h before cerebral edema induction (we have used other treatment schedules but will mainly report results from this group in this paper). All rats were anesthetized, and cerebral edema was produced in the right frontal cortex by applying a freezing probe (−60 °C) to the overlying skull for 1 min. These animals were prepared for study either immediately before or approximately 1 day after cortical freezing by bilateral catheterization of the femoral arteries and veins under halothane – nitrous oxide – oxygen anesthesia. Anesthesia was then stopped, and the rats were encased in plaster casts. Thereafter, the physiological condition of all rats was monitored, and the experiment discarded if an unacceptable physiological state was not maintained. The distribution of two different radiotracers, [^{125}I] RISA and [^{14}C] AIB, was studied at two different times, immediately after and 1 day after cortical freezing. Approximately 1 ml Evans blue in physiological saline was injected IV before the beginning of each experiment. For the RISA studies an IV infusion of a solution containing RISA was begun at the start (t = 0) and was continued in such a way as to maintain a relatively constant level of iodine-125 activity in the plasma for the entire experimental period. The experimental period (namely, the RISA circulation time) was 30 min or 4 h. For the AIB studies, a bolus IV injection of the AIB- containing solution was given at t = 0, and the experiment was terminated 10 min later. For all experiments, numerous carefully timed plasma samples were obtained throughout the experimental period. At the termination of the experiment the rat was decapitated, and the brain was rapidly removed and frozen in liquid Freon cooled to −40 °C.

Radioactivity in the plasma samples was determined by either gamma (^{125}I) or beta (^{14}C) counting; radioactivity in the tissue was measured by quantitative autoradiography as described by Blasberg et al. [1–3]. The latter procedure involves cutting the brain into 20-µm-thick coronal sections in a cryostat at −20 °C and selecting a prescribed number of sections for autoradiographic assay and a matching set of adjacent sections for histological preparation. Set of iodine-125 or carbon-14 standards were included in each autoradiographic exposure. By means of these standards and an image-processing system, images of the distribution within each tissue section of either radioactivity or some function of that radioactivity was produced [2, 4].

Two different functions – the distribution space and the distribution ratio – were determined from the tissue and plasma data. The distribution space was calculated as percentage from the RISA data:

$$\text{RISA space} = (C_b/\bar{C}_p) \times 100 \qquad (1)$$

where C_b is the concentration (cpm/g) of ^{125}I-RISA in the tissue samples and $\bar{C}_p$ is the average ^{125}I concentration (cpm/ml) in the plasma. The distribution ratio (R) was calculated from the AIB data:

$$\mathrm{R} = A/\int_0^{\mathrm{T}} C_p(t)\, dt \qquad (2)$$

where A is the amount of [^{14}C] AIB per gram of brain, T is the experimental duration (in this instance, 10 min), and C_p (t) is the plasma ^{14}C concentration at t.

The histological images were digitized by a video camera system, and these images were accurately overlaid or aligned with the distribution space or distribution ratio images derived from the adjacent tissue sections by an edge-matching routine [3]. The edge of the lesion was outlined on the histological image, and simultaneously a corresponding line was drawn by the image analysis system on the func-

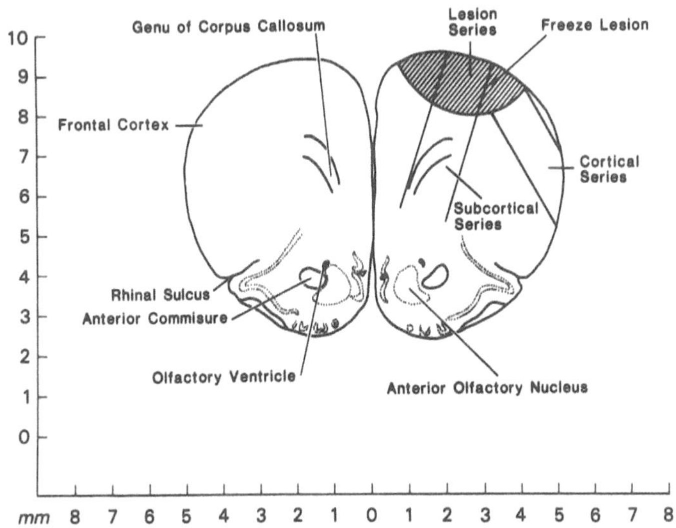

Fig. 1. Diagram of coronal brain section through the widest part of the freeze lesion. The approximate positions of the lesion, cortical, and subcortical sampling series are indicated

tional image. Subsequently, a rectangle was demarcated through the widest part of the lesion from the cortical surface to the lesion margin and into the underlying brain tissue (Fig. 1). This rectangle was divided into a series of thin sclices (usually 0.25 mm thick), enabling the analysis of either the distribution space or the distribution ratio as a function of distance within the lesion (lesion series, Fig. 1) or adjacent to the lesion (subcortical series, Fig. 1). A similar rectangle and function profile over distance was made along the cortical surface in the direction indicated in Fig. 1 (cortical series). Analysis of the images from a series of separate coronal sections yielded profiles running caudal from the edge of the lesion through cortical gray matter in addition; these profiles will also be referred to as cortical.

Results and Discussion

For the sake of brevity, much of the data produced in the course of this study will not be presented. In addition, not all the projected experiments have been performed and analyzed. In accordance with these two considerations, we will only give representative groups of data and hope that these preliminary observations will be substantiated at the conclusion of this investigation.

The RISA distribution spaces within the lesion were identical for the untreated and Dex-treated rats regardless of the experimental period or time after freezing (Fig. 2). The mean RISA spaces of the lesions ranged from 11% to 19% immediately after freezing and from 5% to 7% at 1 day after freezing. Definite conclusions about the pathophysiology and pharmacology of this apparent space change with time cannot be made at present because (a) RISA is probably distributed in both the plasma and the extracellular fluid; (b) the sizes of these two compartments are not known; (c) the rates of blood flow and transcapillary movement are probably much

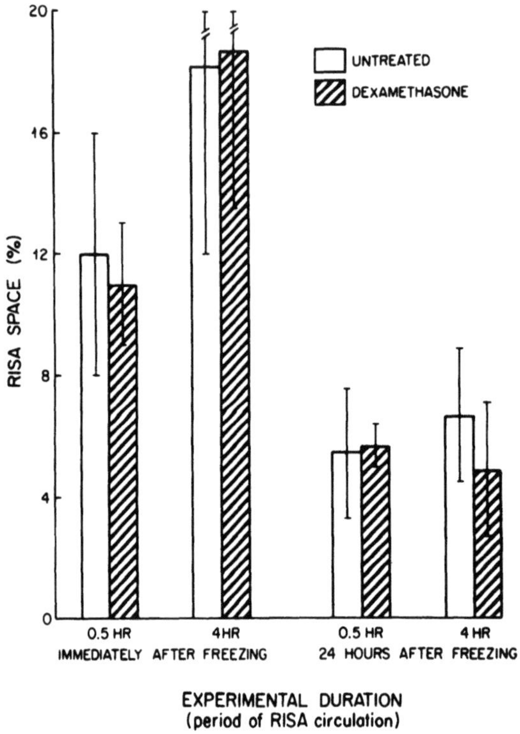

Fig. 2. Mean [^{125}I] RISA space ($\pm$ SD) within the lesion for untreated and dexamethasone-treated animals. Experimental durations and times after the cortical freezing are listed below the *abscissa*

different than normal; and (d) the sizes of these compartments and the rates of these transfer processes may be varying with time after freezing. Nevertheless, these data hint that the distribution spaces and/or rates within the lesion change over the course of the first day after cortical freezing; in addition they clearly indicate that Dex has no significant effect on the blood tissue distribution system for RISA in the lesion.

Outside of the freeze lesion area, Dex definitely changed the distribution of RISA in the 4-h experiments 1 day after freezing (Fig. 3). For both the cortex and the subcortex, the RISA space vs distance curves were higher in the untreated than in the treated rats. The shapes and positions of the two curves for the cortex, however, were different than those for the subcortex. Moreover, the 4-h RISA space data (not presented here) derived from experiments performed immediately after cortical freezing also indicate that Dex had a similar influence on the distribution of RISA in the perilesional tissue within the first several hours of cortical freezing.

Because the intravascular plasma space seems to be fairly small (about 0.5%) and uniform in the cortex outside of the lesion (unpublished data), the space vs distance curve of the untreated rats (Fig. 3, top panel) indicates that there is an appreciable amount of RISA in the interstitium of the cortex up to about 1.0 mm outside of the lesion after 4 h of RISA circulation. The shape of this curve is suggestive of diffusional, and not convective, RISA movement from the lesion into this gray matter area. The cortical space vs distance curve for the Dex-treated rats is only slightly above the vascular plasma space line, indicating that very little RISA has entered

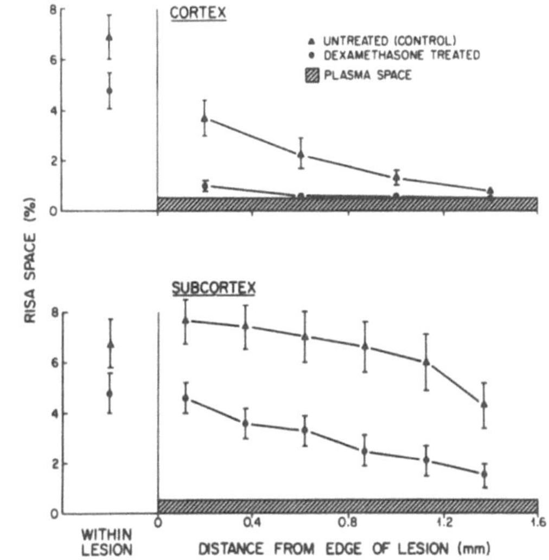

Fig. 3. Mean [^{125}I]RISA space (± SD) at various points within and around the lesion for untreated and dexamethasone-treated rats 1 day after cortical freezing. The experimental duration was 4 h

the interstitium during the 4-h experimental period. As will be more fully developed later, a likely explanation for this finding is that Dex decreases the size of the interstitium which would, in turn, increase the "resistance" to RISA movement into and through the tissue.

The space vs distance curve derived from the 4-h experiments 1 day after freezing show clear differences in RISA distribution between the cortex and subcortex (Fig. 3). Between the untreated groups the subcortical RISA spaces are larger than the cortical spaces, indicating greater movement of RISA into the interstitium of the subcortex than of the cortex. For the Dex-treated rats a similar difference between the cortical and subcortical space vs distance curves were found.

The space vs distance curves in Fig. 3 show that Dex clearly lowers the penetration of RISA into the cortical and subcortical tissue around the lesion and probably affects the transfer of other materials into the perilesional tissue in freeze-injury edema. The two transfer processes which Dex is most likely to affect in this system are diffusion and convection either (a) across the capillaries of the tissue around the lesion or (b) from the capillaries and interstitium of the lesion into the adjacent tissue. Although the appropriate analysis is still incomplete, the data from the 30-min RISA experiments suggest that Dex did not appreciably alter the interstitial uptake of RISA over this short period of time, an observation consistent with the finding just cited of a probable Dex effect on RISA movement from the lesion into the adjacent cortical and subcortical tissue in the 4-h experiments.

As previously mentioned, [^{14}C]AIB experiments of 10 min duration were performed to investigate the effects of Dex on transfer across damaged microvessels. The AIB ratios, defined as the tissue activity divided by the integral of plasma carbon-14 C activity over time (R), in the contralateral brain tissue of these animals was around 2.5×10^{-3} ml g^{-1} min^{-1}. Within the lesion, the AIB ratios ranged from 18 to 45×10^{-3} ml g^{-1} min^{-1} and were unaffected by Dex treatment. For example, Fig. 4 shows that there is no difference in the AIB ratios and ratio profiles (R vs distance) within the lesion (left side of Fig. 4) among the untreated and treated rats

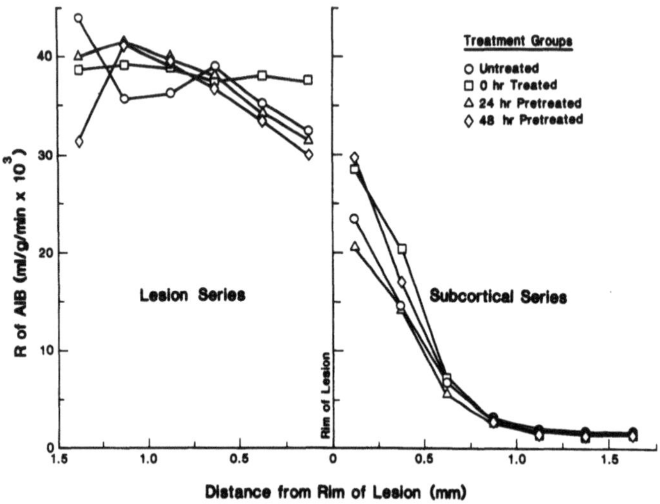

Fig. 4. Mean [^{14}C]AIB distribution ratios (R) at various distances (mm) from the rim of the lesion for untreated and dexamethasone-treated rats. The experiments were begun soon after cortical freezing and were of 10 min duration. The locations of the lesional and subcortical series are indicated in Fig. 1

studied immediately (30 min) after cortical freezing. This lack of a Dex effect on blood-to-tissue transfer within the lesion was not only found with the AIB ratios but also with the RISA spaces (Fig. 2), as previously cited. Accordingly, both these sets of data indicate that Dex does not stabilize or normalize solute transfer across leaky, freeze-damaged microvessels and imply that Dex has little effect on the formation of edema fluid at the microvessels within the lesion. Dexamethasone also did not affect the AIB ratios and ratio profiles of the tissues adjacent to the lesion. For instance, the subcortical AIB ratios of Fig. 4 for all groups are around 25×10^{-3} ml g^{-1} min^{-1} next to the lesion and fall to $2-3 \times 10^{-3}$ ml g^{-1} min^{-1} by 1.0 mm. These and other data certainly indicate that Dex does not appreciably alter the transport processes (blood flow and capillary permeability) and compartments (the vascular space and the surface area and volume of the microvessels) which are involved in the distribution of AIB to the adjacent tissue in the first 10 min following IV administration.

Incidentally, the AIB ratios in the tissue within 0.5 mm of the lesion were always higher than normal (i.e., $2-3 \times 10^{-3}$ ml min^{-1} g^{-1}). This elevation of the AIB ratio may be primarily caused by an artifact of the quantitative autoradiographic technique [6] and may not indicate that the permeability of the capillaries is higher than normal in the tissue immediately around the lesion.

Five points emerge from these preliminary findings. First, Dex does not affect the distribution of RISA and AIB in the tissue directly damaged by freezing; hence this drug probably does not act against this type of edema within the lesion itself. Second, in the 4-h experiments, Dex altered the RISA ratio profiles in the tissue adjacent to the lesion; the change in the shape and position of the subcortical (white matter) profile curve suggests that Dex reduced the convective flow of edema fluid in this region. Third, in the 30-min experiments, the RISA space profiles of the tissue adjacent to the lesion were not appreciably altered by Dex. Fourth, Dex did not detectably affect the 10-min distribution ratios of AIB in the tissue adjacent to the lesion. Fifth, these observations lead to the hypothesis that Dex reduces cerebral edema by increasing the resistance to bulk fluid flow from the leaky vessels and the interstitium of the lesion into the surrounding tissue (in particular, into white matter) and does not act by diminishing the flow of solutes and water across damaged vessels in and around the lesion. Such an increase in resistance could be accomplished either by decreasing the size of the interstitium – probably as a result of cellular swelling – or by changing the structure of the extracellular matrix.

Summary

The effects of dexamethasone (Dex) on the blood-brain distribution of [^{14}C]alpha aminoisobutyric acid (AIB) and [^{125}I]albumin (RISA) was studied in the rat freeze-lesion model of cerebral edema. Untreated and Dex-treated rats were studied by IV administration of either AIB or RISA immediately after or 1 day after localized cortical freezing. The AIB experiments were terminated after 10 min; the RISA experiments were terminated after 30 min or 4 h. Local tissue distribution of AIB and RISA was assessed by quantitative autoradiography. The distribution of both RISA and AIB within the lesion was unaffected by Dex. In the tissue around the lesion, Dex did not alter the distribution of AIB in the 10-min experiments or that of RISA in the 30-min experiments. Dex did, however, diminish the movement of RISA into the adjacent tissue during the 4-h experiments. The intralesional AIB and RISA distribution data plus the perilesional 10-min AIB and 30-min RISA distribution data indicate that Dex does not act by reducing the flow of solutes and water across damaged or leaky vessels in and around the lesion. The 4-h RISA data suggest that Dex alters the structure of the extracellular space in the tissue around the lesion (especially in the white matter) and thereby increases the resistance of the interstitium to the flow of solutes and fluid from the lesion into the adjacent tissue.

Acknowledgements. The authors gratefully acknowledge the technical support of Mr. Ernest Owens, Mr. Roosevelt Hyman, and Ms. Martina McClain plus the secretarial assistance of Ms. Beverly Gabriel.

References

1. Blasberg, R, Gazendem J, Patlak C, Fenstermacher J (1980) Quantitative autoradiographic studies of brain edema and a comparison of multi-isotope autoradiographic techniques. Adv Neurol 28:255–270
2. Blasberg R, Groothuis D, Molnar P (1981) The application of quantitative autoradiographic measurements in experimental brain tumors. Semin Neurol 1:203–223
3. Blasberg R, Molnar P, Groothuis D, Patlak C, Owens E, Fenstermacher J (1985) Concurrent measurements of blood flow and transcapillary transport in ASV-induced experimental brain tumors. J Pharmacol Exp Ther (in press)
4. Goochee C, Rasband W, Sokoloff L (1980) Computerized densitometry and color coding of [^{14}C] deoxyglucose autoradiographs. Ann Neurol 7:359–370
5. Marshall L (1980) Treatment of brain swelling and brain edema in man. Adv Neurol 28:459–469
6. Smith C (1983) Localization of activity-associated changes in metabolism of the central nervous system with the deoxyglucose method: prospects for cellular resolution. In: Barker J, McKelvey J (eds) Current methods in cellular biology. Wiley, New York, pp 270–317

Effect of Dexamethasone on Regional Cerebral Blood Flow and on Serum Protein Extravasation in Experimental Brain Infarcts in Monkeys

A. HARTMANN[1], K.-A. HOSSMANN, Z. CZERNICKI, L. M. BARBOSA-COUTINHO, G. EBHARDT, and J. MENZEL

Key words: Experimental infarcts, dexamethasone, brain edema, rCBF

Introduction

The effect of dexamethasone on brain infarcts has been the subject of numerous clinical and experimental studies [3, 4, 7, 8]. In most experimental investigations no beneficial effect of dexamethasone has been found. However, clinical studies and practice have suggested such an effect [1, 11]. The known experimental studies deal with the early phase of infarct when the vasogenic perifocal edema has not yet developed. On the other hand, a beneficial effect of dexamethasone in stroke patients has been observed many hours and even days after the stroke. Therefore, in the present investigation the effect of dexamethasone treatment on experimental brain infarcts has been studied over a long period.

Materials and Methods

The studies were performed in 33 adult baboons of both sexes, 21 being used for rCBF studies and 12, for serum extravasation studies. In all animals the left middle cerebral artery (MCA) was clipped via the transorbital approach. The technical details are given elsewhere [5]. Figure 1 shows the protocol for the rCBF study.

Among 21 monkeys 8 animals were treated with dexamethasone and the other 13 were untreated. The rCBF studies were performed before clipping, 1 h after clipping, 3 h after, 7 days after, and 28 days after. On each occasion rCBF was measured in three ways: under normal steady state conditions; with hypercapnia, to study the CO_2 reactivity factor; and during slight arterial hypotension to study vascular autoregulation. Dexamethasone was given IM at a dose of 1 mg/kg/day beginning 45 min after clipping up to the 10th day after clipping. Then the dose was reduced to zero until the 13th day.

Protein extravasation was evaluated in 12 animals. The animals were divided into two groups. One group (7 animals) was treated with dexamethasone 1 mg/kg/day, while the other 5 monkeys were not treated. One week after permanent clipping the animals were sacrificed, the brains were removed and fixed in 4% formalin, and the

---

[1] Universitätsnervenklinik, Abt. für Radiologie, Sigmund-Freud-Str. 25, D-5300 Bonn 1

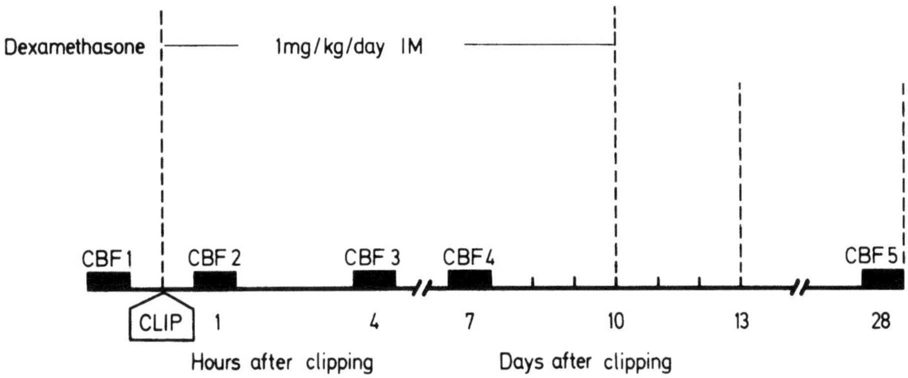

Fig. 1. Protocol of the CBF study. CBF measurements (CBF 1–5) were taken before clipping, 1 and 4 h after clipping and 7 and 28 days after. Dexamethasone was given at a dose of 1 mg/kg/day IM from day 1 to day 10, with subsequent dose reduction until day 13. From day 13 to day 28 no steroids were given

protein extravasation was studied immunologically with normal goat serum, rabbit anti-baboon serum, goat anti-rabbit serum, and the soluble rabbit peroxidase anti-peroxidase complex [2]. The volume of infarcted and edematous brain tissue was determined planimetrically on microphotographs of each coronal slice and expressed as a percentage of the total brain volume [2].

Results

Cerebral Blood Flow

Figure 2a shows the rCBF changes. In the anterior and posterior cerebral artery (ACA/PCA) regions rCBF was significantly higher in the dexamethasone-treated group 7 days after occlusion. The MCA region values were similar in both groups. At 28 days after clipping CBF was higher in all regions in the treated animals. However, a significant increase was observed only in the PCA region.

The CO_2 reactivity studies are shown in Fig. 2b. In all treated animals the values on the 7th and 27th days were significantly higher. The early changes were especially pronounced in the MCA and PCA regions.

Autoregulation increased significantly after 7 days in all treated animals. The autoregulation changes were especially pronounced in the MCA and PCA regions (Fig. 2c).

Morphologic Studies

Brain infarcts were found in the left MCA region in all animals.

In the untreated monkeys the infarcts were surrounded by more severe brain edema. In the animals treated with dexamethasone swelling was less pronounced or absent (Fig. 3).

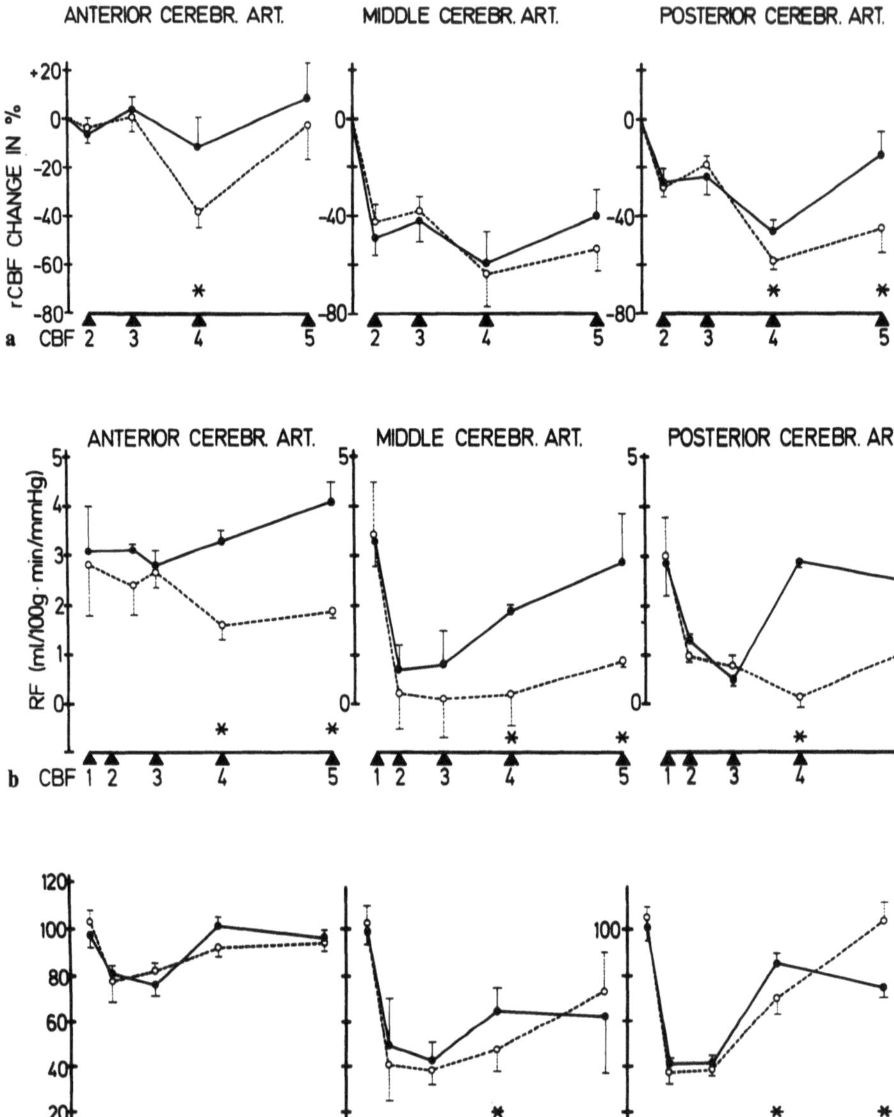

Fig. 2. **a** rCBF, **b** blood gas reactivity, and **c** autoregulation in treated (*solid line*) and nontreated animals (*broken line*). rCBF changes (**a**) are expressed as percentages compared with the actual value in CBF 1 (steady state). Blood gas reactivity (**b**) is expressed as the change in rCBF (ml/100 g/min) per mmHg of $PaCO_2$. Autoregulation (**c**) is expressed as percentage change in rCBF during mild hypotension compared with the actual CBF value recorded at each measurement

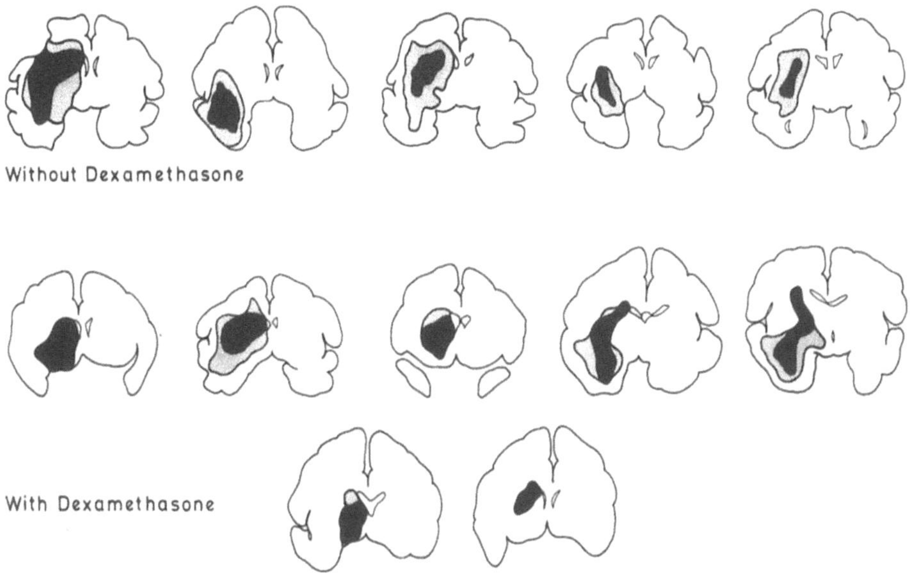

Fig. 3. Distribution and size of infarction (*black area*) and edematous zone (*dotted area*) in untreated and dexamethasone-treated animals

Table 1. Volume of infarct and peri-infarct edema in monkeys 1 week after left middle cerebral artery occlusion

	Infarct (percent hemisphere)	Edema (percent hemisphere)	Serum protein extravasation	
			Optical density (OD)	Volume × OD
Untreated animals (means ± SD)	6.57 ± 4.23	7.83 ± 2.93	0.100 ± 0.057	0.896 ± 0.841
Dexamethasone treatment (means ± SD)	7.95 ± 3.00 NS	2.82 ± 3.06*	0.059 ± 0.030 NS	0.260 ± 0.263 NS

* $P < 0.05$; NS, not significant

The morphometric results are summarized in Table 1. The infarct volume in the two animal groups was not significantly different but the volume of perifocal edema was distinctly larger in the untreated animals.

Discussion

The rCBF values obtained result from two factors: primary ischemia and perifocal edema. In the MCA region the initial decrease in rCBF, impairment of CO_2 reactivity, and changes of autoregulation are caused by the infarct. The changes in other regions, especially the changes after 7 days, are the effect of progressing edema.

The beneficial effect of dexamethasone was observed only in edematous areas when the infarct remained unchanged. The beneficial effect of dexamethasone on vasogenic cerebral edema has been shown by many authors [6, 9], and our own studies have confirmed such an effect.

The morphometric evaluation demonstrated that the rCBF improvement in the dexamethasone group of animals was due to the reduction in the perifocal edema and not to the altered size of the lesion. Such an effect of dexamethasone could explain the discrepancy in the literature between the experimental and clinical studies [1, 3, 8]. The experimental studies are concerned with the early phase of infarct development at a time when there is no evidence of an edema effect. In the clinical studies, however, the steroids are given later and for a longer period and affecting the development of vasogenic edema. The beneficial effect of dexamethasone on brain edema and morphological criteria [11] might be connected with the beneficial effect of steroids on cell metabolism that has recently been reported [10].

Summary

The possible effect of dexamethasone on ischemic brain edema was evaluated in two studies: In monkeys (baboons) with permanent occlusion of the middle cerebral artery regional cerebral blood flow (rCBF) was studied over 4 weeks using the intraarterial xenon-133 technique; in the ischemic territory rCBF was the same after steroids as in untreated control baboons. In the adjacent areas rCBF, autoregulation, and blood gas reactivity were better after dexamethasone on the 7th day. The survival rate at 4 weeks was significantly better in the treated animals.

In 12 animals protein extravasation was tested after 7 days of complete MCA occlusion. Half these animals were treated and the others, not. Extravasation was examined by immunohistochemical means. The size of infarct was the same in both groups, but on the 7th day the volume of peri-infarction edema was significantly larger in the untreated animals. We conclude that high-dose dexamethasone can prevent the spread of edema caused by cerebral ischemia to noninfarcted tissue and also prevent a secondary reduction of rCBF in the perifocal tissue.

References

1. Anderson DC, Cranford RE (1979) Corticosteroids in ischemic stroke. Stroke 10:68–71
2. Barbosa-Coutinho LM, Hartmann A, Hossmann K-A, Rommel T (1984) Effect of dexamethasone on serum protein extravasation in experimental brain infarcts of monkey: an immunohistochemical study. Acta Neuropathol (in press)
3. Bremer AM, Yamada K, West CR (1980) Ischemic cerebral edema in primates: Effects of acetazolamide, phenytoin, sorbitol, dexamethasone, and methylprednisolone on brain water and electrolytes. Neurosurgery 6:149–154
4. Fenske A, Fischer M, Regli F, Hase U (1979) The response of focal ischemic cerebral edema to dexamethasone. J Neurol 220:199–209
5. Hartmann A, Menzel J, Buttinger C, Lange D, Alberti E (1981) Regional cerebral blood flow in the baboon during ischemic cerebral infarction under dexamethasone treatment. Fortschr Neurol Psychiatr 49:380–392

6. Hossmann K-A, Hürter T, Oschlies U (1983) The effect of dexamethasone on serum protein extravasation and edema development in experimental brain tumors of cat. Acta Neuropathol (Berl) 60:223–231
7. Kahn K, Pranzarone G, Newman T (1972) Dexamethasone treatment of experimental cerebral infarction. Neurology 22:406–407
8. Lee MC, Mastri AR, Waltz AG, Loewenson RB (1974) Ineffectiveness of dexamethasone treatment of experimental cerebral infarction. Stroke 5:216–225
9. Pappius HM (1982) Dexamethasone and local cerebral glucose utilization in freeze-traumatized rat brain. Ann Neurol 12:157–162
10. Pappius HM, Wolfe LS (1983) Functional disturbances in brain following injury: search for underlying mechanisms. Neurochem Res 8:63–72
11. Sage JI, van Uitert RL (1982) Clinical benefit of steroids in early postischemic disruption of the blood-brain barrier. Ann Neurol 12:84–85

Distribution, Uptake Kinetics, and Receptor Binding of Glucocorticosteroids in Rat Brain Edema

H. KOSTRON [1], I. MOHSENIPOUR, and G. DAXENBICHLER

Key words: Brain edema, steroids, uptake kinetics, glucocorticoid receptors

Introduction

Gluococorticoids are widely used in the treatment of brain edema associated with brain tumors and with severe head injury. Whereas the first type clearly benefits from treatment with steroids [17], their therapeutic use in head injury still remains controversial [6, 9]. Despite many efforts to elucidate the exact molecular mechanisms of steroid action only partial knowledge has been achieved. Besides the systemic effect on the general metabolism, steroids inhibit the breakdown of the phospholipid layers of cell membranes and subcellular organelles by blocking various phosphatases [13]. Furthermore, the formation of arachidonic acid is inhibited, which is the "second messenger" that otherwise prolongs the postinjury self-destruction process [4]. Certain steroid hormones are taken up both by a specific saturable process into a specific part of the brain and by a nonspecific diffusion-like uptake into all parts of the brain [12]. To our knowledge there are no experimental data available indicating how the uptake kinetics of glucocorticoids change in vasogenic brain edema. Furthermore, GCRs demonstrated in various tissues and tumors are now increasingly being considered for therapeutic applications [3, 8, 14]. Glucocorticoid receptors have also been found in the brain tissue, mainly localized in neurons of the diencephalon [18]. It is still not known what role these receptors play in head injury and whether they are necessary for [^{3}H]dexamethasone ([^{3}H]DM) to take effect.

The object of this study was to find out first, whether there is a homogeneous uptake into all anatomical locations of the rat brain; second, whether there is a preferential uptake of DM into traumatized brain tissue; third, what changes occur in the cellular (glia cells, neurons) and subcellular distribution; and fourth, whether trauma induces the formation of GCR-binding sites.

Methods

Male rats weighing 100–150 g were used throughout the experiments. [^{3}H]DM (0.3 mCi made up with unlabeled DM to a final concentration of 1 mg/kg body weight) was injected via the tail vein 1 h after induction of the cold lesion. All ani-

[1] Clinic for Neurosurgery, University of Innsbruck, Anichstraße 35, A-6020 Innsbruck, Austria

mals were killed by cervical dislocation 30 min after the injection of [^{3}H]DM. The desired tissues were dissected, washed three times in buffer (280 m*M* glucose, 280 m*M* fructose, 10 m*M* KH_2PO_4, pH 6.0), and weighed on an analytical scale. Aliquots of the tissues were dissolved in 2 ml Protosol (NEN, Boston) and counted in a liquid scintillation counter with 12 ml Econofluor (NEN, Boston). Astrocytes and neurons were prepared according to a modified procedure of Farooque et al. [5], which is described in detail elsewhere [11]. The subcellular distribution was determined by sucrose gradient technique and fractionated centrifugation [11]. The protein measurements were carried out according to Lowry.

For the GCR studies the rats were adrenalectomized 4–5 days before the experiments. The animals were maintained on 0.9% sodium chloride and standard laboratory rat chow. The completeness of adrenalectomy was screened by blood sampling before sacrifice of the animals and assay of the plasma corticosterone concentration.

Cold Lesion

The right hemisphere was exposed with a dental drill while the animals were anesthesized with thiopental supplemented with ether. A glass pipet was cooled in liquid nitrogen and was placed on the exposed cortex for 40 s.

Receptor Assay

Samples were homogenized in PMG buffer (20 m*M* Na phosphate, 15 m*M* Na molybdate, 1.5 m*M* EDTA, 5 m*M* monothioglycerol, 3 m*M* Na azide, 10% glycerol, pH 7.5) with an Ultra Turrax (Janke & Kunkel, Germany). Aliquots of the cytosol were incubated for 15 h at 4 °C either with increasing concentrations of [^{3}H]DM alone (total binding) or in the presence of a 200-fold excess of unlabeled DM (nonspecific binding) [1]. The free and protein-bound steroid fractions were separated with dextran-coated charcoal [10]. Specific binding was evaluated by Scatchard plot analysis [15] and related to the protein content of the cytosol. Protein concentration was determined by the Coomassie Blue method [2].

Results

Regional Distribution

In the control animals 26% and 25% of the [^{3}H]DM was found in the right and left hemispheres, respectively. Cerebellum and brainstem contained about the same amounts (24% and 25%, respectively). After induction of the cold lesion the [^{3}H]DM content increased to 40% in the traumatized hemisphere and to 34% in the contralateral hemisphere (Fig. 1). Before the trauma the DM content in the gray and white matter was 6.7 pg/mg and 5.5 pg/mg and after the trauma 8.3 pg/mg and 5.7 pg/mg fresh tissue, respectively. When the brain was removed after various periods of [^{3}H]DM infusion we found a rapid decrease of the [^{3}H]DM content in the brain tis-

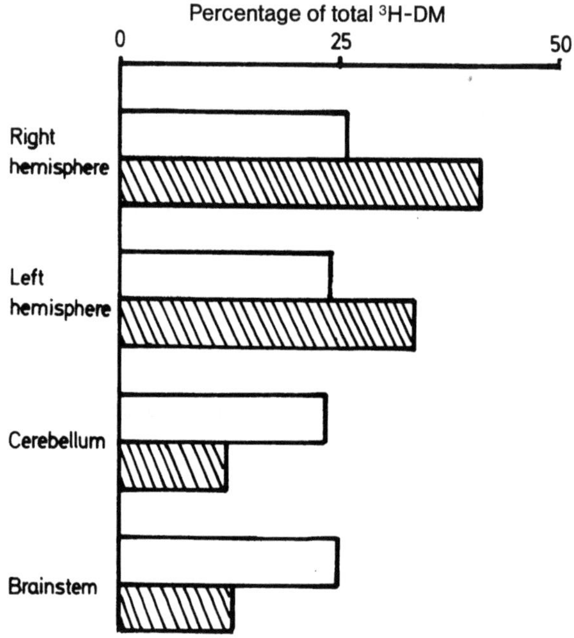

Fig. 1. Regional distribution of [^{3}H]DM in normal rat brain and in rat brain after trauma of the right hemisphere (*hatched bars*). $n=9$ for each data point

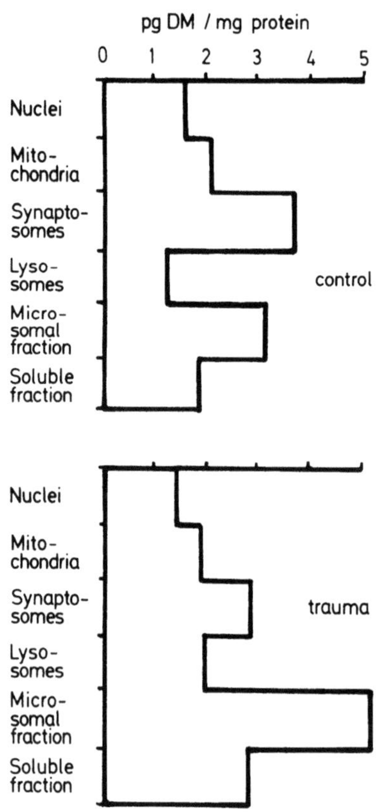

Fig. 2. Subcellular distribution of [^{3}H]DM in normal and traumatized brain cells. $n=8$

sue. After 10 min 74%, after 30 min 13%, and after 60 min 8% of the dexamethasone concentrations found after 2.5 min could be recovered. When the cell suspension was stored for 48 h on ice, 79% of the [^{3}H]DM was released into the medium and 21% retained intracellularly, as against 40% and 60% in normal brain cells, respectively.

Cellular and Subcellular Distribution

In the control hemisphere 75% of the DM was found in astrocytes and 25% in neurons (Fig. 2). After the trauma DM shifted to the neurons and 48% was recovered in the astrocytes and 52% in neurons ($P < 0.02$). In the control hemisphere 12% was bound to nuclei, 15% to mitochondria, 26% to synaptosomes, 9% to lysosomes, and 22% to microsomes, and 13% was found in a soluble, trichloroacetic-acid-precipitable fraction. After the trauma 9% was found in the nuclei, 12% in the mitochondria, 18% in the lysosomes, 32% in microsomes, and 17% in the soluble fraction. [^{3}H]DM was taken up by normal rat brain cells to a level of 5.05 ± 1.34 nmol/min/mg protein. The uptake leveled off at a concentration above 0.1 m*M* DM in the medium and was linear up to 10 min. There was a slight increase in the rate of uptake at 37 °C compared with 4 °C. When [^{3}H]DM was incubated with cells derived from traumatized brain tissue the uptake was concentration dependent and no saturation could be achieved.

Glucocorticoid Receptors

Male rats were adrenalectomized 4–5 days before induction of the cold lesion. The amount of GCRs was the same in the right and left hemispheres. In the experimental animals the brain tissue was assayed for GCRs at different times after cold lesion induction (see Table 1). There was a tendency for the density of receptor sites to increase during the first 24 h, while after the 2nd and 4th days we found exactly the same amount of receptor sites as in the control animals. The contralateral, nontraumatized, hemisphere was also used as a control, and its receptor sites increased in density in parallel with those in the traumatized hemisphere. However, no increase in receptor site density was observed after trauma in animals that had not been adrenalectomized (data not stated), in addition to which a lower level of GCR-

Table 1. Time course of glucocorticoid receptor binding sites after trauma

	Control	1 h	2 h	6 h	12 h	1 day	2 days	4 days
Right hemisphere (cold lesion)	240	238	297	361	322	318	253	242
Left hemisphere (internal control)	254	287	287	344	337	278	194	261

Data were calculated from three animals and are expressed as median values (range 148%–75%) in fmol/mg protein (confidence level 0.94–0.99 [15])

binding sites was detected. The K_d range for GCRs in the adrenalectomized rats was $4-7 \times 10^{-10}$ *M*, whereas that for GCRs in nonadrenalectomized animal cells was $1.5-4.5 \times 10^{-9}$ *M*.

Discussion

These studies were performed to demonstrate the homogeneous uptake of DM in normal rat brain and to examine whether there is preferential uptake of DM into traumatized brain tissue. Furthermore, uptake kinetics were investigated in isolated brain cells, which were then separated into a glial and neuronal fraction. The GCR level was determined in normal and traumatized brain tissue in adrenalectomized rats.

Under normal conditions almost identical DM concentrations were found in all parts of the brain investigated. At 1 h after induction of the cold lesion a significant increase in [^{3}H]DM uptake in the damaged hemisphere was found. Interestingly, the contralateral hemisphere, which served as a control, also showed increased uptake of DM. Recently it has been demonstrated that DM increases cerebral blood flow in cerebral infarction, but also in the contralateral hemisphere. Furthermore, autoregulation was ameliorated [7].

Our results do not indicate conclusively whether the observed uptake into the damaged hemisphere is caused by hyperemia or by an increased cellular uptake itself. In these time course studies the DM content declined rapidly within 30 min. There was no clear difference between the traumatized and contralateral hemisphere. When isolated brain cells were incubated with [^{3}H]DM, we found a concentration and time-dependent uptake, which did not depend on temperature. However, in brain cells derived from traumatized brain the process was not saturable in this way, depending in contrast on the DM concentration in the medium. This diffusion-like uptake might be due to increased membrane permeability, causing DM to enter the intracellular space readily, but obviously it is not connected with proteins, since the DM concentration decreases rapidly when tissue is stored on ice. Another interesting finding in these experiments was the shift of DM to neurons after the trauma. We did not investigate whether this increased uptake into neurons was the cause of the general increase in uptake in traumatized tissue. Subcellular analyses of the DM uptake revealed higher concentration in lysosomal and microsomal structures in the damaged cells than in normal ones. This could explain the protective effect of steroids as an inhibiton of lysosomal enzymes, whereas it remains to be investigated whether the microsomes regain the ability to synthesize proteins faster after steroid administration. The role of GCRs in brain edema was also examined. Our results show a slight increase in the density of GCR sites in traumatized tissue, which was also paralleled by an increase in the contralateral hemisphere. Because of the consistency of our derived data we conclude that trauma produced by cold lesion induces some formation of GCR sites, as already shown for other systems [16]. However, the increase in the density of receptor sites was too slight to be of significant therapeutic value. Noteworthy is the parallel increase of cerebral blood flow, DM concentration, and GCR sites in the contralateral hemisphere, which strongly suggests that neurogenic factors are involved.

This paper demonstrates that DM is preferentially taken up by traumatized brain tissue and by subcellular organelles which are involved in the maintenance of brain cells. The specific uptake of DM gives way to a diffusion-like uptake in the damaged brain cells. The beneficial effect of steroids might be caused by the significant increase in their intracellular concentration and is obviously not due to an increase in GCR binding sites. Our results suggest a high dose of steroids in the treatment of patients suffering from brain edema after head injury.

Acknowledgments. The experiments were partly carried out in the Department of Pharmacology with the kind permission of H. Winkler. The authors wish to thank Ms. Barbara Schmid for excellent technical assistance.

Summary

[^{3}H]Dexamethasone ([^{3}H]DM) is taken up in equal amounts in the two hemispheres containing brainstem and cerebellum of the rat brain. Trauma of the right hemisphere produced by cold lesion resulted in an increased uptake of DM into the lesioned hemisphere. Time course studies revealed a rapid decline in the [^{3}H]DM content. Before induction of the lesion 75% of the [^{3}H]DM was confined to astrocytes and 25% to neurons, while after the trauma 48% of the DM was localized in the astrocytes and 52% in neurons. Subcellularly an accumulation of DM took place in the microsomal, lysosomal, and cytoplasmic fraction of the damaged cells. The suturable process in the normal rat brain is lost to a diffusion-like uptake in the traumatized cells. In adrenalectomized rats glucocorticoid receptors (GCRs) were increased in brain tissue in the contralateral hemisphere also after cold lesion.

The data presented demonstrate a significantly increased accumulation of DM in the traumatized brain tissue, accumulation in neurons, and increased diffusion-like uptake into damaged cells. Glucocorticoid receptors did not change significantly at the trauma site. These results might further explain steroid action at the cellular and subcellular level and suggest the use of high-dose glucocorticoids in the treatment of brain edema following severe head injury also.

References

1. Bichler A, Wiesinger J, Mayr M (1978) Spezifische Glukokortikoidrezeptoraktivität in der Lunge und Corticosteroidgehalt im Plasma neugeborener Kaninchen in der 1. Lebensstunde. Arch Gynäkol 226:307
2. Bradford MM (1976) A rapid and sensitive method for the quantitation of microgram quantities of protein utilizing the principle of protein dye-binding. Anal Biochem 72:248–254
3. Braunschweiger PG, Ting HL, Schiffer LM (1983) Correlation between glucocorticoid receptor content and the antiproliferative effect of dexamethasone in experimental solid tumors. Cancer Res 43:4757–4761
4. Chan PH, Fishman RA (1984) The role of arachidonic acid in vasogenic brain edema. Fed Proc 43:210–213
5. Farooqu M, Norton WT (1978) A modified procedure for isolation of astrocyte and neuron-enriched fractions from rat brain. J Neurochem 31:887–894

6. Gobiet W (1976) The influence of various stages of dexamethasone on intracranial pressure and patients with severe head injury. In: Pappius H, Feindel W (eds) Dynamics of brain edema. Springer, Berlin Heidelberg New York, pp 351–355
7. Hartmann A, Menzel J, Buttinger C, Lange D, Alberti E (1981) The regional cerebral circulation in ischemic cerebral infarction in baboons treated with dexamethasone. Fortschr Neurol Psychiatry 10:380–392
8. Homo-DeLarche (1984) Glucocorticoid receptor and steroid sensitivity in normal and neoplastic human lymphoid tissue: a review. Cancer Res 44:431–437
9. Hoppe E, Christensen L, Christensen KN (1981) The clinical outcome of patients with severe head injuries, treated with high dose dexamethasone, hyperventilation and barbiturates. Neurochirurgia (Stuttg) 24:17–20
10. Korenman SG, Dukes BA (1970) Specific estrogen binding by the cytoplasm of human breast carcinoma. J Clin Endocrinol Metab 30:639
11. Kostron H, Fischer J (1983) Regional, cellular and subcellular distribution of (^{3}H) dexamethasone in rat brain edema. Surg Neurol 20:48–54
12. McEwen BS, Weiss JM, Schwartz LS (1969) Uptake of corticosterone by rat brain and its concentration by certain limbic structures. Brain Res 16:227–241
13. Rehncrona S, Westerberg E, Akesson B, Siesjö BK (1982) Brain cortical fatty acids and phospholipids during and following complete and severe incomplete ischemia. J Neurochem 38:84–93
14. Rengachary SS, Tilzer LL (1981) A study of dexamethasone receptor protein in human gliomas. J Surg 31:447–455
15. Scatchard G (1979) The attractions of proteins for small molecules and ions. Proc Natl Acad Sci USA 51:660–672
16. Schmidt TJ, Litwack G (1982) Activation of the glucocorticoid-receptor complex. J Am Phys 62:1131–1192
17. Yamada K, Ushio Y, Hayakawa T, Arita N, Yamada Y, Mogami H (1983) Effects of methylprednisolone on peritumoral brain edema. A quantitative autoradiographic study. J Neurosurg 59:612–619
18. Yu ZY, Wrange Ö, Boethius J, Gustafson JA, Granholm L (1981) A qualitative comparison of the glucocorticoid receptor in cytosol from human brain and rat brain. Brain Res 223:325–333

Osmotic Dehydrating Agents Reduce Intracranial Pressure After Severe Head Injuries Mainly Through Vasoconstriction *

J. P. MUIZELAAR [1], H. A. LUTZ, and D. P. BECKER

Key words: Mannitol, intracranial pressure, cerebral blood flow, autoregulation, blood viscosity

Introduction

It is generally thought that mannitol and other so-called osmotic agents such as urea and glycerol act through extraction of water from the cerebral extracellular space into the intravascular compartment by induction of a difference in osmotic pressure between the blood and the brain. It has remained unclear, however, whether water is better extracted from edematous brain [1, 24] or from normal brain [6, 10], and there is even evidence that there may be hardly any influence at all exerted upon brain water content according to measurements performed with the very sensitive specific gravity technique [23]. Moreover, a clear relationship between changes in brain water content and intracranial pressure (ICP) has not always been shown with the use of osmotic agents [1, 10, 22].

An unexplained phenomenon has been reported by Bruce and coworkers [4, 13]. They found that mannitol administration in head-injured patients may result in an increase in cerebral blood flow (CBF) without a decrease in ICP; i.e., without a change in cerebral perfusion pressure (CPP) [4, 13], In their publications on this topic it was not mentioned, however, whether this increase in CBF was found only, or mainly, in patients in whom ICP did not decrease, and no statement concerning the status of pressure autoregulation in this particular group of patients was made. Although osmotic agents do not appear to have an influence upon CBF in normal experimental animals [11, 12] they have been found to increase CBF in pathologic conditions [3, 16].

In a previous paper [17] we have shown that IV administration of mannitol in the cat leads to quick changes in blood viscosity, which in turn lead to changes in vessel diameter with concomitant changes in ICP. We postulated that these changes were

---

* The work described in this paper was supported by NIH grant NS-12587 and the Richard Roland Reynolds Neurosurgical Research Laboratory. The tables and parts of the text have already been published elsewhere (Muizelaar JP, Lutz HA, Becker DP (1984) Effect of mannitol on ICP and CBF and correlation with pressure regulation in severely head-injured patients. J Neurosurg 61:700–706) and appears here by permission of the American Association of Neurological Surgeons.

[1] Division of Neurosurgery, Medical College of Virginia, Virginia Commonwealth University, Richmond, Virginia, USA

similar in mechanism to alterations in vessel diameter with blood pressure changes and therefore "blood viscosity autoregulation" would be a new entity in the same category as "pressure autoregulation."

In the present paper, we describe the relationship that exists between the responses of ICP and CBF after mannitol administration and the presence or absence of pressure autoregulation in a group of severely head-injured patients.

Materials and Methods

Patients

Measurements of CBF and ICP were recorded in patients with severe head injury admitted to the neurosurgical intensive care unit of the Medical College of Virginia Hospital in Richmond. We included only patients who were not able to follow simple commands (motor score: localizing or worse) for at least 6 h. These patients are managed in a standard fashion as described earlier [2, 15]. Thus, all the patients in the present study were intubated and received artificial respiration with a mechanical ventilator.

ICP was measured with an intraventricular catheter or with the Richmond bolt [26] and digitally displayed as mean ICP (diastolic + ⅓ pulse pressure). Blood pressure was measured by means of an intraarterial catheter (usually the radial artery) and digitally displayed as systolic, diastolic, and mean (mean arterial blood pressure, MABP = diastolic + ⅓ pulse pressure).

End-expiratory CO_2 was monitored continuously with a Hewlett-Packard capnometer, and during each CBF measurement an arterial blood sample was taken for $PaCO_2$ and other blood gas measurements. All CBF data were reduced to a standard $PaCO_2$ of 34 mmHg by assuming a 3% change in CBF per torr $PaCO_2$ [18], to allow easier comparison of these data with recent literature data [18, 19].

Measurement of CBF

For the measurement of CBF we used the xenon-133 inhalation technique according to Obrist et al. [20]. We have developed a xenon-133 gas delivery and collection system which can be driven by the patient's ventilator but which does not contaminate the ventilator at all with radioactive gas. The CBF system itself consisted of a Harshaw Tasc-5 system with 16 probes (8 over each hemisphere) arrayed concentrically in a Plexiglas helmet.

The patient's head was placed in the helmet and the gas manipulation system was connected; the end-expiratory CO_2 and ICP were then allowed to stabilize. The patient breathed a gas mixture containing 8 mCi xenon-133/liter for 1 min and the washout and air curves were monitored for a further 14 min after that. After any necessary editing of the curves, the computer calculated a number of flow indices. Of these various indices we have only used the CBF infinity in the present paper. The CBF infinity is a combination of fast and slow flow compartments and is not sensitive to slippage [21], which is particularly important in pathologic circumstances and during tests of autoregulation. In this study no large hemispheric or regional differences were found; therefore, we have combined the 16 regional flows into one global CBF curve.

Tests of Pressure Autoregulation

After a baseline CBF measurement had been obtained, the patient's blood pressure was slowly raised with IV administration of phenylephrine in saline (80 mg/500 ml) to a value 30% higher than baseline CPP. This usually took 20 min, and after 5 min of stable higher blood pressure another CBF measurement was performed. On a small number of occasions, in patients with high flows, autoregulation was tested by slowly decreasing blood pressure with trimetaphan camsylate (Arfonad, 500 mg in 500 ml 5% dextrose) to a value 30% lower than baseline CPP. During tests with phenylephrine we often monitored evoked potentials; usually sensory evoked potentials and sometimes visual evoked potentials. However, tests with Arfonad were performed only when simultaneous evoked potential monitoring was available to insure the patient's safety.

Various authors have given different criteria for determining whether pressure autoregulation is intact or not [7–9, 25]. We believe that the key issue in autoregulation is whether or not cerebrovascular resistance (CVR = CPP/CBF) changes in response to pressure changes, and we have defined pressure autoregulation as being intact if $\frac{\Delta\%\ \mathrm{CPP}}{\Delta\%\ \mathrm{CVR}} \leq 2$. Although we realize that autoregulation is not an all-or-nothing phenomenon and can just be slower than normal, be intact within smaller pressure limits, or show smaller adjustments than normal, in the vast majority of cases the value of this equation is either far below the arbitrarily chosen value of 2 (intact autoregulation) or far above 2 (defective autoregulation).

Mannitol Response Test

Mannitol was given only to patients who had not received the drug in the previous 4 h and who seemed unlikely to need it during the next 8 h (stable ICP < 20 mmHg) in order not to jeopardize the blood osmolality. After the blood pressure had been allowed to return to baseline after completion of the pressure autoregulation test, the patient received an IV bolus of mannitol, 0.66 g/kg, in a 20% solution in water over a period of 3 min. The last CBF measurement was performed 25 min later. The ICP at the beginning of this measurement was taken as the "postmannitol ICP."

Results

A total of 42 complete tests, i.e., baseline measurement, pressure autoregulation test, and mannitol response test, were performed in 33 patients. Pressure autoregulation was found to be intact on 28 occasions and defective on 14.

Table 1 shows the incidence of decreases greater than 10% of baseline ICP and the incidence of increases greater than 10% of baseline CBF following mannitol administration in the groups with and without intact pressure autoregulation. The differences between the two groups were statistically significant, with $P < 0.01$ for the ICP data and $P < 0.001$ for the CBF data (chi-square tests). It should be noted that various combinations of ICP and CBF responses could occur in either group; therefore, the sum of the individual responses is larger than the total number in each group.

Table 2 shows the magnitude of ICP changes after mannitol or during phenylephrine or Arfonad in the two administration groups. In the group with intact pressure autoregulation, mannitol decreased ICP by 4.7 mmHg or 27.2%, while in the group without autoregulation this decrease was only 2.3 mmHg or 14.0%. The difference between the decrease in both groups is not statistically significant ($P < 0.3$, unpaired *t*-test). However, the total mean decrease of 2.3 ± 7.0 mmHg in the group without autoregulation was almost completely caused by a single measurement when the baseline ICP had dropped from 37 mmHg to 25 mmHg during phenylephrine ad-

Table 1. Number of changes in ICP and CBF by over 10% of baseline, in groups with intact or defective autoregulation

Response to Mannitol	Pressure autoregulation intact ($n = 28$)	Pressure autoregulation defective ($n = 14$)
Decrease in ICP	24 (86%)	5 (36%)
Increase in CBF	5 (18%)	11 (79%)

The differences between the two groups are statistically significant (ICP: $P < 0.01$; CBF: $P < 0.001$, chi-square tests)

Table 2. Values of ICP (mmHg; mean ± SD) in groups with pressure autoregulation intact and defective

	Autoregulation intact	Autoregulation defective	
	$n = 28$	$n = 14$	$n = 13$ [a]
Baseline ICP	16.9±7.1	16.4±8.0	14.8±5.5
ICP after mannitol	12.3±6.5	14.1±5.8	14.1±6.1
	$n = 25$	$n = 12$	$n = 11$ [a]
Baseline ICP	16.8±7.3	15.8±8.3	13.9±5.5
ICP with phenylephrine	17.2±8.9	16.5±6.4	15.7±6.1
	$n = 3$	$n = 2$	
Baseline ICP	18.7±1.2	19.5±6.4	
ICP with Arfonad	21.3±4.5	13.0±4.2	

[a] Includes one case (no. 9, Table 1) in which ICP had already decreased a great deal before phenylephrine and mannitol administration. Omission of this one case leads to even larger differences in ICP changes in the two groups. The decrease in ICP after mannitol was much larger in the autoregulation-intact group (27.2%) than in the autoregulation-defective group (4.7%, $n = 13$; 14.0%, $n = 14$) and statistically different, if this one case is left out ($P < 0.02$, $n = 13$) but not if we include this one case ($P < 0.3$, $n = 14$, unpaired *t*-tests)

Table 3. Values of CBF (ml/100 g/min, mean ± SD) at a $PaCO_2$ of 34 mmHg in groups with intact and with defective pressure autoregulation

	Autoregulation intact	Autoregulation defective
	$n=28$	$n=14$
Baseline CBF	32.9 ± 10.7	27.9 ± 12.0
CBF after mannitol	32.6 ± 12.2	32.9 ± 11.2
	$n=25$	$n=12$
Baseline CBF	31.3 ± 9.7	24.5 ± 8.1
CBF with phenylephrine	31.4 ± 8.6	35.8 ± 10.2
	$n=3$	$n=2$
Baseline CBF	45.7 ± 11.5	48.5 ± 12.0
CBF with Arfonad	41.3 ± 12.2	37.0 ± 8.5

In the autoregulation-intact group, CBF does not differ significantly from baseline after mannitol or phenylephrine. In the autoregulation-defective group, CBF increased significantly after mannitol ($P<0.002$, paired t-test) and during phenylephrine ($P<0.0001$, paired t-test)

ministration and further to 14 mmHg after mannitol (case no. 9, Table 1). No explanation could be found for this very large decrease, which had already occurred prior to mannitol administration. Omission of this single measurement led to a mean reduction in ICP of only 0.7 ± 4.0 mmHg or 4.7% in the nonautoregulating group. The difference between this decrease and that in the autoregulating group is statistically significant ($P<0.02$, unpaired t-test).

Table 3 shows the magnitude of CBF changes after mannitol or during phenylephrine or Arfonad administration. It is clear that with autoregulation intact no change in CBF occurred after mannitol administration or during phenylephrine-induced high blood pressure. On admission of Arfonad a small (9.6%) decrease in CBF occurred, but CVR also dropped considerably (23%), showing that autoregulation was indeed intact.

In the group without autoregulation, administration of mannitol caused a 17.9% increase in CBF, which was statistically different from baseline CBF in these cases ($P<0.002$, paired t-test). Although mannitol administration often caused a small, transient increase in blood pressure, the CPP (CPP, CPP = MABP-ICP) at the time of the baseline CBF measurement in the non-autoregulating group was 90.1 ± 21.3 mmHg, and at the time of the mannitol CBF measurement it was 89.4 ± 25.3 mmHg. Thus, the increase in CBF certainly cannot be explained by a change in CPP in the non-autoregulating group.

Discussion

The present results show that the effects of IV mannitol administration of ICP and CBF are interdependent and, in turn, dependent upon the autoregulatory status of the brain. If pressure autoregulation is intact, mannitol causes ICP to decrease while

CBF remains equal. If pressure autoregulation is not intact the decrease in ICP is much smaller, but CBF increases after mannitol.

These findings are in complete agreement with the results and conclusions from earlier experiments carried out in normal cats [17]. In those experiments, it was shown that mannitol first caused a large decrease in blood viscosity and later a large "rebound" increase in viscosity. Through a cranial window we observed with this decreased viscosity a constriction of pial arterioles similar in degree to that brought about by vigorous hyperventilation. The rebound increase in viscosity was accompanied by a large increase in vessel diameter. ICP correlated extremely well with the vessel diameter changes. It was postulated that the vessel diameter changes were autoregulatory in nature. The present paper has shown that when pressure autoregulation is defective no vasoconstriction occurs after the administration of mannitol, so that only a small ICP decrease will follow but CBF will be increased. Thus, blood viscosity autoregulation is closely related to pressure autoregulation and they probably share the same mechanism. Admittedly, blood viscosity measurements were not included in the present investigation, but blood viscosity decrease is a very constant finding in humans after mannitol administration [5].

Another explanation for the lack of ICP decrease with mannitol in the non-autoregulating group would be that in such cases the blood brain barrier is so severely compromised that mannitol immediately enters the brain and no osmotic gradient exists between blood and brain. There are several arguments against this explanation. Severe vasogenic edema might be expected in such cases, with high ICP. However, the ICP was similar in the group with and without autoregulation. Moreover, with such a severely compromised blood brain barrier a higher blood pressure should lead to a quick increase in cerebral edema with concomitant rise in ICP, but this did not happen in our tests of autoregulation with phenylephrine. Finally, such an explanation could not explain why CBF increases in the absence of ICP changes. Thus, although we do not deny that decrease in brain water content and possibly also in the amount of cerebrospinal fluid plays a role in the ICP decrease with osmotic agents, the autoregulatory vasoconstriction also seems to be important. With vasoconstriction present the ICP decreased by 27.2%; with no vasoconstriction present the decrease was only 4.7% (if we leave out the one measurement in which ICP had already dropped substantially before the mannitol administration).

Recently, Albright et al. have described the effects of IV mannitol, furosemide, albumin, and furosemide/albumin administration on brain water content and ICP in dogs with vasogenic edema in one hemisphere following a cold lesion [1]. All these treatments decreased ICP, except albumin alone, even though this drug was nearly as effective as mannitol in dehydrating the brain. Albumin alone dehydrated the brain more than furosemide or the furosemide/albumin combination, but nevertheless lacked the effect of the latter two treatments on ICP. It is of interest to note that albumin administration has also failed to improve CBF or reduce infarct size in a stroke model [14]. Although it was shown in this last investigation that albumin administration reduced the hematocrit, the lack of effect on CBF in the territory of the occluded middle cerebral artery probably must be explained by a lack of effect on blood viscosity. Blood viscosity measurements or erythrocyte deformability measurements were not performed, however. Further studies on the effects of albumin on blood viscosity are needed, because the disappointing findings in studies on ICP and CBF may share the same mechanism: no reduction of blood viscosity.

The present findings also resolve the question as to why mannitol does not increase CBF in normal animals [11, 12] but sometimes does so after injury [3] or in stroke victims [16]. Several explanations have been put forward for this increase. One was that mannitol increased cardiac output, which somehow leads to an increase in CBF in the traumatized brain [3]. Mizukami and Tarawa [16] measured CBF in stroke patients in whom ICP was kept constant at zero by ventricular drainage. They explained the increase in CBF in the areas with low flows after glycerol by assuming that glycerol decreased cerebral edema in the compromised region which would lead to an improvement in the microcirculation despite the constant intracranial pressure. It now seems clear that the increased CBF was caused by decreased blood viscosity with lack of autoregulatory vasoconstriction in the low flow areas.

In the experiments of Wood et al. [27], in which blood viscosity was lowered with low-molecular-weight dextran in dogs with focal cerebral ischemia, surprisingly an increase in ICP was found. We cannot offer an explanation for these findings, which are in complete contradiction to our own, nor can the authors themselves (J. H. Wood, personal communication). Nevertheless, we feel there is a need to investigate the possibility of controlling high ICP by blood viscosity manipulation with drugs with longer lasting action and fewer side effects than osmotic agents, such as dextran or fluorocarbon blood substitutes. It also appears that, because maintaining low blood viscosity is equally important as decreasing brain water content in the management of high ICP, the fluid management of head-injured patients needs further investigation. It may be necessary to restrict patients' fluid intake to control cerebral edema; it may be necessary to give them large amounts of fluids to keep blood viscosity low; or it may be best to maintain normovolemia.

In conclusion, this paper offers an explanation for some poorly understood effects of osmotic agents on CBF. It also makes it likely that vasoconstriction is an effect additional to the cerebral dehydration resulting from the use of osmotic agents to reduce ICP.

Summary

Intravenous mannitol or urea causes vasoconstriction in response to blood viscosity decrease in cats. This is presumably due to the same mechanism as the vasoconstriction seen during blood pressure increases with intact autoregulation. We proposed that ICP decrease with administration of osmotic agents is mainly due to this vasoconstriction and occurs only with autoregulation intact. In severely head-injured patients CBF was measured by means of xenon-133 inhalation, autoregulation was tested by raising blood pressure with phenylephrine, and ICP and CBF were measured again 25 min after an IV bolus of 0.6 g/kg mannitol. Autoregulation was intact on 28 occasions (group A) and defective on 14 (group B). With mannitol we found an ICP decrease in group A on 24 occasions (86%) and in group B on 4 (36%) ($P < 0.01$). In group A, CBF was increased 5 times (18%), and in group B, 11 times (79%) ($P < 0.001$). The mean ICP decrease was 27.2% in group A and 4.7% in group B ($P < 0.02$). The mean CBF increase was −1% in group A and 17.9% in group B ($P < 0.001$). These results confirm that ICP and/or CBF changes after mannitol are interdependent and, in turn, dependent on the autoregulatory status of the brain. They can be completely explained by the occurrence of vasoconstriction (ICP↓, CBF unchanged) or by the lack thereof (CBF↑, ICP unchanged). For management of acute ICP increases vasoconstriction through blood viscosity decrease is more important than "dehydration" of the brain. We advocate not restricting the patient's fluid intake, as this would lead to increased blood viscosity.

Acknowledgments. The authors wish to thank Ms Joyce Baskerville and Mrs. Rae Spivey for their secretarial assistance in the preparation of this manuscript, and Dr. Sung Choi for statistical calculations.

References

1. Albright AL, Latchaw RE, Robinson AG (1984) Intracranial and systemic effects of osmotic and oncotic therapy in experimental cerebral edema. J Neurosurg 60:481–489
2. Becker DP, Miller JD, Ward JD, et al. (1977) The outcome from severe head injury with early diagnosis and intensive management. J Neurosurg 47:491–502
3. Brown FD, Johns L, Jaffar JJ, et al. (1979) Detailed monitoring of the effects of mannitol following experimental head injury. J Neurosurg 50:423–432
4. Bruce DA, Langfitt TW, Miller JD, et al. (1973) Regional cerebral blood flow, intracranial pressure, and brain metabolism in comatose patients. J Neurosurg 38:131–144
5. Burke AM, Quest DO, Chien S, et al. (1981) The effects of mannitol on blood viscosity. J Neurosurg 55:550–553
6. Clasen RA, Cooke PM, Pandolfi S, et al. (1965) Hypertonic urea in experimental cerebral edema. Arch Neurol 12:424–434
7. Enevoldsen EM, Cold G, Jensen FT, et al. (1976) Dynamic changes in regional CBF, intraventricular pressure, CSF, pH and lactate levels during the acute phase of head injury. J Neurosurg 44:191–214
8. Enevoldsen FM, Jensen FT (1978) Autoregulation and CO_2 responses of cerebral blood flow in patients with acute severe head injury. J Neurosurg 48:689–703
9. Fieschi C, Battistini N, Beduschi A, et al. (1974) Regional cerebral blood flow and intraventricular pressure in acute head injuries. J Neurol Neurosurg Psychiatry 37:1378–1388
10. Guisado R, Arieff AI, Massry SG (1976) Effects of glycerol administration on experimental brain edema. Neurology 26:69–75
11. Johnston IH, Harper AM (1973) The effect of mannitol on cerebral blood flow. An experimental study. J Neurosurg 38:461–471
12. Kassell NF, Baumann KW, Mitchon PW, et al. (1982) The effects of high dose mannitol on cerebral blood flow in dogs with normal intracranial pressure. Stroke 13:59–61
13. Langfitt TW (1982) Increased intracranial pressure and the cerebral circulation. In: Youmans JR (ed) Neurological surgery, 2nd edn, vol 2. Saunders, Philadelphia, pp 905–910
14. Little JR, Slugg RM, Latchaw JP, et al. (1981) Treatment of acute focal cerebral ischemia with concentrated albumin. Neurosurgery 9:552–558
15. Miller JD, Butterworth JF, Gudeman SK, et al. (1981) Further experience in the management of severe head injury. J Neurosurg 54:289–299
16. Mizukami M, Tazawa T (1983) Theoretical background for surgical treatment in hypertensive intracerebral hemorrhage. In: Mizukami M, Kanaya H, Kogure K, et al. (eds) Hypertensive intracerebral hemorrhage. Raven, New York, pp 239–247
17. Muizelaar JP, Wei EP, Kontos HE, et al. (1983) Mannitol causes compensatory cerebral vasoconstriction and vasodilation in response to blood viscosity changes. J Neurosurg 59:822–828

18. Obrist WD, Gennarelli TA, Segawa H, et al. (1979) Relation of cerebral blood flow to neurological status and outcome in head-injured patients. J Neurosurg 51:292–300
19. Obrist WD, Langfitt TW, Jaggi JL, et al. (1985) Cerebral blood flow and metabolism in comatose patients with acute head injury: relation to intracranial hypertension. J Neurosurg (in press)
20. Obrist WD, Thompson HK, Wang HS, et al. (1975) Regional cerebral blood flow estimated by ^{133}xenon inhalation. Stroke 6:245–256
21. Obrist WD, Wilkinson WE (1980) The non-invasive Xe-133 method: evaluation of CBF indices. In: Bes A, Geraud G (eds) Cerebral circulation. Excerpta Medica, Amsterdam, pp 119–124
22. Reed DJ, Woodbury DM (1962) Effect of hypertonic urea on cerebrospinal fluid pressure and brain volume. J Physiol (Lond) 164:252–264
23. Takagi H, Saito T, Kitahara T, et al. (1983) The mechanism of the ICP reducing effect of mannitol. In: Ishii S, Nagai H, Brock M (eds) Intracranial pressure V. Springer, Berlin, pp 729–733
24. Takagi H, Shapiro K, Marmarou A, et al. (1981) Microgravimetric analysis of human brain tissue. Correlation with computerized tomography scanning. J Neurosurg 54:797–801
25. Tweed WA, Overgaard J (1975) Disturbed regulation of CBF after acute brain injury with particular reference to the effects of MIVP and CPP. In: Langfitt TW, McHenry LC, Reivich M, et al. (eds) Cerebral circulation and metabolism. Springer, Berlin, pp 245–248
26. Vries JK, Becker DP, Young HF (1973) A subarachnoid screw for monitoring intracranial pressure. Technical note. J Neurosurg 39:416–419
27. Wood JH, Simeone FA, Fink EA, et al. (1983) Hypervolemic hemodilution in experimental focal cerebral ischemia. Elevation of cardiac output, regional cortical blood flow, and ICP after intravascular volume expansion with low molecular weight dextran. J Neurosurg 59:500–509

Cerebrovascular Effect of Mannitol

L. M. AUER [1], and K. HASELSBERGER

Key words: Mannitol, pial vessels, ICP, cat

Introduction

The present study was designed to investigate a hypothesized [6] cerebrovascular effect of mannitol, i.e., a reduction of intracranial pressure (ICP) via cerebral blood volume. Since the cerebral veins have received little attention in recent decades though a major proportion of blood volume is known to be located in the veins [5], special attention was paid to the reaction of pial veins. Mannitol is clinically used mainly as a drug to reduce elevated ICP; therefore, cerebrovascular reactions to mannitol should be investigated during increased ICP.

Materials and Methods

The investigations were performed in cats during barbiturate anesthesia and controlled ventilation with $N_2O : O_2$ 3 : 1. Mean arterial pressure (MAP) and intracranial pressure (ICP) were continuously monitored, and arterial blood gases were frequently checked. Pial vessels were investigated with the aid of a closed parietal cranial window by means of a Leitz intravital microscope and a multichannel videoangiometer [2].

In six animals, 1 g/kg mannitol was infused IV over 15 min in resting conditions of all parameters; six animals were used as controls. In a second series, ICP was elevated by cisternal infusion of mock CSF to a level of 20 mmHg and mannitol treatment was performed as in group 1; again, six sham-treated animals served as controls.

Results

With initially normal ICP, mannitol caused a 34% decrease of ICP within the 15 min of administration; during the subsequent 10 min ICP fell to 66% below levels in the control group. Thereafter, ICP returned to normal within 30 min. The pial arteries showed a very modest tendency to constrict during mannitol infusion, whereas dila-

[1] Universitätsklinik für Neurochirurgie, Auenbruggerplatz 20, A-8036 Graz

tation by roughly 4% was observed in controls; this 5% constriction relative to controls was significant ($P < 0.0005$). Pial veins remained unreactive during mannitol infusion and in the control group, whereas very minor dilatation was noted during 30 min after mannitol [4].

When ICP was initially elevated it was consistently reduced by mannitol, falling to a minimum level of 10%–15% below controls during the administration period (Fig. 1). In these circumstances, pial veins showed a reduction in caliber by several percentage points during mannitol infusion (Fig. 2), especially the small veins,

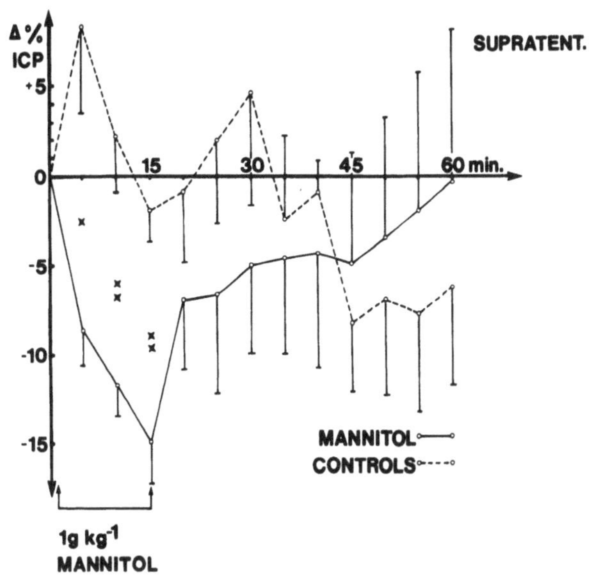

Fig. 1. Supratentorial ICP recorded via a subarachnoid catheter in the cranial window during and after mannitol administration, indicated as percentage of the pretreatment level of 20 mmHg achieved by mock CSF infusion. * $P < 0.05$; ** $P < 0.005$

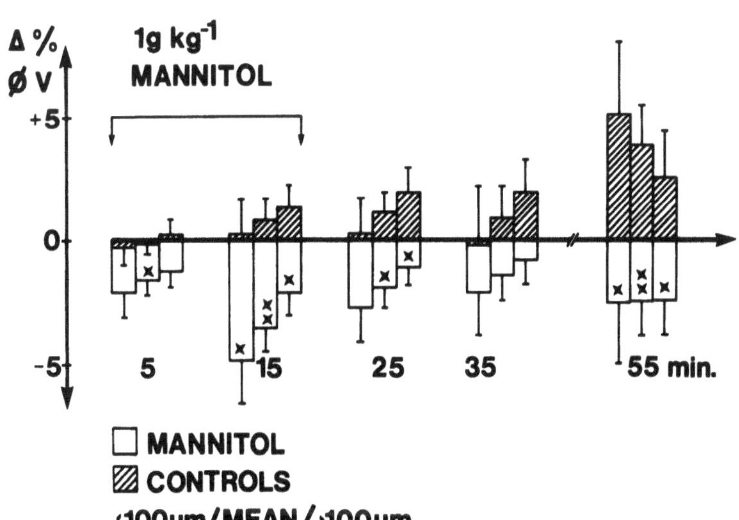

Fig. 2. Variations in pial venous calibers (øV) as percentages of pretreatment calibers. *Left bars,* caliber changes of vessels up to 100 µm resting diameter; *right bars,* large vessels above 100 µm resting diameter; *center bars,* average reaction. * $P < 0.05$; ** $P < 0.005$

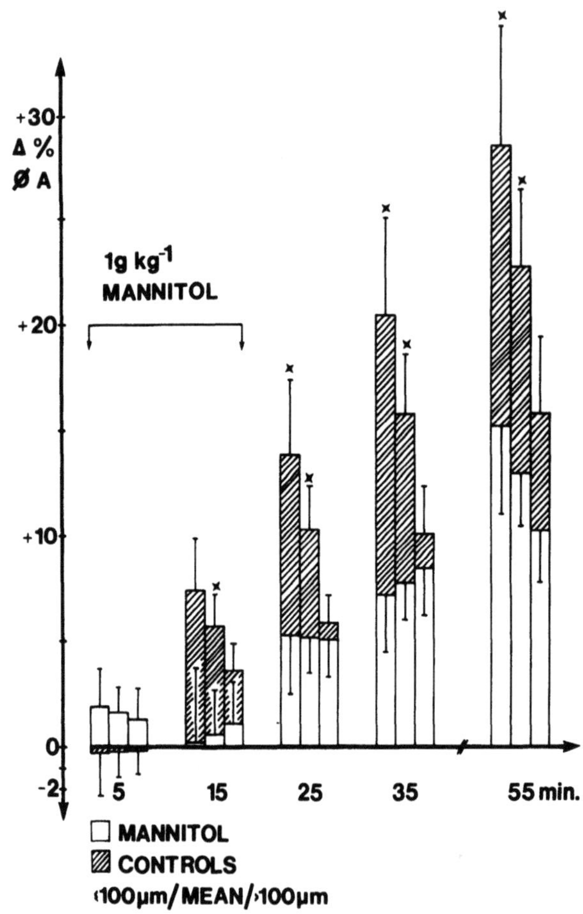

Fig. 3. Reaction of pial arteries (oA) as percentages of resting calibers. Mannitol seems to suppress the dilatation of pial arteries observed in controls

which were 5% narrower than control veins by the end of mannitol treatment. This effect persisted for the next 30 min, though to a lesser extent. Pial arteries showed a consistent dilatation in the control group, rising to over 12% above the resting caliber during the first 25 min. This behavior was not observed in pial arteries of mannitol-treated animals, which remained unresponsive for the duration of the treatment and did not start to dilate significantly also until 5 min after mannitol treatment was complete (Fig. 3). Pial arterial diameters were thus 5% smaller than control diameters after 15 min, and as much as 8% smaller after 20 min.

Discussion

In accordance with previous observations [6], the present data show that IV mannitol is able to reduce the pial arterial blood volume. In addition, the present study shows this effect in the circumstances of elevated ICP; decreased venous calibers were also observed during mannitol infusion. Since 70%–80% of the blood volume is located in the veins [5], the behavior of veins can be assumed to be even more important than arterial reactions in ICP reduction by mannitol via cerebral blood volume. The response of pial arteries, like the degree of ICP reduction, was markedly smaller, probably as a consequence of lower mannitol concentrations in the present series. The possible explanations for this cerebrovascular effect of mannitol has been discussed in detail elsewhere [4]; the present data do not allow the assumption of autoregulative vasoconstriction due to decreased blood viscosity and consecutively rising CBF, because similar hematocrit changes to those recorded in other investigations [6] were seen in this study, together with different arterial reactions in the different series.

Arterial dilatation as a consequence of rising ICP, both with elevation of CSF pressure and with developing brain edema, has been a consistent observation in previous studies [3]; it can be explained by smooth muscle relaxation with rising perivascular pressure. Provided that mannitol constricts predilated vessels to the same extent as it prevents arterial dilatation during rising ICP, it can be assumed that a moderate proportion of the ICP-reducing effect of mannitol is due to a direct cerebrovascular constricting effect which may become more significant with rising initial level of ICP according to the volume–pressure relationship. The major effect of mannitol, however, still seems to remain its osmotic effect on brain bulk, as has been determined in edematous brain [1].

Summary

Reactions of pial arteries and veins during IV administration of 1 g/kg mannitol over 15 min in conditions of normal and elevated initial intracranial pressure (ICP) were investigated in cats under barbiturate and nitrous oxide anesthesia. Treatment under resting conditions caused a 66% reduction in ICP (all values relative to controls); mannitol caused a 7% constriction of pial arteries, veins remaining unreactive. When mannitol was given in a situation of increased ICP (cisternal infusion of mock CSF), ICP was reduced by about 15%; pial arteries constricted by 5%, pial veins by 4%.

From these data it is concluded that mannitol at the indicated dose exerts a modest effect on cerebral blood volume during both normal and increased ICP; the dominant ICP-reducing action of mannitol seems to remain its osmotic effect.

References

1. Albright AL, Latchaw RE, Robinson AG (1984) Intracranial and systemic effects of osmotic and oncotic therapy in experimental cerebral edema. J Neurosurg 60:481–489
2. Auer LM, Haydn F (1979) Multichannel videoangiometry for continuous measurement of pial microvessels. Acta Neurol Scand 60, Suppl 72:208–209
3. Auer LM, MacKenzie ET (1984) Physiology of the cerebral venous system. In: Kapp JP, Schmidek HH (eds) The cerebral venous system and its disorders. Grune Stratton, Orlando, pp 169–227
4. Auer LM, Haselsberger K (1985) The effect of intravenous mannitol on cat pial arteries and veins during normal and elevated intracranial pressure. J Neurosurg (in press)
5. Mellander S, Johansson BB (1968) Control of resistance, exchange and capacitance vessels in the peripheral circulation. Pharm Rev 20:117–196
6. Muizelaar JP, Wei EP, Kontos HA, Becker DP (1983) Mannitol causes compensatory cerebral vasoconstriction and vasodilation in response to blood viscosity changes. J Neurosurg 59:822–828

Effects of Sympathectomy on Brain Edema

LIN SHINN-ZONG[1], SHIH CHUN-JEN, LIN MAO-TSUN, and TSAI SHIH-HAN

Key words: Sympathectomy, brain edema, heat stroke, ganglionectomy

Introduction

The adrenergic nerves innervating the cerebral artery are believed to originate from the superior cervical ganglia, and their preganglionic outflow, from the lateral horn of the spinal cord. In a recent study we also demonstrated that the adrenergic nerves innervating the middle cerebral artery originated solely in the ipsilateral superior cervical ganglion, by applying horseradish peroxidase (HRP) to the wall of the middle cerebral artery. Stimulation of the cervical sympathetic trunk or superior cervical ganglia causes vasoconstriction of the cerebral vessels [2]. In contrast, superior cervical ganglionectomy and cervical sympathetic preganglionic excision each caused an increase in cerebral blood flow [1, 4, 10].

In this study, we attempted to assess the possible therapeutic effects of preganglionic or postganglionic sympathetic denervation of the cerebral vessels on brain edema formation produced by induction of cold injury in the cerebral cortex or the development of heat stroke in rats in response to external heat stress.

Materials and Methods

Adult male Sprague-Dawley rats weighing between 250 and 300 g were used in all experiments. The operations were performed via a midline incision in the neck with the animals in sodium pentobarbital anesthesia (6 mg/100 g). Three types of operation were performed under operative microscopy. In one group postganglionic sympathectomy with bilateral extirpation of the superior cervical ganglia was performed. For preganglionic sympathectomy bilateral section of the sympathetic trunks was performed 2–3 mm below the superior cervical ganglia. In the sham-operated group all steps in the above operation were performed except that the sympathetic nerves were left intact. Two weeks after the operation, the animals were subjected to experimentation.

---

[1] Department of Surgery, National Defense Medical Center and Tri-Service General Hospital, Taipei, Taiwan, Republic of China

Induction of Brain Edema

Brain edema was induced by cold injury to the cerebral cortex. After local anesthesia with 2% xylocaine, a 60-mm^2 plate attached to a brass cup filled with dry ice-acetone (–50 °C) was applied to the intact skull on the right frontoparietal bone area and left for 2 min. Brain edema was assessed 3 h after the cold injury by measuring brain water content, which was determined by difference after drying at 95 °C for 4 h to a constant weight.

Production of Heat Stroke

Heat stroke was induced by exposing the animals to an ambient temperature of 41 °C. The occurrence of loss of sensation, decreased muscle tone, and unconsciousness was taken as the onset of heat stroke [9]. At the time of the onset of heat stroke, the comatose animals were immediately removed to a chamber maintained at 24 °C. The interval between the onset of heat stroke and death was recorded as the duration of survival after heat stroke.

Results

Experimentally Induced Brain Edema

Table 1 shows the effects of preganglionic or postganglionic sympathectomy on brain edema induced by cold injury. It was found that the brain edema formation was significantly inhibited or prevented by the pretreatment with preganglionic sympathectomy ($P < 0.05$; one-way analysis of variance). In contrast, the brain edema was significantly exacerbated by pretreatment of the animals with postganglionic sympathectomy ($P < 0.05$; one-way analysis of variance).

Experimentally Induced Heat Stroke

The latencies for the onset of heat stroke were found to be 30.2 ± 0.8, 37.5 ± 1.2 and 20.4 ± 0.1 min, respectively, for the sham-operated, preganglionically sympathec-

Table 1. The water contents of both hemispheres of eight sham-operated control rats, eight preganglionically sympathectomized rats, and eight postganglionically sympathectomized rats

Treatments	Water contact (%) of the hemisphere	
	Left side	Right side
1. Sham operation	79.6 ± 0.1	84.0 ± 0.2
2. Preganglionic sympathectomy	79.6 ± 0.1	82.1 ± 0.1*
3. Postganglionic sympathectomy	79.8 ± 0.1	85.2 ± 0.1*

* $P < 0.05$ (one-way analysis of variance) against corresponding control values (after sham operation). Values are expressed as means ± SEM

Table 2. Time to reach coma and the survival time of eight sham-operated control rats, eight preganglionically sympathectomized rats, and eight postganglionically sympathectomized rats in response to a heat stress

Treatment	Time to reach coma (min; mean ± SEM)	Survival time (min; mean ± SEM)
1. Sham operation	30.2 ± 0.8	36.8 ± 1.1
2. Preganglionic sympathectomy	37.5 ± 1.2*	62.1 ± 1.6*
3. Postganglionic sympathectomy	20.4 ± 0.7*	24.3 ± 0.8*

* $P < 0.05$ (one-way analysis of variance) against corresponding control values (after sham operation)

tomized and postganglionically sympathectomized rats. Meanwhile, the preganglionically sympathectomized animals survived longer than those subjected to sham operation. On the other hand, the postganglionically sympathectomized rats had a shorter survival time than the sham-operated animals. The data are summarized in Table 2.

Discussion

The acute effects of superior cervical ganglionectomy have been shown to cause an increase in cerebral blood flow and volume [1, 5]. These may be due to reduced vascular tone, which occurs when a sufficient amount of noradrenaline has disappeared from the degenerating nerves [3]. However, the cerebral blood flow and volume returned to normal levels a week postoperatively [1, 5]. At this stage, the denervated adrenergic vascular receptors developed supersensitivity to circulating catecholamines [7]. On the other hand, preganglionic sympathetic denervation of the cerebral vessels results in an increased cerebral blood volume and vasodilatation consequent on reduced activation of the nerve terminals in the vasculature [3, 4]. The present experiments were performed on animals 2 weeks after the operations. The denervated adrenergic vascular receptors of the postganglionically sympathectomized animals may have resulted in a supersensitivity to catecholamines. For the preganglionically sympathectomized animals the cerebral vascular response may be reduced, probably reflecting lowered activity in the postganglionic neurons after deprivation of afferent innervation. The present results showed that the formation of experimental brain edema was inhibited by preganglionic sympathectomy, while postganglionic sympathectomy exacerbated brain edema formation. This may be due to the increased sensitivity of the denervated vascular bed to the external cold stimulation.

Our recent results have demonstrated that at the onset of heat stroke the comatose animals showed higher levels of intracranial pressure and cerebral water content and lower levels of mean arterial pressure. Brain edema, intracranial hypertension, and decreased mean arterial pressure can cause cerebral ischemia leading to neurologic damage and then the onset of heat stroke. The present results also show that the preganglionically sympathectomized animals had a longer latency and a longer survival time in heat stroke, whereas the postganglionically sympathectomized animals had a shorter latency and a shorter survival time in heat stroke. Thus, it appears that the potential benefit of preganglionic sympathectomy in the prevention of heat stroke may be due to the increased cerebral blood flow after lowering of the postganglionic neuronal activity. On the other hand, the supersensitized adrenergic vascular receptors may be responsible for the exaggeration of the effects of heat stroke in the postganglionically sympathectomized rats.

In fact, the contention is supported by several clinical findings reported by many investigators. For example, postganglionic sympathectomy was shown to have little therapeutic effect on most cases of cerebral vasospasm following aneurysmal rupture [6]. However, a bilateral stellectomy, which constitutes a preganglionic sympathectomy, caused decreased cerebral vascular resistance in patients [8].

In summary, the present results demonstrate that preganglionic sympathectomy, but not postganglionic sympathectomy, inhibits the formation or development of brain edema or heat stroke.

Summary

In the present study, the effects of superior cervical ganglionectomy on brain edema induced by cold injury or heat stroke were assessed in rats. The animals were subjected to either preganglionic or postganglionic sympathectomy 2 weeks prior to the experiments. Brain edema was induced by cold injury to the cerebral cortex. Preganglionic sympathectomy significantly inhibited the formation of brain edema. In contrast, postganglionic sympathectomy exacerbated the formation of brain edema. In the second series of experiments, heat stroke was produced by exposing the rats to an ambient temperature of 41 °C. It was found that both the latency for the onset of heat stroke and the survival time of comatose animals which had undergone preganglionic sympathectomy were greatly prolonged. On the other hand, postganglionic sympathectomy greatly shortened both the latency of onset of heat stroke and the survival time after the onset of heat stroke. The present results demonstrate that preganglionic sympathectomy has inhibitory effects on the formation or development of brain edema and heat stroke.

References

1. Alborch E, Gomez B, Godofredo D, Marin J, Lluch S (1977) Cerebral blood flow and vascular reactivity after removal of the superior cervical ganglion in the goat. Circ Res 41:278–282
2. Edvinsson L, Mackenzie ET (1977) Amine mechanisms in the cerebral circulation. Pharmacol Rev 28:285–348
3. Edvinsson L, Owman CH, Rosengren E, West KA (1972) Concentration of noradrenaline in pial vessels, choroid plexus, and iris during two weeks after sympathetic ganglionectomy or decentralization. Acta Physiol Scand 85:201–206
4. Edvinsson L, Owman CH, West KA (1972) Sympathetic influence of cerebral blood volume; time-dependent effect of decentralization of the superior cervical ganglia in mice. Experientia 28:790–791
5. Edvinsson L, Nielsen KC, Owman CH, West KA (1973) Evidence of vasoconstrictor sympathetic nerves in brain vessels of mice. Neurology 23:73–77

6. Kodama N, Hori S, Kamiyama K, Mizoi K, Suzuki J (1980) Cervical sympathectomy for cerebral vasospasm after aneurysm rupture. In: Wilkins RH (ed) Cerebral arterial spasm. Williams and Wilkins, Baltimore, pp 680–684
7. Langer SZ, Draskoczy PR, Trendelenburg U (1967) Time course of the development of super sensitivity to various amines in the nictating membrane of the pithed cat after denervation or decentralization. J Pharmacol Exp Ther 157:255–273
8. Shenkin HA, Cabieses F, Van Den Noordt G (1951) The effect of bilateral stellectomy upon the cerebral circulation of man. J Clin Invest 30:90–93
9. Shih CJ, Lin MT, Tsai SH (1984) Experimental study on the pathogenesis of heat stroke. J Neurosurg 60:1246–1252
10. Tomita M, Gotoh F, Tanahashi N, Kobari M (1982) Ipsilateral increase in CBV by unilateral severing of the cervical sympathetic preganglionic fiber in cats. In: Heistad DD, Marcus ML (ed) Cerebral blood flow: effect of nerves and neurotransmitters. Elsevier/North-Holland, Amsterdam, pp 403–408

Index of Key Words

Index of Authors

MIX
Papier aus verantwortungsvollen Quellen
Paper from responsible sources
FSC® C105338

If you have any concerns about our products,
you can contact us on
ProductSafety@springernature.com

In case Publisher is established outside the EU,
the EU authorized representative is:
Springer Nature Customer Service Center GmbH
Europaplatz 3, 69115 Heidelberg, Germany

Printed by Libri Plureos GmbH
in Hamburg, Germany